Lippincott Atlas of Anatomy,Second Edition

LWW 解剖图谱 第二版

主　编　〔美〕托马斯·格斯特 (Thomas R. Gest)

主　译　欧阳钧

译　者（按姓氏笔画排序）

毕振宇　孙培栋　李庆涛　李鉴轶　张美超

钱　蕾　温广明　廖　华　樊继宏　戴景兴

Wolters Kluwer Health　北京科学技术出版社

著作权合同登记号　图字：01-2021-2345

图书在版编目（CIP）数据

LWW 解剖图谱：第二版 /（美）托马斯·格斯特
（Thomas R. Gest）主编；欧阳钧主译 . —北京：北京
科学技术出版社，2021.7（2023.5重印）
书名原文：Lippincott Atlas of Anatomy, 2/E
ISBN 978-7-5714-1208-1

Ⅰ.①L… Ⅱ.①托… ②欧… Ⅲ.①人体解剖学–图
谱 Ⅳ.①R322-64

中国版本图书馆CIP数据核字（2020）第214243号

本书中提供了正确的适应证、不良反应和用药方法，但这些都有改变的可能。强烈希望读者阅读本书提到的药物的生产厂家所提供在包装上的信息。作者、编辑、出版人、发行商不对任何错误或忽略负责，不对应用本书中的信息后可能造成的任何结果负责，也不会对出版物内容进行明确或不明确的承诺。作者、编辑、出版人、发行商对与本出版物相关的人身或财产伤害不承担任何责任。

责任编辑：杨　帆	网　　址：www.bkydw.cn
责任校对：贾　荣	印　　刷：北京捷迅佳彩印刷有限公司
图文制作：北京永诚天地艺术设计有限公司	开　　本：889 mm × 1194 mm　1/16
责任印制：吕　越	字　　数：360千字
出 版 人：曾庆宇	印　　张：29.5
出版发行：北京科学技术出版社	版　　次：2021年7月第1版
社　　址：北京西直门南大街16号	印　　次：2023年5月第2次印刷
邮政编码：100035	ISBN 978-7-5714-1208-1
电　　话：0086-10-66135495（总编室） 　　　　　0086-10-66113227（发行部）	

定　　价：298.00元

感谢北京科学技术出版社和欧阳钧教授，在他们的策划组织下，邀请了一批学者，翻译了由 LWW 公司出版的原创性图谱的第 2 版，为医学生提供了珍贵的参考资料。

人体解剖学是一门形态科学，形态学的学习方法，若加以通俗的概括，就是"百闻不如一见"。直观性很强的图谱就是"工欲善其事，必先利其器"中重要的"器"之一。"兼听则明"，开放改革的事实证明，这是社会发展的正确道路；闭关锁国，视野狭窄是无法成就伟业的。尽管我国在近 40 多年来，在解剖学领域，出版过大批解剖学图谱，取得过许多光辉的成就。但"寸有所长，尺有所短"，就以这部《LWW 解剖学图谱》为例：虚实结合、循序渐进、由浅入深、由此及彼、令人身历其境，熟识毗邻，有其独特的优点，是教学经验与绘画艺术高度统一的珍品。在学习和借鉴国外教辅参考书时，我们当然不要搞"近寺人家不重僧，远来和尚好看经"；但"一目之视也，不若二目之视也；一耳之听也，不若二耳之听也"。辩证的法则，就是"扬长补短"，是要通中法外，舍短取长，这也是我们应当采取的态度。

我作为在解剖学教学园地里耕耘了一辈子的老园丁，深知园艺创新培育的功力，是善于引进，善于结合，因时制宜，因地制宜。在引进一个新品种后，要举一反三，触类旁通，要像"深处种菱浅种稻，不深不浅种荷花"那样灵巧适应，才能发挥引进新品种的最高效益。"物竞天择，适者生存"，在前沿性学科不断萌发，医学教育时数又不允许无限期延长的现实情况下，翻译出版 LWW 公司出版的原创性解剖学教学参考图谱，有其现实意义，是为之序。

中国解剖学会原名誉理事长

中国工程院院士

钟世镇

2021 年春于广州

　　解剖学图谱是医学生的重要参考工具书。作为解剖学老师，我们使用过许多国内外经典的解剖学图谱，或是实物照片，或是艺术绘图，百花斗艳，各具特色。2009 年翻译了威科公司出版的原创性图谱《LWW 解剖学图谱》，转眼间 10 年飞逝，很高兴继续有机会参与第 2 版图谱的翻译出版。

　　在众多的解剖学图谱当中，《LWW 解剖学图谱》的编写、绘图和设计都具有独到之处。全书按照身体部位分区编撰目录，按照表面解剖、浅层结构、深层结构的逻辑顺序安排插图，同时插图也兼顾了局部解剖学的教学需要。作者匠心独具、虚实结合，采用全新的理念绘制这部图谱。应用色彩、明暗、阴影、虚像等技巧，能够充分调动读者的感官注意力，可以有效地提高医学生的学习效率。第 2 版继续秉承了为医学生提供精炼、简约、重点突出，并且高效实用的参考图谱的初衷，修改和补充了部分插图，增加了肌学表格，以方便医学生查阅和复习。

　　"他山之石，可以攻玉"，感谢北京科学技术出版社慧眼识珠，在众多的教辅工具书中，选择了这部有高度实用价值的图谱翻译出版。第 1 版发行以来，受到中国医学生们的喜爱和欢迎，现在出版社又在第一时间推出威科公司创新团队带来的第 2 版，希望这本图谱能成为你学习人体解剖学的好助手。

欧阳钧

2021 年 4 月于南方医科大学

目　录

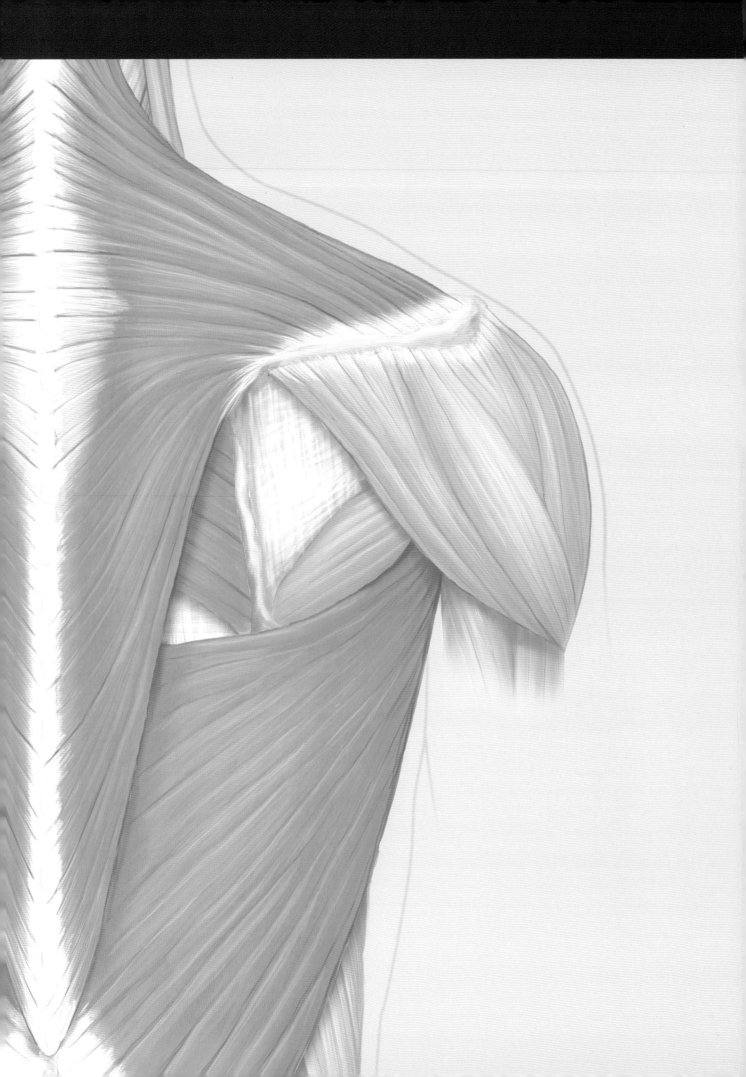

第一章 背部

CHAPTER 1 | **THE BACK**

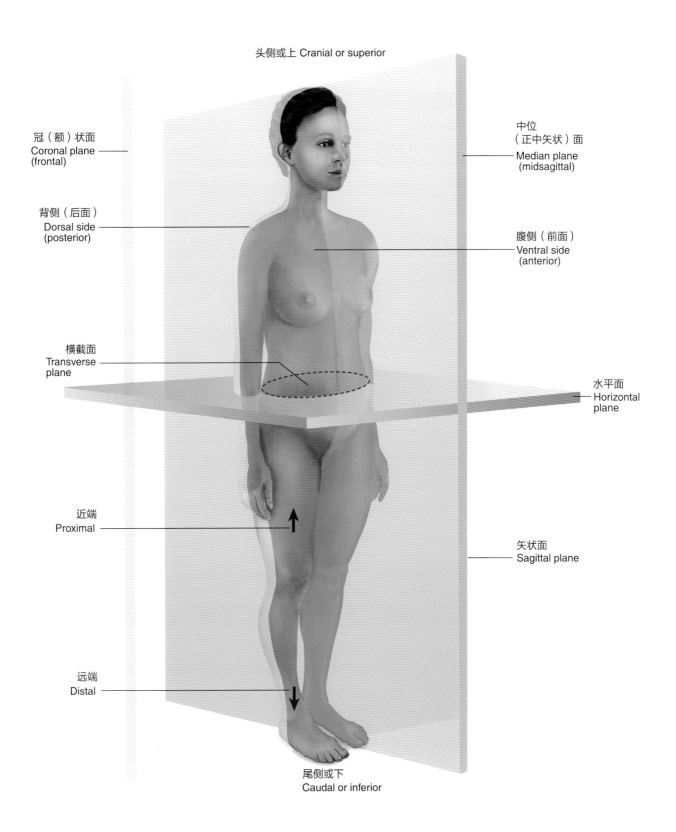

头侧或上 Cranial or superior

冠（额）状面
Coronal plane
(frontal)

中位
（正中矢状）面
Median plane
(midsagittal)

背侧（后面）
Dorsal side
(posterior)

腹侧（前面）
Ventral side
(anterior)

横截面
Transverse
plane

水平面
Horizontal
plane

近端
Proximal

矢状面
Sagittal plane

远端
Distal

尾侧或下
Caudal or inferior

图 1-02　背部可触及的结构　Palpable Features of the Back

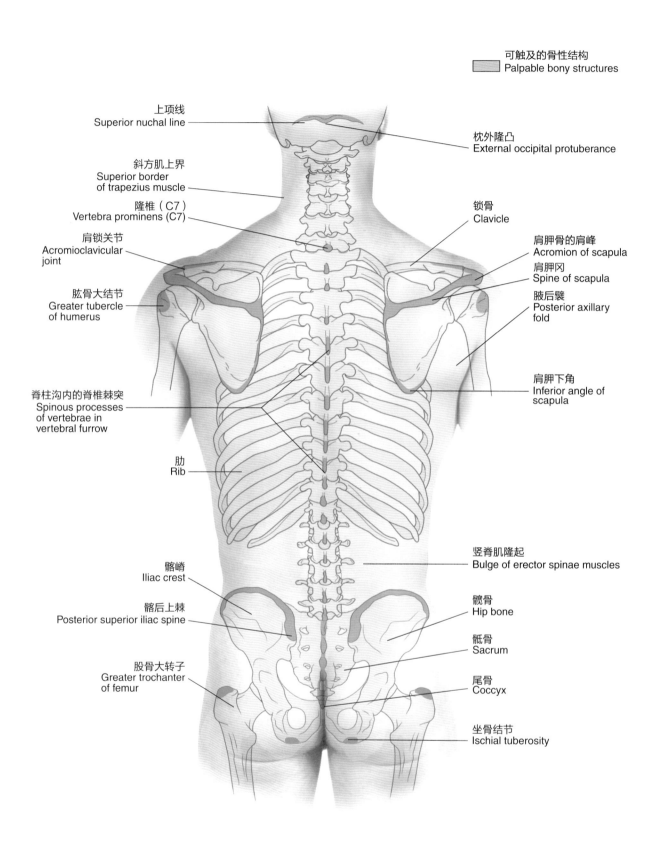

可触及的骨性结构
Palpable bony structures

上项线
Superior nuchal line

枕外隆凸
External occipital protuberance

斜方肌上界
Superior border
of trapezius muscle

隆椎（C7）
Vertebra prominens (C7)

锁骨
Clavicle

肩锁关节
Acromioclavicular
joint

肩胛骨的肩峰
Acromion of scapula

肩胛冈
Spine of scapula

肱骨大结节
Greater tubercle
of humerus

腋后襞
Posterior axillary
fold

肩胛下角
Inferior angle of
scapula

脊柱沟内的脊椎棘突
Spinous processes
of vertebrae in
vertebral furrow

肋
Rib

竖脊肌隆起
Bulge of erector spinae muscles

髂嵴
Iliac crest

髂后上棘
Posterior superior iliac spine

髋骨
Hip bone

骶骨
Sacrum

股骨大转子
Greater trochanter
of femur

尾骨
Coccyx

坐骨结节
Ischial tuberosity

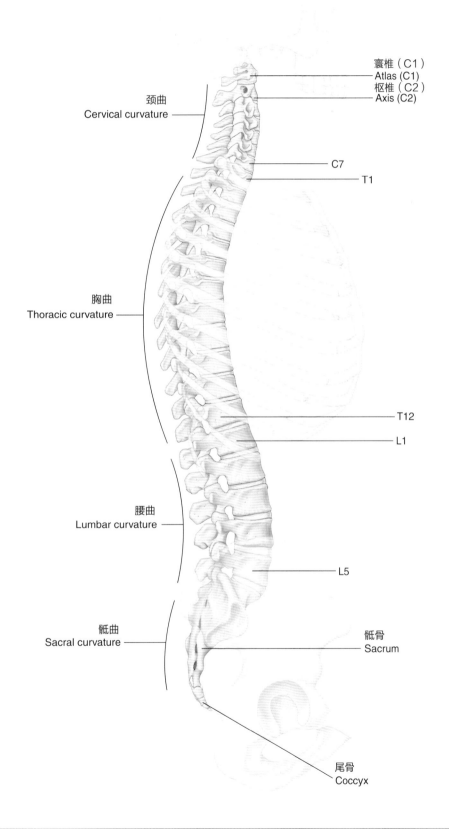

颈曲
Cervical curvature

寰椎（C1）
Atlas (C1)
枢椎（C2）
Axis (C2)

C7

T1

胸曲
Thoracic curvature

T12

L1

腰曲
Lumbar curvature

L5

骶曲
Sacral curvature

骶骨
Sacrum

尾骨
Coccyx

图 1-04　颈椎　Cervical Vertebrae

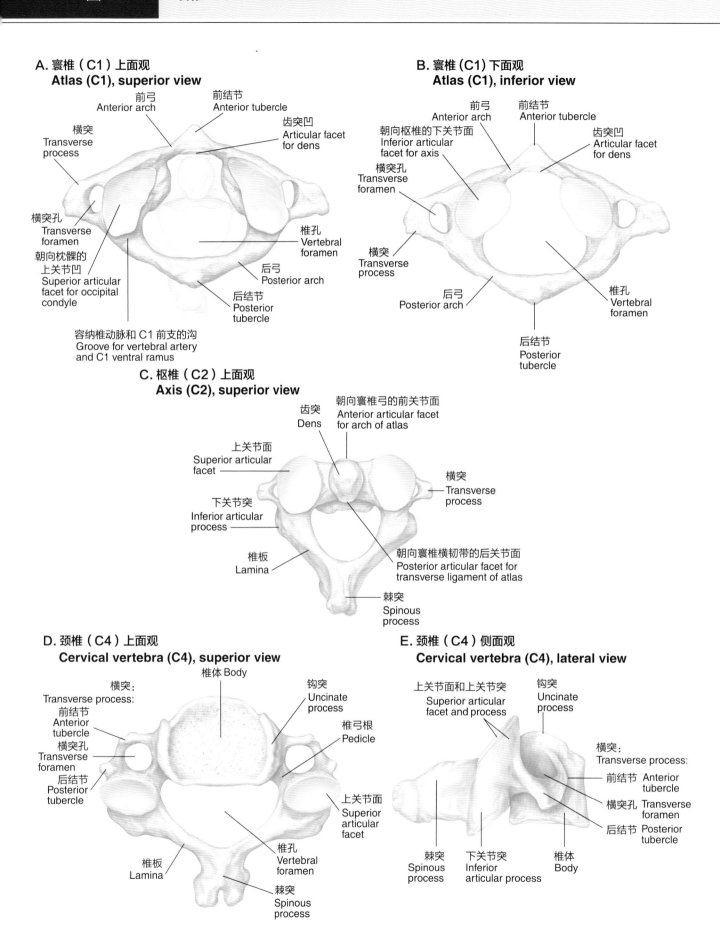

A. 寰椎（C1）上面观
Atlas (C1), superior view

横突
Transverse process

前弓
Anterior arch

前结节
Anterior tubercle

齿突凹
Articular facet for dens

横突孔
Transverse foramen

朝向枕髁的上关节凹
Superior articular facet for occipital condyle

椎孔
Vertebral foramen

后弓
Posterior arch

后结节
Posterior tubercle

容纳椎动脉和 C1 前支的沟
Groove for vertebral artery and C1 ventral ramus

B. 寰椎（C1）下面观
Atlas (C1), inferior view

前弓
Anterior arch

前结节
Anterior tubercle

朝向枢椎的下关节面
Inferior articular facet for axis

齿突凹
Articular facet for dens

横突孔
Transverse foramen

横突
Transverse process

后弓
Posterior arch

椎孔
Vertebral foramen

后结节
Posterior tubercle

C. 枢椎（C2）上面观
Axis (C2), superior view

齿突
Dens

朝向寰椎弓的前关节面
Anterior articular facet for arch of atlas

上关节面
Superior articular facet

横突
Transverse process

下关节突
Inferior articular process

椎板
Lamina

朝向寰椎横韧带的后关节面
Posterior articular facet for transverse ligament of atlas

棘突
Spinous process

D. 颈椎（C4）上面观
Cervical vertebra (C4), superior view

横突：
Transverse process:

前结节
Anterior tubercle

横突孔
Transverse foramen

后结节
Posterior tubercle

椎体 Body

钩突
Uncinate process

椎弓根
Pedicle

上关节面
Superior articular facet

椎板
Lamina

椎孔
Vertebral foramen

棘突
Spinous process

E. 颈椎（C4）侧面观
Cervical vertebra (C4), lateral view

上关节面和上关节突
Superior articular facet and process

钩突
Uncinate process

横突：
Transverse process:

前结节 Anterior tubercle

横突孔 Transverse foramen

后结节 Posterior tubercle

棘突
Spinous process

下关节突
Inferior articular process

椎体
Body

A. 侧面观
Lateral view

B. 颈椎 X 线片，侧面观
Radiograph of cervical vertebrae, lateral view

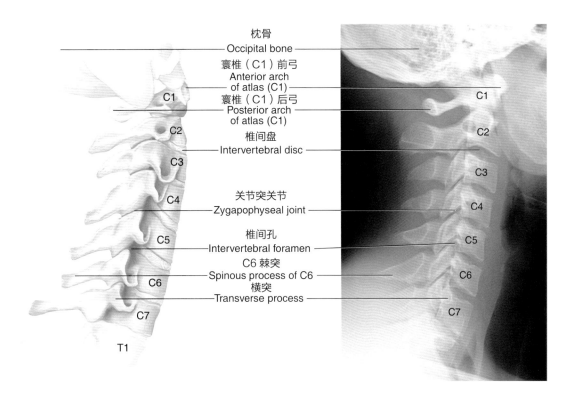

枕骨
Occipital bone

寰椎（C1）前弓
Anterior arch
of atlas (C1)

寰椎（C1）后弓
Posterior arch
of atlas (C1)

椎间盘
Intervertebral disc

关节突关节
Zygapophyseal joint

椎间孔
Intervertebral foramen

C6 棘突
Spinous process of C6

横突
Transverse process

C. 后面观
Posterior view

D. 颈椎 X 线片，后面观
Radiograph of cervical vertebrae, posterior view

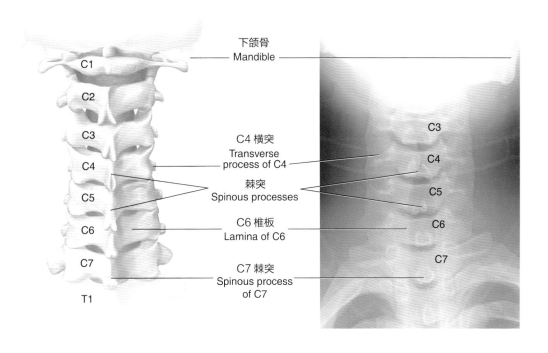

下颌骨
Mandible

C4 横突
Transverse
process of C4

棘突
Spinous processes

C6 椎板
Lamina of C6

C7 棘突
Spinous process
of C7

图 1-06　胸椎和腰椎　Thoracic and Lumbar Vertebrae

A. 胸椎（T6）上面观
Thoracic vertebra (T6), superior view

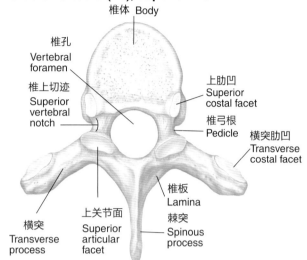

椎体 Body
椎孔 Vertebral foramen
椎上切迹 Superior vertebral notch
上肋凹 Superior costal facet
椎弓根 Pedicle
横突肋凹 Transverse costal facet
椎板 Lamina
横突 Transverse process
上关节面 Superior articular facet
棘突 Spinous process

B. 胸椎（T6）侧面观
Thoracic vertebra (T6), lateral view

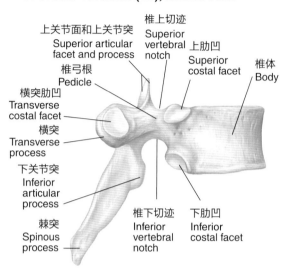

上关节面和上关节突 Superior articular facet and process
椎上切迹 Superior vertebral notch
上肋凹 Superior costal facet
椎体 Body
椎弓根 Pedicle
横突肋凹 Transverse costal facet
横突 Transverse process
下关节突 Inferior articular process
棘突 Spinous process
椎下切迹 Inferior vertebral notch
下肋凹 Inferior costal facet

C. 椎间盘上面观
Intervertebral disc, superior view

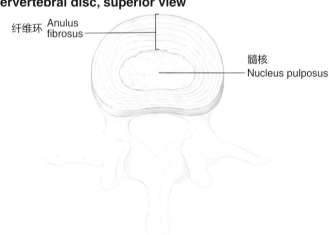

纤维环 Anulus fibrosus
髓核 Nucleus pulposus

D. 腰椎（L3）上面观
Lumbar vertebra (L3), superior view

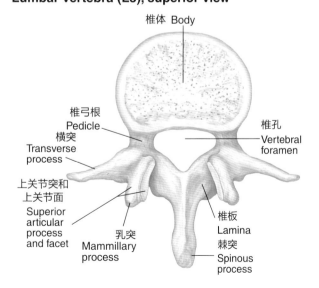

椎体 Body
椎弓根 Pedicle
横突 Transverse process
椎孔 Vertebral foramen
上关节突和上关节面 Superior articular process and facet
乳突 Mammillary process
椎板 Lamina
棘突 Spinous process

E. 腰椎（L3）侧面观
Lumbar vertebra (L3), lateral view

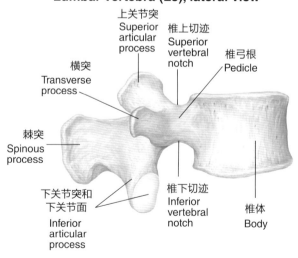

上关节突 Superior articular process
椎上切迹 Superior vertebral notch
椎弓根 Pedicle
横突 Transverse process
棘突 Spinous process
下关节突和下关节面 Inferior articular process
椎下切迹 Inferior vertebral notch
椎体 Body

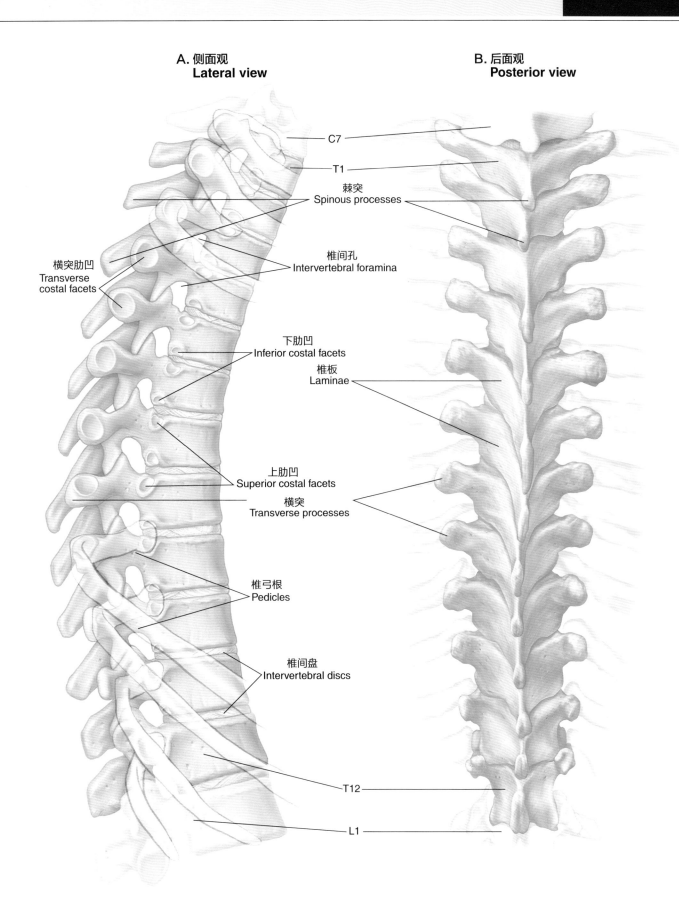

A. 侧面观
Lateral view

B. 后面观
Posterior view

C7

T1

棘突
Spinous processes

椎间孔
Intervertebral foramina

横突肋凹
Transverse
costal facets

下肋凹
Inferior costal facets

椎板
Laminae

上肋凹
Superior costal facets

横突
Transverse processes

椎弓根
Pedicles

椎间盘
Intervertebral discs

T12

L1

图 1-08　腰椎关节　Articulated Lumbar Vertebrae

A. 侧面观
Lateral view

B. 腰椎 X 线片，侧面观
Radiograph of lumbar vertebrae, lateral view

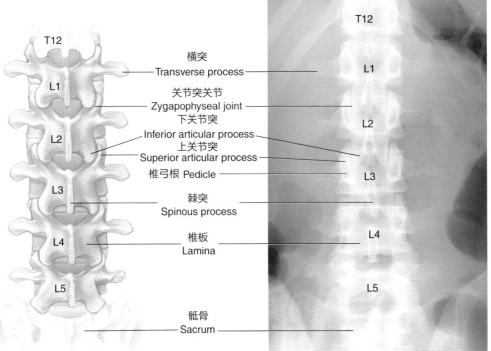

下关节突
Inferior articular process

上关节突
Superior articular process

椎弓根
Pedicle

椎间盘
Intervertebral disc

棘突
Spinous process

椎下切迹
Inferior vertebral notch

椎间孔
Intervertebral foramen

椎上切迹
Superior vertebral notch

L4 横突
Transverse process of L4

椎体
Body

骶骨
Sacrum

T12
L1
L2
L3
L4
L5

C. 后面观
Posterior view

D. 腰椎 X 线片，后面观
Radiograph of lumbar vertebrae, posterior view

横突
Transverse process

关节突关节
Zygapophyseal joint

下关节突
Inferior articular process

上关节突
Superior articular process

椎弓根 Pedicle

棘突
Spinous process

椎板
Lamina

骶骨
Sacrum

T12
L1
L2
L3
L4
L5

A. 前面观
Anterior view

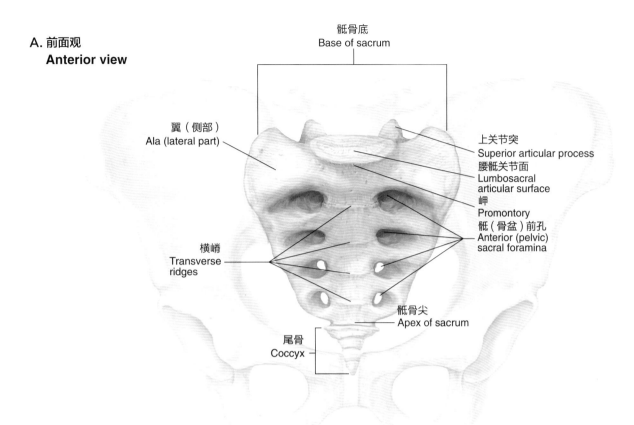

骶骨底
Base of sacrum

翼（侧部）
Ala (lateral part)

上关节突
Superior articular process

腰骶关节面
Lumbosacral articular surface

岬
Promontory

骶（骨盆）前孔
Anterior (pelvic) sacral foramina

横嵴
Transverse ridges

骶骨尖
Apex of sacrum

尾骨
Coccyx

B. 后面观
Posterior view

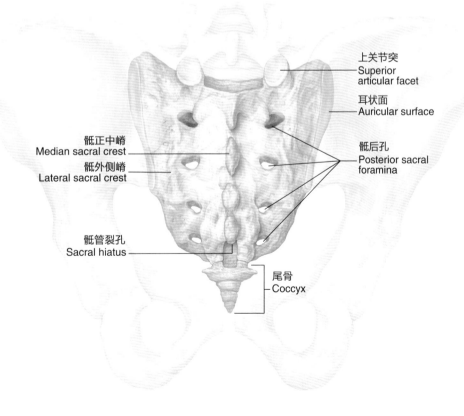

上关节突
Superior articular facet

耳状面
Auricular surface

骶正中嵴
Median sacral crest

骶外侧嵴
Lateral sacral crest

骶后孔
Posterior sacral foramina

骶管裂孔
Sacral hiatus

尾骨
Coccyx

图 1-10　颈椎韧带　Ligaments of the Cervical Vertebrae

A. 侧面观
Lateral view

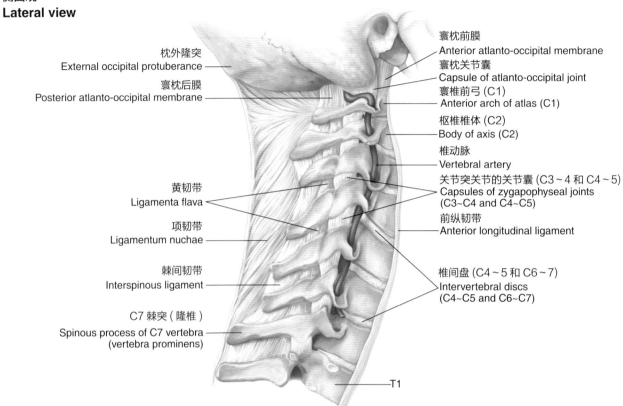

枕外隆突
External occipital protuberance

寰枕后膜
Posterior atlanto-occipital membrane

黄韧带
Ligamenta flava

项韧带
Ligamentum nuchae

棘间韧带
Interspinous ligament

C7 棘突（隆椎）
Spinous process of C7 vertebra
(vertebra prominens)

寰枕前膜
Anterior atlanto-occipital membrane

寰枕关节囊
Capsule of atlanto-occipital joint

寰椎前弓 (C1)
Anterior arch of atlas (C1)

枢椎椎体 (C2)
Body of axis (C2)

椎动脉
Vertebral artery

关节突关节的关节囊 (C3～4 和 C4～5)
Capsules of zygapophyseal joints
(C3~C4 and C4~C5)

前纵韧带
Anterior longitudinal ligament

椎间盘 (C4～5 和 C6～7)
Intervertebral discs
(C4~C5 and C6~C7)

T1

B. 后面观
Posterior view

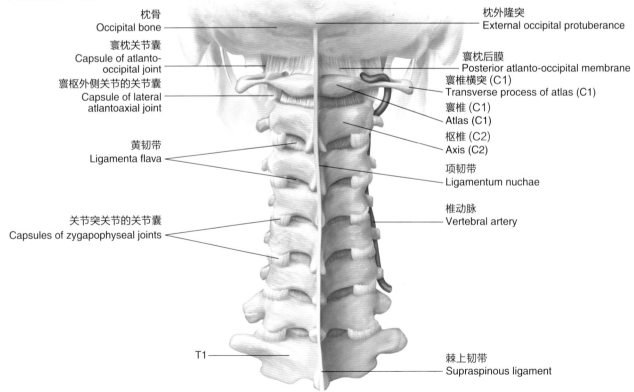

枕骨
Occipital bone

寰枕关节囊
Capsule of atlanto-
occipital joint

寰枢外侧关节的关节囊
Capsule of lateral
atlantoaxial joint

黄韧带
Ligamenta flava

关节突关节的关节囊
Capsules of zygapophyseal joints

T1

枕外隆突
External occipital protuberance

寰枕后膜
Posterior atlanto-occipital membrane

寰椎横突 (C1)
Transverse process of atlas (C1)

寰椎 (C1)
Atlas (C1)

枢椎 (C2)
Axis (C2)

项韧带
Ligamentum nuchae

椎动脉
Vertebral artery

棘上韧带
Supraspinous ligament

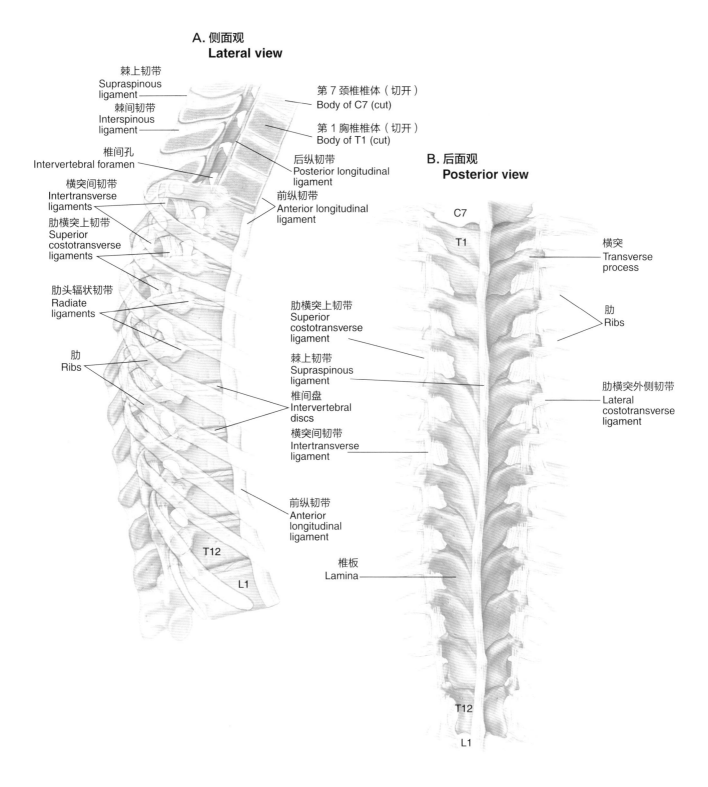

A. 侧面观
Lateral view

棘上韧带
Supraspinous ligament

棘间韧带
Interspinous ligament

椎间孔
Intervertebral foramen

横突间韧带
Intertransverse ligaments

肋横突上韧带
Superior costotransverse ligaments

肋头辐状韧带
Radiate ligaments

肋
Ribs

第 7 颈椎椎体（切开）
Body of C7 (cut)

第 1 胸椎椎体（切开）
Body of T1 (cut)

后纵韧带
Posterior longitudinal ligament

前纵韧带
Anterior longitudinal ligament

B. 后面观
Posterior view

肋横突上韧带
Superior costotransverse ligament

棘上韧带
Supraspinous ligament

椎间盘
Intervertebral discs

横突间韧带
Intertransverse ligament

前纵韧带
Anterior longitudinal ligament

T12

L1

C7

T1

横突
Transverse process

肋
Ribs

肋横突外侧韧带
Lateral costotransverse ligament

椎板
Lamina

T12

L1

图 1-12　腰椎和骶骨韧带　Ligaments of the Lumbar Vertebrae and Sacrum

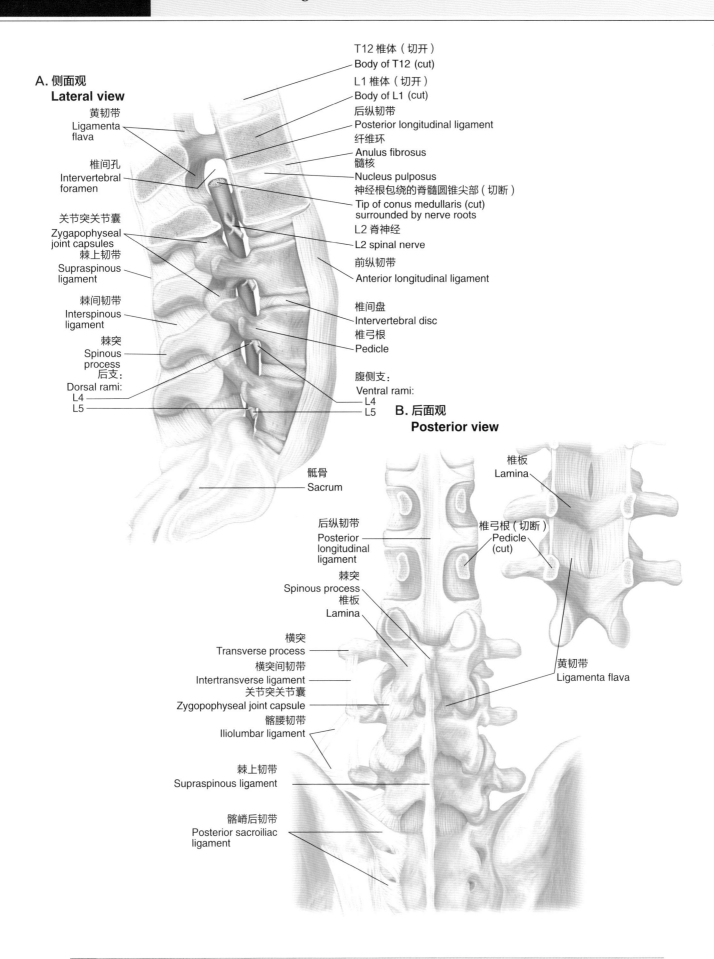

A. 侧面观
Lateral view

黄韧带
Ligamenta
flava

椎间孔
Intervertebral
foramen

关节突关节囊
Zygapophyseal
joint capsules

棘上韧带
Supraspinous
ligament

棘间韧带
Interspinous
ligament

棘突
Spinous
process

后支：
Dorsal rami:
L4
L5

T12 椎体（切开）
Body of T12 (cut)

L1 椎体（切开）
Body of L1 (cut)

后纵韧带
Posterior longitudinal ligament

纤维环
Anulus fibrosus

髓核
Nucleus pulposus

神经根包绕的脊髓圆锥尖部（切断）
Tip of conus medullaris (cut)
surrounded by nerve roots

L2 脊神经
L2 spinal nerve

前纵韧带
Anterior longitudinal ligament

椎间盘
Intervertebral disc

椎弓根
Pedicle

腹侧支：
Ventral rami:
L4
L5

B. 后面观
Posterior view

骶骨
Sacrum

后纵韧带
Posterior
longitudinal
ligament

棘突
Spinous process

椎板
Lamina

横突
Transverse process

横突间韧带
Intertransverse ligament

关节突关节囊
Zygopophyseal joint capsule

髂腰韧带
Iliolumbar ligament

棘上韧带
Supraspinous ligament

髂嵴后韧带
Posterior sacroiliac
ligament

椎板
Lamina

椎弓根（切断）
Pedicle
(cut)

黄韧带
Ligamenta flava

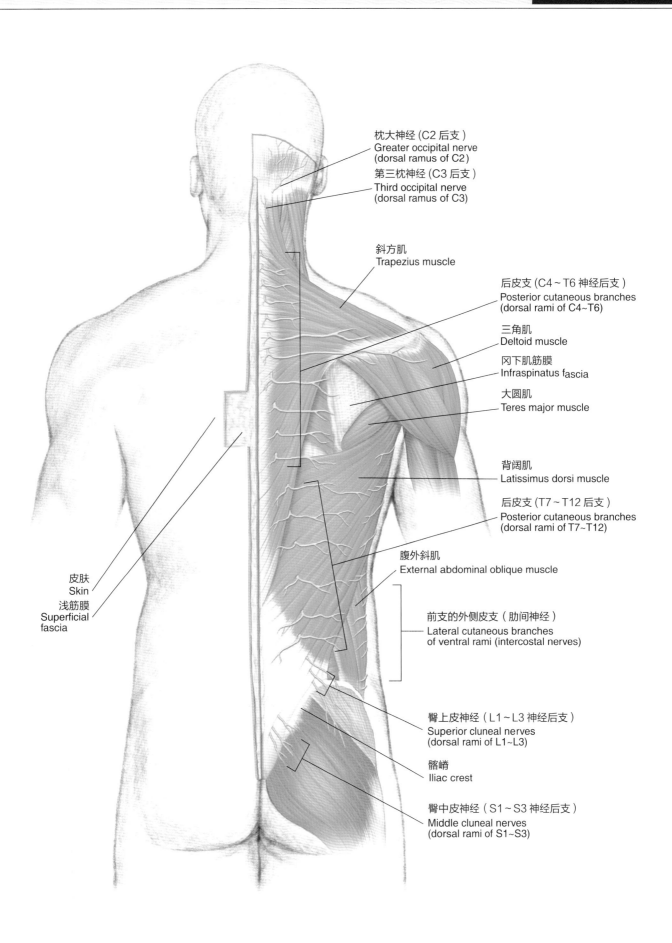

枕大神经 (C2 后支)
Greater occipital nerve
(dorsal ramus of C2)

第三枕神经 (C3 后支)
Third occipital nerve
(dorsal ramus of C3)

斜方肌
Trapezius muscle

后皮支 (C4 ~ T6 神经后支)
Posterior cutaneous branches
(dorsal rami of C4~T6)

三角肌
Deltoid muscle

冈下肌筋膜
Infraspinatus fascia

大圆肌
Teres major muscle

背阔肌
Latissimus dorsi muscle

后皮支 (T7 ~ T12 后支)
Posterior cutaneous branches
(dorsal rami of T7~T12)

腹外斜肌
External abdominal oblique muscle

前支的外侧皮支（肋间神经）
Lateral cutaneous branches
of ventral rami (intercostal nerves)

臀上皮神经（L1 ~ L3 神经后支)
Superior cluneal nerves
(dorsal rami of L1~L3)

髂嵴
Iliac crest

臀中皮神经（S1 ~ S3 神经后支)
Middle cluneal nerves
(dorsal rami of S1~S3)

皮肤
Skin

浅筋膜
Superficial
fascia

背部皮肤神经支配　**Cutaneous innervation of the black**

图 1-14　　背部浅层肌　Superficial Muscles of the Back

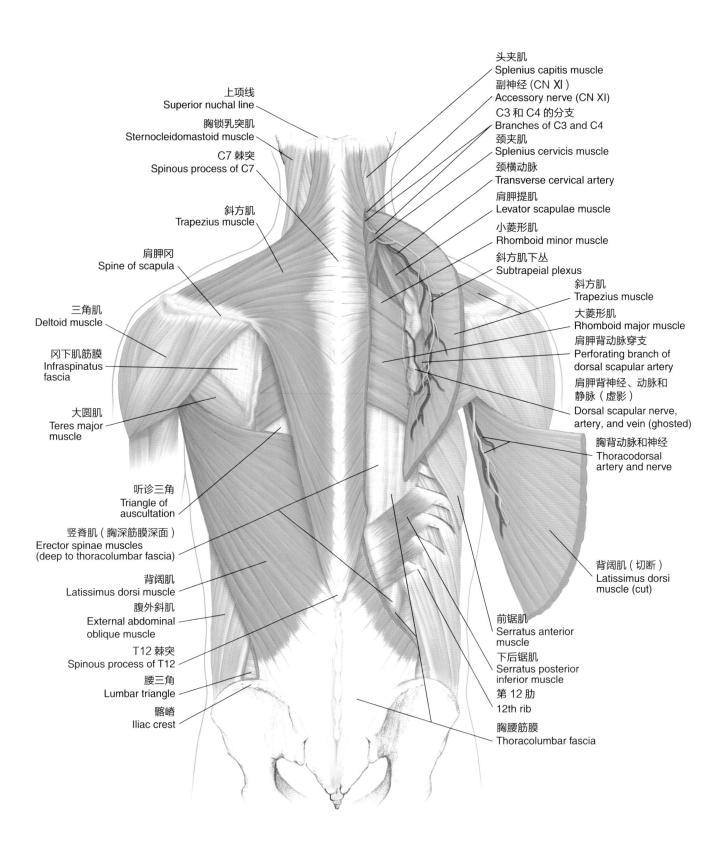

上项线
Superior nuchal line

胸锁乳突肌
Sternocleidomastoid muscle

C7 棘突
Spinous process of C7

斜方肌
Trapezius muscle

肩胛冈
Spine of scapula

三角肌
Deltoid muscle

冈下肌筋膜
Infraspinatus fascia

大圆肌
Teres major muscle

听诊三角
Triangle of auscultation

竖脊肌（胸深筋膜深面）
Erector spinae muscles (deep to thoracolumbar fascia)

背阔肌
Latissimus dorsi muscle

腹外斜肌
External abdominal oblique muscle

T12 棘突
Spinous process of T12

腰三角
Lumbar triangle

髂嵴
Iliac crest

头夹肌
Splenius capitis muscle

副神经（CN XI）
Accessory nerve (CN XI)

C3 和 C4 的分支
Branches of C3 and C4

颈夹肌
Splenius cervicis muscle

颈横动脉
Transverse cervical artery

肩胛提肌
Levator scapulae muscle

小菱形肌
Rhomboid minor muscle

斜方肌下丛
Subtrapeial plexus

斜方肌
Trapezius muscle

大菱形肌
Rhomboid major muscle

肩胛背动脉穿支
Perforating branch of dorsal scapular artery

肩胛背神经、动脉和静脉（虚影）
Dorsal scapular nerve, artery, and vein (ghosted)

胸背动脉和神经
Thoracodorsal artery and nerve

背阔肌（切断）
Latissimus dorsi muscle (cut)

前锯肌
Serratus anterior muscle

下后锯肌
Serratus posterior inferior muscle

第 12 肋
12th rib

胸腰筋膜
Thoracolumbar fascia

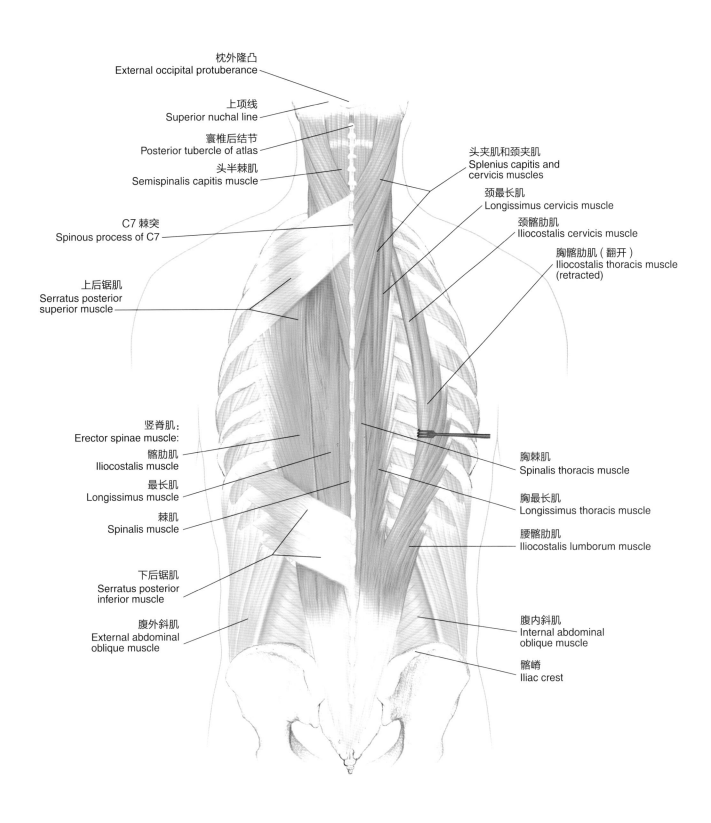

枕外隆凸
External occipital protuberance

上项线
Superior nuchal line

寰椎后结节
Posterior tubercle of atlas

头半棘肌
Semispinalis capitis muscle

C7 棘突
Spinous process of C7

上后锯肌
Serratus posterior
superior muscle

竖脊肌：
Erector spinae muscle:

髂肋肌
Iliocostalis muscle

最长肌
Longissimus muscle

棘肌
Spinalis muscle

下后锯肌
Serratus posterior
inferior muscle

腹外斜肌
External abdominal
oblique muscle

头夹肌和颈夹肌
Splenius capitis and
cervicis muscles

颈最长肌
Longissimus cervicis muscle

颈髂肋肌
Iliocostalis cervicis muscle

胸髂肋肌（翻开）
Iliocostalis thoracis muscle
(retracted)

胸棘肌
Spinalis thoracis muscle

胸最长肌
Longissimus thoracis muscle

腰髂肋肌
Iliocostalis lumborum muscle

腹内斜肌
Internal abdominal
oblique muscle

髂嵴
Iliac crest

图 1-16 背部深层肌，深层解剖 Deep Back Muscles, Deeper Dissection

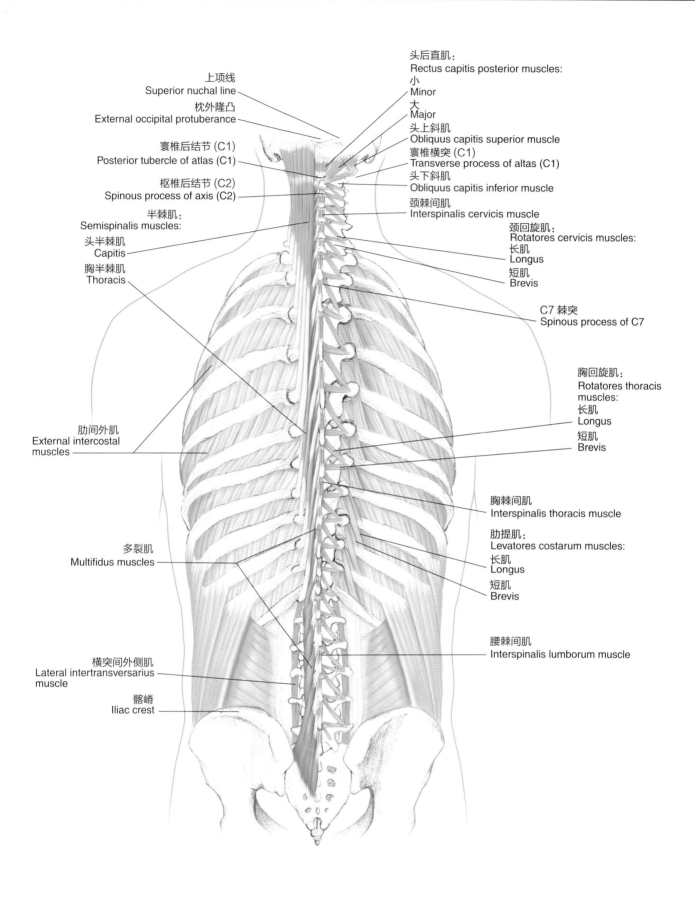

上项线
Superior nuchal line

枕外隆凸
External occipital protuberance

寰椎后结节 (C1)
Posterior tubercle of atlas (C1)

枢椎后结节 (C2)
Spinous process of axis (C2)

半棘肌：
Semispinalis muscles:

头半棘肌
Capitis

胸半棘肌
Thoracis

肋间外肌
External intercostal
muscles

多裂肌
Multifidus muscles

横突间外侧肌
Lateral intertransversarius
muscle

髂嵴
Iliac crest

头后直肌：
Rectus capitis posterior muscles:
小
Minor
大
Major

头上斜肌
Obliquus capitis superior muscle

寰椎横突 (C1)
Transverse process of altas (C1)

头下斜肌
Obliquus capitis inferior muscle

颈棘间肌
Interspinalis cervicis muscle

颈回旋肌：
Rotatores cervicis muscles:
长肌
Longus
短肌
Brevis

C7 棘突
Spinous process of C7

胸回旋肌：
Rotatores thoracis
muscles:
长肌
Longus
短肌
Brevis

胸棘间肌
Interspinalis thoracis muscle

肋提肌：
Levatores costarum muscles:
长肌
Longus
短肌
Brevis

腰棘间肌
Interspinalis lumborum muscle

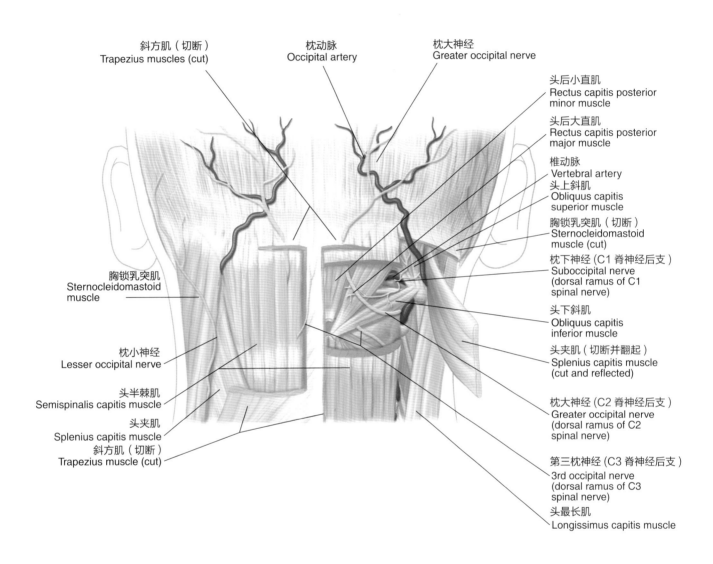

斜方肌（切断）
Trapezius muscles (cut)

枕动脉
Occipital artery

枕大神经
Greater occipital nerve

头后小直肌
Rectus capitis posterior
minor muscle

头后大直肌
Rectus capitis posterior
major muscle

椎动脉
Vertebral artery

头上斜肌
Obliquus capitis
superior muscle

胸锁乳突肌（切断）
Sternocleidomastoid
muscle (cut)

枕下神经 (C1 脊神经后支)
Suboccipital nerve
(dorsal ramus of C1
spinal nerve)

头下斜肌
Obliquus capitis
inferior muscle

头夹肌（切断并翻起）
Splenius capitis muscle
(cut and reflected)

枕大神经 (C2 脊神经后支)
Greater occipital nerve
(dorsal ramus of C2
spinal nerve)

第三枕神经 (C3 脊神经后支)
3rd occipital nerve
(dorsal ramus of C3
spinal nerve)

头最长肌
Longissimus capitis muscle

胸锁乳突肌
Sternocleidomastoid
muscle

枕小神经
Lesser occipital nerve

头半棘肌
Semispinalis capitis muscle

头夹肌
Splenius capitis muscle

斜方肌（切断）
Trapezius muscle (cut)

图 1-18　典型的脊神经组成　Pattern of a Typical Spinal Nerve

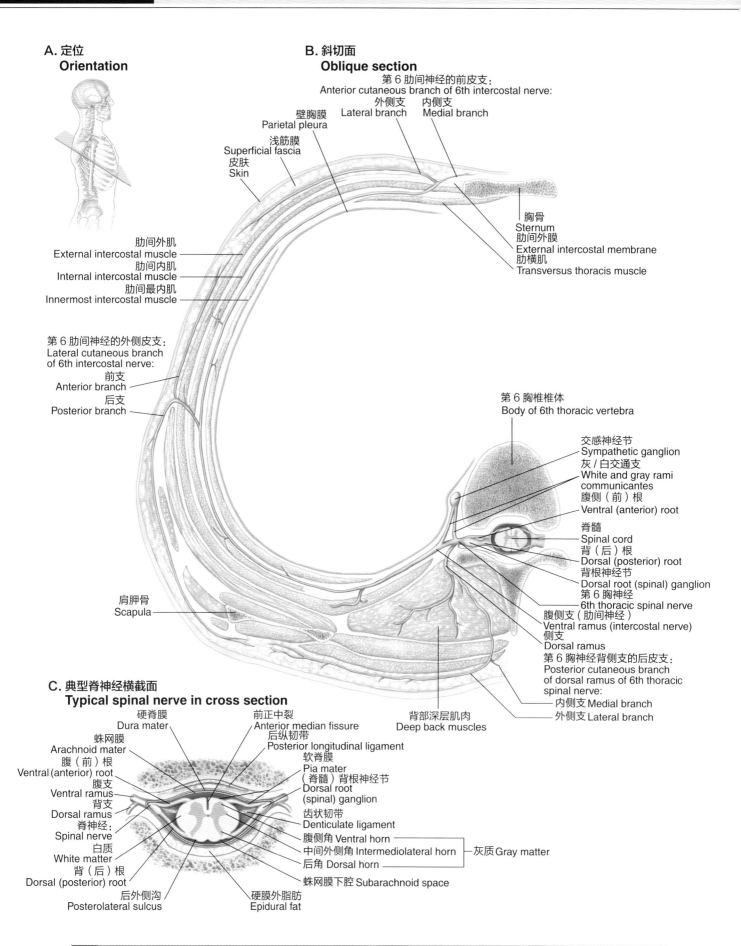

A. 定位
Orientation

B. 斜切面
Oblique section

第 6 肋间神经的前皮支：
Anterior cutaneous branch of 6th intercostal nerve:
外侧支
Lateral branch
内侧支
Medial branch

壁胸膜
Parietal pleura

浅筋膜
Superficial fascia
皮肤
Skin

胸骨
Sternum
肋间外膜
External intercostal membrane
肋横肌
Transversus thoracis muscle

肋间外肌
External intercostal muscle
肋间内肌
Internal intercostal muscle
肋间最内肌
Innermost intercostal muscle

第 6 肋间神经的外侧皮支：
Lateral cutaneous branch
of 6th intercostal nerve:
前支
Anterior branch
后支
Posterior branch

第 6 胸椎椎体
Body of 6th thoracic vertebra

交感神经节
Sympathetic ganglion
灰／白交通支
White and gray rami
communicantes
腹侧（前）根
Ventral (anterior) root
脊髓
Spinal cord
背（后）根
Dorsal (posterior) root
背根神经节
Dorsal root (spinal) ganglion
第 6 胸神经
6th thoracic spinal nerve
腹侧支（肋间神经）
Ventral ramus (intercostal nerve)
侧支
Dorsal ramus
第 6 胸神经背侧支的后皮支：
Posterior cutaneous branch
of dorsal ramus of 6th thoracic
spinal nerve:
内侧支 Medial branch
外侧支 Lateral branch

肩胛骨
Scapula

背部深层肌肉
Deep back muscles

C. 典型脊神经横截面
Typical spinal nerve in cross section

硬脊膜
Dura mater

蛛网膜
Arachnoid mater
腹（前）根
Ventral (anterior) root
腹支
Ventral ramus
背支
Dorsal ramus
脊神经：
Spinal nerve:
白质
White matter
背（后）根
Dorsal (posterior) root

后外侧沟
Posterolateral sulcus

前正中裂
Anterior median fissure
后纵韧带
Posterior longitudinal ligament
软脊膜
Pia mater
（脊髓）背根神经节
Dorsal root
(spinal) ganglion
齿状韧带
Denticulate ligament
腹侧角 Ventral horn
中间外侧角 Intermediolateral horn
后角 Dorsal horn
蛛网膜下腔 Subarachnoid space

硬膜外脂肪
Epidural fat

灰质 Gray matter

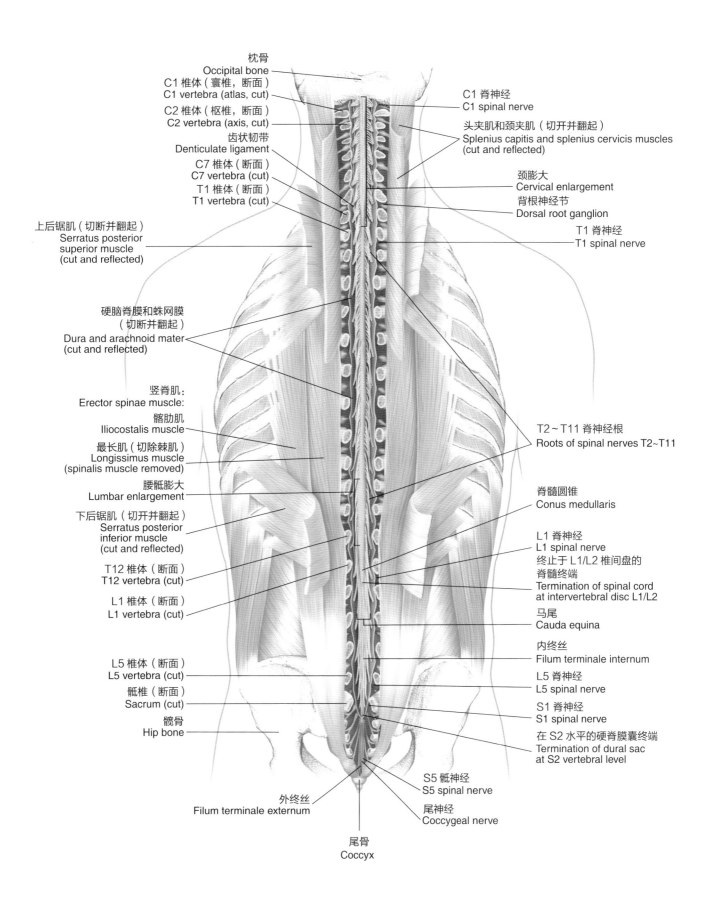

枕骨
Occipital bone

C1 椎体（寰椎，断面）
C1 vertebra (atlas, cut)

C2 椎体（枢椎，断面）
C2 vertebra (axis, cut)

齿状韧带
Denticulate ligament

C7 椎体（断面）
C7 vertebra (cut)

T1 椎体（断面）
T1 vertebra (cut)

上后锯肌（切断并翻起）
Serratus posterior
superior muscle
(cut and reflected)

硬脑脊膜和蛛网膜
（切断并翻起）
Dura and arachnoid mater
(cut and reflected)

竖脊肌：
Erector spinae muscle:

髂肋肌
Iliocostalis muscle

最长肌（切除棘肌）
Longissimus muscle
(spinalis muscle removed)

腰骶膨大
Lumbar enlargement

下后锯肌（切开并翻起）
Serratus posterior
inferior muscle
(cut and reflected)

T12 椎体（断面）
T12 vertebra (cut)

L1 椎体（断面）
L1 vertebra (cut)

L5 椎体（断面）
L5 vertebra (cut)

骶椎（断面）
Sacrum (cut)

髋骨
Hip bone

外终丝
Filum terminale externum

尾骨
Coccyx

C1 脊神经
C1 spinal nerve

头夹肌和颈夹肌（切开并翻起）
Splenius capitis and splenius cervicis muscles
(cut and reflected)

颈膨大
Cervical enlargement

背根神经节
Dorsal root ganglion

T1 脊神经
T1 spinal nerve

T2~T11 脊神经根
Roots of spinal nerves T2~T11

脊髓圆锥
Conus medullaris

L1 脊神经
L1 spinal nerve
终止于 L1/L2 椎间盘的
脊髓终端
Termination of spinal cord
at intervertebral disc L1/L2

马尾
Cauda equina

内终丝
Filum terminale internum

L5 脊神经
L5 spinal nerve

S1 脊神经
S1 spinal nerve

在 S2 水平的硬脊膜囊终端
Termination of dural sac
at S2 vertebral level

S5 骶神经
S5 spinal nerve

尾神经
Coccygeal nerve

图 1-20   脊髓上部 **Superior Portion of the Spinal Cord**

A. 定位
Orientation

B. 剖面图
Dissection

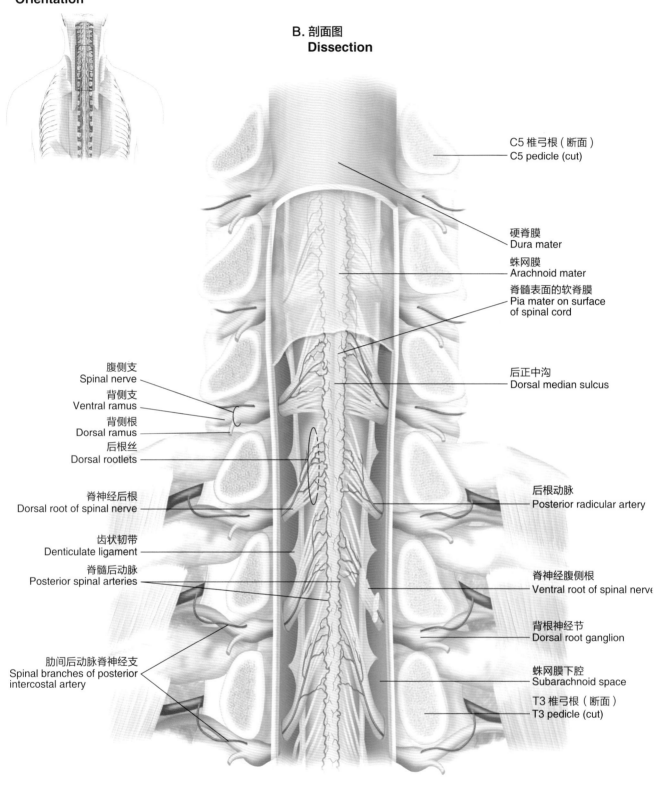

C5 椎弓根（断面）
C5 pedicle (cut)

硬脊膜
Dura mater

蛛网膜
Arachnoid mater

脊髓表面的软脊膜
Pia mater on surface
of spinal cord

后正中沟
Dorsal median sulcus

后根动脉
Posterior radicular artery

脊神经腹侧根
Ventral root of spinal nerve

背根神经节
Dorsal root ganglion

蛛网膜下腔
Subarachnoid space

T3 椎弓根（断面）
T3 pedicle (cut)

腹侧支
Spinal nerve

背侧支
Ventral ramus

背侧根
Dorsal ramus

后根丝
Dorsal rootlets

脊神经后根
Dorsal root of spinal nerve

齿状韧带
Denticulate ligament

脊髓后动脉
Posterior spinal arteries

肋间后动脉脊神经支
Spinal branches of posterior
intercostal artery

A. 定位
Orientation

B. 剖面图
Dissection

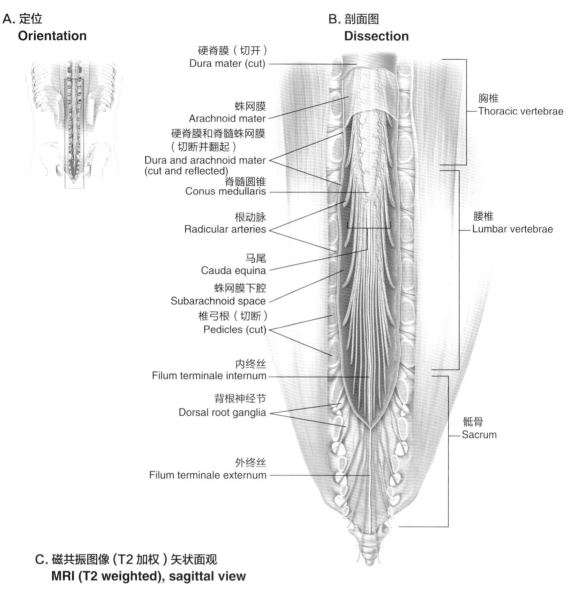

硬脊膜（切开）
Dura mater (cut)

蛛网膜
Arachnoid mater

硬脊膜和脊髓蛛网膜
（切断并翻起）
Dura and arachnoid mater
(cut and reflected)

脊髓圆锥
Conus medullaris

根动脉
Radicular arteries

马尾
Cauda equina

蛛网膜下腔
Subarachnoid space

椎弓根（切断）
Pedicles (cut)

内终丝
Filum terminale internum

背根神经节
Dorsal root ganglia

外终丝
Filum terminale externum

胸椎
Thoracic vertebrae

腰椎
Lumbar vertebrae

骶骨
Sacrum

C. 磁共振图像（T2 加权）矢状面观
MRI (T2 weighted), sagittal view

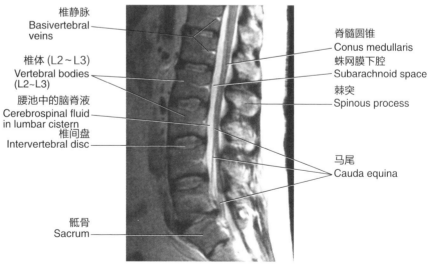

椎静脉
Basivertebral
veins

椎体（L2～L3）
Vertebral bodies
(L2~L3)

腰池中的脑脊液
Cerebrospinal fluid
in lumbar cistern

椎间盘
Intervertebral disc

骶骨
Sacrum

脊髓圆锥
Conus medullaris

蛛网膜下腔
Subarachnoid space

棘突
Spinous process

马尾
Cauda equina

图 1-22　　脊髓血供前面观　Blood Supply of the Spinal Cord, Anterior View

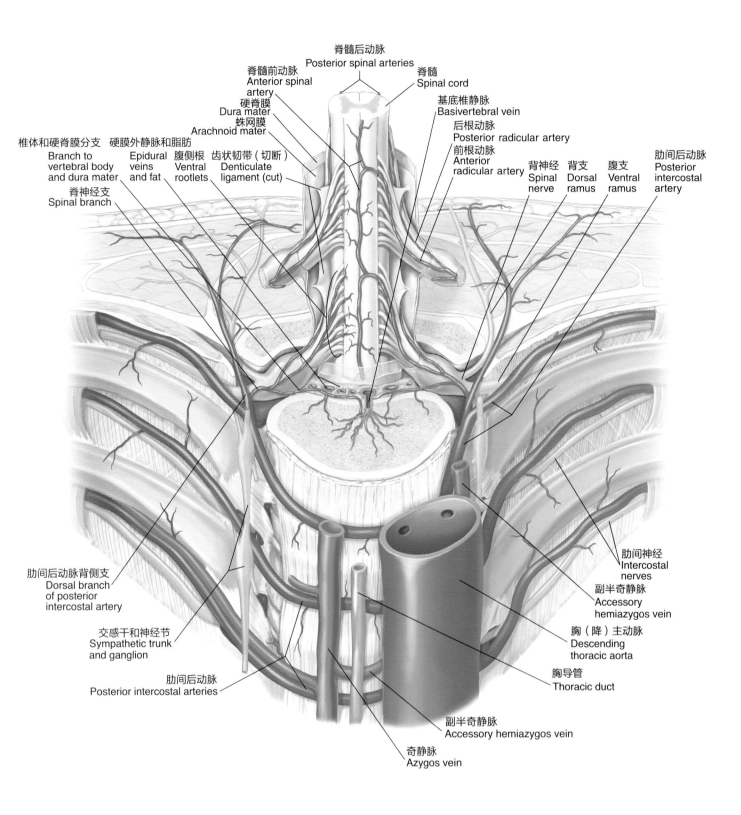

脊髓后动脉
Posterior spinal arteries

脊髓前动脉
Anterior spinal
artery

硬脊膜
Dura mater

蛛网膜
Arachnoid mater

脊髓
Spinal cord

基底椎静脉
Basivertebral vein

后根动脉
Posterior radicular artery

前根动脉
Anterior
radicular artery

椎体和硬脊膜分支　硬膜外静脉和脂肪
Branch to　　　　Epidural
vertebral body　　veins
and dura mater　　and fat

腹侧根　齿状韧带（切断）
Ventral　Denticulate
rootlets　ligament (cut)

背神经　背支　腹支
Spinal　Dorsal　Ventral
nerve　ramus　ramus

肋间后动脉
Posterior
intercostal
artery

脊神经支
Spinal branch

肋间神经
Intercostal
nerves

副半奇静脉
Accessory
hemiazygos vein

胸（降）主动脉
Descending
thoracic aorta

胸导管
Thoracic duct

肋间后动脉背侧支
Dorsal branch
of posterior
intercostal artery

交感干和神经节
Sympathetic trunk
and ganglion

肋间后动脉
Posterior intercostal arteries

副半奇静脉
Accessory hemiazygos vein

奇静脉
Azygos vein

A. 矢状观
Sagittal view

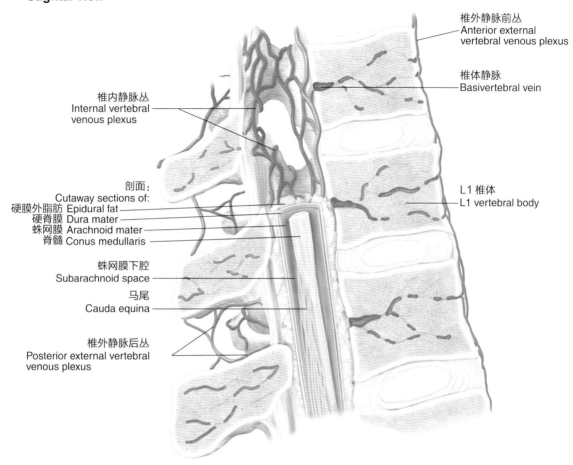

椎外静脉前丛
Anterior external
vertebral venous plexus

椎体静脉
Basivertebral vein

椎内静脉丛
Internal vertebral
venous plexus

剖面：
Cutaway sections of:
硬膜外脂肪 Epidural fat
硬脊膜 Dura mater
蛛网膜 Arachnoid mater
脊髓 Conus medullaris

L1 椎体
L1 vertebral body

蛛网膜下腔
Subarachnoid space

马尾
Cauda equina

椎外静脉后丛
Posterior external vertebral
venous plexus

B. 上面观
Superior view

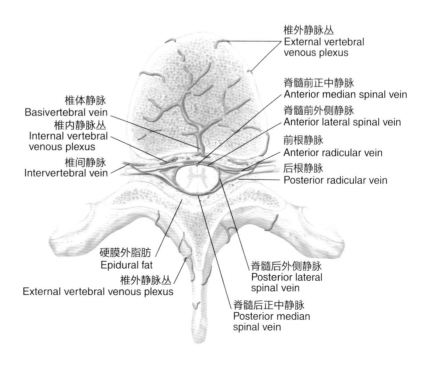

椎外静脉丛
External vertebral
venous plexus

脊髓前正中静脉
Anterior median spinal vein

脊髓前外侧静脉
Anterior lateral spinal vein

椎体静脉
Basivertebral vein

椎内静脉丛
Internal vertebral
venous plexus

椎间静脉
Intervertebral vein

前根静脉
Anterior radicular vein

后根静脉
Posterior radicular vein

硬膜外脂肪
Epidural fat

椎外静脉丛
External vertebral venous plexus

脊髓后外侧静脉
Posterior lateral
spinal vein

脊髓后正中静脉
Posterior median
spinal vein

图 1-24　皮区　**Dermatomes**

A. 前面观
Anterior view

B. 后面观
Posterior view

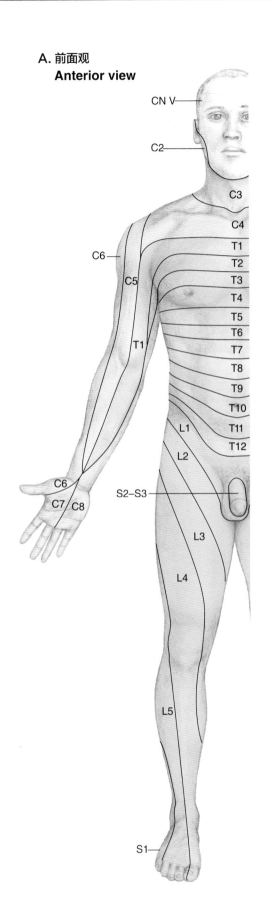

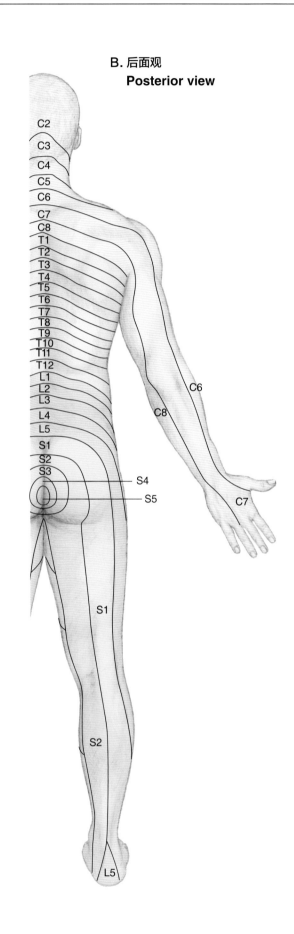

背部肌群：浅层						
名称	**起点**	**止点**	**主要作用**	**神经支配**	**动脉**	**注释**
背阔肌（图 1-14）	T7 至骶骨棘突、髂嵴的后 1/3、下 3~4 肋、有时起于肩胛骨下角	结节间沟的底	后伸和向内旋转上臂，并内收上臂	来自臂丛后束的胸背神经（C7，C8）	胸背动脉	止点肌腱扭转因此肌纤维起点最高而止点最低
肩胛提肌（图 1-14）	C1~C4 横突	肩胛骨内侧缘自上角至肩胛冈	上提肩胛骨	肩胛背神经（C5）；肌的上半部分还接受 C3 和 C4 的分支	肩胛背动脉	肩胛提肌是按其功能命名
大菱形肌（图 1-14）	T2~T5 棘突	肩胛冈以下的肩胛骨内侧缘	拉肩胛骨向内，上提和下旋肩胛骨	肩胛背神经（C5）	肩胛背动脉	按形态命名
小菱形肌（图 1-14）	项韧带下端、C7 和 T1 棘突	肩胛冈内侧缘的肩胛冈根部	拉肩胛骨向内，上提和下旋肩胛骨	肩胛背神经（C5）	肩胛背动脉	按形态命名
斜方肌（图 1-14）	上项线的内侧 1/3、枕外隆凸、项韧带，C7~T12 棘突	锁骨外 1/3 肩峰内侧，肩胛冈上嵴，肩胛冈结节	上提和降肩胛骨（取决于哪一部分肌收缩）；向上旋转肩胛骨；拉肩胛骨向内	运动：脊副神经（XI），本体感觉：C3~C4	颈横动脉	按形态命名；斜方肌在发育过程中自起点水平（颈部）连同其神经和动脉一起迁移至最终的位置，是发育过程中骨骼肌迁移的一个典型

背部肌群：中层						
名称	**起点**	**止点**	**主要作用**	**神经支配**	**动脉**	**注释**
下后锯肌	胸腰筋膜、T11~T12 和 L1~L2 棘突	第 9~12 肋，肋角外侧	下拉肋	T9~T12 脊神经腹侧主支的分支	最下肋间后动脉，肋下动脉，第 1、2 腰动脉	呼吸肌，接受脊神经前支支配，胚胎来源与肋间肌相关而非深层背肌
上后锯肌	项韧带、C7 和 T1~T3 棘突	第 1~4 肋，肋角外侧	上提肋	T1~T4 脊神经腹侧主支的分支	第 1~4 肋间后动脉	呼吸肌，接受脊神经前支支配，胚胎来源与肋间肌相关而非深层背肌

背部肌群：深层

名称	起点	止点	主要作用	神经支配	动脉	注释
竖脊肌（图1-15）	髂嵴、骶骨、椎骨的横突、棘突和棘上韧带	肋角、椎骨的横突、棘突和颅骨后面	后伸和侧弯躯干、颈和头	C1~S5脊神经背侧主支的节段支配	由以下动脉节段供应：颈深动脉、肋间后动脉、腰动脉	竖脊肌分为3个肌柱：外侧的髂肋肌、中间的最长肌和内侧的棘肌；每个柱都有许多不同的命名部分
髂肋肌	髂嵴和骶骨	肋角	后伸和侧弯躯干和颈	C4~S5脊神经背侧主支	由以下动脉节段供应：颈深动脉、肋间后动脉、腰动脉	竖脊肌的最外侧部分；可进一步分为腰部、胸部和颈部
棘间肌	棘突上缘	上位椎体棘突下缘	后伸躯干和颈	C1~L5脊神经背侧主支	由以下动脉节段供应：颈深动脉、肋间后动脉、腰动脉	这些是小且不重要的肌肉
横突间肌	横突上缘	上位椎体横突下缘	侧弯躯干和颈	C1~L5脊神经背侧主支	由以下动脉节段供应：颈深动脉、肋间后动脉、腰动脉	这些是小而不重要的肌肉
最长肌	下位椎骨横突	上位椎体横突和乳突	后伸和侧弯躯干、颈和头	C1~S1脊神经背侧主支	由以下动脉节段供应：颈深动脉、肋间后动脉、腰动脉	竖脊肌的中间部分；可进一步分为胸部、颈部和头部
多裂肌	骶骨、C3~L5横突	起点上2~4个水平的椎体棘突	后伸和侧弯躯干和颈，向对侧转头	C1~L5脊神经背侧主支	由以下动脉节段供应：颈深动脉、肋间后动脉、腰动脉	半棘肌、多裂肌和回旋肌组成横突棘肌群
头下斜肌	枢椎棘突	寰椎横突	向同侧转头	枕下神经（C1背侧主支）	枕动脉	枕大神经（C2脊神经背侧主支）走行于头下斜肌下缘的上方
头上斜肌	寰椎横突	枕骨的下项线上方	后伸头，向同侧转头	枕下神经（C1背侧主支）	枕动脉	头上斜肌和头后大直肌构成枕下三角
头后大直肌	枢椎棘突	下项线	后伸头，向同侧转头	枕下神经（C1背侧主支）	枕动脉	无
头后小直肌	寰椎后结节	下项线内侧	后伸头	枕下神经（C1背侧主支）	枕动脉	头后小直肌位于头后大直肌深面，止点靠近内侧

续表

背部肌群：深层						
名称	起点	止点	主要作用	神经支配	动脉	注释
回旋肌	横突	长回旋肌：起点上方2个椎骨的棘突短回旋肌：起点上方1个椎骨的棘突	将脊柱向对侧旋转	C1~L5脊神经背侧主支	由以下动脉节段供应：颈深动脉、肋间后动脉、腰动脉	半棘肌、多裂肌和回旋肌组成横突棘肌群
半棘肌	C7~T12横突	头半棘肌：颅骨后面上下项线之间；颈半棘肌和胸半棘肌：起点上方4~6个椎体的棘突	后伸躯干并协同侧弯和向对侧旋转躯干	C1~T12脊神经背侧主支	由以下动脉节段供应：颈深动脉、肋间后动脉、腰动脉	根据其止点分3部分命名：头半棘肌、颈半棘肌和胸半棘肌；半棘肌、多裂肌和回旋肌组成横突棘肌群
棘肌	下位椎骨棘突	上位椎骨棘突和颅底	后伸和侧弯躯干和颈	C2~L3脊神经背侧主支	由以下动脉节段供应：颈深动脉、肋间后动脉、腰动脉	竖脊肌的最内侧部：可进一步分为胸部、颈部和头部
夹肌	项韧带和C7~T6棘突	头夹肌：乳突和上项线外侧；颈夹肌：C1~C3后结节	后伸和侧弯躯干、颈和头；向同侧转头	C2~C6脊神经背侧主支	由以下动脉节段供应：颈深动脉、肋间后动脉	夹肌意为包扎；因其的宽阔扁平的形状得名
头夹肌	项韧带C7~T6棘突	乳突和上项线外侧端	后伸和侧弯颈和头；向同侧转头	C2~C6脊神经背侧主支	由以下动脉节段供应：颈深动脉、肋间后动脉	因其形态命名：夹肌意为包扎，头指肌的止点
颈夹肌	项韧带C7~T6棘突	C1~C3横突后结节	后伸和侧弯颈和头；向同侧转头	C2~C6脊神经背侧主支	由以下动脉节段供应：颈深动脉、肋间后动脉	因其形态命名：夹肌意为包扎，颈指肌的止点

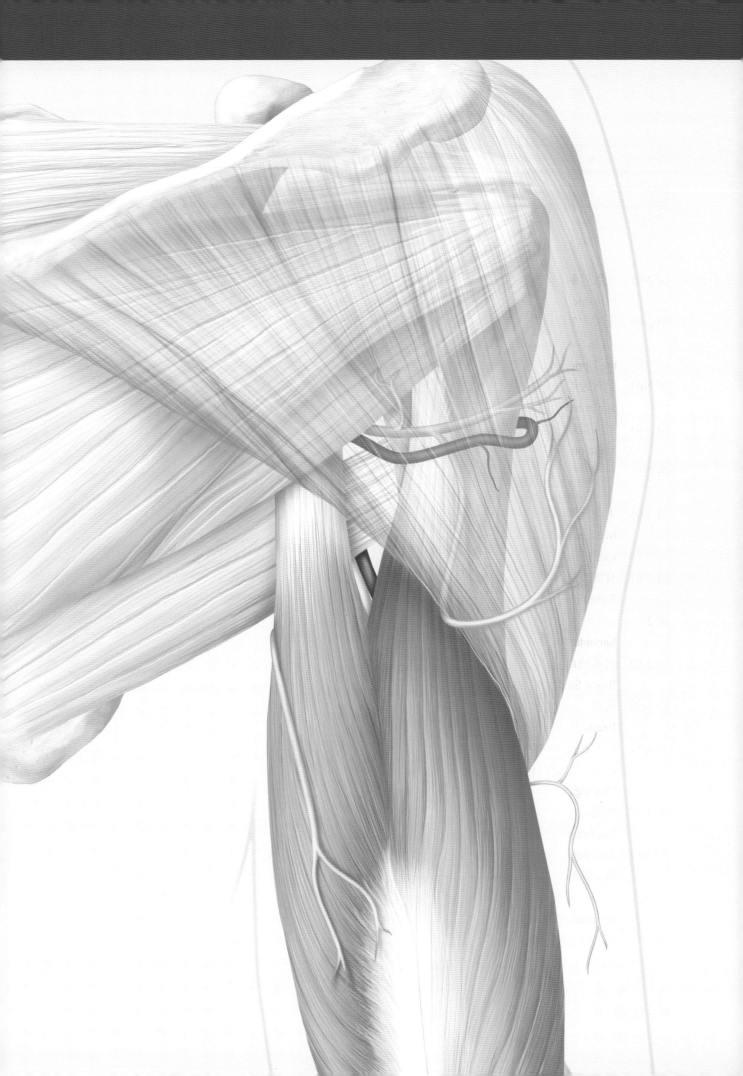

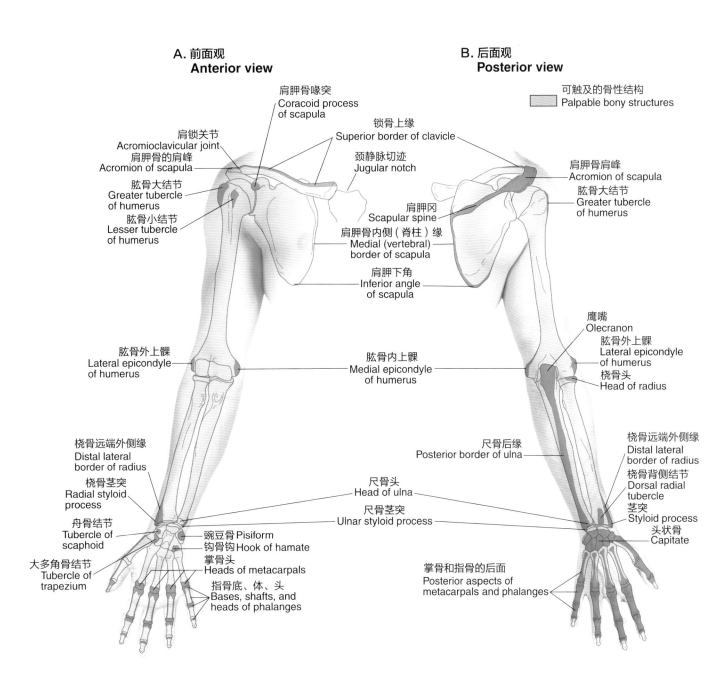

A. 前面观
Anterior view

B. 后面观
Posterior view

肩胛骨喙突
Coracoid process
of scapula

锁骨上缘
Superior border of clavicle

颈静脉切迹
Jugular notch

可触及的骨性结构
Palpable bony structures

肩锁关节
Acromioclavicular joint
肩胛骨的肩峰
Acromion of scapula

肱骨大结节
Greater tubercle
of humerus

肱骨小结节
Lesser tubercle
of humerus

肩胛冈
Scapular spine

肩胛骨内侧（脊柱）缘
Medial (vertebral)
border of scapula

肩胛下角
Inferior angle
of scapula

肩胛骨肩峰
Acromion of scapula

肱骨大结节
Greater tubercle
of humerus

肱骨外上髁
Lateral epicondyle
of humerus

肱骨内上髁
Medial epicondyle
of humerus

鹰嘴
Olecranon

肱骨外上髁
Lateral epicondyle
of humerus

桡骨头
Head of radius

桡骨远端外侧缘
Distal lateral
border of radius

桡骨茎突
Radial styloid
process

舟骨结节
Tubercle of
scaphoid

大多角骨结节
Tubercle of
trapezium

豌豆骨 Pisiform
钩骨钩 Hook of hamate
掌骨头
Heads of metacarpals
指骨底、体、头
Bases, shafts, and
heads of phalanges

尺骨后缘
Posterior border of ulna

尺骨头
Head of ulna

尺骨茎突
Ulnar styloid process

掌骨和指骨的后面
Posterior aspects of
metacarpals and phalanges

桡骨远端外侧缘
Distal lateral
border of radius

桡骨背侧结节
Dorsal radial
tubercle

茎突
Styloid process

头状骨
Capitate

A. 前面观
Anterior view

B. 后面观
Posterior view

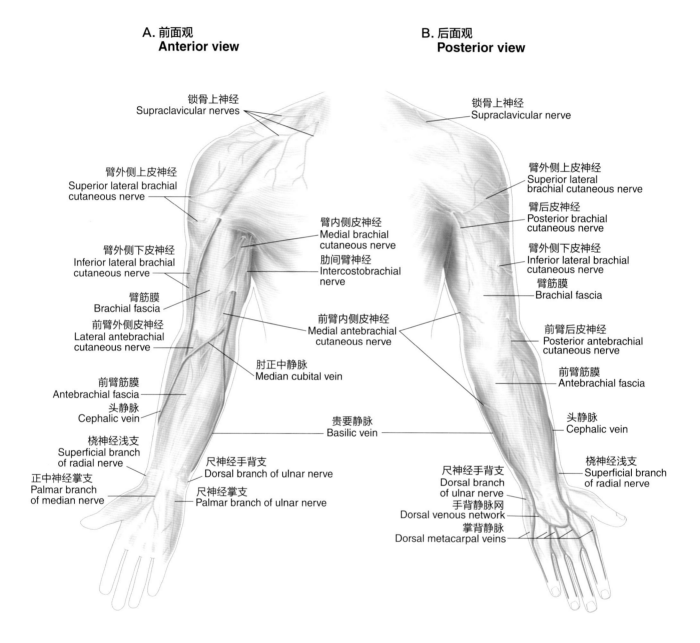

锁骨上神经
Supraclavicular nerves

臂外侧上皮神经
Superior lateral brachial
cutaneous nerve

臂内侧皮神经
Medial brachial
cutaneous nerve

肋间臂神经
Intercostobrachial
nerve

臂外侧下皮神经
Inferior lateral brachial
cutaneous nerve

臂筋膜
Brachial fascia

前臂外侧皮神经
Lateral antebrachial
cutaneous nerve

前臂内侧皮神经
Medial antebrachial
cutaneous nerve

肘正中静脉
Median cubital vein

前臂筋膜
Antebrachial fascia

头静脉
Cephalic vein

贵要静脉
Basilic vein

桡神经浅支
Superficial branch
of radial nerve

尺神经手背支
Dorsal branch of ulnar nerve

正中神经掌支
Palmar branch
of median nerve

尺神经掌支
Palmar branch of ulnar nerve

锁骨上神经
Supraclavicular nerve

臂外侧上皮神经
Superior lateral
brachial cutaneous nerve

臂后皮神经
Posterior brachial
cutaneous nerve

臂外侧下皮神经
Inferior lateral brachial
cutaneous nerve

臂筋膜
Brachial fascia

前臂后皮神经
Posterior antebrachial
cutaneous nerve

前臂筋膜
Antebrachial fascia

头静脉
Cephalic vein

桡神经浅支
Superficial branch
of radial nerve

尺神经手背支
Dorsal branch
of ulnar nerve

手背静脉网
Dorsal venous network

掌背静脉
Dorsal metacarpal veins

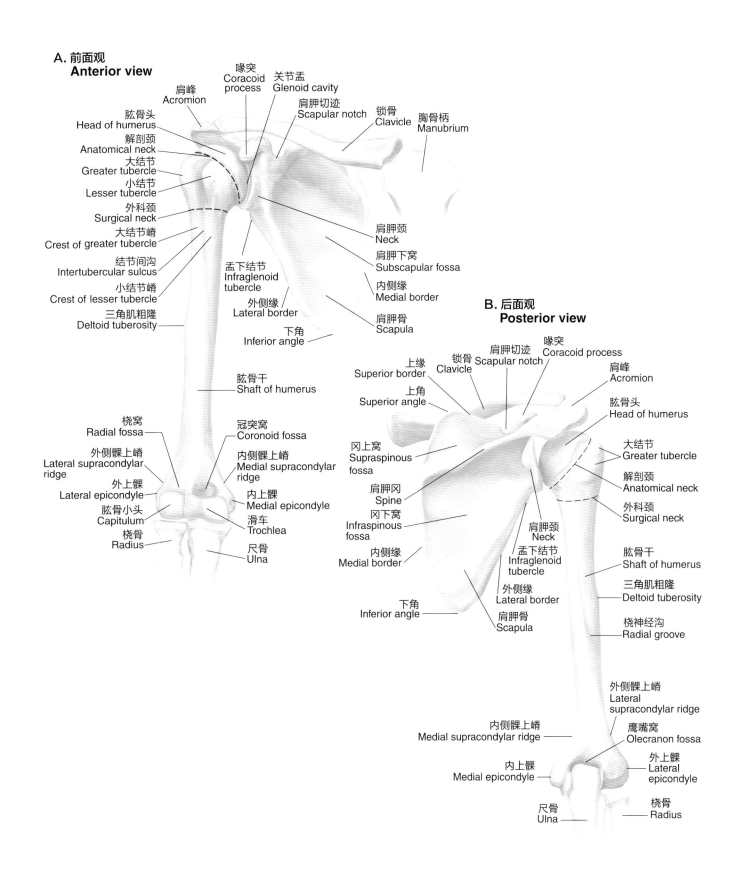

A. 前面观
Anterior view

喙突
Coracoid
process

关节盂
Glenoid cavity

肩胛切迹
Scapular notch

锁骨
Clavicle

胸骨柄
Manubrium

肩峰
Acromion

肱骨头
Head of humerus

解剖颈
Anatomical neck

大结节
Greater tubercle

小结节
Lesser tubercle

外科颈
Surgical neck

大结节嵴
Crest of greater tubercle

结节间沟
Intertubercular sulcus

小结节嵴
Crest of lesser tubercle

三角肌粗隆
Deltoid tuberosity

盂下结节
Infraglenoid
tubercle

外侧缘
Lateral border

下角
Inferior angle

肩胛颈
Neck

肩胛下窝
Subscapular fossa

内侧缘
Medial border

肩胛骨
Scapula

肱骨干
Shaft of humerus

桡窝
Radial fossa

冠突窝
Coronoid fossa

外侧髁上嵴
Lateral supracondylar
ridge

内侧髁上嵴
Medial supracondylar
ridge

外上髁
Lateral epicondyle

内上髁
Medial epicondyle

肱骨小头
Capitulum

滑车
Trochlea

桡骨
Radius

尺骨
Ulna

B. 后面观
Posterior view

上缘
Superior border

锁骨
Clavicle

肩胛切迹
Scapular notch

喙突
Coracoid process

肩峰
Acromion

上角
Superior angle

肱骨头
Head of humerus

冈上窝
Supraspinous
fossa

大结节
Greater tubercle

肩胛冈
Spine

解剖颈
Anatomical neck

冈下窝
Infraspinous
fossa

外科颈
Surgical neck

肩胛颈
Neck

内侧缘
Medial border

盂下结节
Infraglenoid
tubercle

肱骨干
Shaft of humerus

外侧缘
Lateral border

三角肌粗隆
Deltoid tuberosity

下角
Inferior angle

肩胛骨
Scapula

桡神经沟
Radial groove

外侧髁上嵴
Lateral
supracondylar ridge

内侧髁上嵴
Medial supracondylar ridge

鹰嘴窝
Olecranon fossa

内上髁
Medial epicondyle

外上髁
Lateral
epicondyle

尺骨
Ulna

桡骨
Radius

A. 前面观
Anterior view

B. 后面观
Posterior view

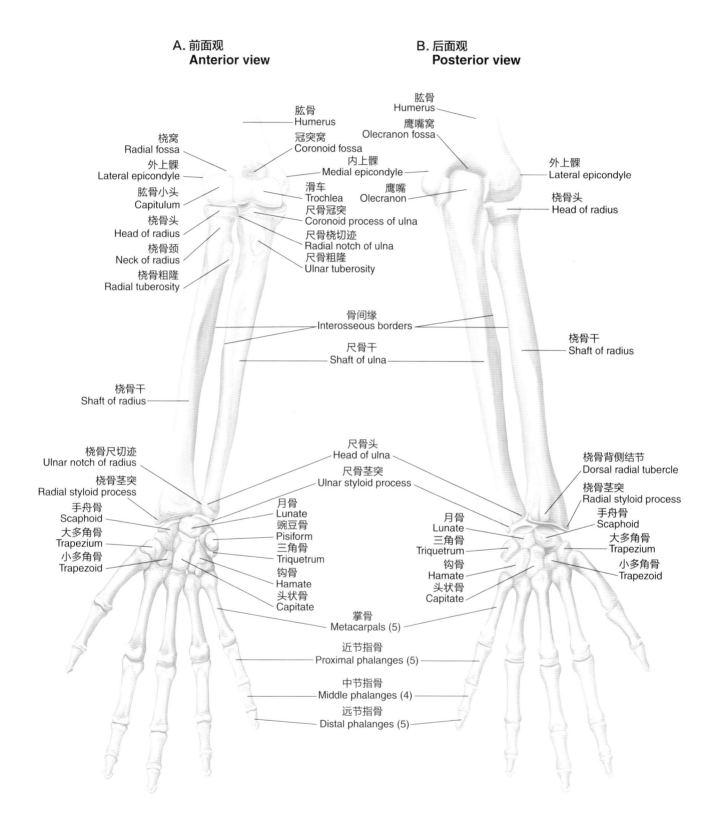

肱骨
Humerus

桡窝
Radial fossa

冠突窝
Coronoid fossa

外上髁
Lateral epicondyle

内上髁
Medial epicondyle

肱骨小头
Capitulum

滑车
Trochlea

桡骨头
Head of radius

尺骨冠突
Coronoid process of ulna

桡骨颈
Neck of radius

尺骨桡切迹
Radial notch of ulna

桡骨粗隆
Radial tuberosity

尺骨粗隆
Ulnar tuberosity

肱骨
Humerus

鹰嘴窝
Olecranon fossa

外上髁
Lateral epicondyle

鹰嘴
Olecranon

桡骨头
Head of radius

骨间缘
Interosseous borders

尺骨干
Shaft of ulna

桡骨干
Shaft of radius

桡骨干
Shaft of radius

桡骨尺切迹
Ulnar notch of radius

桡骨茎突
Radial styloid process

手舟骨
Scaphoid

大多角骨
Trapezium

小多角骨
Trapezoid

尺骨头
Head of ulna

尺骨茎突
Ulnar styloid process

月骨
Lunate

豌豆骨
Pisiform

三角骨
Triquetrum

钩骨
Hamate

头状骨
Capitate

桡骨背侧结节
Dorsal radial tubercle

桡骨茎突
Radial styloid process

手舟骨
Scaphoid

大多角骨
Trapezium

小多角骨
Trapezoid

月骨
Lunate

三角骨
Triquetrum

钩骨
Hamate

头状骨
Capitate

掌骨
Metacarpals (5)

近节指骨
Proximal phalanges (5)

中节指骨
Middle phalanges (4)

远节指骨
Distal phalanges (5)

A. 右肩，前面观
Right shoulder, anterior view

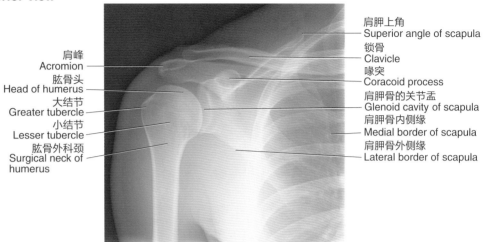

肩胛上角
Superior angle of scapula

锁骨
Clavicle

喙突
Coracoid process

肩胛骨的关节盂
Glenoid cavity of scapula

肩胛骨内侧缘
Medial border of scapula

肩胛骨外侧缘
Lateral border of scapula

肩峰
Acromion

肱骨头
Head of humerus

大结节
Greater tubercle

小结节
Lesser tubercle

肱骨外科颈
Surgical neck of humerus

B. 右肘，前面观
Right elbow, anterior view

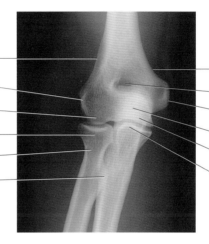

外侧髁上嵴
Lateral supracondylar ridge

外上髁
Lateral epicondyle

肱骨小头
Capitulum

桡骨头
Head of radius

桡骨颈
Neck of radius

桡骨粗隆
Radial tuberosity

内侧髁上嵴
Medial supracondylar ridge

冠突窝
Coronoid fossa

内上髁
Medial epicondyle

鹰嘴
Olecranon

滑车
Trochlea

尺骨冠突
Coronoid process of ulna

C. 右腕和手，前面观
Right wrist and hand, anterior view

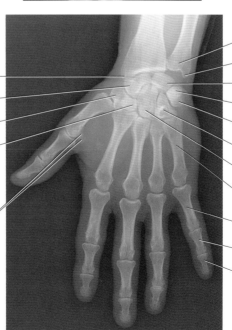

桡骨茎突
Radial styloid process

手舟骨
Scaphoid

大多角骨
Trapezium

小多角骨
Trapezoid

籽骨
Sesamoid bones

尺骨头
Head of ulna

尺骨茎突
Ulnar styloid process

月骨
Lunate

豌豆骨
Pisiform

三角骨
Triquetrum

钩骨
Hamate

头状骨
Capitate

掌骨（5 块）
Metacarpals (5)

近节指骨（5 块）
Proximal phalanges (5)

中节指骨（4 块）
Middle phalanges (4)

远节指骨（5 块）
Distal phalanges (5)

图 2-06　上肢近端肌肉附着点　Muscle Attachments of the Proximal Upper Limb

A. 前面观
Anterior view

肱二头肌（长头）
Biceps brachii muscle (long head)

斜方肌
Trapezius muscle

喙肱肌和肱二头肌
（短头）共同起点
Coracobrachialis muscle and
biceps brachii muscle (short head)
shared origin

三角肌
Deltoid muscle

胸小肌
Pectoralis minor muscle

肩胛舌骨肌
Omohyoid muscle

冈上肌
Supraspinatus muscle

肩胛下肌
Subscapularis muscle

胸大肌
Pectoralis major muscle

背阔肌
Latissimus dorsi muscle

大圆肌
Teres major muscle

三角肌
Deltoid muscle

喙肱肌
Coracobrachialis muscle

前锯肌
Serratus anterior muscle

肩胛下肌
Subscapularis muscle

肱三头肌（长头）
Triceps brachii muscle
(long head)

肱肌
Brachialis muscle

肱桡肌
Brachioradialis muscle

桡侧腕长伸肌
Extensor carpi radialis
longus muscle

旋前圆肌（肱骨头）
Pronator teres muscle (humeral head)

屈肌总腱
Common flexor tendon

伸肌总腱
Common extensor tendon

肱二头肌
Biceps brachii muscle

肱肌
Brachialis muscle

肌肉附着点
Muscle attachments
起点 Origins
止点 Insertions

B. 后面观
Posterior view

肱二头肌（长头）
Biceps brachii muscle (long head)

斜方肌
Trapezius muscle

三角肌
Deltoid muscle

冈上肌
Supraspinatus muscle

肩胛提肌
Levator scapulae muscle

小菱形肌
Rhomboid minor muscle

小圆肌
Teres minor muscle

冈下肌
Infraspinatus muscle

大菱形肌
Rhomboid major muscle

大圆肌
Teres major muscle

背阔肌
Latissimus dorsi muscle*

冈上肌
Supraspinatus muscle

冈下肌
Infraspinatus muscle

小圆肌
Teres minor muscle

肱三头肌（外侧头）
Triceps brachii muscle
(lateral head)

三角肌
Deltoid muscle

肱肌
Brachialis muscle

肱三头肌（内侧头）
Triceps brachii muscle
(medial head)

肱三头肌（长头）
Triceps
brachii
muscle
(long head)

伸肌总腱
Common
extensor
tendon

肘肌
Anconeus muscle

肱三头肌
Triceps brachii muscle

屈肌总腱
Common flexor tendon

53% 人群有小束起于此
*Small slip of origin in 53% of cases

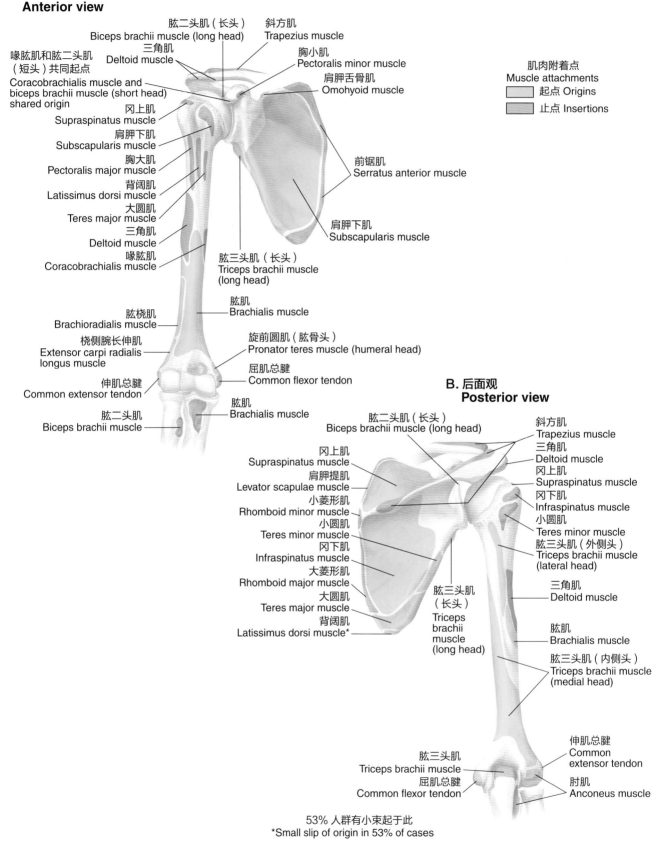

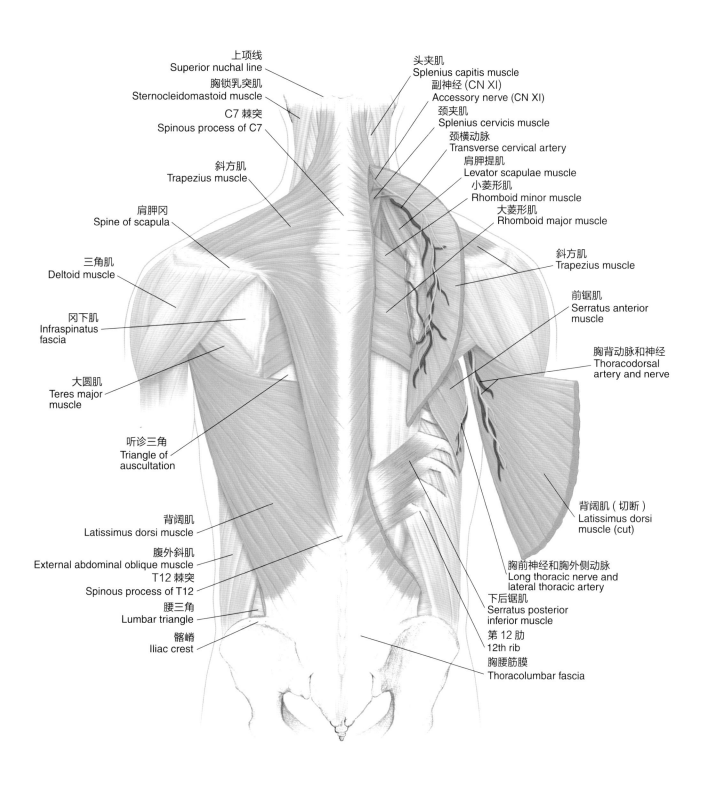

上项线
Superior nuchal line

胸锁乳突肌
Sternocleidomastoid muscle

C7 棘突
Spinous process of C7

斜方肌
Trapezius muscle

肩胛冈
Spine of scapula

三角肌
Deltoid muscle

冈下肌
Infraspinatus fascia

大圆肌
Teres major muscle

听诊三角
Triangle of auscultation

背阔肌
Latissimus dorsi muscle

腹外斜肌
External abdominal oblique muscle

T12 棘突
Spinous process of T12

腰三角
Lumbar triangle

髂嵴
Iliac crest

头夹肌
Splenius capitis muscle

副神经 (CN XI)
Accessory nerve (CN XI)

颈夹肌
Splenius cervicis muscle

颈横动脉
Transverse cervical artery

肩胛提肌
Levator scapulae muscle

小菱形肌
Rhomboid minor muscle

大菱形肌
Rhomboid major muscle

斜方肌
Trapezius muscle

前锯肌
Serratus anterior muscle

胸背动脉和神经
Thoracodorsal artery and nerve

背阔肌（切断）
Latissimus dorsi muscle (cut)

胸前神经和胸外侧动脉
Long thoracic nerve and lateral thoracic artery

下后锯肌
Serratus posterior inferior muscle

第 12 肋
12th rib

胸腰筋膜
Thoracolumbar fascia

图 2-08　肩肌　Shoulder Muscles

A. 浅层
Superficial view

肩胛舌骨肌（切断）
Omohyoid muscle (cut)

肩胛上动脉和神经
Suprascapular
nerve and artery

斜方肌（切断）
Trapezius muscle (cut)

冈上肌
Supraspinatus muscle

肩峰
Acromion

肩胛提肌（切断）
Levator scapulae
muscle (cut)

三角肌（切断并翻起）
Deltoid muscle (cut and reflected)

肌腱：
Tendons of:
冈上肌 Supraspinatus muscle
冈下肌 Infraspinatus muscle
小圆肌 Teres minor muscle

小菱形肌（切断）
Rhomboid minor
muscle (cut)

肩胛背动脉和神经
Dorsal scapular
artery and nerve

肩胛冈
Spine of scapula

冈下肌
Infraspinatus
muscle

腋神经和旋肱后动脉
Axillary nerve and
posterior circumflex
humeral artery

桡神经和肱深动脉
Radial nerve and
deep brachial artery

大菱形肌（切断）
Rhomboid
major muscle
(cut)

肱三头肌外侧头
Lateral head of
triceps brachii
muscle

大圆肌
Teres major muscle

背阔肌（切断）
Latissimus dorsi
muscle (cut)

肱三头肌长头
Long head of
triceps brachii muscle

B. 深层
Deep view

斜方肌（切断）
Trapezius muscle (cut)

肩胛舌骨肌（切断）
Omohyoid muscle (cut)

冈上肌
Supraspinatus muscle

肩胛上动脉和神经
Suprascapular nerve and artery

肩峰
Acromion

三角肌（切断并翻起）
Deltoid muscle
(cut and reflected)

肌腱：
Tendons of:
冈上肌 Supraspinatus muscle
冈下肌 Infraspinatus muscle
小圆肌 Teres minor muscle

肩胛提肌（切断）
Levator scapulae
muscle (cut)

小菱形肌（切断）
Rhomboid minor
muscle (cut)

肩胛冈
Spine of scapula

冈下肌（切断）
Infraspinatus
muscle (cut)

肩胛背动脉和神经
Dorsal scapular
artery and nerve

大菱形肌（切断）
Rhomboid major
muscle (cut)

旋肩胛动脉（穿三边孔）
Circumflex scapular artery
(seen through triangular space)

大圆肌
Teres major muscle

臂外侧上皮神经
Superior lateral
brachial cutaneous
nerve

腋神经和旋肱后动脉（穿四边孔）
Axillary nerve and posterior
circumflex humeral artery
(passing through
quadrangular space)

桡神经和肱深动脉
Radial nerve and
deep brachial artery

肱三头肌外侧头
Lateral head of
triceps brachii muscle

背阔肌（切断）
Latissimus dorsi
muscle (cut)

肱三头肌长头
Long head of
triceps brachii muscle

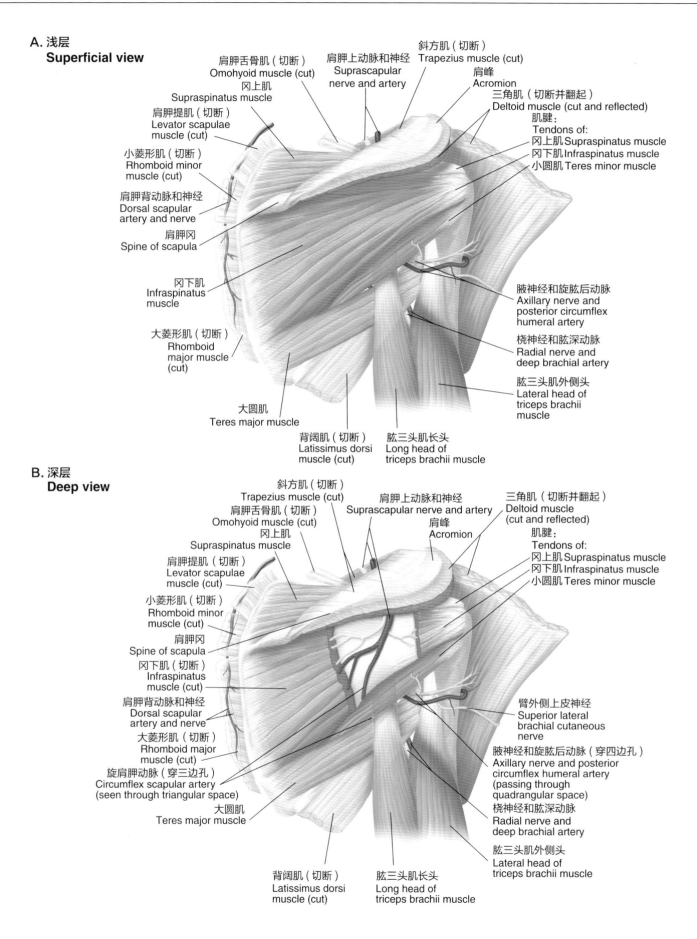

A. 动脉
Arteries

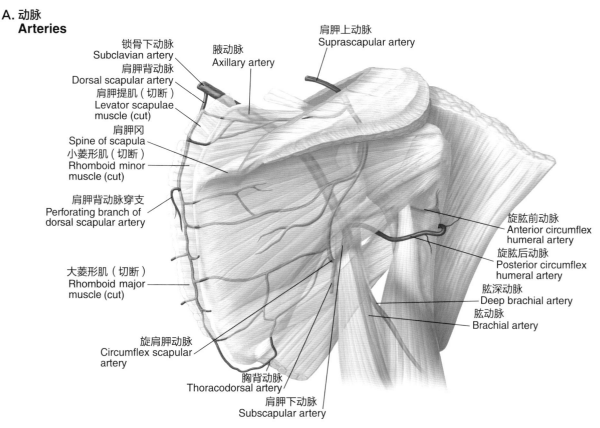

锁骨下动脉
Subclavian artery

肩胛背动脉
Dorsal scapular artery

肩胛提肌（切断）
Levator scapulae muscle (cut)

肩胛冈
Spine of scapula

小菱形肌（切断）
Rhomboid minor muscle (cut)

肩胛背动脉穿支
Perforating branch of dorsal scapular artery

大菱形肌（切断）
Rhomboid major muscle (cut)

旋肩胛动脉
Circumflex scapular artery

腋动脉
Axillary artery

肩胛上动脉
Suprascapular artery

旋肱前动脉
Anterior circumflex humeral artery

旋肱后动脉
Posterior circumflex humeral artery

肱深动脉
Deep brachial artery

肱动脉
Brachial artery

胸背动脉
Thoracodorsal artery

肩胛下动脉
Subscapular artery

B. 造影
Angiogram

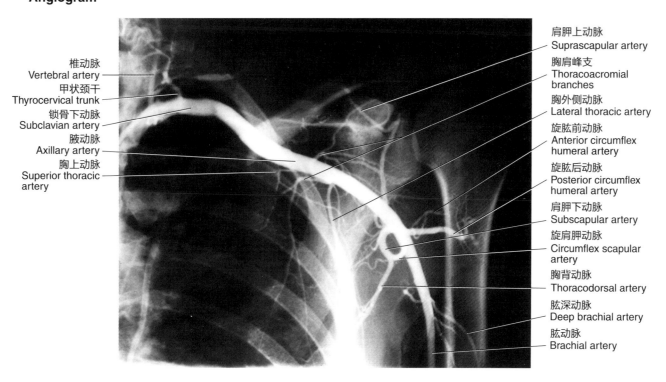

椎动脉
Vertebral artery

甲状颈干
Thyrocervical trunk

锁骨下动脉
Subclavian artery

腋动脉
Axillary artery

胸上动脉
Superior thoracic artery

肩胛上动脉
Suprascapular artery

胸肩峰支
Thoracoacromial branches

胸外侧动脉
Lateral thoracic artery

旋肱前动脉
Anterior circumflex humeral artery

旋肱后动脉
Posterior circumflex humeral artery

肩胛下动脉
Subscapular artery

旋肩胛动脉
Circumflex scapular artery

胸背动脉
Thoracodorsal artery

肱深动脉
Deep brachial artery

肱动脉
Brachial artery

图 2-10 乳腺 Breast

A. 前面观
Anterior view

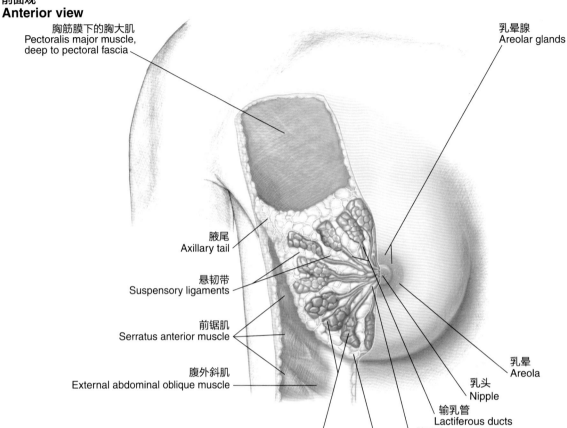

胸筋膜下的胸大肌
Pectoralis major muscle,
deep to pectoral fascia

乳晕腺
Areolar glands

腋尾
Axillary tail

悬韧带
Suspensory ligaments

前锯肌
Serratus anterior muscle

腹外斜肌
External abdominal oblique muscle

乳晕
Areola

乳头
Nipple

输乳管
Lactiferous ducts

输乳窦
Lactiferous sinus

小叶
Lobes

脂肪
Fat

B. 矢状面
Sagittal section

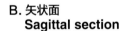
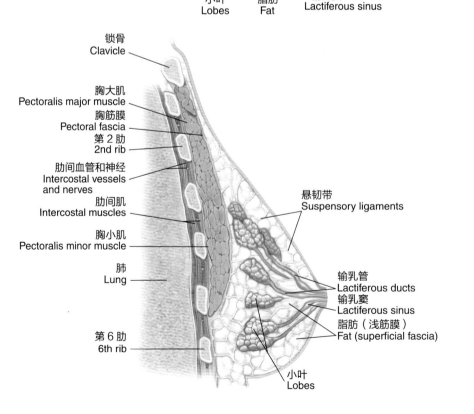

锁骨
Clavicle

胸大肌
Pectoralis major muscle

胸筋膜
Pectoral fascia

第 2 肋
2nd rib

肋间血管和神经
Intercostal vessels
and nerves

肋间肌
Intercostal muscles

胸小肌
Pectoralis minor muscle

肺
Lung

第 6 肋
6th rib

悬韧带
Suspensory ligaments

输乳管
Lactiferous ducts

输乳窦
Lactiferous sinus

脂肪（浅筋膜）
Fat (superficial fascia)

小叶
Lobes

A. 动脉 Arteries

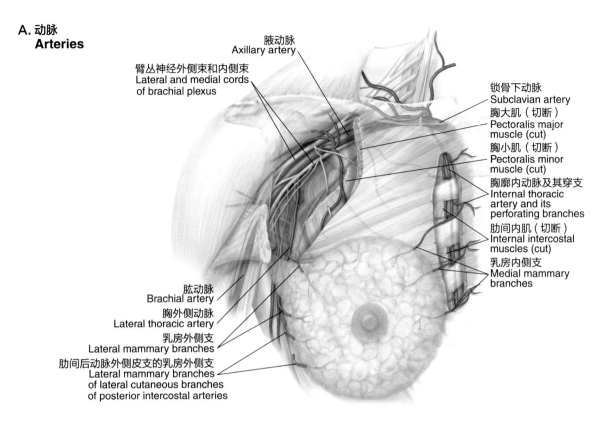

腋动脉
Axillary artery

臂丛神经外侧束和内侧束
Lateral and medial cords
of brachial plexus

锁骨下动脉
Subclavian artery

胸大肌（切断）
Pectoralis major
muscle (cut)

胸小肌（切断）
Pectoralis minor
muscle (cut)

胸廓内动脉及其穿支
Internal thoracic
artery and its
perforating branches

肋间内肌（切断）
Internal intercostal
muscles (cut)

乳房内侧支
Medial mammary
branches

肱动脉
Brachial artery

胸外侧动脉
Lateral thoracic artery

乳房外侧支
Lateral mammary branches

肋间后动脉外侧皮支的乳房外侧支
Lateral mammary branches
of lateral cutaneous branches
of posterior intercostal arteries

B. 淋巴回流 Lymphatic drainage

中央淋巴结
Central axillary nodes

腋外侧（肱骨）淋巴结
Lateral axillary
(humeral) nodes

腋尖淋巴结
Apical axillary nodes

锁骨下干
Subclavian trunk

胸大肌（切断）
Pectoralis major
muscle (cut)

胸小肌（切断）
Pectoralis minor
muscle (cut)

中央淋巴结
Interpectoral nodes

引流至胸骨旁淋巴结
Drainage to
parasternal nodes

胸骨旁淋巴结
Parasternal nodes

腋后（肩胛下）淋巴结
Posterior axillary
(subscapular) nodes

腋前（胸部）淋巴结
Anterior axillary
(pectoral) nodes

引流至对侧乳腺
Drainage to
opposite breast

引流至膈下淋巴结和肝
Drainage to inferior
phrenic nodes and liver

乳晕下淋巴丛
Subareolar lymphatic plexus

图 2-12　胸肌　Pectoral Muscles

A. 浅层解剖
Superficial dissection

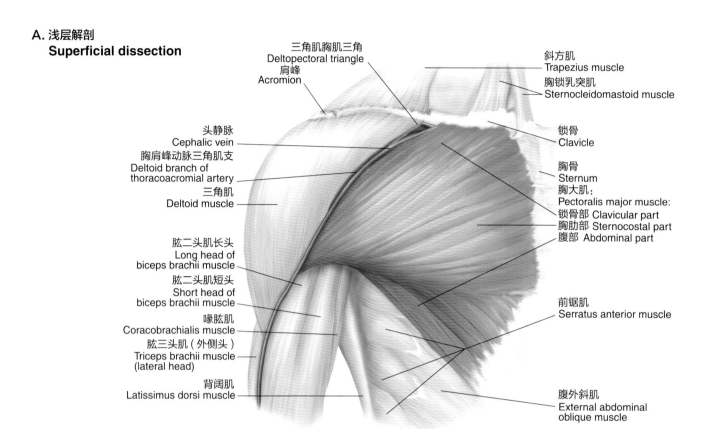

三角肌胸肌三角
Deltopectoral triangle
肩峰
Acromion

斜方肌
Trapezius muscle

胸锁乳突肌
Sternocleidomastoid muscle

锁骨
Clavicle

头静脉
Cephalic vein

胸肩峰动脉三角肌支
Deltoid branch of
thoracoacromial artery

三角肌
Deltoid muscle

胸骨
Sternum
胸大肌：
Pectoralis major muscle:
锁骨部 Clavicular part
胸肋部 Sternocostal part
腹部 Abdominal part

肱二头肌长头
Long head of
biceps brachii muscle

肱二头肌短头
Short head of
biceps brachii muscle

喙肱肌
Coracobrachialis muscle

肱三头肌（外侧头）
Triceps brachii muscle
(lateral head)

背阔肌
Latissimus dorsi muscle

前锯肌
Serratus anterior muscle

腹外斜肌
External abdominal
oblique muscle

B. 深层解剖
Deep dissection

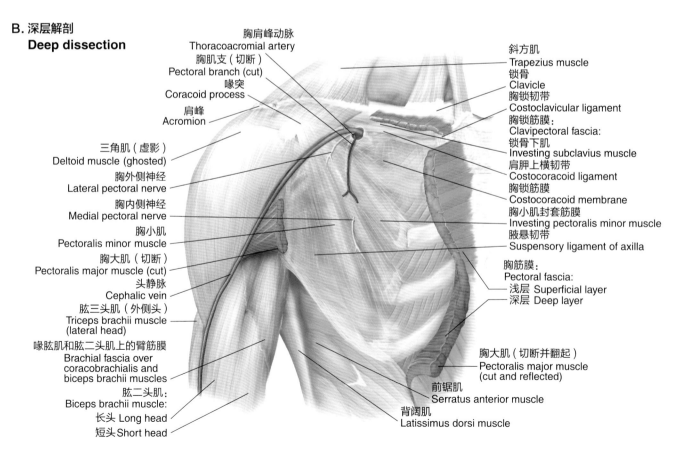

胸肩峰动脉
Thoracoacromial artery
胸肌支（切断）
Pectoral branch (cut)
喙突
Coracoid process
肩峰
Acromion

斜方肌
Trapezius muscle
锁骨
Clavicle
胸锁韧带
Costoclavicular ligament
胸锁筋膜：
Clavipectoral fascia:
锁骨下肌
Investing subclavius muscle
肩胛上横韧带
Costocoracoid ligament
胸锁筋膜
Costocoracoid membrane
胸小肌封套筋膜
Investing pectoralis minor muscle
腋悬韧带
Suspensory ligament of axilla

三角肌（虚影）
Deltoid muscle (ghosted)

胸外侧神经
Lateral pectoral nerve

胸内侧神经
Medial pectoral nerve

胸小肌
Pectoralis minor muscle

胸大肌（切断）
Pectoralis major muscle (cut)

头静脉
Cephalic vein

肱三头肌（外侧头）
Triceps brachii muscle
(lateral head)

喙肱肌和肱二头肌上的臂筋膜
Brachial fascia over
coracobrachialis and
biceps brachii muscles

肱二头肌：
Biceps brachii muscle:
长头 Long head
短头 Short head

胸筋膜：
Pectoral fascia:
浅层 Superficial layer
深层 Deep layer

胸大肌（切断并翻起）
Pectoralis major muscle
(cut and reflected)

前锯肌
Serratus anterior muscle

背阔肌
Latissimus dorsi muscle

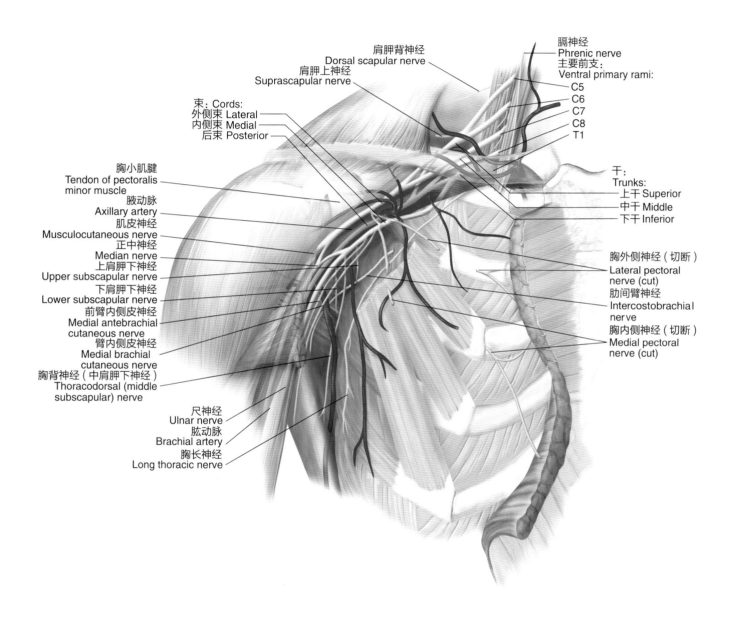

肩胛背神经
Dorsal scapular nerve
肩胛上神经
Suprascapular nerve

膈神经
Phrenic nerve
主要前支：
Ventral primary rami:
C5
C6
C7
C8
T1

束：Cords:
外侧束 Lateral
内侧束 Medial
后束 Posterior

干：
Trunks:
上干 Superior
中干 Middle
下干 Inferior

胸小肌腱
Tendon of pectoralis
minor muscle
腋动脉
Axillary artery
肌皮神经
Musculocutaneous nerve
正中神经
Median nerve
上肩胛下神经
Upper subscapular nerve
下肩胛下神经
Lower subscapular nerve
前臂内侧皮神经
Medial antebrachial
cutaneous nerve
臂内侧皮神经
Medial brachial
cutaneous nerve
胸背神经（中肩胛下神经）
Thoracodorsal (middle
subscapular) nerve

胸外侧神经（切断）
Lateral pectoral
nerve (cut)
肋间臂神经
Intercostobrachial
nerve
胸内侧神经（切断）
Medial pectoral
nerve (cut)

尺神经
Ulnar nerve
肱动脉
Brachial artery
胸长神经
Long thoracic nerve

图 2-14　臂丛示意图　Brachial Plexus Schema

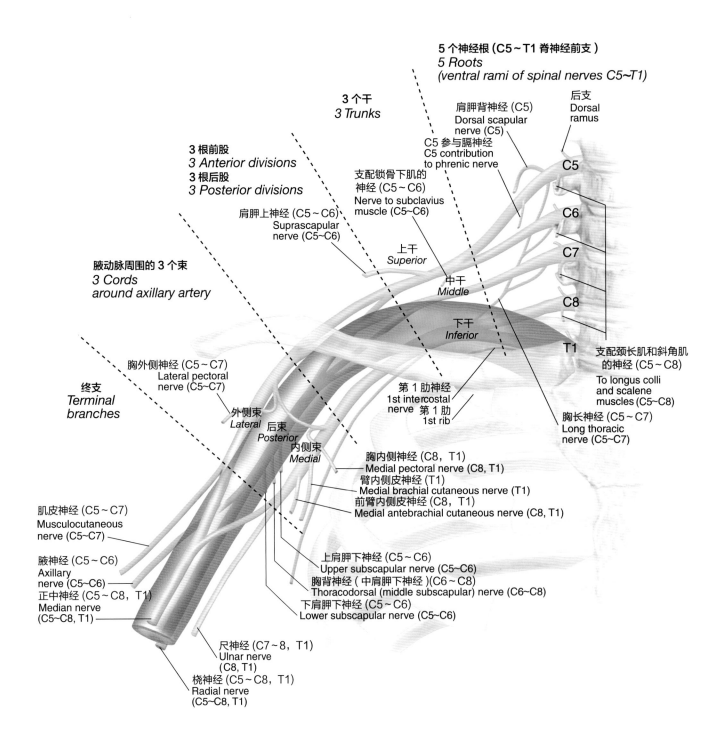

5 个神经根 (C5 ～ T1 脊神经前支)
5 Roots
(ventral rami of spinal nerves C5~T1)

3 个干
3 Trunks

肩胛背神经 (C5)
Dorsal scapular
nerve (C5)

后支
Dorsal
ramus

C5 参与膈神经
C5 contribution
to phrenic nerve

3 根前股
3 Anterior divisions
3 根后股
3 Posterior divisions

支配锁骨下肌的
神经 (C5 ～ C6)
Nerve to subclavius
muscle (C5~C6)

C5

肩胛上神经 (C5 ～ C6)
Suprascapular
nerve (C5~C6)

C6

C7

上干
Superior

C8

腋动脉周围的 3 个束
3 Cords
around axillary artery

中干
Middle

下干
Inferior

T1

支配颈长肌和斜角肌
的神经 (C5 ～ C8)
To longus colli
and scalene
muscles (C5~C8)

胸外侧神经 (C5 ～ C7)
Lateral pectoral
nerve (C5~C7)

第 1 肋神经
1st intercostal
nerve 第 1 肋
1st rib

胸长神经 (C5 ～ C7)
Long thoracic
nerve (C5~C7)

终支
Terminal
branches

外侧束
Lateral

后束
Posterior

内侧束
Medial

胸内侧神经 (C8，T1)
Medial pectoral nerve (C8, T1)
臂内侧皮神经 (T1)
Medial brachial cutaneous nerve (T1)
前臂内侧皮神经 (C8，T1)
Medial antebrachial cutaneous nerve (C8, T1)

肌皮神经 (C5 ～ C7)
Musculocutaneous
nerve (C5~C7)

腋神经 (C5 ～ C6)
Axillary
nerve (C5~C6)
正中神经 (C5 ～ C8，T1)
Median nerve
(C5~C8, T1)

上肩胛下神经 (C5 ～ C6)
Upper subscapular nerve (C5~C6)
胸背神经 (中肩胛下神经)(C6 ～ C8)
Thoracodorsal (middle subscapular) nerve (C6~C8)
下肩胛下神经 (C5 ～ C6)
Lower subscapular nerve (C5~C6)

尺神经 (C7 ～ 8，T1)
Ulnar nerve
(C8, T1)
桡神经 (C5 ～ C8，T1)
Radial nerve
(C5~C8, T1)

A. 解剖
Dissection

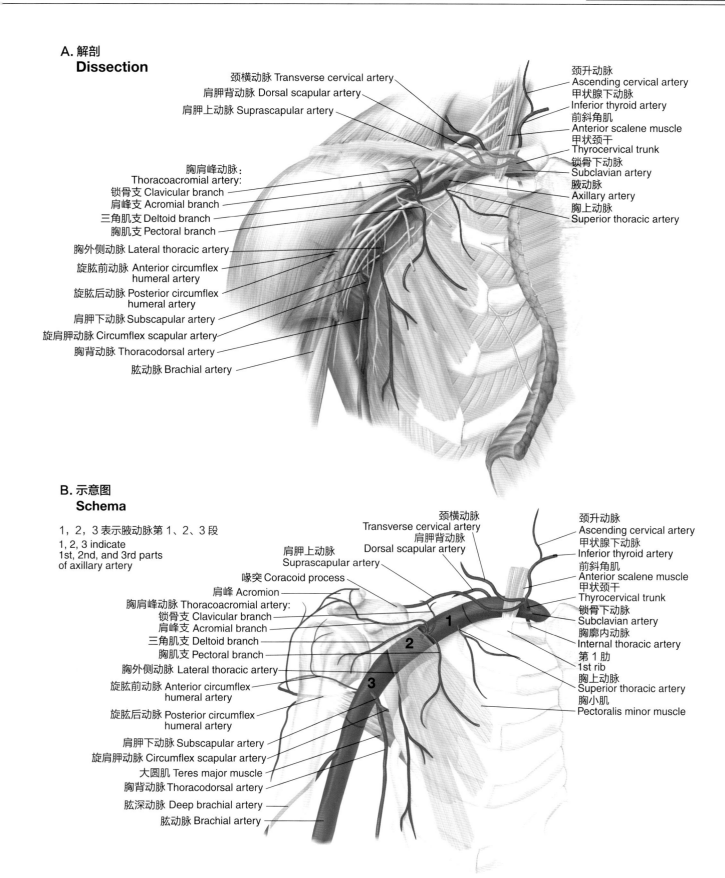

颈横动脉 Transverse cervical artery
肩胛背动脉 Dorsal scapular artery
肩胛上动脉 Suprascapular artery

胸肩峰动脉：
Thoracoacromial artery:
锁骨支 Clavicular branch
肩峰支 Acromial branch
三角肌支 Deltoid branch
胸肌支 Pectoral branch
胸外侧动脉 Lateral thoracic artery
旋肱前动脉 Anterior circumflex humeral artery
旋肱后动脉 Posterior circumflex humeral artery
肩胛下动脉 Subscapular artery
旋肩胛动脉 Circumflex scapular artery
胸背动脉 Thoracodorsal artery
肱动脉 Brachial artery

颈升动脉
Ascending cervical artery
甲状腺下动脉
Inferior thyroid artery
前斜角肌
Anterior scalene muscle
甲状颈干
Thyrocervical trunk
锁骨下动脉
Subclavian artery
腋动脉
Axillary artery
胸上动脉
Superior thoracic artery

B. 示意图
Schema

1，2，3 表示腋动脉第 1、2、3 段
1, 2, 3 indicate
1st, 2nd, and 3rd parts
of axillary artery

颈横动脉
Transverse cervical artery
肩胛背动脉
Dorsal scapular artery
肩胛上动脉
Suprascapular artery
喙突 Coracoid process
肩峰 Acromion
胸肩峰动脉 Thoracoacromial artery:
锁骨支 Clavicular branch
肩峰支 Acromial branch
三角肌支 Deltoid branch
胸肌支 Pectoral branch
胸外侧动脉 Lateral thoracic artery
旋肱前动脉 Anterior circumflex humeral artery
旋肱后动脉 Posterior circumflex humeral artery
肩胛下动脉 Subscapular artery
旋肩胛动脉 Circumflex scapular artery
大圆肌 Teres major muscle
胸背动脉 Thoracodorsal artery
肱深动脉 Deep brachial artery
肱动脉 Brachial artery

颈升动脉
Ascending cervical artery
甲状腺下动脉
Inferior thyroid artery
前斜角肌
Anterior scalene muscle
甲状颈干
Thyrocervical trunk
锁骨下动脉
Subclavian artery
胸廓内动脉
Internal thoracic artery
第 1 肋
1st rib
胸上动脉
Superior thoracic artery
胸小肌
Pectoralis minor muscle

图 2-16　肩袖肌　**Rotator Cuff Muscles**

A. 后面观
Posterior view

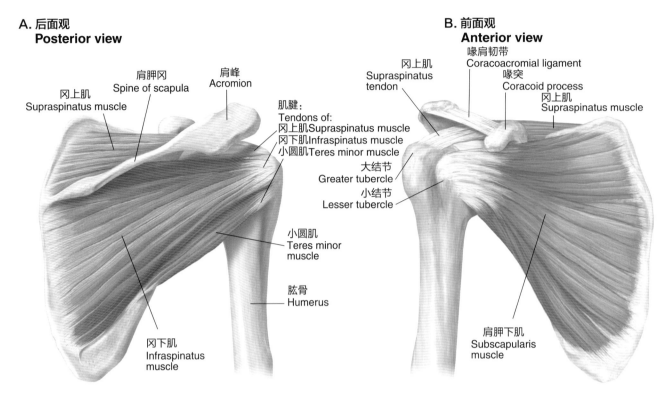

冈上肌
Supraspinatus muscle

肩胛冈
Spine of scapula

肩峰
Acromion

肌腱：
Tendons of:
冈上肌 Supraspinatus muscle
冈下肌 Infraspinatus muscle
小圆肌 Teres minor muscle

小圆肌
Teres minor muscle

肱骨
Humerus

冈下肌
Infraspinatus muscle

B. 前面观
Anterior view

冈上肌
Supraspinatus tendon

喙肩韧带
Coracoacromial ligament

喙突
Coracoid process

冈上肌
Supraspinatus muscle

大结节
Greater tubercle

小结节
Lesser tubercle

肩胛下肌
Subscapularis muscle

C. 上外侧观
Superolateral view

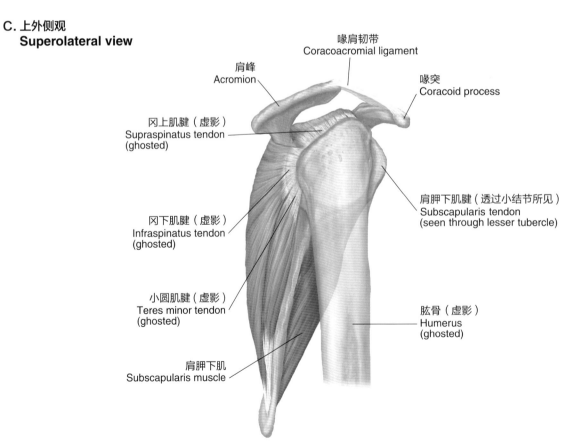

肩峰
Acromion

喙肩韧带
Coracoacromial ligament

喙突
Coracoid process

冈上肌腱（虚影）
Supraspinatus tendon (ghosted)

肩胛下肌腱（透过小结节所见）
Subscapularis tendon (seen through lesser tubercle)

冈下肌腱（虚影）
Infraspinatus tendon (ghosted)

小圆肌腱（虚影）
Teres minor tendon (ghosted)

肱骨（虚影）
Humerus (ghosted)

肩胛下肌
Subscapularis muscle

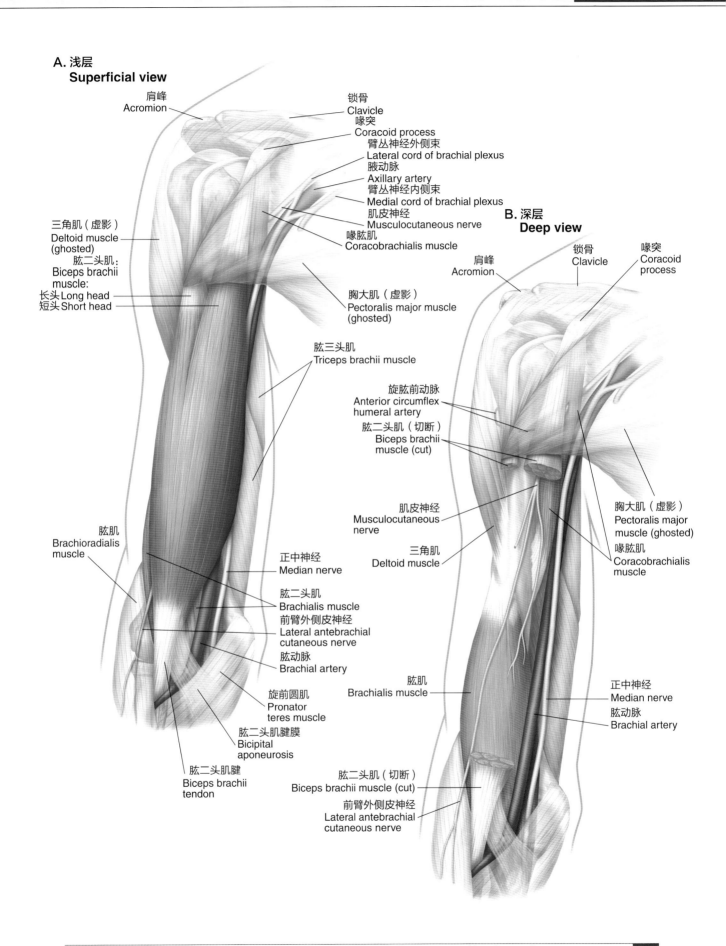

A. 浅层
Superficial view

肩峰
Acromion

锁骨
Clavicle

喙突
Coracoid process

臂丛神经外侧束
Lateral cord of brachial plexus

腋动脉
Axillary artery

臂丛神经内侧束
Medial cord of brachial plexus

肌皮神经
Musculocutaneous nerve

喙肱肌
Coracobrachialis muscle

三角肌（虚影）
Deltoid muscle
(ghosted)

肱二头肌：
Biceps brachii
muscle:

长头 Long head
短头 Short head

胸大肌（虚影）
Pectoralis major muscle
(ghosted)

肱三头肌
Triceps brachii muscle

B. 深层
Deep view

肩峰
Acromion

锁骨
Clavicle

喙突
Coracoid
process

旋肱前动脉
Anterior circumflex
humeral artery

肱二头肌（切断）
Biceps brachii
muscle (cut)

肌皮神经
Musculocutaneous
nerve

三角肌
Deltoid muscle

胸大肌（虚影）
Pectoralis major
muscle (ghosted)

喙肱肌
Coracobrachialis
muscle

肱肌
Brachioradialis
muscle

正中神经
Median nerve

肱二头肌
Brachialis muscle

前臂外侧皮神经
Lateral antebrachial
cutaneous nerve

肱动脉
Brachial artery

旋前圆肌
Pronator
teres muscle

肱二头肌腱膜
Bicipital
aponeurosis

肱二头肌腱
Biceps brachii
tendon

肱肌
Brachialis muscle

正中神经
Median nerve

肱动脉
Brachial artery

肱二头肌（切断）
Biceps brachii muscle (cut)

前臂外侧皮神经
Lateral antebrachial
cutaneous nerve

图 2-18　臂肌后群　Muscles of the Posterior Arm

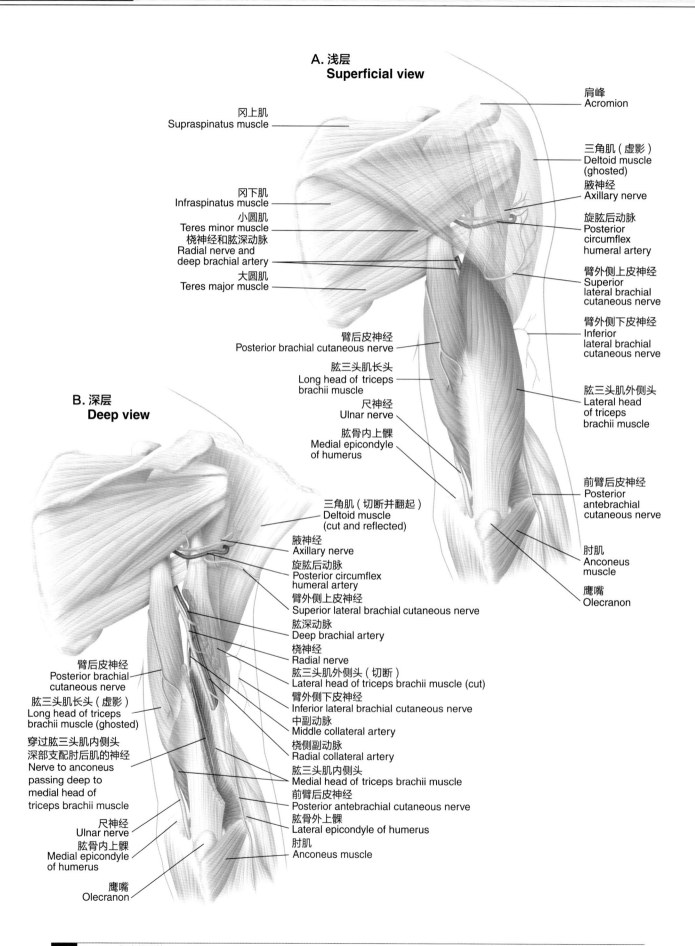

A. 浅层
Superficial view

冈上肌
Supraspinatus muscle

冈下肌
Infraspinatus muscle

小圆肌
Teres minor muscle

桡神经和肱深动脉
Radial nerve and
deep brachial artery

大圆肌
Teres major muscle

肩峰
Acromion

三角肌（虚影）
Deltoid muscle
(ghosted)

腋神经
Axillary nerve

旋肱后动脉
Posterior
circumflex
humeral artery

臂外侧上皮神经
Superior
lateral brachial
cutaneous nerve

臂外侧下皮神经
Inferior
lateral brachial
cutaneous nerve

臂后皮神经
Posterior brachial cutaneous nerve

肱三头肌长头
Long head of triceps
brachii muscle

尺神经
Ulnar nerve

肱骨内上髁
Medial epicondyle
of humerus

肱三头肌外侧头
Lateral head
of triceps
brachii muscle

前臂后皮神经
Posterior
antebrachial
cutaneous nerve

肘肌
Anconeus
muscle

鹰嘴
Olecranon

B. 深层
Deep view

三角肌（切断并翻起）
Deltoid muscle
(cut and reflected)

腋神经
Axillary nerve

旋肱后动脉
Posterior circumflex
humeral artery

臂外侧上皮神经
Superior lateral brachial cutaneous nerve

肱深动脉
Deep brachial artery

桡神经
Radial nerve

肱三头肌外侧头（切断）
Lateral head of triceps brachii muscle (cut)

臂外侧下皮神经
Inferior lateral brachial cutaneous nerve

中副动脉
Middle collateral artery

桡侧副动脉
Radial collateral artery

肱三头肌内侧头
Medial head of triceps brachii muscle

前臂后皮神经
Posterior antebrachial cutaneous nerve

肱骨外上髁
Lateral epicondyle of humerus

肘肌
Anconeus muscle

臂后皮神经
Posterior brachial
cutaneous nerve

肱三头肌长头（虚影）
Long head of triceps
brachii muscle (ghosted)

穿过肱三头肌内侧头
深部支配肘后肌的神经
Nerve to anconeus
passing deep to
medial head of
triceps brachii muscle

尺神经
Ulnar nerve

肱骨内上髁
Medial epicondyle
of humerus

鹰嘴
Olecranon

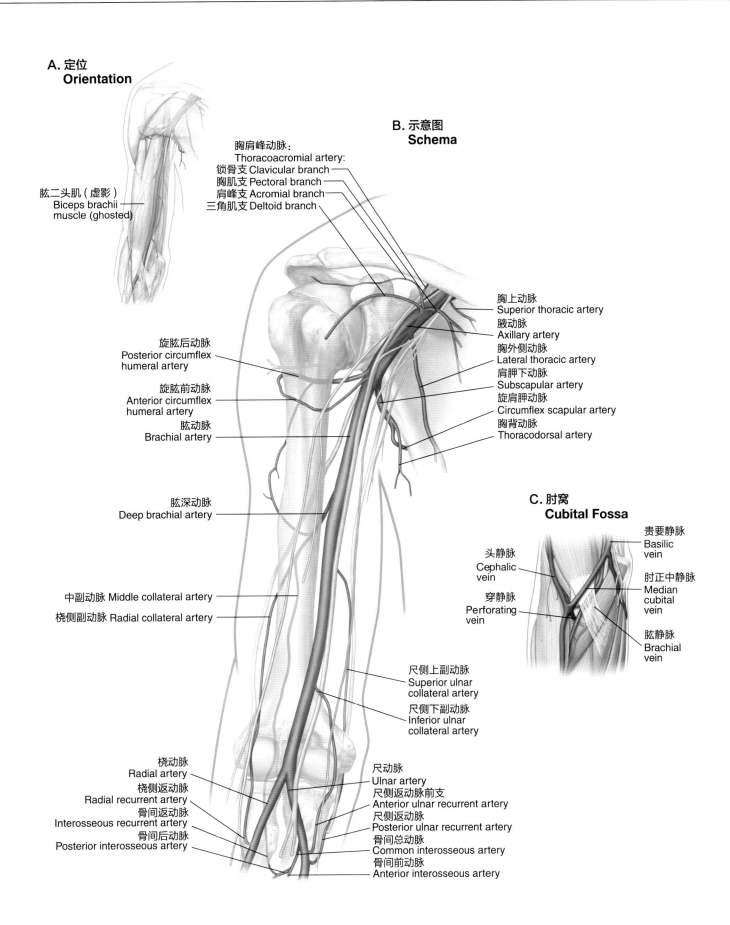

A. 定位
Orientation

B. 示意图
Schema

肱二头肌（虚影）
Biceps brachii
muscle (ghosted)

胸肩峰动脉：
Thoracoacromial artery:
锁骨支 Clavicular branch
胸肌支 Pectoral branch
肩峰支 Acromial branch
三角肌支 Deltoid branch

胸上动脉
Superior thoracic artery
腋动脉
Axillary artery
胸外侧动脉
Lateral thoracic artery
肩胛下动脉
Subscapular artery
旋肩胛动脉
Circumflex scapular artery
胸背动脉
Thoracodorsal artery

旋肱后动脉
Posterior circumflex
humeral artery

旋肱前动脉
Anterior circumflex
humeral artery

肱动脉
Brachial artery

肱深动脉
Deep brachial artery

C. 肘窝
Cubital Fossa

中副动脉 Middle collateral artery
桡侧副动脉 Radial collateral artery

头静脉
Cephalic
vein

穿静脉
Perforating
vein

贵要静脉
Basilic
vein

肘正中静脉
Median
cubital
vein

肱静脉
Brachial
vein

尺侧上副动脉
Superior ulnar
collateral artery
尺侧下副动脉
Inferior ulnar
collateral artery

桡动脉
Radial artery
桡侧返动脉
Radial recurrent artery
骨间返动脉
Interosseous recurrent artery
骨间后动脉
Posterior interosseous artery

尺动脉
Ulnar artery
尺侧返动脉前支
Anterior ulnar recurrent artery
尺侧返动脉
Posterior ulnar recurrent artery
骨间总动脉
Common interosseous artery
骨间前动脉
Anterior interosseous artery

图 2-20　臂的神经　Nerves of the Arm

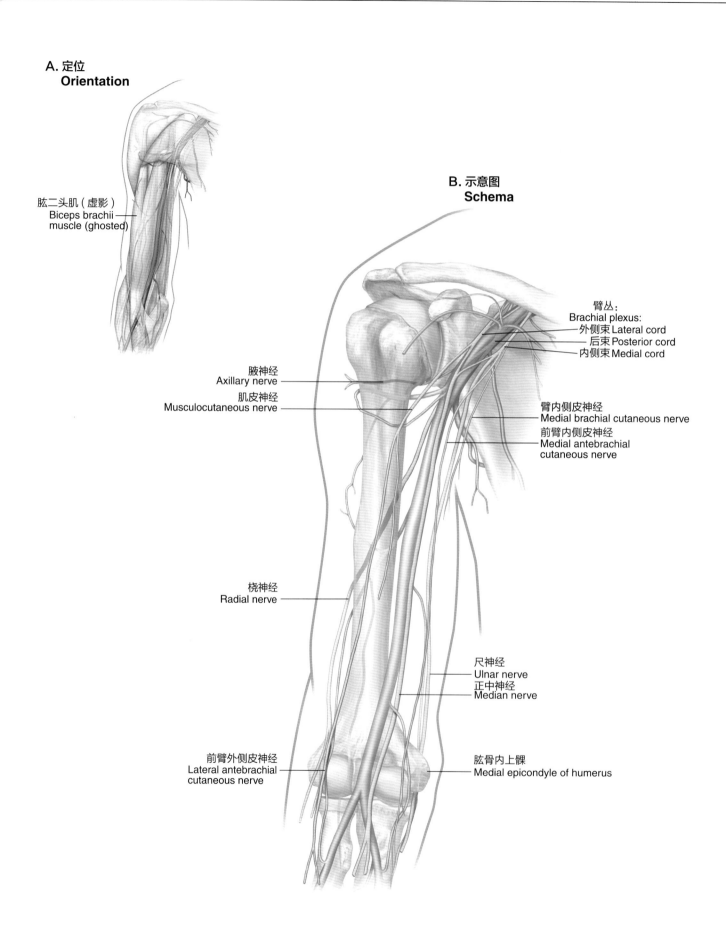

A. 定位
Orientation

肱二头肌（虚影）
Biceps brachii
muscle (ghosted)

B. 示意图
Schema

臂丛：
Brachial plexus:
外侧束 Lateral cord
后束 Posterior cord
内侧束 Medial cord

腋神经
Axillary nerve

肌皮神经
Musculocutaneous nerve

臂内侧皮神经
Medial brachial cutaneous nerve

前臂内侧皮神经
Medial antebrachial
cutaneous nerve

桡神经
Radial nerve

尺神经
Ulnar nerve

正中神经
Median nerve

前臂外侧皮神经
Lateral antebrachial
cutaneous nerve

肱骨内上髁
Medial epicondyle of humerus

肌肉附着点
Muscle attachments
起点Origins
止点Insertions

肱桡肌
Brachioradialis muscle

桡侧腕长伸肌
Extensor carpi radialis longus muscle

由桡侧腕短伸肌、指伸肌、小指伸肌、尺侧腕伸肌共起形成的伸肌总腱
Common extensor tendon shared by:
Extensor carpi radialis brevis muscle
Extensor digitorum muscle
Extensor digiti minimi muscle
Extensor carpi ulnaris muscle

肱肌
Brachialis muscle

旋前圆肌（肱骨头）
Pronator teres muscle (humeral head)

由桡侧腕屈肌、掌长肌、尺侧腕屈肌、指浅屈肌的肌腱（肱尺头）共起形成的屈肌总腱
Common flexor tendon shared by:
Flexor carpi radialis muscle
Palmaris longus muscle
Flexor carpi ulnaris muscle
Flexor digitorum superficialis muscle (humeroulnar head)

肱肌
Brachialis muscle

肱二头肌
Biceps brachii muscle

旋后肌
Supinator muscle

指浅屈肌（肱尺头）
Flexor digitorum superficialis muscle (humeroulnar head)

旋前圆肌（尺骨头）
Pronator teres muscle (ulnar head)

指浅屈肌（桡骨头）
Flexor digitorum superficialis muscle (radial head)

指深屈肌
Flexor digitorum profundus muscle

旋前圆肌
Pronator teres muscle

拇长屈肌
Flexor pollicis longus muscle

桡骨
Radius

旋前方肌
Pronator quadratus muscle

旋前方肌
Pronator quadratus muscle

尺骨
Ulna

肱桡肌
Brachioradialis muscle

拇长展肌
Abductor pollicis longus muscle

尺侧腕屈肌
Flexor carpi ulnaris muscle

桡侧腕屈肌
Flexor carpi radialis muscle

拇长屈肌
Flexor pollicis longus muscle

指浅屈肌
Flexor digitorum superficialis muscle

指深屈肌
Flexor digitorum profundus muscle

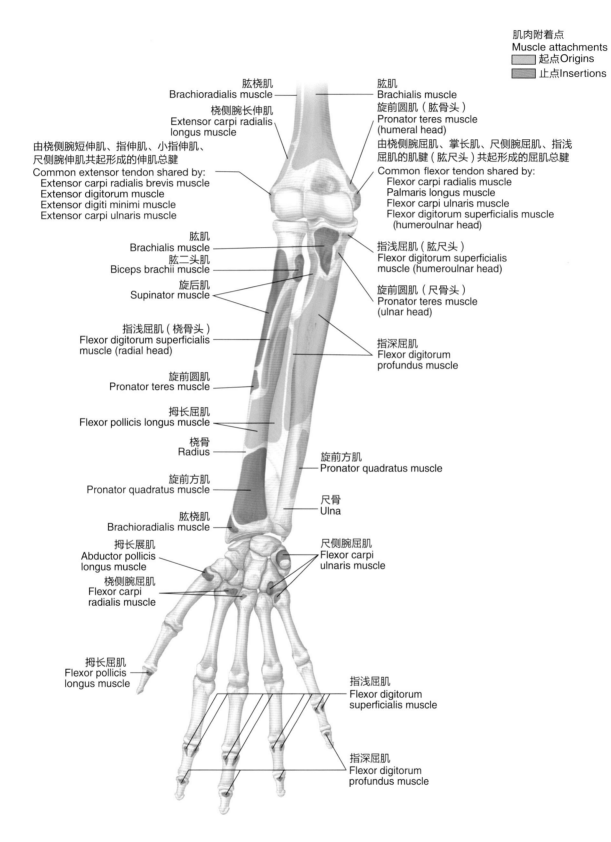

肌肉附着点
Muscle attachments
起点 Origins
止点 Insertions

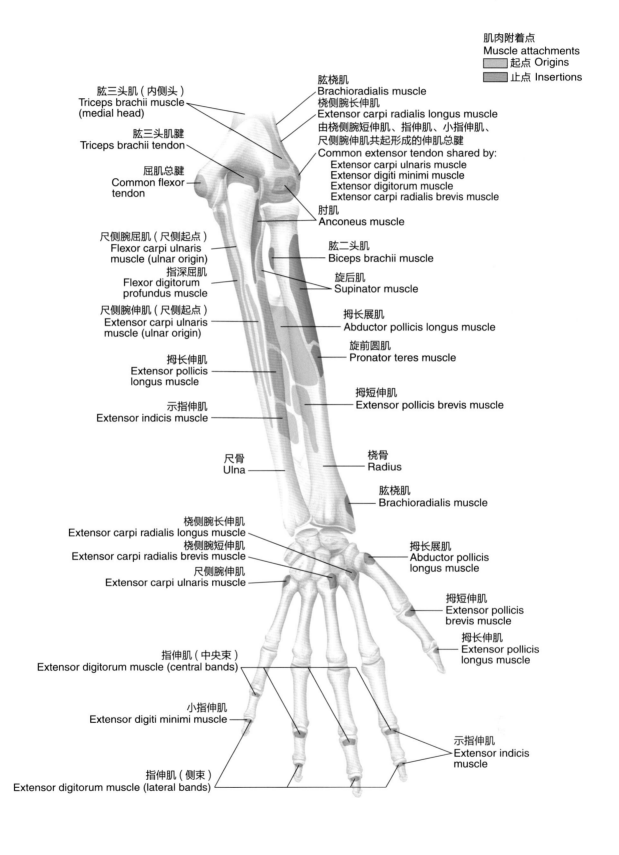

肱三头肌（内侧头）
Triceps brachii muscle
(medial head)

肱三头肌腱
Triceps brachii tendon

屈肌总腱
Common flexor
tendon

尺侧腕屈肌（尺侧起点）
Flexor carpi ulnaris
muscle (ulnar origin)

指深屈肌
Flexor digitorum
profundus muscle

尺侧腕伸肌（尺侧起点）
Extensor carpi ulnaris
muscle (ulnar origin)

拇长伸肌
Extensor pollicis
longus muscle

示指伸肌
Extensor indicis muscle

尺骨
Ulna

桡侧腕长伸肌
Extensor carpi radialis longus muscle

桡侧腕短伸肌
Extensor carpi radialis brevis muscle

尺侧腕伸肌
Extensor carpi ulnaris muscle

指伸肌（中央束）
Extensor digitorum muscle (central bands)

小指伸肌
Extensor digiti minimi muscle

指伸肌（侧束）
Extensor digitorum muscle (lateral bands)

肱桡肌
Brachioradialis muscle
桡侧腕长伸肌
Extensor carpi radialis longus muscle
由桡侧腕短伸肌、指伸肌、小指伸肌、
尺侧腕伸肌共起形成的伸肌总腱
Common extensor tendon shared by:
Extensor carpi ulnaris muscle
Extensor digiti minimi muscle
Extensor digitorum muscle
Extensor carpi radialis brevis muscle

肘肌
Anconeus muscle

肱二头肌
Biceps brachii muscle

旋后肌
Supinator muscle

拇长展肌
Abductor pollicis longus muscle

旋前圆肌
Pronator teres muscle

拇短伸肌
Extensor pollicis brevis muscle

桡骨
Radius

肱桡肌
Brachioradialis muscle

拇长展肌
Abductor pollicis
longus muscle

拇短伸肌
Extensor pollicis
brevis muscle

拇长伸肌
Extensor pollicis
longus muscle

示指伸肌
Extensor indicis
muscle

前臂前群肌，浅层解剖
Muscles of the Anterior Forearm, Superficial Dissection

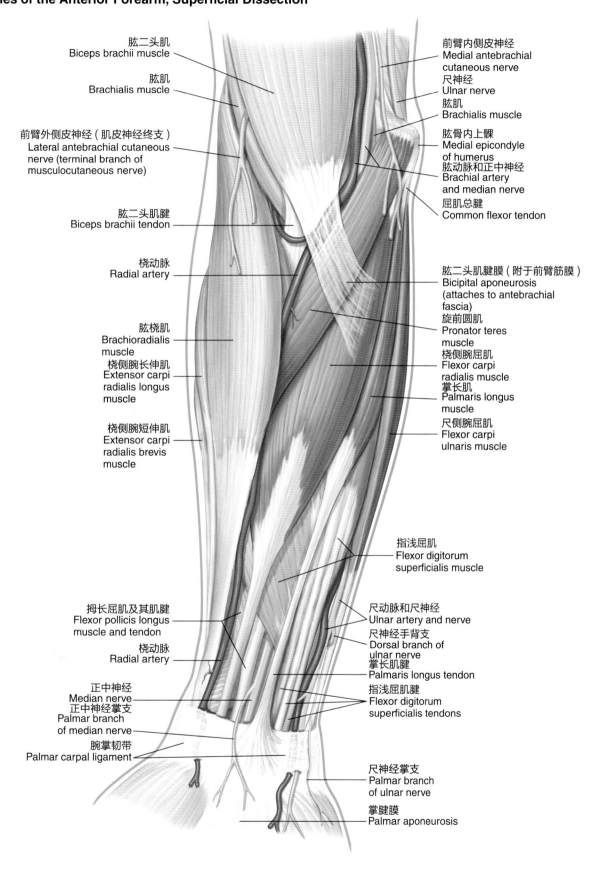

肱二头肌
Biceps brachii muscle

肱肌
Brachialis muscle

前臂外侧皮神经（肌皮神经终支）
Lateral antebrachial cutaneous
nerve (terminal branch of
musculocutaneous nerve)

肱二头肌腱
Biceps brachii tendon

桡动脉
Radial artery

肱桡肌
Brachioradialis
muscle

桡侧腕长伸肌
Extensor carpi
radialis longus
muscle

桡侧腕短伸肌
Extensor carpi
radialis brevis
muscle

拇长屈肌及其肌腱
Flexor pollicis longus
muscle and tendon

桡动脉
Radial artery

正中神经
Median nerve
正中神经掌支
Palmar branch
of median nerve

腕掌韧带
Palmar carpal ligament

前臂内侧皮神经
Medial antebrachial
cutaneous nerve
尺神经
Ulnar nerve
肱肌
Brachialis muscle

肱骨内上髁
Medial epicondyle
of humerus
肱动脉和正中神经
Brachial artery
and median nerve
屈肌总腱
Common flexor tendon

肱二头肌腱膜（附于前臂筋膜）
Bicipital aponeurosis
(attaches to antebrachial
fascia)
旋前圆肌
Pronator teres
muscle
桡侧腕屈肌
Flexor carpi
radialis muscle
掌长肌
Palmaris longus
muscle
尺侧腕屈肌
Flexor carpi
ulnaris muscle

指浅屈肌
Flexor digitorum
superficialis muscle

尺动脉和尺神经
Ulnar artery and nerve
尺神经手背支
Dorsal branch of
ulnar nerve
掌长肌腱
Palmaris longus tendon
指浅屈肌腱
Flexor digitorum
superficialis tendons

尺神经掌支
Palmar branch
of ulnar nerve

掌腱膜
Palmar aponeurosis

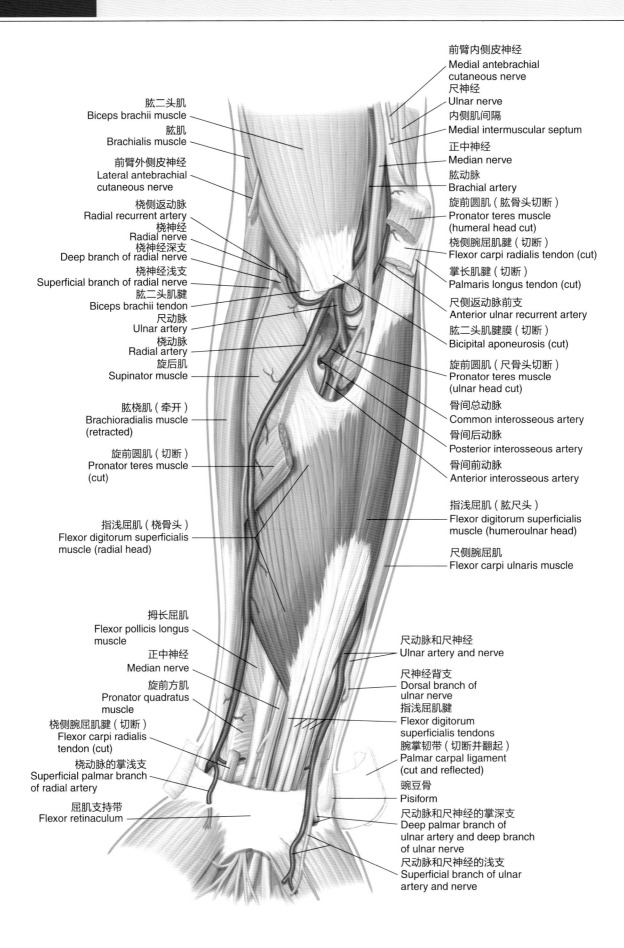

前臂内侧皮神经
Medial antebrachial cutaneous nerve
尺神经
Ulnar nerve
内侧肌间隔
Medial intermuscular septum
正中神经
Median nerve
肱动脉
Brachial artery
旋前圆肌（肱骨头切断）
Pronator teres muscle (humeral head cut)
桡侧腕屈肌腱（切断）
Flexor carpi radialis tendon (cut)
掌长肌腱（切断）
Palmaris longus tendon (cut)
尺侧返动脉前支
Anterior ulnar recurrent artery
肱二头肌腱膜（切断）
Bicipital aponeurosis (cut)
旋前圆肌（尺骨头切断）
Pronator teres muscle (ulnar head cut)
骨间总动脉
Common interosseous artery
骨间后动脉
Posterior interosseous artery
骨间前动脉
Anterior interosseous artery
指浅屈肌（肱尺头）
Flexor digitorum superficialis muscle (humeroulnar head)
尺侧腕屈肌
Flexor carpi ulnaris muscle
尺动脉和尺神经
Ulnar artery and nerve
尺神经背支
Dorsal branch of ulnar nerve
指浅屈肌腱
Flexor digitorum superficialis tendons
腕掌韧带（切断并翻起）
Palmar carpal ligament (cut and reflected)
豌豆骨
Pisiform
尺动脉和尺神经的掌深支
Deep palmar branch of ulnar artery and deep branch of ulnar nerve
尺动脉和尺神经的浅支
Superficial branch of ulnar artery and nerve

肱二头肌
Biceps brachii muscle
肱肌
Brachialis muscle
前臂外侧皮神经
Lateral antebrachial cutaneous nerve
桡侧返动脉
Radial recurrent artery
桡神经
Radial nerve
桡神经深支
Deep branch of radial nerve
桡神经浅支
Superficial branch of radial nerve
肱二头肌腱
Biceps brachii tendon
尺动脉
Ulnar artery
桡动脉
Radial artery
旋后肌
Supinator muscle
肱桡肌（牵开）
Brachioradialis muscle (retracted)
旋前圆肌（切断）
Pronator teres muscle (cut)
指浅屈肌（桡骨头）
Flexor digitorum superficialis muscle (radial head)
拇长屈肌
Flexor pollicis longus muscle
正中神经
Median nerve
旋前方肌
Pronator quadratus muscle
桡侧腕屈肌腱（切断）
Flexor carpi radialis tendon (cut)
桡动脉的掌浅支
Superficial palmar branch of radial artery
屈肌支持带
Flexor retinaculum

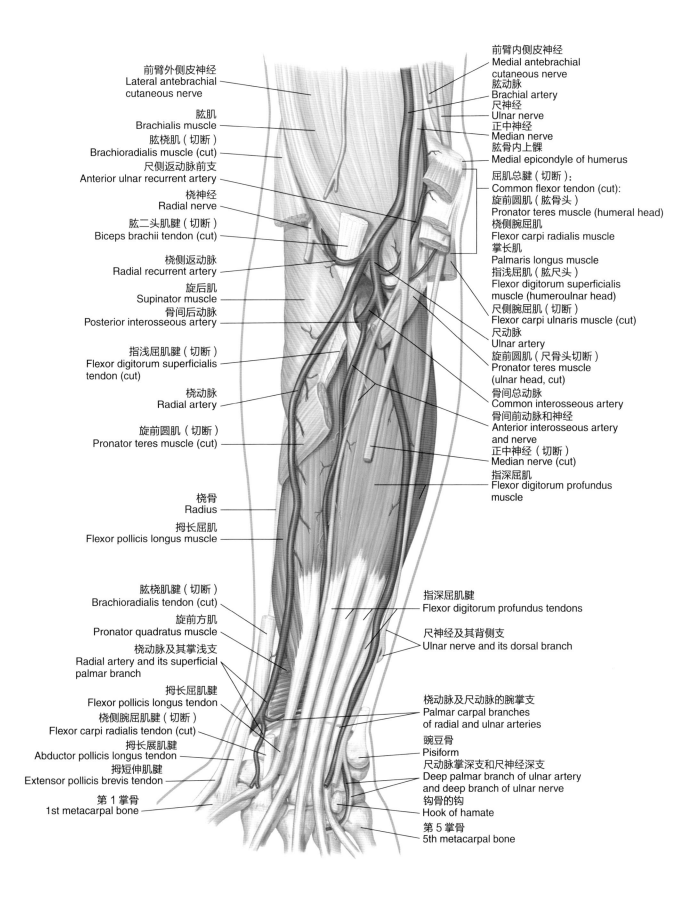

前臂外侧皮神经
Lateral antebrachial
cutaneous nerve

肱肌
Brachialis muscle

肱桡肌（切断）
Brachioradialis muscle (cut)

尺侧返动脉前支
Anterior ulnar recurrent artery

桡神经
Radial nerve

肱二头肌腱（切断）
Biceps brachii tendon (cut)

桡侧返动脉
Radial recurrent artery

旋后肌
Supinator muscle

骨间后动脉
Posterior interosseous artery

指浅屈肌腱（切断）
Flexor digitorum superficialis
tendon (cut)

桡动脉
Radial artery

旋前圆肌（切断）
Pronator teres muscle (cut)

桡骨
Radius

拇长屈肌
Flexor pollicis longus muscle

肱桡肌腱（切断）
Brachioradialis tendon (cut)

旋前方肌
Pronator quadratus muscle

桡动脉及其掌浅支
Radial artery and its superficial
palmar branch

拇长屈肌腱
Flexor pollicis longus tendon

桡侧腕屈肌腱（切断）
Flexor carpi radialis tendon (cut)

拇长展肌腱
Abductor pollicis longus tendon

拇短伸肌腱
Extensor pollicis brevis tendon

第 1 掌骨
1st metacarpal bone

前臂内侧皮神经
Medial antebrachial
cutaneous nerve

肱动脉
Brachial artery

尺神经
Ulnar nerve

正中神经
Median nerve

肱骨内上髁
Medial epicondyle of humerus

屈肌总腱（切断）：
Common flexor tendon (cut):

旋前圆肌（肱骨头）
Pronator teres muscle (humeral head)

桡侧腕屈肌
Flexor carpi radialis muscle

掌长肌
Palmaris longus muscle

指浅屈肌（肱尺头）
Flexor digitorum superficialis
muscle (humeroulnar head)

尺侧腕屈肌（切断）
Flexor carpi ulnaris muscle (cut)

尺动脉
Ulnar artery

旋前圆肌（尺骨头切断）
Pronator teres muscle
(ulnar head, cut)

骨间总动脉
Common interosseous artery

骨间前动脉和神经
Anterior interosseous artery
and nerve

正中神经（切断）
Median nerve (cut)

指深屈肌
Flexor digitorum profundus
muscle

指深屈肌腱
Flexor digitorum profundus tendons

尺神经及其背侧支
Ulnar nerve and its dorsal branch

桡动脉及尺动脉的腕掌支
Palmar carpal branches
of radial and ulnar arteries

豌豆骨
Pisiform

尺动脉掌深支和尺神经深支
Deep palmar branch of ulnar artery
and deep branch of ulnar nerve

钩骨的钩
Hook of hamate

第 5 掌骨
5th metacarpal bone

图 2-26　前臂前侧动脉　Arteries of the Anterior Forearm

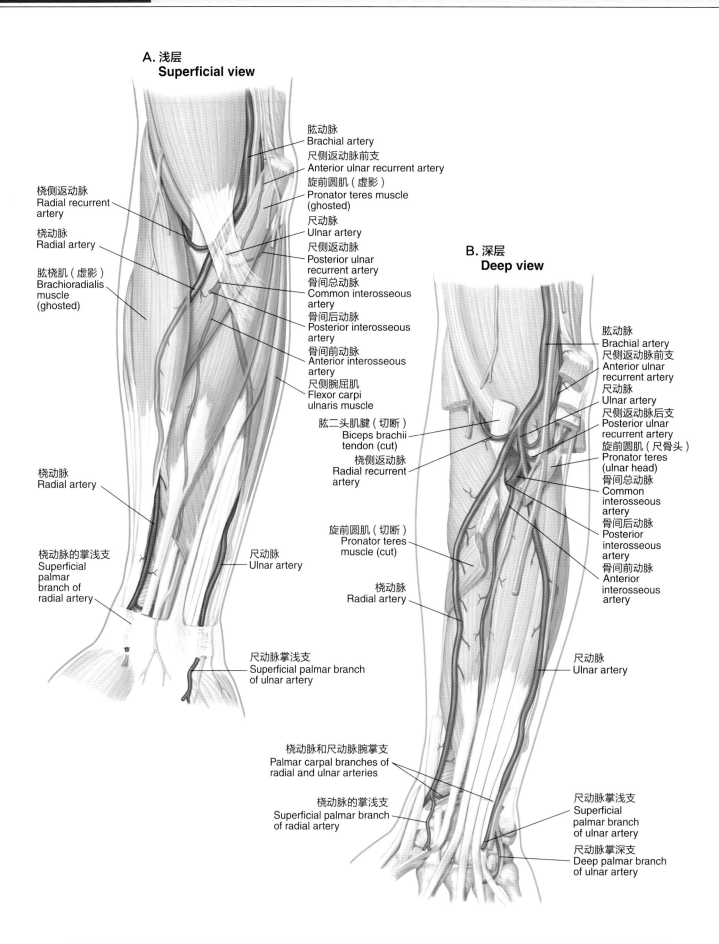

A. 浅层
Superficial view

肱动脉
Brachial artery

尺侧返动脉前支
Anterior ulnar recurrent artery

旋前圆肌（虚影）
Pronator teres muscle (ghosted)

尺动脉
Ulnar artery

尺侧返动脉
Posterior ulnar recurrent artery

骨间总动脉
Common interosseous artery

骨间后动脉
Posterior interosseous artery

骨间前动脉
Anterior interosseous artery

尺侧腕屈肌
Flexor carpi ulnaris muscle

桡侧返动脉
Radial recurrent artery

桡动脉
Radial artery

肱桡肌（虚影）
Brachioradialis muscle (ghosted)

桡动脉
Radial artery

桡动脉的掌浅支
Superficial palmar branch of radial artery

尺动脉
Ulnar artery

尺动脉掌浅支
Superficial palmar branch of ulnar artery

B. 深层
Deep view

肱动脉
Brachial artery

尺侧返动脉前支
Anterior ulnar recurrent artery

尺动脉
Ulnar artery

尺侧返动脉后支
Posterior ulnar recurrent artery

旋前圆肌（尺骨头）
Pronator teres (ulnar head)

骨间总动脉
Common interosseous artery

骨间后动脉
Posterior interosseous artery

骨间前动脉
Anterior interosseous artery

肱二头肌腱（切断）
Biceps brachii tendon (cut)

桡侧返动脉
Radial recurrent artery

旋前圆肌（切断）
Pronator teres muscle (cut)

桡动脉
Radial artery

尺动脉
Ulnar artery

桡动脉和尺动脉腕掌支
Palmar carpal branches of radial and ulnar arteries

桡动脉的掌浅支
Superficial palmar branch of radial artery

尺动脉掌浅支
Superficial palmar branch of ulnar artery

尺动脉掌深支
Deep palmar branch of ulnar artery

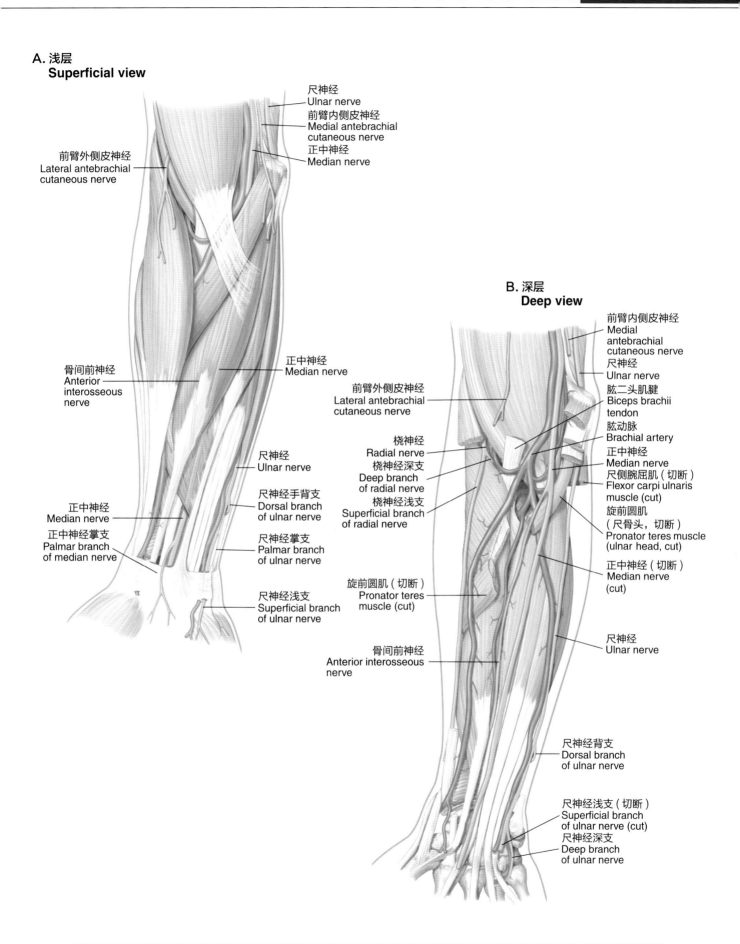

A. 浅层
Superficial view

尺神经
Ulnar nerve

前臂内侧皮神经
Medial antebrachial
cutaneous nerve

正中神经
Median nerve

前臂外侧皮神经
Lateral antebrachial
cutaneous nerve

骨间前神经
Anterior interosseous nerve

正中神经
Median nerve

尺神经
Ulnar nerve

尺神经手背支
Dorsal branch
of ulnar nerve

正中神经
Median nerve

尺神经掌支
Palmar branch
of ulnar nerve

正中神经掌支
Palmar branch
of median nerve

尺神经浅支
Superficial branch
of ulnar nerve

B. 深层
Deep view

前臂内侧皮神经
Medial
antebrachial
cutaneous nerve

尺神经
Ulnar nerve

肱二头肌腱
Biceps brachii
tendon

肱动脉
Brachial artery

正中神经
Median nerve

尺侧腕屈肌（切断）
Flexor carpi ulnaris
muscle (cut)

旋前圆肌
（尺骨头，切断）
Pronator teres muscle
(ulnar head, cut)

正中神经（切断）
Median nerve
(cut)

尺神经
Ulnar nerve

前臂外侧皮神经
Lateral antebrachial
cutaneous nerve

桡神经
Radial nerve

桡神经深支
Deep branch
of radial nerve

桡神经浅支
Superficial branch
of radial nerve

旋前圆肌（切断）
Pronator teres
muscle (cut)

骨间前神经
Anterior interosseous
nerve

尺神经背支
Dorsal branch
of ulnar nerve

尺神经浅支（切断）
Superficial branch
of ulnar nerve (cut)

尺神经深支
Deep branch
of ulnar nerve

图 2-28　前臂神经横断面　Nerves of the Forearm in Cross Section

A. 定位
Orientation

图 B 所在平面
Plane of section B

图 C 所在平面
Plane of section C

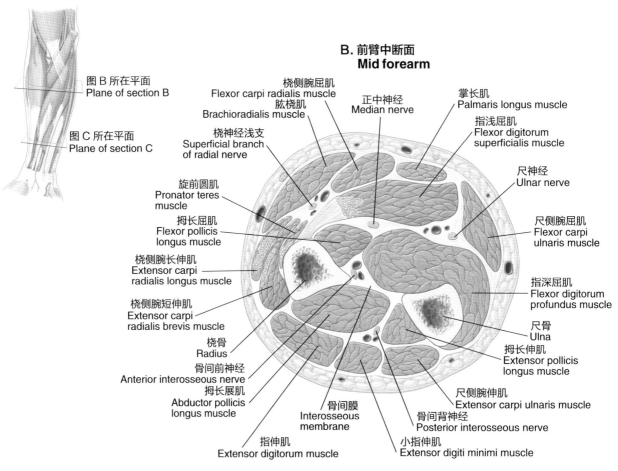

B. 前臂中断面
Mid forearm

桡侧腕屈肌
Flexor carpi radialis muscle
肱桡肌
Brachioradialis muscle

正中神经
Median nerve

掌长肌
Palmaris longus muscle

指浅屈肌
Flexor digitorum superficialis muscle

桡神经浅支
Superficial branch of radial nerve

尺神经
Ulnar nerve

旋前圆肌
Pronator teres muscle

尺侧腕屈肌
Flexor carpi ulnaris muscle

拇长屈肌
Flexor pollicis longus muscle

指深屈肌
Flexor digitorum profundus muscle

桡侧腕长伸肌
Extensor carpi radialis longus muscle

尺骨
Ulna

桡侧腕短伸肌
Extensor carpi radialis brevis muscle

拇长伸肌
Extensor pollicis longus muscle

桡骨
Radius

尺侧腕伸肌
Extensor carpi ulnaris muscle

骨间前神经
Anterior interosseous nerve
拇长展肌
Abductor pollicis longus muscle

骨间膜
Interosseous membrane

骨间背神经
Posterior interosseous nerve

指伸肌
Extensor digitorum muscle

小指伸肌
Extensor digiti minimi muscle

C. 前臂远端断面
Distal forearm

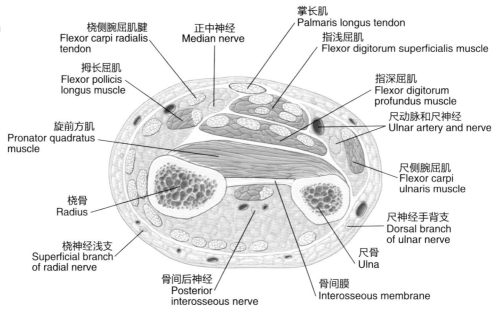

桡侧腕屈肌腱
Flexor carpi radialis tendon

正中神经
Median nerve

掌长肌
Palmaris longus tendon

指浅屈肌
Flexor digitorum superficialis muscle

拇长屈肌
Flexor pollicis longus muscle

指深屈肌
Flexor digitorum profundus muscle

旋前方肌
Pronator quadratus muscle

尺动脉和尺神经
Ulnar artery and nerve

尺侧腕屈肌
Flexor carpi ulnaris muscle

桡骨
Radius

尺神经手背支
Dorsal branch of ulnar nerve

桡神经浅支
Superficial branch of radial nerve

尺骨
Ulna

骨间后神经
Posterior interosseous nerve

骨间膜
Interosseous membrane

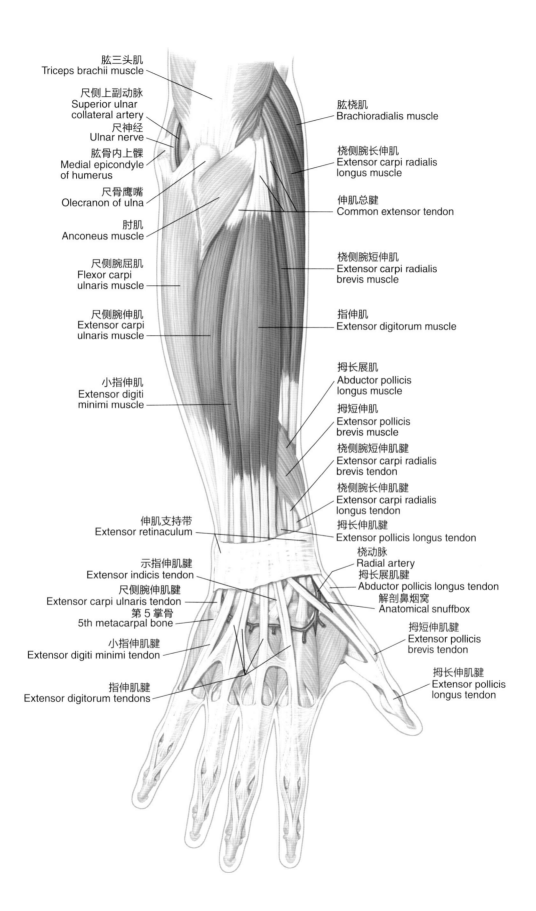

肱三头肌
Triceps brachii muscle

尺侧上副动脉
Superior ulnar collateral artery

尺神经
Ulnar nerve

肱骨内上髁
Medial epicondyle of humerus

尺骨鹰嘴
Olecranon of ulna

肘肌
Anconeus muscle

尺侧腕屈肌
Flexor carpi ulnaris muscle

尺侧腕伸肌
Extensor carpi ulnaris muscle

小指伸肌
Extensor digiti minimi muscle

伸肌支持带
Extensor retinaculum

示指伸肌腱
Extensor indicis tendon

尺侧腕伸肌腱
Extensor carpi ulnaris tendon

第 5 掌骨
5th metacarpal bone

小指伸肌腱
Extensor digiti minimi tendon

指伸肌腱
Extensor digitorum tendons

肱桡肌
Brachioradialis muscle

桡侧腕长伸肌
Extensor carpi radialis longus muscle

伸肌总腱
Common extensor tendon

桡侧腕短伸肌
Extensor carpi radialis brevis muscle

指伸肌
Extensor digitorum muscle

拇长展肌
Abductor pollicis longus muscle

拇短伸肌
Extensor pollicis brevis muscle

桡侧腕短伸肌腱
Extensor carpi radialis brevis tendon

桡侧腕长伸肌腱
Extensor carpi radialis longus tendon

拇长伸肌腱
Extensor pollicis longus tendon

桡动脉
Radial artery

拇长展肌腱
Abductor pollicis longus tendon

解剖鼻烟窝
Anatomical snuffbox

拇短伸肌腱
Extensor pollicis brevis tendon

拇长伸肌腱
Extensor pollicis longus tendon

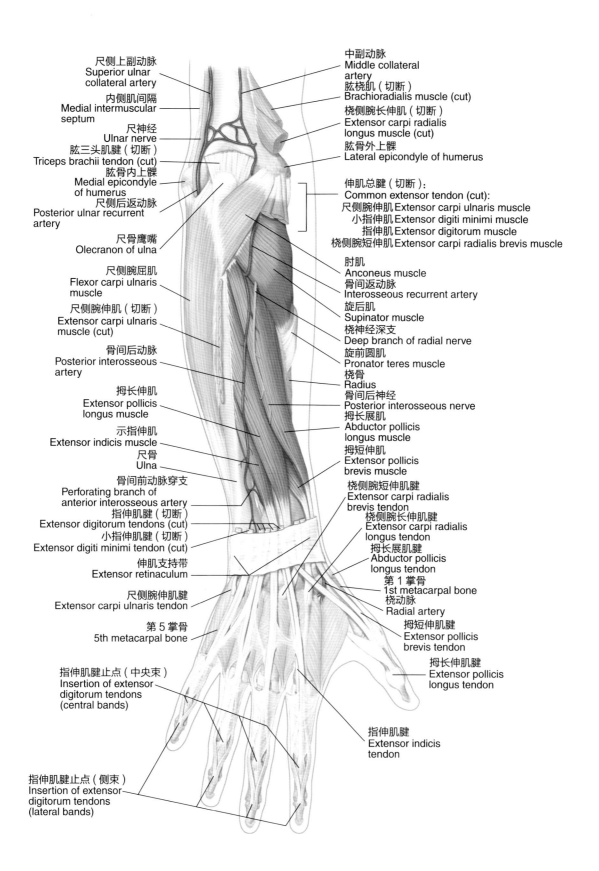

尺侧上副动脉
Superior ulnar collateral artery

内侧肌间隔
Medial intermuscular septum

尺神经
Ulnar nerve

肱三头肌腱（切断）
Triceps brachii tendon (cut)

肱骨内上髁
Medial epicondyle of humerus

尺侧后返动脉
Posterior ulnar recurrent artery

尺骨鹰嘴
Olecranon of ulna

尺侧腕屈肌
Flexor carpi ulnaris muscle

尺侧腕伸肌（切断）
Extensor carpi ulnaris muscle (cut)

骨间后动脉
Posterior interosseous artery

拇长伸肌
Extensor pollicis longus muscle

示指伸肌
Extensor indicis muscle

尺骨
Ulna

骨间前动脉穿支
Perforating branch of anterior interosseous artery

指伸肌腱（切断）
Extensor digitorum tendons (cut)

小指伸肌腱（切断）
Extensor digiti minimi tendon (cut)

伸肌支持带
Extensor retinaculum

尺侧腕伸肌腱
Extensor carpi ulnaris tendon

第 5 掌骨
5th metacarpal bone

指伸肌腱止点（中央束）
Insertion of extensor digitorum tendons (central bands)

指伸肌腱止点（侧束）
Insertion of extensor digitorum tendons (lateral bands)

中副动脉
Middle collateral artery

肱桡肌（切断）
Brachioradialis muscle (cut)

桡侧腕长伸肌（切断）
Extensor carpi radialis longus muscle (cut)

肱骨外上髁
Lateral epicondyle of humerus

伸肌总腱（切断）：
Common extensor tendon (cut):
尺侧腕伸肌 Extensor carpi ulnaris muscle
小指伸肌 Extensor digiti minimi muscle
指伸肌 Extensor digitorum muscle
桡侧腕短伸肌 Extensor carpi radialis brevis muscle

肘肌
Anconeus muscle

骨间返动脉
Interosseous recurrent artery

旋后肌
Supinator muscle

桡神经深支
Deep branch of radial nerve

旋前圆肌
Pronator teres muscle

桡骨
Radius

骨间后神经
Posterior interosseous nerve

拇长展肌
Abductor pollicis longus muscle

拇短伸肌
Extensor pollicis brevis muscle

桡侧腕短伸肌腱
Extensor carpi radialis brevis tendon

桡侧腕长伸肌腱
Extensor carpi radialis longus tendon

拇长展肌腱
Abductor pollicis longus tendon

第 1 掌骨
1st metacarpal bone

桡动脉
Radial artery

拇短伸肌腱
Extensor pollicis brevis tendon

拇长伸肌腱
Extensor pollicis longus tendon

指伸肌腱
Extensor indicis tendon

A. 骨
Bones

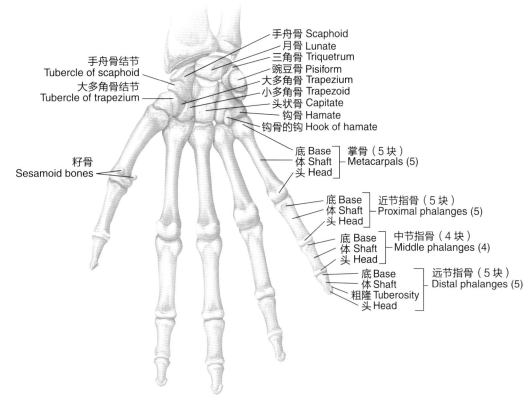

手舟骨 Scaphoid
月骨 Lunate
三角骨 Triquetrum
豌豆骨 Pisiform
大多角骨 Trapezium
小多角骨 Trapezoid
头状骨 Capitate
钩骨 Hamate
钩骨的钩 Hook of hamate

手舟骨结节
Tubercle of scaphoid
大多角骨结节
Tubercle of trapezium

籽骨
Sesamoid bones

底 Base
体 Shaft — 掌骨（5 块）
头 Head   Metacarpals (5)

底 Base — 近节指骨（5 块）
体 Shaft   Proximal phalanges (5)
头 Head

底 Base — 中节指骨（4 块）
体 Shaft   Middle phalanges (4)
头 Head

底 Base
体 Shaft — 远节指骨（5 块）
粗隆 Tuberosity   Distal phalanges (5)
头 Head

B. 肌肉附着点
Muscle attachments

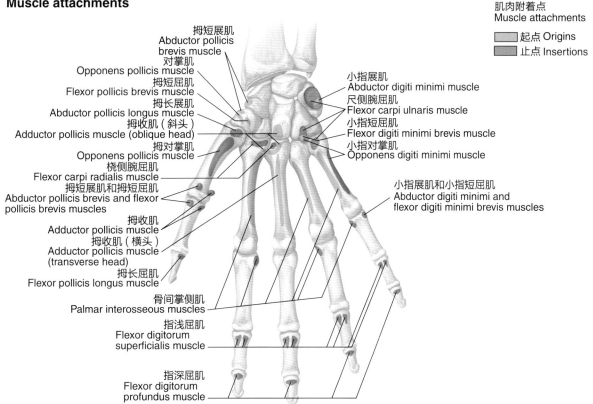

肌肉附着点
Muscle attachments
起点 Origins
止点 Insertions

拇短展肌
Abductor pollicis
brevis muscle
对掌肌
Opponens pollicis muscle
拇短屈肌
Flexor pollicis brevis muscle
拇长展肌
Abductor pollicis longus muscle
拇收肌（斜头）
Adductor pollicis muscle (oblique head)
拇对掌肌
Opponens pollicis muscle
桡侧腕屈肌
Flexor carpi radialis muscle
拇短展肌和拇短屈肌
Abductor pollicis brevis and flexor
pollicis brevis muscles
拇收肌
Adductor pollicis muscle
拇收肌（横头）
Adductor pollicis muscle
(transverse head)
拇长屈肌
Flexor pollicis longus muscle
骨间掌侧肌
Palmar interosseous muscles
指浅屈肌
Flexor digitorum
superficialis muscle
指深屈肌
Flexor digitorum
profundus muscle

小指展肌
Abductor digiti minimi muscle
尺侧腕屈肌
Flexor carpi ulnaris muscle
小指短屈肌
Flexor digiti minimi brevis muscle
小指对掌肌
Opponens digiti minimi muscle

小指展肌和小指短屈肌
Abductor digiti minimi and
flexor digiti minimi brevis muscles

A. 骨
Bones

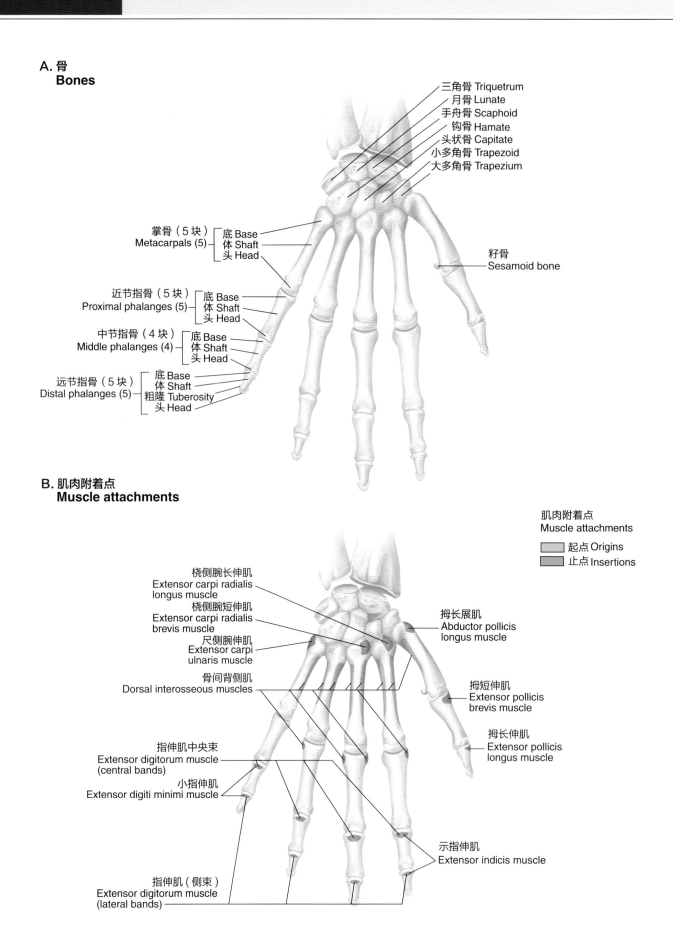

三角骨 Triquetrum
月骨 Lunate
手舟骨 Scaphoid
钩骨 Hamate
头状骨 Capitate
小多角骨 Trapezoid
大多角骨 Trapezium

掌骨（5 块）
Metacarpals (5)
底 Base
体 Shaft
头 Head

籽骨
Sesamoid bone

近节指骨（5 块）
Proximal phalanges (5)
底 Base
体 Shaft
头 Head

中节指骨（4 块）
Middle phalanges (4)
底 Base
体 Shaft
头 Head

远节指骨（5 块）
Distal phalanges (5)
底 Base
体 Shaft
粗隆 Tuberosity
头 Head

B. 肌肉附着点
Muscle attachments

肌肉附着点
Muscle attachments
□ 起点 Origins
□ 止点 Insertions

桡侧腕长伸肌
Extensor carpi radialis longus muscle

桡侧腕短伸肌
Extensor carpi radialis brevis muscle

尺侧腕伸肌
Extensor carpi ulnaris muscle

骨间背侧肌
Dorsal interosseous muscles

拇长展肌
Abductor pollicis longus muscle

拇短伸肌
Extensor pollicis brevis muscle

拇长伸肌
Extensor pollicis longus muscle

指伸肌中央束
Extensor digitorum muscle (central bands)

小指伸肌
Extensor digiti minimi muscle

示指伸肌
Extensor indicis muscle

指伸肌（侧束）
Extensor digitorum muscle (lateral bands)

A. 解剖 Dissection

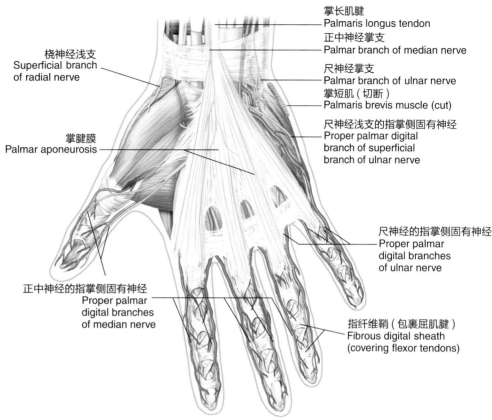

掌长肌腱
Palmaris longus tendon

正中神经掌支
Palmar branch of median nerve

尺神经掌支
Palmar branch of ulnar nerve

掌短肌（切断）
Palmaris brevis muscle (cut)

尺神经浅支的指掌侧固有神经
Proper palmar digital branch of superficial branch of ulnar nerve

尺神经的指掌侧固有神经
Proper palmar digital branches of ulnar nerve

指纤维鞘（包裹屈肌腱）
Fibrous digital sheath (covering flexor tendons)

桡神经浅支
Superficial branch of radial nerve

掌腱膜
Palmar aponeurosis

正中神经的指掌侧固有神经
Proper palmar digital branches of median nerve

B. 神经支配区域 Nerve territories

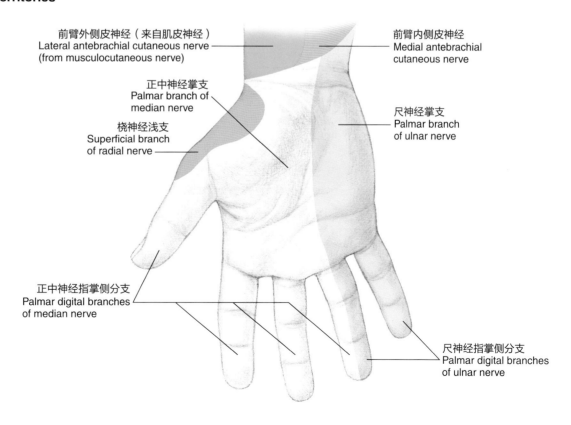

前臂外侧皮神经（来自肌皮神经）
Lateral antebrachial cutaneous nerve (from musculocutaneous nerve)

前臂内侧皮神经
Medial antebrachial cutaneous nerve

正中神经掌支
Palmar branch of median nerve

尺神经掌支
Palmar branch of ulnar nerve

桡神经浅支
Superficial branch of radial nerve

正中神经指掌侧分支
Palmar digital branches of median nerve

尺神经指掌侧分支
Palmar digital branches of ulnar nerve

A. 浅层解剖
Superficial dissection

桡动脉 Radial artery

桡侧滑囊 Radial bursa

桡动脉掌浅支 Superficial palmar branch of radial artery

屈肌支持带 Flexor retinaculum

拇短展肌 Abductor pollicis brevis muscle

拇对掌肌 Opponens pollicis muscle

正中神经回返支 Recurrent branch of median nerve

拇短屈肌 Flexor pollicis brevis muscle

第 1 蚓状肌 1st lumbrical muscle

鱼际腱膜（切断）Thenar fascia (cut)

拇收肌 Adductor pollicis muscle

指纤维鞘 Fibrous digital sheath

正中神经 Median nerve

尺动脉和尺神经 Ulnar artery and nerve

尺动脉掌深支 Deep palmar branch of ulnar artery

尺神经深支 Deep branch of ulnar nerve

小指展肌 Abductor digiti minimi muscle

尺神经浅支 Superficial branch of ulnar nerve

小指短屈肌 Flexor digiti minimi brevis muscle

尺侧滑膜囊 Ulnar bursa

小鱼际筋膜（切断）Hypothenar fascia (cut)

掌浅弓 Superficial palmar arch

掌指总动脉和神经 Common palmar digital arteries and nerves

掌腱膜（翻开）Palmar aponeurosis (reflected)

指掌侧固有神经和动脉 Proper palmar digital nerves and arteries

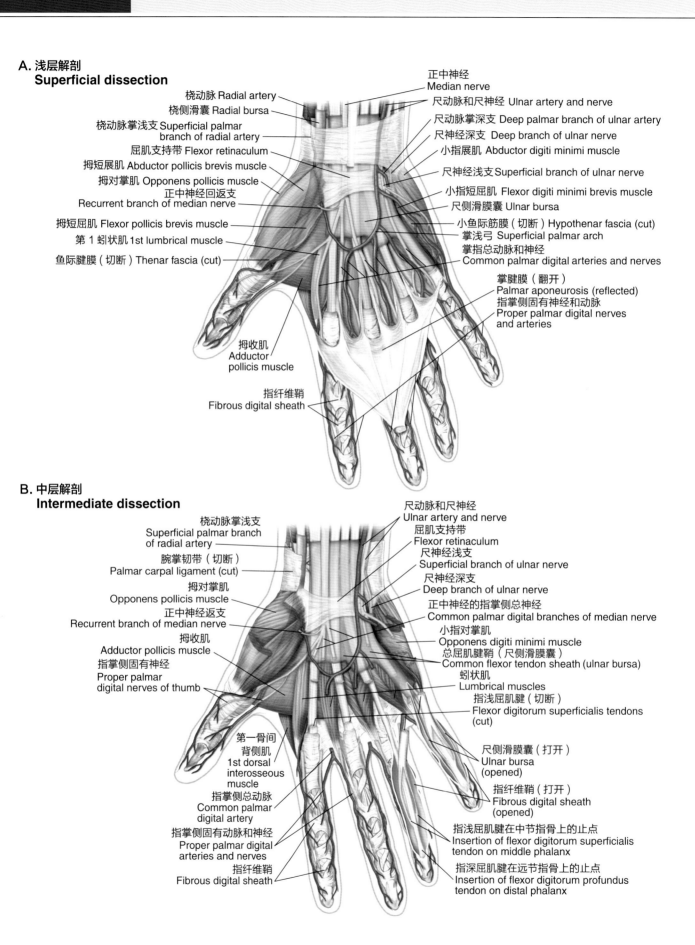

B. 中层解剖
Intermediate dissection

桡动脉掌浅支 Superficial palmar branch of radial artery

腕掌韧带（切断）Palmar carpal ligament (cut)

拇对掌肌 Opponens pollicis muscle

正中神经返支 Recurrent branch of median nerve

拇收肌 Adductor pollicis muscle

指掌侧固有神经 Proper palmar digital nerves of thumb

第一骨间背侧肌 1st dorsal interosseous muscle

指掌侧总动脉 Common palmar digital artery

指掌侧固有动脉和神经 Proper palmar digital arteries and nerves

指纤维鞘 Fibrous digital sheath

尺动脉和尺神经 Ulnar artery and nerve

屈肌支持带 Flexor retinaculum

尺神经浅支 Superficial branch of ulnar nerve

尺神经深支 Deep branch of ulnar nerve

正中神经的指掌侧总神经 Common palmar digital branches of median nerve

小指对掌肌 Opponens digiti minimi muscle

总屈肌腱鞘（尺侧滑膜囊）Common flexor tendon sheath (ulnar bursa)

蚓状肌 Lumbrical muscles

指浅屈肌腱（切断）Flexor digitorum superficialis tendons (cut)

尺侧滑膜囊（打开）Ulnar bursa (opened)

指纤维鞘（打开）Fibrous digital sheath (opened)

指浅屈肌腱在中节指骨上的止点 Insertion of flexor digitorum superficialis tendon on middle phalanx

指深屈肌腱在远节指骨上的止点 Insertion of flexor digitorum profundus tendon on distal phalanx

A. 深层解剖
Deep dissection

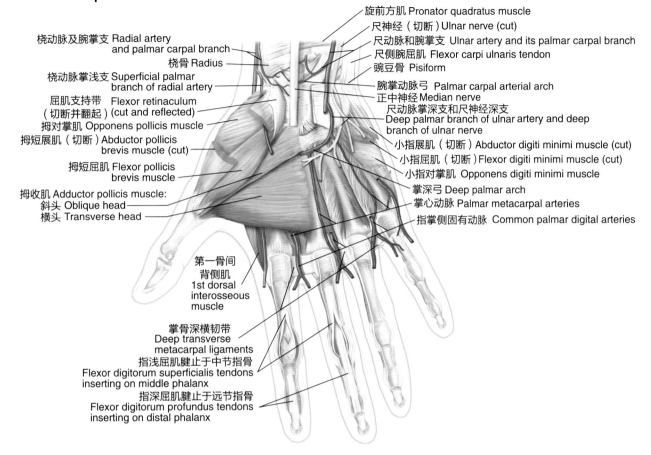

桡动脉及腕掌支 Radial artery and palmar carpal branch

桡骨 Radius

桡动脉掌浅支 Superficial palmar branch of radial artery

屈肌支持带 Flexor retinaculum（切断并翻起）(cut and reflected)

拇对掌肌 Opponens pollicis muscle

拇短展肌（切断）Abductor pollicis brevis muscle (cut)

拇短屈肌 Flexor pollicis brevis muscle

拇收肌 Adductor pollicis muscle:
斜头 Oblique head
横头 Transverse head

旋前方肌 Pronator quadratus muscle

尺神经（切断）Ulnar nerve (cut)

尺动脉和腕掌支 Ulnar artery and its palmar carpal branch

尺侧腕屈肌 Flexor carpi ulnaris tendon

豌豆骨 Pisiform

腕掌动脉弓 Palmar carpal arterial arch

正中神经 Median nerve

尺动脉掌深支和尺神经深支 Deep palmar branch of ulnar artery and deep branch of ulnar nerve

小指展肌（切断）Abductor digiti minimi muscle (cut)

小指屈肌（切断）Flexor digiti minimi muscle (cut)

小指对掌肌 Opponens digiti minimi muscle

掌深弓 Deep palmar arch

掌心动脉 Palmar metacarpal arteries

指掌侧固有动脉 Common palmar digital arteries

第一骨间背侧肌 1st dorsal interosseous muscle

掌骨深横韧带 Deep transverse metacarpal ligaments

指浅屈肌腱止于中节指骨 Flexor digitorum superficialis tendons inserting on middle phalanx

指深屈肌腱止于远节指骨 Flexor digitorum profundus tendons inserting on distal phalanx

B. 骨间掌侧肌
Palmar interosseous muscles

C. 骨间背侧肌
Dorsal interosseous muscles

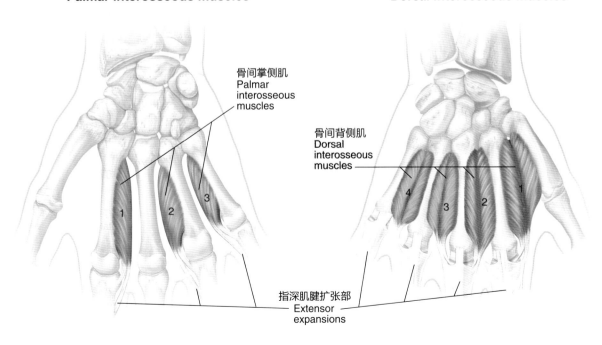

骨间掌侧肌 Palmar interosseous muscles

骨间背侧肌 Dorsal interosseous muscles

指深肌腱扩张部 Extensor expansions

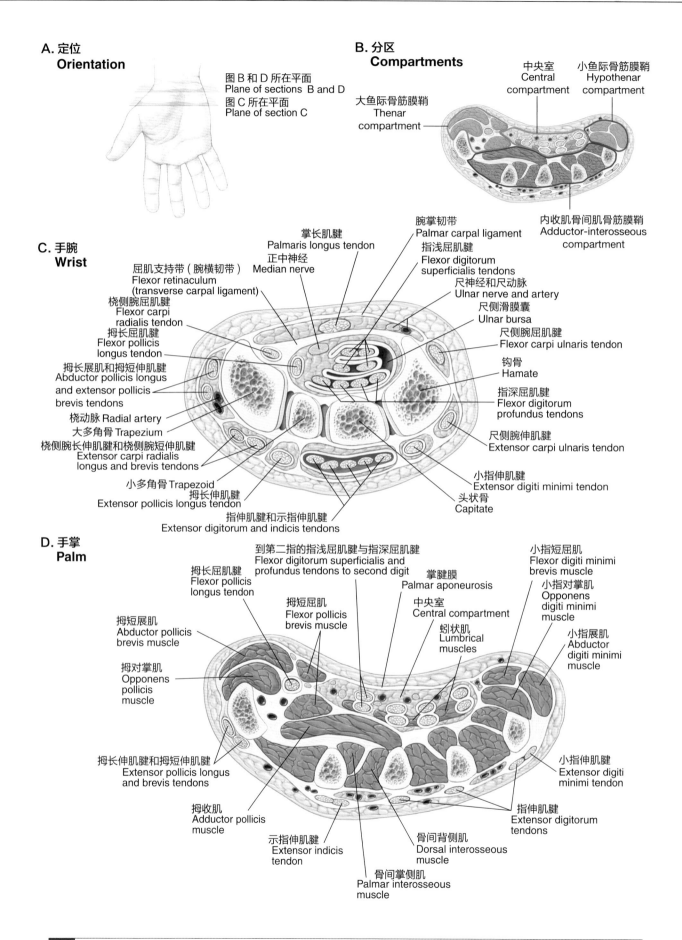

A. 定位
Orientation

图 B 和 D 所在平面
Plane of sections B and D
图 C 所在平面
Plane of section C

B. 分区
Compartments

中央室
Central compartment

小鱼际骨筋膜鞘
Hypothenar compartment

大鱼际骨筋膜鞘
Thenar compartment

内收肌骨间肌骨筋膜鞘
Adductor-interosseous compartment

C. 手腕
Wrist

掌长肌腱
Palmaris longus tendon

腕掌韧带
Palmar carpal ligament

指浅屈肌腱
Flexor digitorum superficialis tendons

屈肌支持带（腕横韧带）
Flexor retinaculum (transverse carpal ligament)

正中神经
Median nerve

桡侧腕屈肌腱
Flexor carpi radialis tendon

尺神经和尺动脉
Ulnar nerve and artery

尺侧滑膜囊
Ulnar bursa

拇长屈肌腱
Flexor pollicis longus tendon

尺侧腕屈肌腱
Flexor carpi ulnaris tendon

拇长展肌和拇短伸肌腱
Abductor pollicis longus and extensor pollicis brevis tendons

钩骨
Hamate

指深屈肌腱
Flexor digitorum profundus tendons

桡动脉 Radial artery
大多角骨 Trapezium

尺侧腕伸肌腱
Extensor carpi ulnaris tendon

桡侧腕长伸肌腱和桡侧腕短伸肌腱
Extensor carpi radialis longus and brevis tendons

小指伸肌腱
Extensor digiti minimi tendon

小多角骨 Trapezoid
拇长伸肌腱
Extensor pollicis longus tendon

头状骨
Capitate

指伸肌腱和示指伸肌腱
Extensor digitorum and indicis tendons

D. 手掌
Palm

到第二指的指浅屈肌腱与指深屈肌腱
Flexor digitorum superficialis and profundus tendons to second digit

小指短屈肌
Flexor digiti minimi brevis muscle

拇长屈肌腱
Flexor pollicis longus tendon

掌腱膜
Palmar aponeurosis

小指对掌肌
Opponens digiti minimi muscle

拇短屈肌
Flexor pollicis brevis muscle

中央室
Central compartment

拇短展肌
Abductor pollicis brevis muscle

蚓状肌
Lumbrical muscles

小指展肌
Abductor digiti minimi muscle

拇对掌肌
Opponens pollicis muscle

拇长伸肌腱和拇短伸肌腱
Extensor pollicis longus and brevis tendons

小指伸肌腱
Extensor digiti minimi tendon

拇收肌
Adductor pollicis muscle

指伸肌腱
Extensor digitorum tendons

示指伸肌腱
Extensor indicis tendon

骨间背侧肌
Dorsal interosseous muscle

骨间掌侧肌
Palmar interosseous muscle

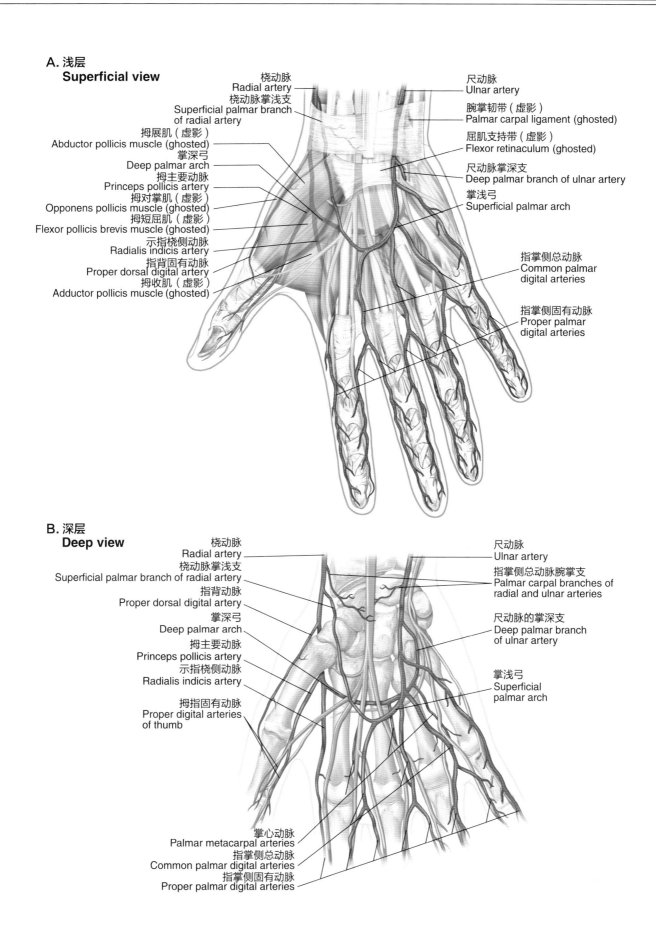

A. 浅层
Superficial view

桡动脉
Radial artery

桡动脉掌浅支
Superficial palmar branch
of radial artery

拇展肌（虚影）
Abductor pollicis muscle (ghosted)

掌深弓
Deep palmar arch

拇主要动脉
Princeps pollicis artery

拇对掌肌（虚影）
Opponens pollicis muscle (ghosted)

拇短屈肌（虚影）
Flexor pollicis brevis muscle (ghosted)

示指桡侧动脉
Radialis indicis artery

指背固有动脉
Proper dorsal digital artery

拇收肌（虚影）
Adductor pollicis muscle (ghosted)

尺动脉
Ulnar artery

腕掌韧带（虚影）
Palmar carpal ligament (ghosted)

屈肌支持带（虚影）
Flexor retinaculum (ghosted)

尺动脉掌深支
Deep palmar branch of ulnar artery

掌浅弓
Superficial palmar arch

指掌侧总动脉
Common palmar
digital arteries

指掌侧固有动脉
Proper palmar
digital arteries

B. 深层
Deep view

桡动脉
Radial artery

桡动脉掌浅支
Superficial palmar branch of radial artery

指背动脉
Proper dorsal digital artery

掌深弓
Deep palmar arch

拇主要动脉
Princeps pollicis artery

示指桡侧动脉
Radialis indicis artery

拇指固有动脉
Proper digital arteries
of thumb

尺动脉
Ulnar artery

指掌侧总动脉腕掌支
Palmar carpal branches of
radial and ulnar arteries

尺动脉的掌深支
Deep palmar branch
of ulnar artery

掌浅弓
Superficial
palmar arch

掌心动脉
Palmar metacarpal arteries

指掌侧总动脉
Common palmar digital arteries

指掌侧固有动脉
Proper palmar digital arteries

图 2-38　手的神经　Nerves of the Hand

A. 前面观
Anterior view

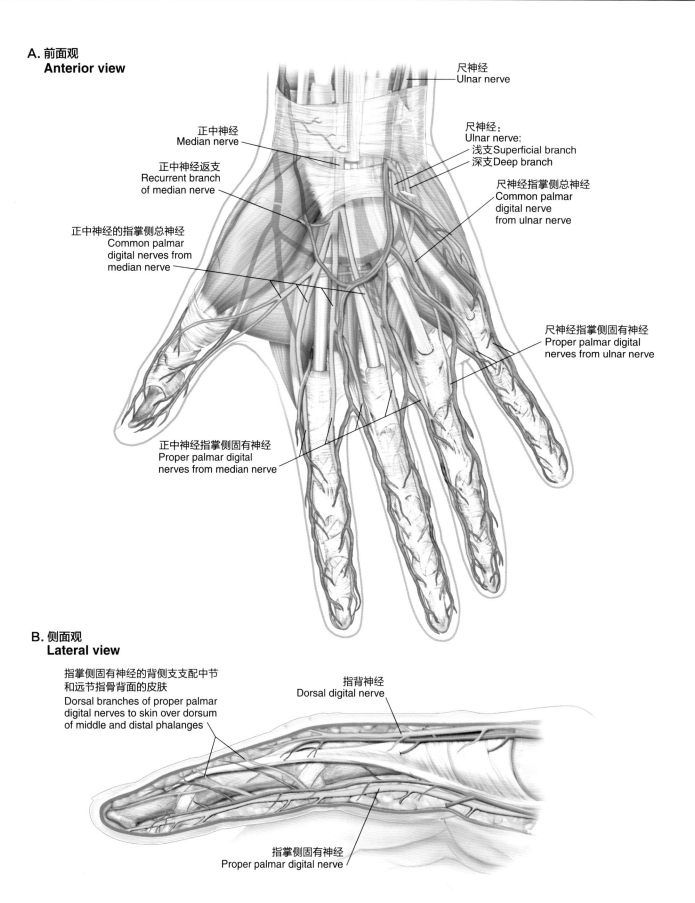

尺神经
Ulnar nerve

正中神经
Median nerve

正中神经返支
Recurrent branch
of median nerve

尺神经：
Ulnar nerve:
浅支 Superficial branch
深支 Deep branch

尺神经指掌侧总神经
Common palmar
digital nerve
from ulnar nerve

正中神经的指掌侧总神经
Common palmar
digital nerves from
median nerve

尺神经指掌侧固有神经
Proper palmar digital
nerves from ulnar nerve

正中神经指掌侧固有神经
Proper palmar digital
nerves from median nerve

B. 侧面观
Lateral view

指掌侧固有神经的背侧支支配中节
和远节指骨背面的皮肤
Dorsal branches of proper palmar
digital nerves to skin over dorsum
of middle and distal phalanges

指背神经
Dorsal digital nerve

指掌侧固有神经
Proper palmar digital nerve

A. 解剖
Dissection

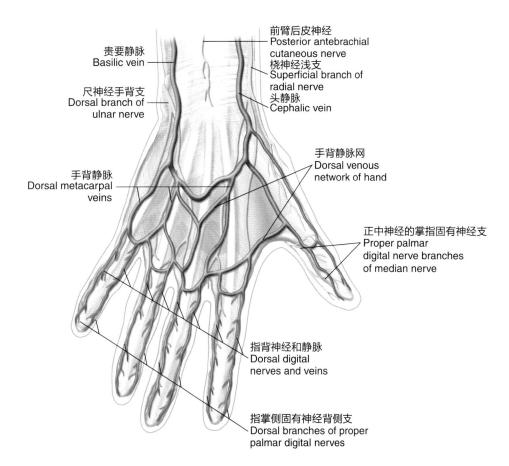

贵要静脉
Basilic vein

尺神经手背支
Dorsal branch of
ulnar nerve

手背静脉
Dorsal metacarpal
veins

前臂后皮神经
Posterior antebrachial
cutaneous nerve

桡神经浅支
Superficial branch of
radial nerve

头静脉
Cephalic vein

手背静脉网
Dorsal venous
network of hand

正中神经的掌指固有神经支
Proper palmar
digital nerve branches
of median nerve

指背神经和静脉
Dorsal digital
nerves and veins

指掌侧固有神经背侧支
Dorsal branches of proper
palmar digital nerves

B. 神经支配区域
Nerve territories

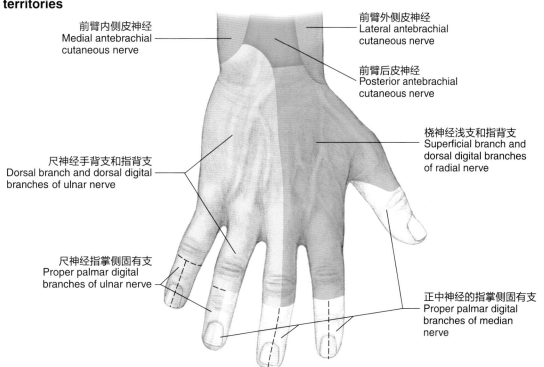

前臂内侧皮神经
Medial antebrachial
cutaneous nerve

尺神经手背支和指背支
Dorsal branch and dorsal digital
branches of ulnar nerve

尺神经指掌侧固有支
Proper palmar digital
branches of ulnar nerve

前臂外侧皮神经
Lateral antebrachial
cutaneous nerve

前臂后皮神经
Posterior antebrachial
cutaneous nerve

桡神经浅支和指背支
Superficial branch and
dorsal digital branches
of radial nerve

正中神经的指掌侧固有支
Proper palmar digital
branches of median
nerve

A. 解剖
Dissection

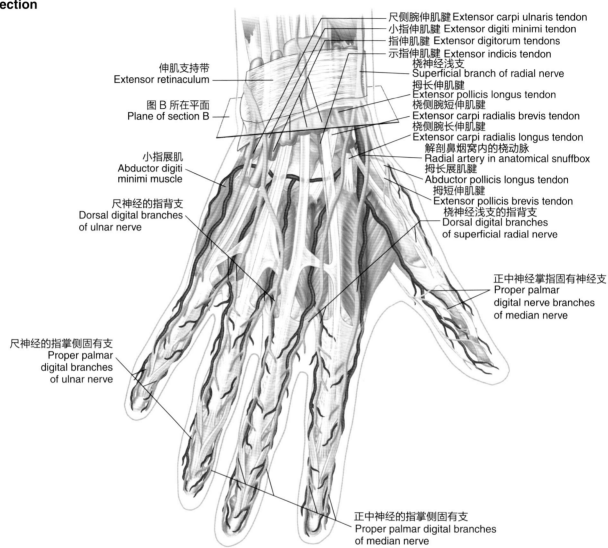

尺侧腕伸肌腱 Extensor carpi ulnaris tendon
小指伸肌腱 Extensor digiti minimi tendon
指伸肌腱 Extensor digitorum tendons
示指伸肌腱 Extensor indicis tendon
桡神经浅支 Superficial branch of radial nerve
拇长伸肌腱 Extensor pollicis longus tendon
桡侧腕短伸肌腱 Extensor carpi radialis brevis tendon
桡侧腕长伸肌腱 Extensor carpi radialis longus tendon
解剖鼻烟窝内的桡动脉 Radial artery in anatomical snuffbox
拇长展肌腱 Abductor pollicis longus tendon
拇短伸肌腱 Extensor pollicis brevis tendon
桡神经浅支的指背支 Dorsal digital branches of superficial radial nerve
正中神经掌指固有神经支 Proper palmar digital nerve branches of median nerve

伸肌支持带 Extensor retinaculum
图 B 所在平面 Plane of section B
小指展肌 Abductor digiti minimi muscle
尺神经的指背支 Dorsal digital branches of ulnar nerve
尺神经的指掌侧固有支 Proper palmar digital branches of ulnar nerve
正中神经的指掌侧固有支 Proper palmar digital branches of median nerve

B. 通过腕部的横断面
Cross section through the wrist

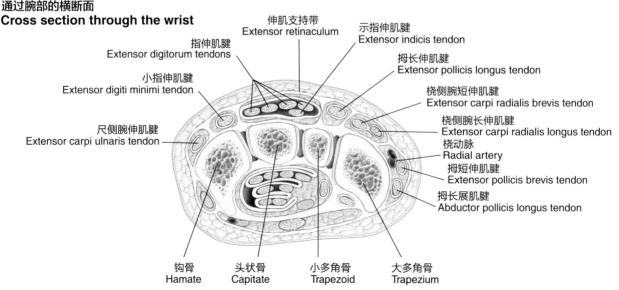

伸肌支持带 Extensor retinaculum
示指伸肌腱 Extensor indicis tendon
指伸肌腱 Extensor digitorum tendons
小指伸肌腱 Extensor digiti minimi tendon
拇长伸肌腱 Extensor pollicis longus tendon
桡侧腕短伸肌腱 Extensor carpi radialis brevis tendon
尺侧腕伸肌腱 Extensor carpi ulnaris tendon
桡侧腕长伸肌腱 Extensor carpi radialis longus tendon
桡动脉 Radial artery
拇短伸肌腱 Extensor pollicis brevis tendon
拇长展肌腱 Abductor pollicis longus tendon

钩骨 Hamate
头状骨 Capitate
小多角骨 Trapezoid
大多角骨 Trapezium

A. 解剖
Dissection

桡骨背侧结节
Dorsal radial tubercle

指伸肌腱
Extensor digitorum tendons

桡神经浅支
Superficial branch of radial nerve

桡侧腕短伸肌腱
Extensor carpi radialis brevis tendon

示指伸肌腱
Extensor indicis tendon

拇长伸肌腱
Extensor pollicis longus tendon

解剖鼻烟窝内的桡动脉
Radial artery in anatomical snuffbox

拇长展肌腱
Abductor pollicis longus tendon

桡侧腕长伸肌腱
Extensor carpi radialis longus tendon

拇短伸肌腱
Extensor pollicis brevis tendon

骨间背侧肌
Dorsal interosseous muscles

伸肌支持带（切断）
Extensor retinaculum (cut)

尺神经手背支
Dorsal branch of ulnar nerve

尺侧腕伸肌腱
Extensor carpi ulnaris tendon

小指伸肌腱
Extensor digiti minimi tendon

小指展肌
Abductor digiti minimi muscle

腕背侧弓
Dorsal carpal arch

掌背动脉
Dorsal metacarpal arteries

指背动脉
Dorsal digital arteries

尺神经手背支的指背支
Dorsal digital branches of dorsal branch of ulnar nerve

尺神经指掌侧固有支的背侧支和指掌侧固有动脉
Dorsal branches of proper palmar digital branches of ulnar nerve and proper palmar digital arteries

桡神经浅支的指背侧支
Dorsal digital branches of superficial branch of radial nerve

正中神经指掌侧固有支的指背侧支和指掌侧固有动脉
Dorsal branches of proper palmar digital branches of median nerve and proper palmar digital arteries

B. 右示指伸指肌腱扩张部
Extensor expansion, right index finger

掌骨
Metacarpal bone

骨间掌侧肌
Palmar interosseous muscle

示指伸肌腱
Extensor indicis tendon

伸指肌腱扩张部
Extensor expansion

中央束（到中节指骨底）
Central band (to base of middle phalanx)

远端指间关节囊
Distal interphalangeal joint capsule

第一骨间背侧肌
First dorsal interosseous muscle

第 1 蚓状肌
First lumbrical muscle

指伸肌腱
Extensor digitorum tendon

侧束（到远节指骨底）
Lateral bands (to base of distal phalanx)

图 2-42　　上肢近端关节　Joints of the Proximal Upper Limb

A. 解剖 Dissection

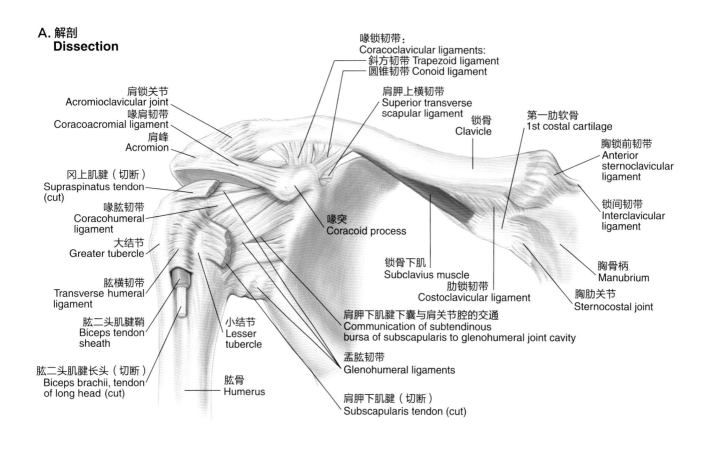

喙锁韧带:
Coracoclavicular ligaments:
斜方韧带 Trapezoid ligament
圆锥韧带 Conoid ligament

肩胛上横韧带
Superior transverse
scapular ligament

锁骨
Clavicle

第一肋软骨
1st costal cartilage

胸锁前韧带
Anterior
sternoclavicular
ligament

锁间韧带
Interclavicular
ligament

胸骨柄
Manubrium

胸肋关节
Sternocostal joint

肩锁关节
Acromioclavicular joint

喙肩韧带
Coracoacromial ligament

肩峰
Acromion

冈上肌腱（切断）
Supraspinatus tendon
(cut)

喙肱韧带
Coracohumeral
ligament

大结节
Greater tubercle

肱横韧带
Transverse humeral
ligament

肱二头肌腱鞘
Biceps tendon
sheath

肱二头肌腱长头（切断）
Biceps brachii, tendon
of long head (cut)

喙突
Coracoid process

锁骨下肌
Subclavius muscle

肋锁韧带
Costoclavicular ligament

肩胛下肌腱下囊与肩关节腔的交通
Communication of subtendinous
bursa of subscapularis to glenohumeral joint cavity

盂肱韧带
Glenohumeral ligaments

肩胛下肌腱（切断）
Subscapularis tendon (cut)

小结节
Lesser
tubercle

肱骨
Humerus

B. 肩关节，冠状面 Shoulder joint, coronal section

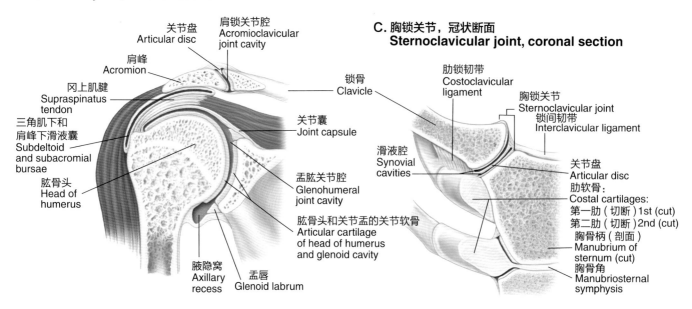

关节盘
Articular disc

肩锁关节腔
Acromioclavicular
joint cavity

肩峰
Acromion

冈上肌腱
Supraspinatus
tendon

三角肌下和
肩峰下滑液囊
Subdeltoid
and subacromial
bursae

肱骨头
Head of
humerus

腋隐窝
Axillary
recess

盂唇
Glenoid labrum

锁骨
Clavicle

关节囊
Joint capsule

盂肱关节腔
Glenohumeral
joint cavity

肱骨头和关节盂的关节软骨
Articular cartilage
of head of humerus
and glenoid cavity

C. 胸锁关节，冠状断面 Sternoclavicular joint, coronal section

肋锁韧带
Costoclavicular
ligament

胸锁关节
Sternoclavicular joint
锁间韧带
Interclavicular ligament

滑液腔
Synovial
cavities

关节盘
Articular disc

肋软骨:
Costal cartilages:
第一肋（切断）1st (cut)
第二肋（切断）2nd (cut)
胸骨柄（剖面）
Manubrium of
sternum (cut)
胸骨角
Manubriosternal
symphysis

A. 前面观
Anterior view

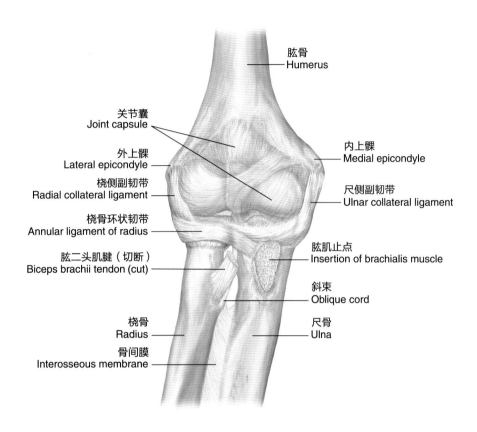

肱骨
Humerus

关节囊
Joint capsule

外上髁
Lateral epicondyle

桡侧副韧带
Radial collateral ligament

桡骨环状韧带
Annular ligament of radius

肱二头肌腱（切断）
Biceps brachii tendon (cut)

桡骨
Radius

骨间膜
Interosseous membrane

内上髁
Medial epicondyle

尺侧副韧带
Ulnar collateral ligament

肱肌止点
Insertion of brachialis muscle

斜束
Oblique cord

尺骨
Ulna

B. 外侧面观
Lateral view

C. 内侧面观
Medial view

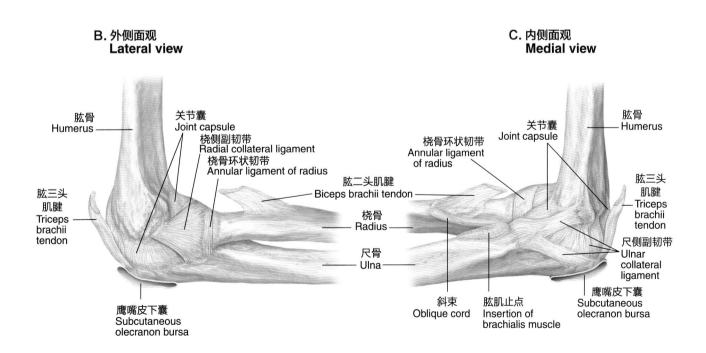

肱骨
Humerus

关节囊
Joint capsule

桡侧副韧带
Radial collateral ligament

桡骨环状韧带
Annular ligament of radius

肱三头肌腱
Triceps brachii tendon

肱二头肌腱
Biceps brachii tendon

桡骨
Radius

尺骨
Ulna

鹰嘴皮下囊
Subcutaneous olecranon bursa

桡骨环状韧带
Annular ligament of radius

关节囊
Joint capsule

肱骨
Humerus

肱三头肌腱
Triceps brachii tendon

尺侧副韧带
Ulnar collateral ligament

鹰嘴皮下囊
Subcutaneous olecranon bursa

斜束
Oblique cord

肱肌止点
Insertion of brachialis muscle

图 2-44   腕关节   **Joints of the Wrist**

A. 前面观
Anterior view

桡骨
Radius

尺骨
Ulna

骨间膜
Interosseous membrane

桡尺掌侧韧带
Palmar radioulnar ligament

月骨
Lunate

桡腕掌侧韧带
Palmar radiocarpal ligament

尺侧副韧带
Ulnar collateral ligament

桡侧副韧带
Radial collateral ligament

尺侧腕屈肌腱（切断）
Flexor carpi ulnaris tendon (cut)

手舟骨结节
Tubercle of scaphoid

豌豆骨
Pisiform

大多角骨结节
Tubercle of trapezium

豆钩韧带
Pisohamate ligament

屈肌支持带附着点（切断）
Attachment of flexor retinaculum (cut)

屈肌支持带附着点（切断）
Attachment of flexor retinaculum (cut)

拇指腕掌关节关节囊
Articular capsule of carpometacarpal joint of thumb

钩骨的钩
Hook of hamate

掌骨掌侧韧带
Palmar metacarpal ligaments

头状骨
Capitate

腕掌掌侧韧带
Palmar carpometacarpal ligaments

1 2 3 4 5

掌骨 Metacarpal bones

B. 后面观
Posterior view

尺骨
Ulna

桡骨
Radius

骨间膜
Interosseous membrane

桡腕背侧韧带
Dorsal radiocarpal ligament

桡尺背侧韧带
Dorsal radioulnar ligament

月骨（被韧带覆盖）
Lunate (covered by ligament)

尺腕背侧韧带
Dorsal ulnocarpal ligament

手舟骨
Scaphoid

尺侧副韧带
Ulnar collateral ligament

桡侧副韧带
Radial collateral ligament

腕骨间背侧韧带
Dorsal intercarpal ligament

三角骨
Triquetrum

大多角骨
Trapezium

钩骨
Hamate

小多角骨
Trapezoid

腕掌背侧韧带
Dorsal carpometacarpal ligaments

头状骨
Capitate

第一掌骨
1st metacarpal

掌骨背侧韧带
Dorsal metacarpal ligaments

C. 冠状断面，后面观
Coronal section, posterior view

桡尺远侧关节
Distal radioulnar joint

桡尺远侧关节关节盘
Articular disc of distal radioulnar joint

尺侧副韧带
Ulnar collateral ligament

掌骨间关节
Interosseous intercarpal ligaments

腕骨间骨间韧带
Intermetacarpal joints

腕（桡腕）关节
Wrist (radiocarpal) joint

桡侧副韧带
Radial collateral ligament

腕中关节
Midcarpal joint

腕掌关节
Carpometacarpal joints

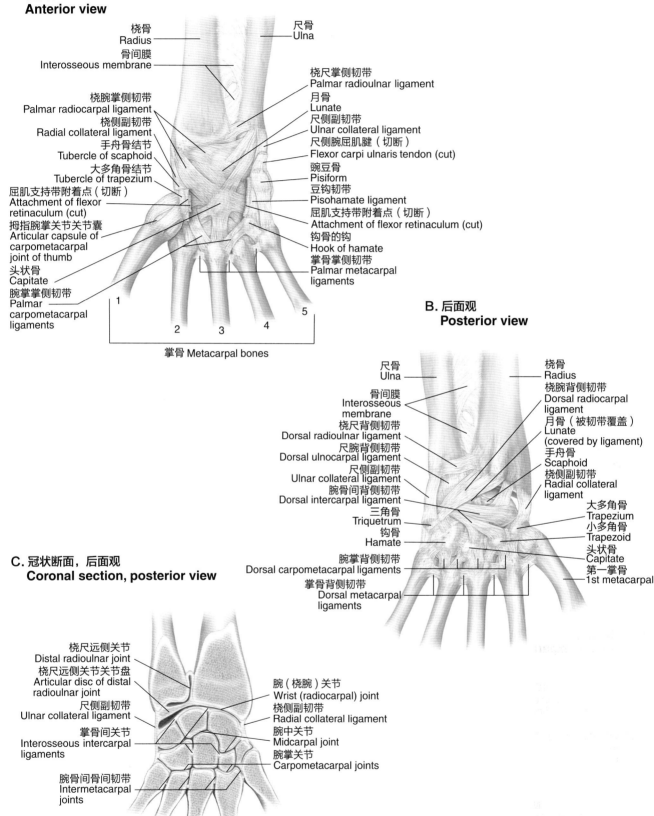

A. 前面观
Anterior view

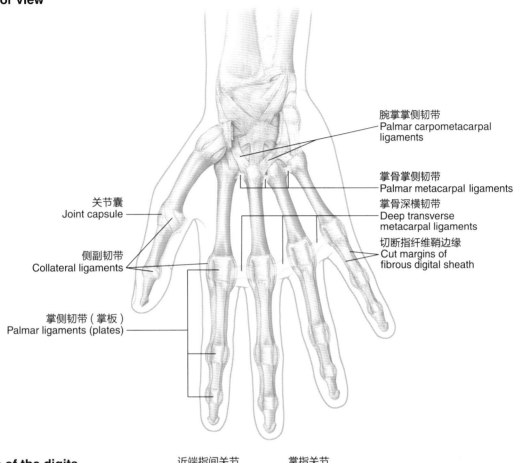

腕掌掌侧韧带
Palmar carpometacarpal
ligaments

掌骨掌侧韧带
Palmar metacarpal ligaments

掌骨深横韧带
Deep transverse
metacarpal ligaments

切断指纤维鞘边缘
Cut margins of
fibrous digital sheath

关节囊
Joint capsule

侧副韧带
Collateral ligaments

掌侧韧带（掌板）
Palmar ligaments (plates)

B. 指关节
Joints of the digits

远端指间关节
Distal
interphalangeal
joint

近端指间关节
Proximal
interphalangeal
joint

掌指关节
Metacarpophalangeal
joint

掌骨
Metacarpal bone

侧副韧带
Collateral ligaments

关节囊
Joint capsule

掌侧韧带（掌板）
Palmar ligament (plate)

C. 伸指肌腱扩张部
Extensor expansion

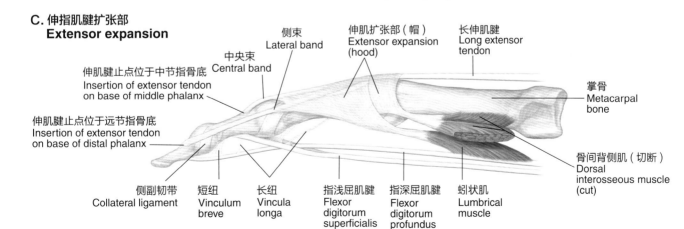

侧束
Lateral band

伸肌扩张部（帽）
Extensor expansion
(hood)

长伸肌腱
Long extensor
tendon

中央束
Central band

伸肌腱止点位于中节指骨底
Insertion of extensor tendon
on base of middle phalanx

掌骨
Metacarpal
bone

伸肌腱止点位于远节指骨底
Insertion of extensor tendon
on base of distal phalanx

骨间背侧肌（切断）
Dorsal
interosseous muscle
(cut)

侧副韧带
Collateral ligament

短纽
Vinculum
breve

长纽
Vincula
longa

指浅屈肌腱
Flexor
digitorum
superficialis
tendon

指深屈肌腱
Flexor
digitorum
profundus
tendon

蚓状肌
Lumbrical
muscle

图 2-46　上肢的动脉　Arteries of the Upper Limb

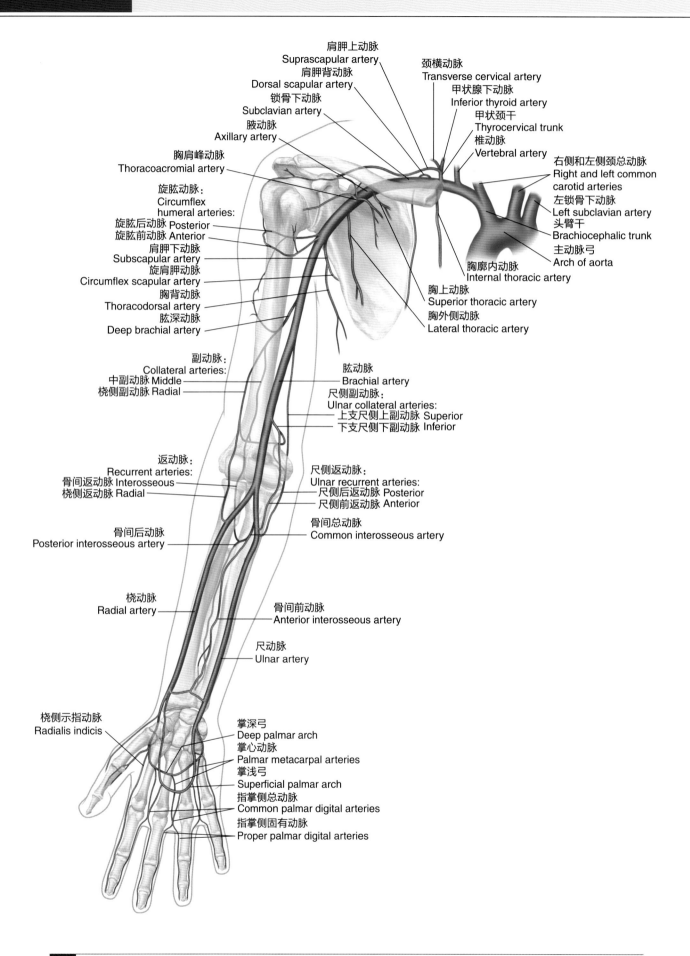

肩胛上动脉
Suprascapular artery
肩胛背动脉
Dorsal scapular artery
锁骨下动脉
Subclavian artery
腋动脉
Axillary artery
胸肩峰动脉
Thoracoacromial artery
旋肱动脉：
Circumflex
humeral arteries:
旋肱后动脉 Posterior
旋肱前动脉 Anterior
肩胛下动脉
Subscapular artery
旋肩胛动脉
Circumflex scapular artery
胸背动脉
Thoracodorsal artery
肱深动脉
Deep brachial artery

颈横动脉
Transverse cervical artery
甲状腺下动脉
Inferior thyroid artery
甲状颈干
Thyrocervical trunk
椎动脉
Vertebral artery

右侧和左侧颈总动脉
Right and left common
carotid arteries
左锁骨下动脉
Left subclavian artery
头臂干
Brachiocephalic trunk
主动脉弓
Arch of aorta

胸廓内动脉
Internal thoracic artery
胸上动脉
Superior thoracic artery
胸外侧动脉
Lateral thoracic artery

副动脉：
Collateral arteries:
中副动脉 Middle
桡侧副动脉 Radial

肱动脉
Brachial artery
尺侧副动脉：
Ulnar collateral arteries:
上支尺侧上副动脉 Superior
下支尺侧下副动脉 Inferior

返动脉：
Recurrent arteries:
骨间返动脉 Interosseous
桡侧返动脉 Radial

尺侧返动脉：
Ulnar recurrent arteries:
尺侧后返动脉 Posterior
尺侧前返动脉 Anterior

骨间后动脉
Posterior interosseous artery

骨间总动脉
Common interosseous artery

桡动脉
Radial artery

骨间前动脉
Anterior interosseous artery

尺动脉
Ulnar artery

桡侧示指动脉
Radialis indicis

掌深弓
Deep palmar arch
掌心动脉
Palmar metacarpal arteries
掌浅弓
Superficial palmar arch
指掌侧总动脉
Common palmar digital arteries
指掌侧固有动脉
Proper palmar digital arteries

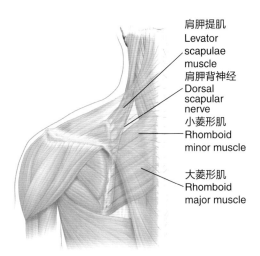

肩胛提肌
Levator
scapulae
muscle

肩胛背神经
Dorsal
scapular
nerve

小菱形肌
Rhomboid
minor muscle

大菱形肌
Rhomboid
major muscle

A. 肩胛背神经
Dorsal scapular nerve

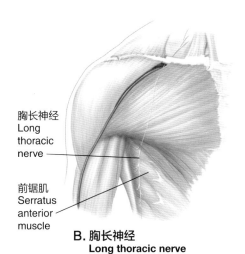

胸长神经
Long
thoracic
nerve

前锯肌
Serratus
anterior
muscle

B. 胸长神经
Long thoracic nerve

肩胛上神经
Suprascapular nerve

肩胛下神经
Supraspinatus muscle

冈下肌
Infraspinatus
muscle

C. 肩胛上神经
Suprascapular nerve

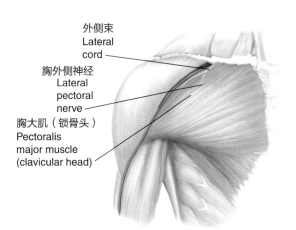

外侧束
Lateral
cord

胸外侧神经
Lateral
pectoral
nerve

胸大肌（锁骨头）
Pectoralis
major muscle
(clavicular head)

D. 胸外侧神经
Lateral pectoral nerve

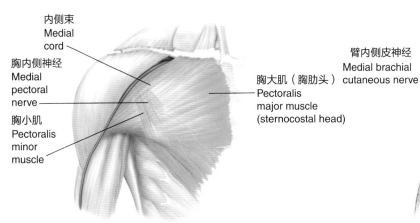

内侧束
Medial
cord

胸内侧神经
Medial
pectoral
nerve

胸小肌
Pectoralis
minor
muscle

胸大肌（胸肋头）
Pectoralis
major muscle
(sternocostal head)

E. 胸内侧神经
Medial pectoral nerve

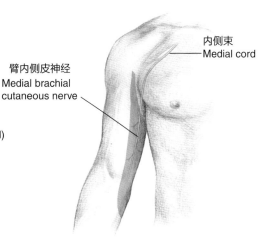

臂内侧皮神经
Medial brachial
cutaneous nerve

内侧束
Medial cord

F. 臂内侧皮神经和肋间臂皮神经
Medial brachial cutaneous and
intercostobrachial cutaneous nerves

图 2-48　臂丛神经的分支，总结Ⅱ　Branches of the Brachial Plexus, Summary Ⅱ

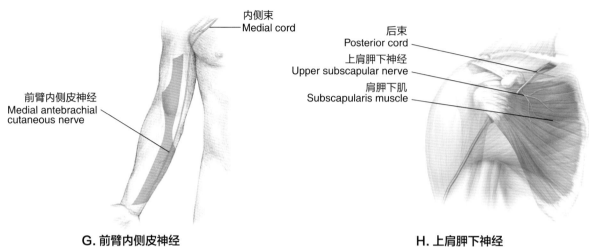

内侧束
Medial cord

前臂内侧皮神经
Medial antebrachial
cutaneous nerve

后束
Posterior cord

上肩胛下神经
Upper subscapular nerve

肩胛下肌
Subscapularis muscle

G. 前臂内侧皮神经
Medial antebrachial cutaneous nerve

H. 上肩胛下神经
Upper subscapular nerve

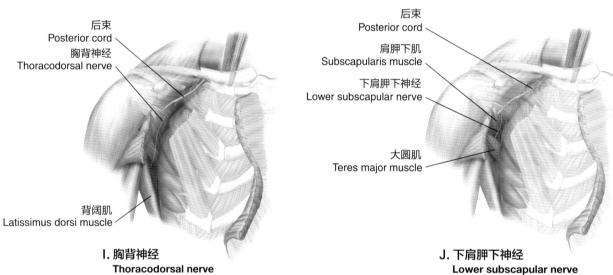

后束
Posterior cord

胸背神经
Thoracodorsal nerve

背阔肌
Latissimus dorsi muscle

后束
Posterior cord

肩胛下肌
Subscapularis muscle

下肩胛下神经
Lower subscapular nerve

大圆肌
Teres major muscle

I. 胸背神经
Thoracodorsal nerve

J. 下肩胛下神经
Lower subscapular nerve

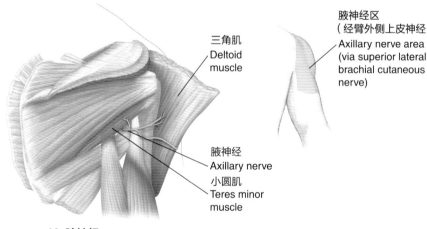
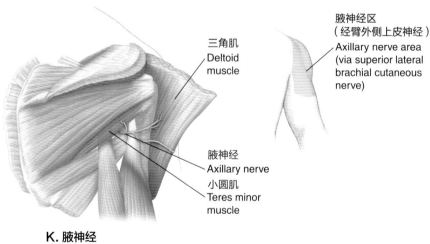

三角肌
Deltoid
muscle

腋神经
Axillary nerve

小圆肌
Teres minor
muscle

腋神经区
（经臂外侧上皮神经）
Axillary nerve area
(via superior lateral
brachial cutaneous
nerve)

K. 腋神经
Axillary nerve

A. 前面观
Anterior view

臂丛：
Brachial plexus:

外侧束 Lateral cord
后束 Posterior cord
内侧束 Medial cord

肌皮神经（C5~C7）
Musculocutaneous nerve
(C5~C7)

喙肱肌
Coracobrachialis muscle

肱二头肌（切断）
Biceps brachii muscle (cut)

前臂外侧皮神经
Lateral antebrachial
cutaneous nerve

肱肌
Brachialis muscle

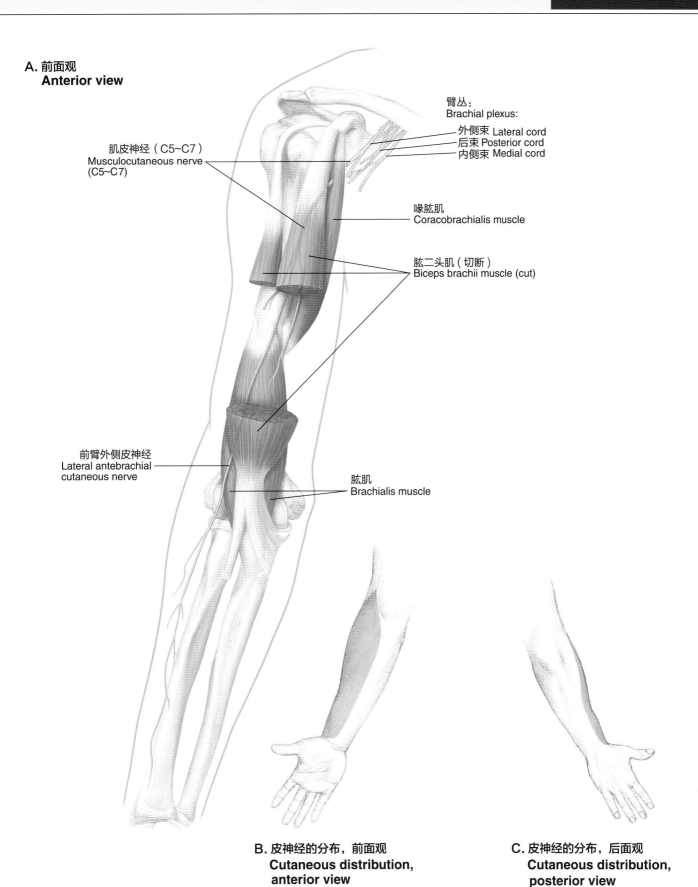

B. 皮神经的分布，前面观
**Cutaneous distribution,
anterior view**

C. 皮神经的分布，后面观
**Cutaneous distribution,
posterior view**

图 2-50　正中神经　Median Nerve

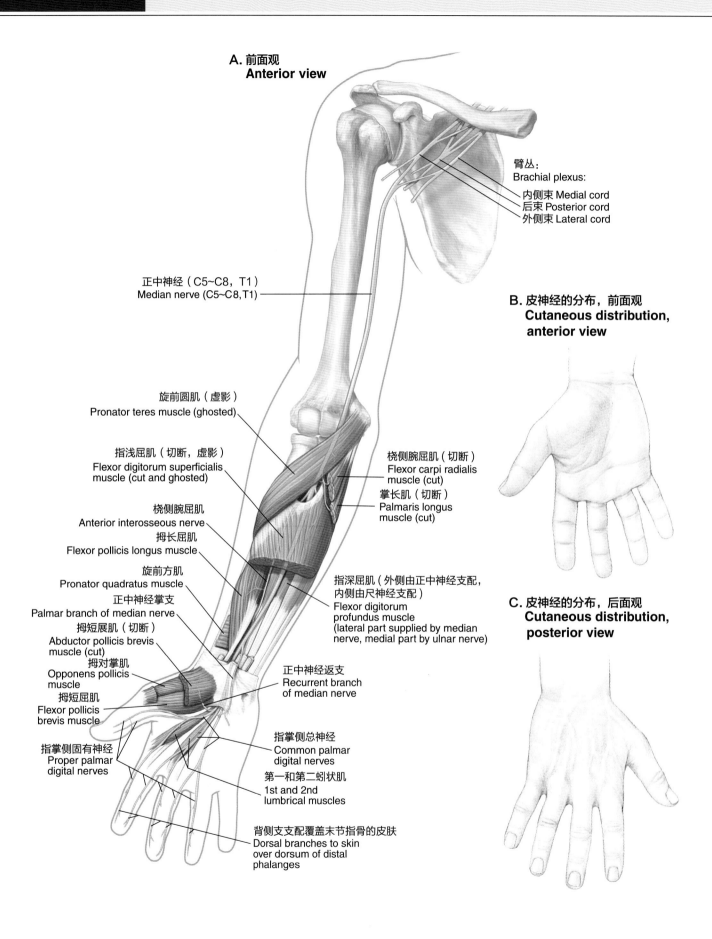

A. 前面观
Anterior view

臂丛：
Brachial plexus:

内侧束 Medial cord
后束 Posterior cord
外侧束 Lateral cord

正中神经（C5~C8，T1）
Median nerve (C5~C8,T1)

B. 皮神经的分布，前面观
Cutaneous distribution, anterior view

旋前圆肌（虚影）
Pronator teres muscle (ghosted)

指浅屈肌（切断，虚影）
Flexor digitorum superficialis muscle (cut and ghosted)

桡侧腕屈肌（切断）
Flexor carpi radialis muscle (cut)

掌长肌（切断）
Palmaris longus muscle (cut)

桡侧腕屈肌
Anterior interosseous nerve

拇长屈肌
Flexor pollicis longus muscle

旋前方肌
Pronator quadratus muscle

正中神经掌支
Palmar branch of median nerve

拇短展肌（切断）
Abductor pollicis brevis muscle (cut)

拇对掌肌
Opponens pollicis muscle

拇短屈肌
Flexor pollicis brevis muscle

指深屈肌（外侧由正中神经支配，内侧由尺神经支配）
Flexor digitorum profundus muscle (lateral part supplied by median nerve, medial part by ulnar nerve)

C. 皮神经的分布，后面观
Cutaneous distribution, posterior view

正中神经返支
Recurrent branch of median nerve

指掌侧总神经
Common palmar digital nerves

第一和第二蚓状肌
1st and 2nd lumbrical muscles

指掌侧固有神经
Proper palmar digital nerves

背侧支支配覆盖末节指骨的皮肤
Dorsal branches to skin over dorsum of distal phalanges

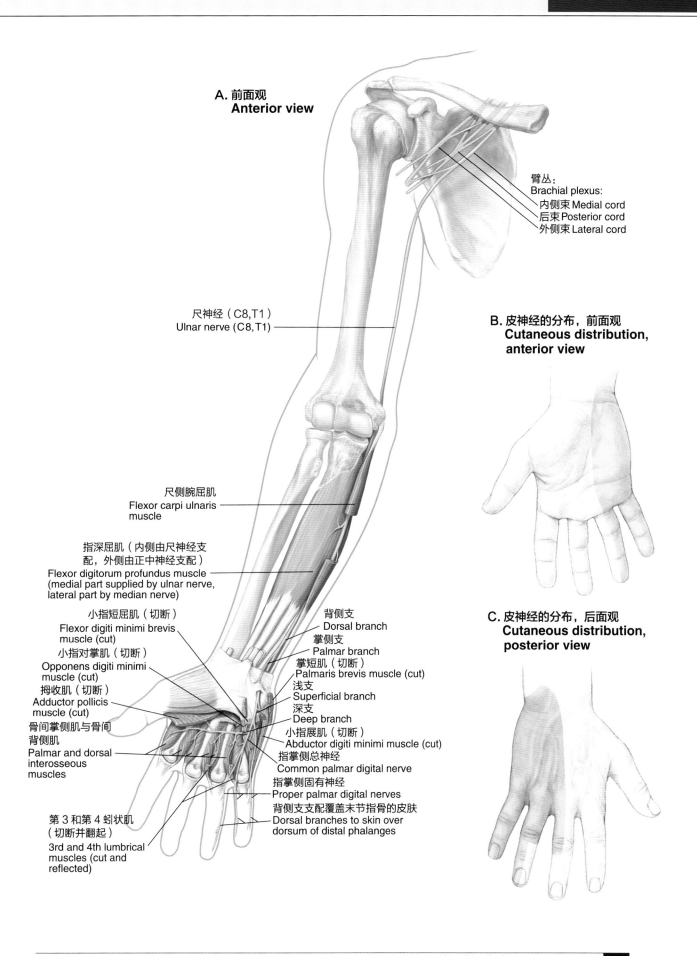

A. 前面观
Anterior view

臂丛：
Brachial plexus:
内侧束 Medial cord
后束 Posterior cord
外侧束 Lateral cord

尺神经（C8,T1）
Ulnar nerve (C8,T1)

B. 皮神经的分布，前面观
Cutaneous distribution, anterior view

尺侧腕屈肌
Flexor carpi ulnaris muscle

指深屈肌（内侧由尺神经支配，外侧由正中神经支配）
Flexor digitorum profundus muscle (medial part supplied by ulnar nerve, lateral part by median nerve)

C. 皮神经的分布，后面观
Cutaneous distribution, posterior view

小指短屈肌（切断）
Flexor digiti minimi brevis muscle (cut)

小指对掌肌（切断）
Opponens digiti minimi muscle (cut)

拇收肌（切断）
Adductor pollicis muscle (cut)

骨间掌侧肌与骨间背侧肌
Palmar and dorsal interosseous muscles

背侧支
Dorsal branch
掌侧支
Palmar branch
掌短肌（切断）
Palmaris brevis muscle (cut)
浅支
Superficial branch
深支
Deep branch
小指展肌（切断）
Abductor digiti minimi muscle (cut)
指掌侧总神经
Common palmar digital nerve
指掌侧固有神经
Proper palmar digital nerves
背侧支支配覆盖末节指骨的皮肤
Dorsal branches to skin over dorsum of distal phalanges

第 3 和第 4 蚓状肌（切断并翻起）
3rd and 4th lumbrical muscles (cut and reflected)

图 2-52　桡神经　Radial Nerve

A. 后面观
Posterior view

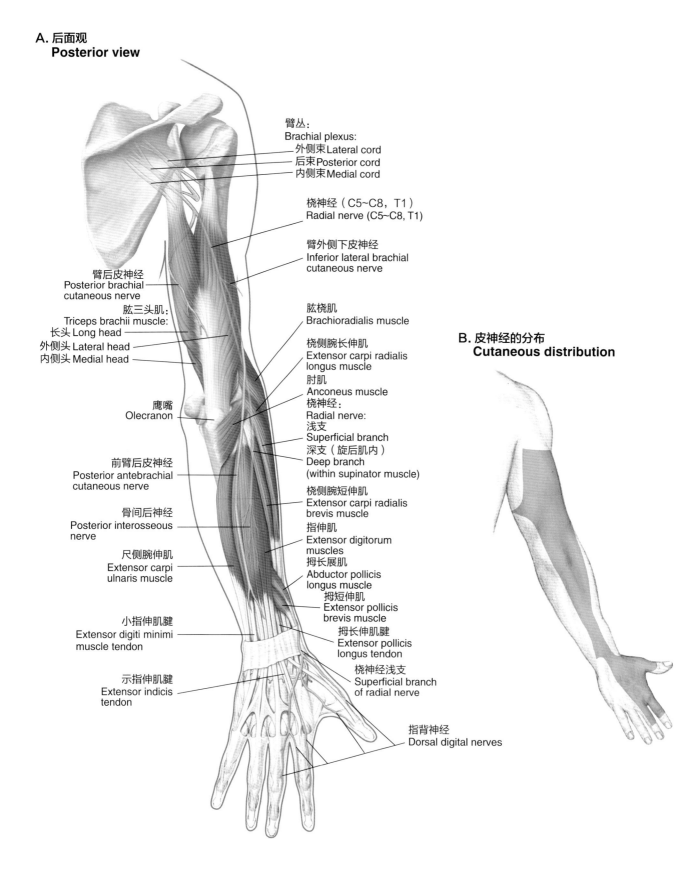

臂丛：
Brachial plexus:
外侧束 Lateral cord
后束 Posterior cord
内侧束 Medial cord

桡神经（C5~C8，T1）
Radial nerve (C5~C8, T1)

臂外侧下皮神经
Inferior lateral brachial
cutaneous nerve

臂后皮神经
Posterior brachial
cutaneous nerve

肱三头肌：
Triceps brachii muscle:
长头 Long head
外侧头 Lateral head
内侧头 Medial head

鹰嘴
Olecranon

前臂后皮神经
Posterior antebrachial
cutaneous nerve

骨间后神经
Posterior interosseous
nerve

尺侧腕伸肌
Extensor carpi
ulnaris muscle

小指伸肌腱
Extensor digiti minimi
muscle tendon

示指伸肌腱
Extensor indicis
tendon

肱桡肌
Brachioradialis muscle

桡侧腕长伸肌
Extensor carpi radialis
longus muscle

肘肌
Anconeus muscle
桡神经：
Radial nerve:
浅支
Superficial branch
深支（旋后肌内）
Deep branch
(within supinator muscle)

桡侧腕短伸肌
Extensor carpi radialis
brevis muscle

指伸肌
Extensor digitorum
muscles
拇长展肌
Abductor pollicis
longus muscle

拇短伸肌
Extensor pollicis
brevis muscle

拇长伸肌腱
Extensor pollicis
longus tendon

桡神经浅支
Superficial branch
of radial nerve

指背神经
Dorsal digital nerves

B. 皮神经的分布
Cutaneous distribution

A. 前面观
Anterior view

锁骨上神经（发自颈丛）
Supraclavicular nerves
(from cervical plexus)

臂外侧上皮神经（发自腋神经）
Superior lateral brachial cutaneous
nerve (from axillary nerve)

臂外侧下皮神经（发自桡神经）
Inferior lateral brachial cutaneous
nerve (from radial nerve)

臂内侧皮神经（发自内侧束）和
肋间臂神经（发自第二肋间神经）
Medial brachial cutaneous
nerve (from medial cord)
and intercostobrachial nerve
(from 2nd intercostal nerve)

前臂内侧皮神经（发自内侧束）
Medial antebrachial
cutaneous nerve
(from medial cord)

前臂外侧皮神经（发自肌皮神经）
Lateral antebrachial cutaneous nerve
(from musculocutaneous nerve)

桡神经浅支
Superficial branch
of radial nerve

正中神经掌支
Palmar branch
of median nerve

尺神经掌支
Palmar branch
of ulnar nerve

正中神经指掌支
Palmar digital branches
of median nerve

尺神经指掌支
Palmar digital branches
of ulnar nerve

B. 后面观
Posterior view

臂内侧皮神经（发自内侧束）和
肋间臂神经（发自第二肋间神经）
Medial brachial cutaneous
nerve (from medial cord)
and intercostobrachial nerve
(from 2nd intercostal nerve)

臂外侧上皮神经（发自腋神经）
Superior lateral brachial
cutaneous nerve
(from axillary nerve)

臂后皮神经（发自桡神经）
Posterior brachial cutaneous
nerve (from radial nerve)

臂外侧下皮神经（发自桡神经）
Inferior lateral brachial
cutaneous nerve
(from radial nerve)

前臂后皮神经（发自桡神经）
Posterior antebrachial cutaneous
nerve (from radial nerve)

前臂外侧皮神经（发自肌皮神经）
Lateral antebrachial cutaneous
nerve (from musculocutaneous nerve)

桡神经浅支
Superficial branch
of radial nerve

前臂内侧皮神经
（发自内侧束）
Medial antebrachial
cutaneous nerve
(from medial cord)

尺神经手背支
Dorsal branch
of ulnar nerve

尺神经指掌支
Palmar digital branches
of ulnar nerve

正中神经指掌支
Palmar digital branches
of median nerve

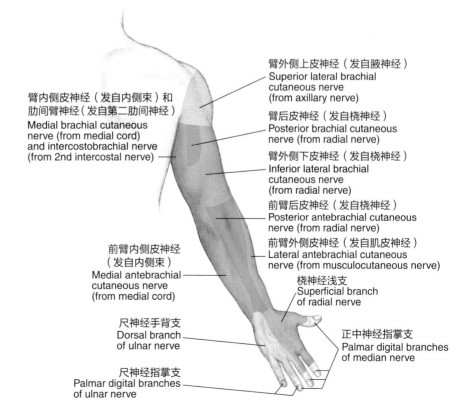

图 2-54　上肢神经支配的皮区　**Dermatomes of the Upper Limb**

A. 后面观
Posterior view

B. 前面观
Anterior view

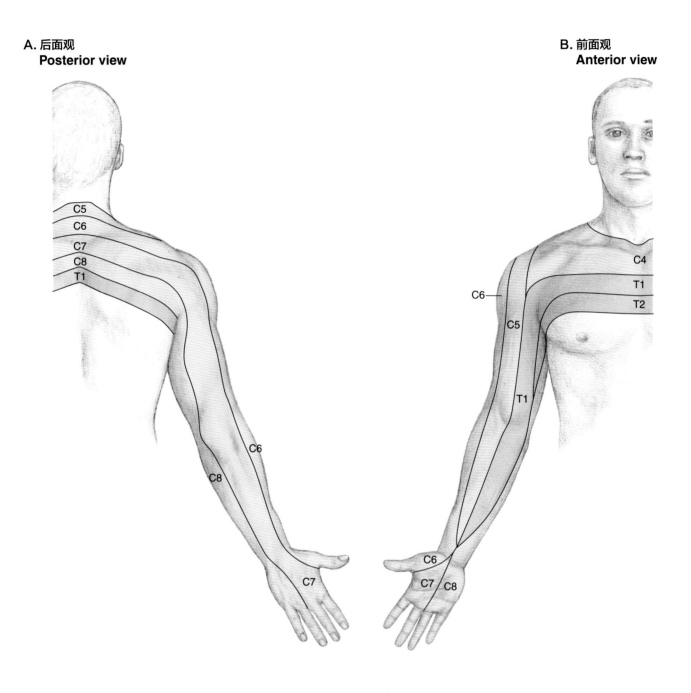

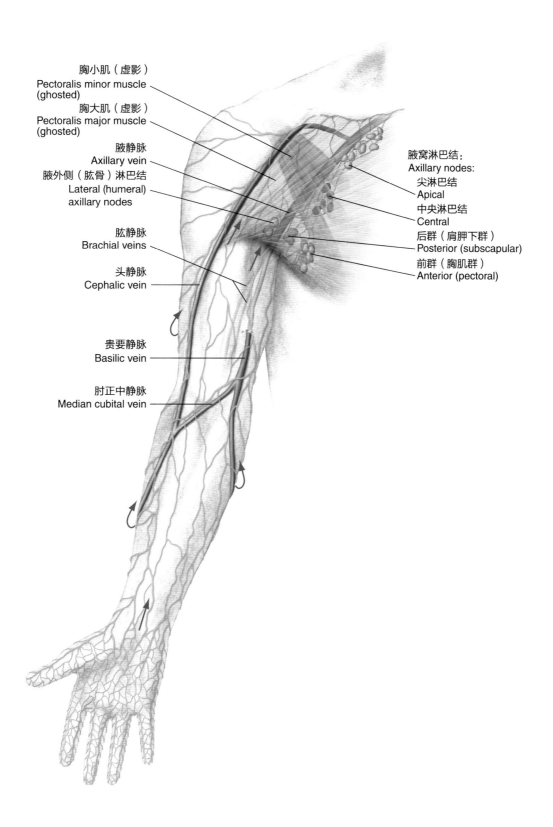

胸小肌（虚影）
Pectoralis minor muscle
(ghosted)

胸大肌（虚影）
Pectoralis major muscle
(ghosted)

腋静脉
Axillary vein

腋外侧（肱骨）淋巴结
Lateral (humeral)
axillary nodes

肱静脉
Brachial veins

头静脉
Cephalic vein

贵要静脉
Basilic vein

肘正中静脉
Median cubital vein

腋窝淋巴结：
Axillary nodes:

尖淋巴结
Apical

中央淋巴结
Central

后群（肩胛下群）
Posterior (subscapular)

前群（胸肌群）
Anterior (pectoral)

上肢肌

名称	起点	止点	主要作用	神经支配	动脉	注释
胸大肌 （图 2-12）	锁骨内侧 1/3、胸骨柄、胸骨体、第 2~6 肋软骨，有时起于上腹壁的腹直肌鞘	肱骨大结节嵴	屈曲、内收和内旋上臂	胸内和胸外侧神经（C5~T1）	胸肩峰动脉的胸肌支	前方的深筋膜不与乳腺筋膜愈合，如果粘连是指示乳腺疾病的重要临床体征
胸小肌 （图 2-12 和图 2-47）	第 3~5 肋	肩胛骨的喙突	拉肩胛骨向前内下方	胸内侧神经（C8、T1）	胸肩峰动脉的胸肌支	胸内侧神经的肌支通常穿过胸小肌进入胸大肌
前锯肌 （图 4-07）	第 1~8 肋或第 9 肋	肩胛骨内侧缘的肋面	拉肩胛骨向前，下方的肌纤维旋肩胛骨向上	胸长神经（来自 C5~C7 腹侧支）	胸外侧动脉	胸长神经损伤会导致翼状肩胛骨（肩胛骨内侧缘离开胸后壁，看起来像天使的翅膀）
三角肌 （图 2-07）	锁骨外侧 1/3、肩胛冈嵴的下唇	肱骨的三角肌粗隆	外展上臂；前部肌纤维屈曲和内旋上臂；后部肌纤维后伸和外旋上臂	腋神经（C5、C6）发自臂丛后束	旋肱后动脉；胸肩峰动脉的三角肌支	三角肌是上臂的主要外展肌，但是由于欠缺机制不能启动这个动作，需要冈上肌的辅助
大圆肌 （图 2-07 和图 2-08）	肩胛骨下角背面	肱骨小结节嵴	内收、内旋上臂，辅助上臂后伸	肩胛下神经（C5、C6）发自臂丛后束	胸背动脉和旋肩胛动脉	大圆肌止于背阔肌腱旁，辅助背阔肌功能
冈上肌 （图 2-08 和图 2-16）	冈上窝	肱骨大结节（最高点）	外展上臂（启动外展）	肩胛上神经（C5、C6）发自臂丛上干	肩胛上动脉	冈上肌启动上臂外展，然后三角肌完成这个动作
冈下肌 （图 2-08 和图 2-16）	冈下窝	肱骨大结节（中份）	外旋上臂	肩胛上神经	肩胛上动脉和旋肩胛动脉	冈下肌、冈上肌、小圆肌和肩胛下肌构成肩袖肌
小圆肌 （图 2-08 和图 2-16）	肩胛骨外侧缘上 2/3	肱骨大结节（最低点）	外旋上臂	腋神经	旋肩胛动脉	在外展和屈曲上臂时将肱骨头固定于关节盂
肩胛下肌 （图 2-08 和图 2-16）	肩胛骨肋面的内侧 2/3（肩胛下窝）	肱骨小结节	内旋上臂；辅助后伸上臂	上、下肩胛下神经（C5、C6）	腋动脉	肩胛下肌、冈上肌、冈下肌和小圆肌构成肩袖肌
肱二头肌 （图 2-17）	短头：喙突尖；长头：肱骨的盂上结节	桡骨粗隆	屈前臂，屈上臂（长头），旋后	肌皮神经（C5、C6）	肱动脉	肘关节屈曲时的强大旋后肌
肱肌 （图 2-17）	肱骨下 1/3 前面和肌间隔	尺骨粗隆	屈前臂	肌皮神经（C5、C6）	肱动脉	强大的屈肌
喙肱肌 （图 2-17）	肩胛骨的喙突	肱骨干中份内侧	屈曲和内收上臂	肌皮神经（C5、C6）	肱动脉	肌皮神经穿过喙肱肌进入其他上臂屈肌
肱三头肌 （图 2-18）	长头：肩胛骨的盂下结节；外侧头：肱骨后外侧外侧肌间隔；内侧头：肱骨下半的后内侧面	尺骨鹰嘴	后伸前臂；长头后伸和外展上臂	桡神经	肱深动脉	肱三头肌长头分隔三边孔和四边孔（大圆肌、小圆肌和肱骨有其他边界）

上肢肌

名称	起点	止点	主要作用	神经支配	动脉	注释
肘肌 （图 2-18）	外上髁	尺骨上 1/4 和鹰嘴外侧	伸前臂	桡神经发出的肘肌神经	中副动脉和骨间返动脉	
肱桡肌 （图 2-29）	肱骨外上髁嵴的上 2/3	桡骨茎突基底外侧	屈曲肘关节并付诸旋前和旋后	桡神经	桡侧返动脉	虽然肱桡肌受支配伸肌的神经（桡神经）支配，但是其主要功能是屈肘；其中立位居于旋前和旋后之间
桡侧腕长伸肌 （图 2-29）	肱骨外上髁嵴的下 1/3	第 2 掌骨（底）背面	伸腕；手外展	桡神经	桡动脉	与桡侧腕短伸肌和桡侧腕屈肌一起外展手
桡侧腕短伸肌 （图 2-29）	伸肌总腱（肱骨外上髁）	第 3 掌骨（底）背面	伸腕；手外展	桡神经深支	桡动脉	与桡侧腕长伸肌和桡侧腕屈肌一起外展手
尺侧腕伸肌 （图 2-29）	伸肌总腱和尺骨后缘的中间一半	第 5 掌骨底内侧	伸腕；手内收	桡神经深支	尺动脉	与尺侧腕屈肌一起内收手
小指伸肌 （图 2-29）	伸肌总腱（肱骨外上髁）	加入指伸肌的第 5 指肌腱止于指背腱膜	伸第 5 指的掌指关节、近侧指间关节和远侧指间关节	桡神经深支	骨间返动脉	小指伸肌出现于指伸肌的最尺侧部
指伸肌 （图 2-29）	伸肌总腱（肱骨外上髁）	第 2~5 指背腱膜	伸第 2~5 指的掌指关节、近侧指间关节和远侧指间关节	桡神经深支	骨间返动脉和骨间后动脉	指背腱膜借中央束止于中节指骨底，外侧束和内侧束止于远节指骨
拇长展肌 （图 2-30）	桡骨后面的中 1/3，骨间膜，尺骨后外侧中部	第 1 指骨底桡侧	在掌指关节外展拇指	桡神经深支	骨间后动脉	拇长展肌和拇短伸肌腱构成解剖鼻烟窝的外侧界
拇短伸肌 （图 2-30）	桡骨远端后面和骨间膜	拇指近节指骨底	在掌指关节伸拇指	桡神经深支	骨间后动脉	拇短伸肌和拇长展肌腱构成解剖鼻烟窝的外侧界，窝内可扪及桡动脉搏动
拇长伸肌 （图 2-30）	尺骨后外侧中部和骨间膜	拇指远节指骨底	在掌指关节伸拇指	桡神经深支	骨间后动脉	拇长伸肌绕过桡骨背结节；形成解剖鼻烟窝的内侧界，窝内可扪及桡动脉搏动
示指伸肌 （图 2-30）	尺骨远端后外侧面和骨间膜	加入指伸肌的第 2 指肌腱止于指背腱膜	在掌指关节、近侧指间关节和远侧指间关节伸示指	桡神经深支	骨间后动脉	示指伸肌位于前臂伸肌深层，小指伸肌位于伸肌浅层
桡侧腕屈肌 （图 2-23）	肱骨内上髁的屈肌总腱	第 2、3 掌骨底	屈腕和手外展	正中神经	尺动脉	与桡侧腕长伸肌和桡侧腕短伸肌一起外展手
尺侧腕屈肌 （图 2-23）	尺骨后缘上 2/3 和鹰嘴内侧缘的屈肌总腱（和尺骨头）	豌豆骨、钩骨钩、第 5 掌骨底	屈腕和手外展	尺神经	尺动脉	尺神经穿过尺侧腕屈肌的两个头之间

续表

上肢肌

名称	起点	止点	主要作用	神经支配	动脉	注释
指浅屈肌（图2-24）	肱尺头：屈肌总腱；桡骨头：桡骨中1/3	第2~5指中节指骨干	屈掌指关节和近侧指间关节	正中神经	尺动脉	正中神经在前臂远端走行于指浅屈肌深面
指深屈肌（图2-25）	尺骨后缘、尺骨近侧2/3内侧缘、骨间膜	第2~5指远节指骨底	屈掌指关节、近侧指间关节和远侧指间关节	正中神经的骨间前支（桡侧半）；尺神经(尺侧半)	尺动脉、骨间前动脉	尺神经支配的指深屈肌部分作用于第4指和第5指
拇长屈肌（图2-25）	桡骨前面和骨间膜	拇指远节指骨底	屈拇指掌指关节和指间关节	正中神经的骨间前支	骨间前动脉	拇长屈肌腱与指长屈肌腱和正中神经一起穿过腕管
旋前方肌（图2-25）	尺骨远端1/4前面内侧	桡骨远端1/4前面	前臂旋前	正中神经的骨间前支	骨间前动脉	旋前方肌是前臂最深层肌，与旋前圆肌功能相同神经支配相同
掌长肌（图2-23）	肱骨内上髁	屈肌支持带远侧半和掌腱膜	屈腕和紧张掌腱膜	正中神经（C7和C8）	尺动脉	掌长肌是腕部寻找正中神经的标志
旋前圆肌（图2-23和图2-24）	屈肌总腱和（尺骨头）尺骨冠突内侧	桡骨干中点外侧面	前臂旋前	正中神经	尺动脉、尺前返动脉	正中神经在旋前圆肌的2个头之间穿过
旋后肌（图2-30）	肱骨外上髁、旋后肌嵴、尺骨窝、桡侧副韧带、环状韧带	桡骨近端1/3外侧	前臂旋后	桡神经深支	骨间返动脉	桡神经深支穿过旋后肌进入前臂后骨筋膜鞘
小指展肌（手）（图2-35）	豌豆骨	第5指的近节指骨底尺侧	外展第5指	尺神经深支	尺动脉	小指展肌、小指短屈肌和小指对掌肌位于手的小鱼际骨筋膜鞘
拇短展肌（图2-34）	屈肌支持带、舟状骨、大多角骨	第1指的近节指骨底	外展拇指	正中神经返支	桡动脉掌浅支	拇短展肌、拇短屈肌和拇对掌肌位于手的大鱼际骨筋膜鞘内
拇收肌（图2-35）	斜头：头状骨和第2、第3掌骨底；横头：第3掌骨体	拇指近节指骨底	内收拇指	尺神经深支	掌深弓动脉	掌深弓和尺神经深支穿过拇收肌的两个头，拇收肌位于收肌－骨间骨筋膜鞘
拇短伸肌	骨间膜和桡骨远端后面	拇指近节指骨底	在掌指关节伸拇指	桡神经深支	骨间后动脉	拇短伸肌腱和拇长伸肌腱构成解剖鼻烟窝的外侧界，窝内可扪及桡动脉搏动
小指短屈肌（手）（图2-34）	钩骨钩和屈肌支持带	第5指近节指骨	屈第5指掌指关节和指间关节	尺神经深支	尺动脉	小指短屈肌、小指对掌肌位于手的小鱼际骨筋膜鞘内
拇短屈肌（图2-34）	屈肌支持带、大多角骨	第1指近节指骨	屈拇指掌指关节和指间关节	正中神经返支	桡动脉掌浅支	拇短屈肌、拇收肌和拇对掌肌位于手的大鱼际骨筋膜内

上肢肌						
名称	起点	止点	主要作用	神经支配	动脉	注释
骨间背侧肌（手）（图2-35）	4块肌，每块起于相邻两块掌骨体	第2~4指骨近节指骨底，第2指骨指背腱膜外侧，第3指骨指背腱膜内外两侧和第4指骨指背腱膜内侧	屈第2~4指掌指关节，伸近侧和远侧指间关节，外展第2~4指（手指的外展定义为远离第3指中线的运动）	尺神经深支	掌背动脉和浅掌动脉	双羽肌；记住骨间背侧肌外展，骨间掌侧肌内收，你就可以分辨它们必须止于何处才能完成这个功能
骨间掌侧肌（图2-35）	3（或4）块肌，起于第1、2、4和5掌骨（第1骨间掌侧肌通常与拇收肌融合）	近节指骨底，第1、2指骨指背腱膜内侧，第4、5指骨指背腱膜外侧	屈第1、2、4和5指掌指关节，伸近侧和远侧指间关节，内收第1、2、4和5指（手指内收运动的定义以第3指中线为参照）	尺神经深支	浅掌动脉	半羽肌；记住骨间掌侧肌内收，骨间背侧肌外展，你就可以分辨出它们必须止于何处才能完成这个功能
蚓状肌（手）（图2-34）	第2~5指指深屈肌腱	第2~5指近节指骨桡侧的指背腱膜	第2~5指屈掌指关节，伸近侧和远侧指间关节	正中神经的指掌侧总神经（桡侧2块）和尺神经深支（尺侧2块）	掌浅弓动脉	蚓状肌起自指深屈肌腱且与深肌腱的神经支配模式一致（尺神经和正中神经各支配一半）
小指对掌肌（图2-35）	钩骨钩和屈肌支持带	第5掌骨干	第5指对掌	尺神经深支	尺动脉	对掌是指第15掌骨绕其骨干长轴的旋转运动；小指对掌肌、小指收肌和小指短屈肌位于手的小鱼际骨筋膜鞘内
拇对掌肌（图2-35）	屈肌支持带、大多角骨	第1掌骨体	拇指对掌	正中神经返支	桡动脉的掌浅支	对掌是指第1掌骨绕其骨干长轴的旋转运动；拇对掌肌、拇收肌和拇短屈肌位于手的大鱼际骨筋膜鞘
掌短肌（图2-33）	覆盖小鱼际隆起的筋膜	靠近手尺侧缘的掌部皮肤	将手尺侧缘的皮肤拉向掌中央	尺神经浅支	尺动脉	掌短肌可改善抓握能力

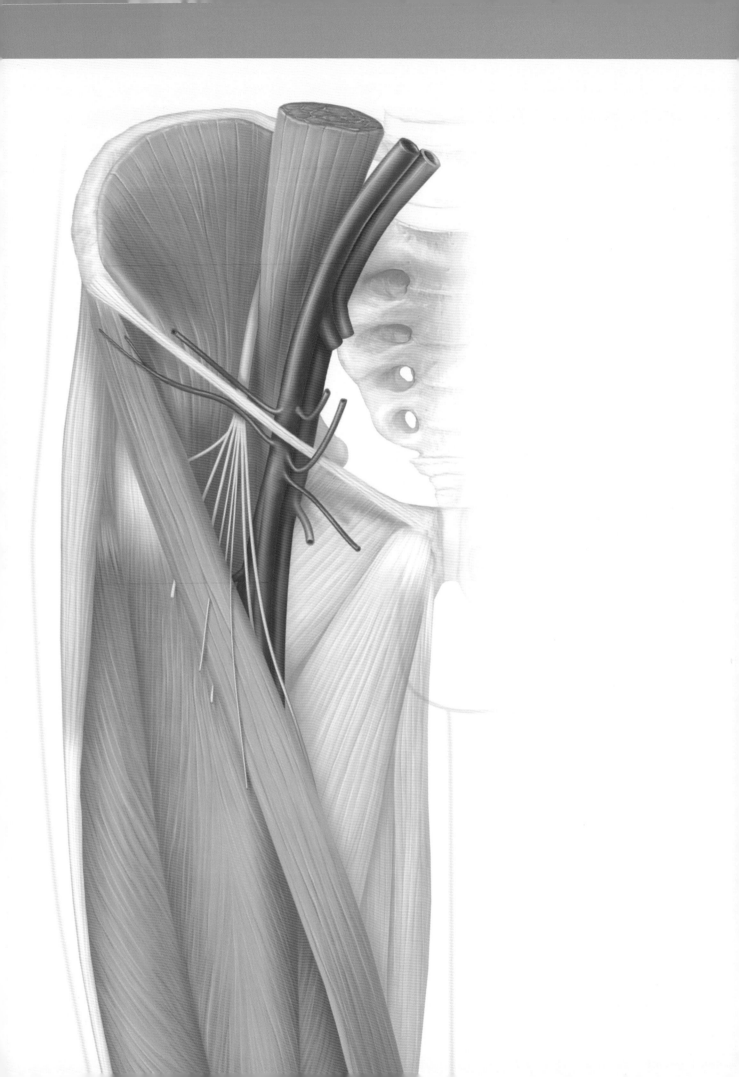

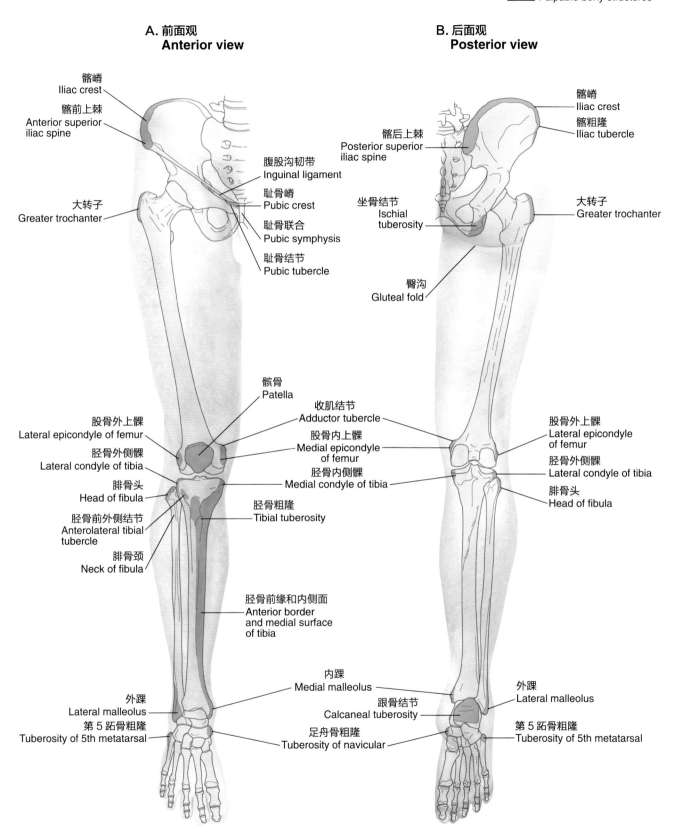

可触及的骨性结构
Palpable bony structures

A. 前面观
Anterior view

B. 后面观
Posterior view

髂嵴
Iliac crest

髂前上棘
Anterior superior iliac spine

腹股沟韧带
Inguinal ligament

耻骨嵴
Pubic crest

大转子
Greater trochanter

耻骨联合
Pubic symphysis

耻骨结节
Pubic tubercle

髂嵴
Iliac crest

髂粗隆
Iliac tubercle

髂后上棘
Posterior superior iliac spine

坐骨结节
Ischial tuberosity

大转子
Greater trochanter

臀沟
Gluteal fold

髌骨
Patella

收肌结节
Adductor tubercle

股骨外上髁
Lateral epicondyle of femur

股骨内上髁
Medial epicondyle of femur

胫骨外侧髁
Lateral condyle of tibia

胫骨内侧髁
Medial condyle of tibia

腓骨头
Head of fibula

胫骨粗隆
Tibial tuberosity

胫骨前外侧结节
Anterolateral tibial tubercle

腓骨颈
Neck of fibula

股骨外上髁
Lateral epicondyle of femur

胫骨外侧髁
Lateral condyle of tibia

腓骨头
Head of fibula

胫骨前缘和内侧面
Anterior border and medial surface of tibia

内踝
Medial malleolus

外踝
Lateral malleolus

第 5 跖骨粗隆
Tuberosity of 5th metatarsal

跟骨结节
Calcaneal tuberosity

足舟骨粗隆
Tuberosity of navicular

外踝
Lateral malleolus

第 5 跖骨粗隆
Tuberosity of 5th metatarsal

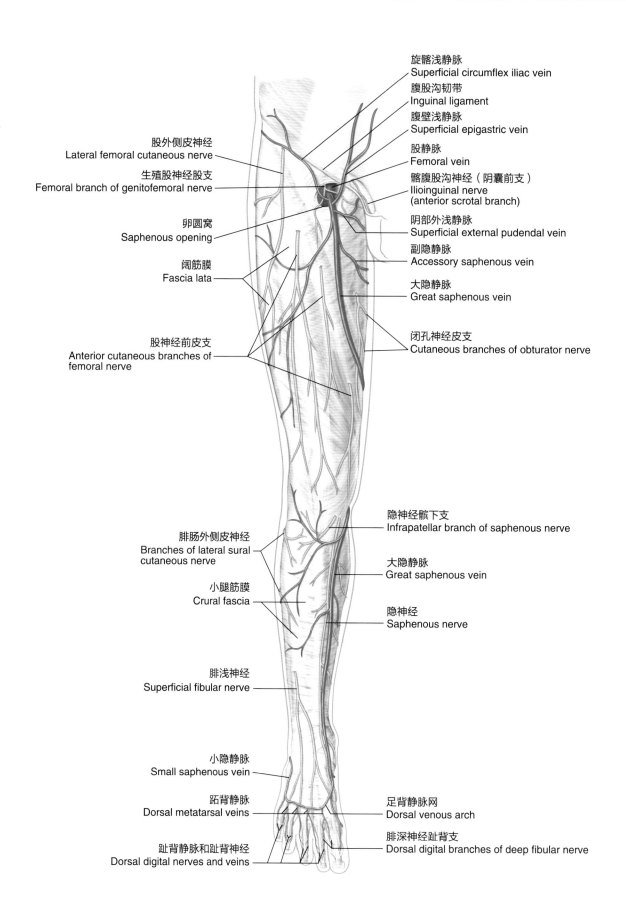

旋髂浅静脉
Superficial circumflex iliac vein

腹股沟韧带
Inguinal ligament

腹壁浅静脉
Superficial epigastric vein

股静脉
Femoral vein

髂腹股沟神经（阴囊前支）
Ilioinguinal nerve
(anterior scrotal branch)

阴部外浅静脉
Superficial external pudendal vein

副隐静脉
Accessory saphenous vein

大隐静脉
Great saphenous vein

闭孔神经皮支
Cutaneous branches of obturator nerve

隐神经髌下支
Infrapatellar branch of saphenous nerve

大隐静脉
Great saphenous vein

隐神经
Saphenous nerve

足背静脉网
Dorsal venous arch

腓深神经趾背支
Dorsal digital branches of deep fibular nerve

股外侧皮神经
Lateral femoral cutaneous nerve

生殖股神经股支
Femoral branch of genitofemoral nerve

卵圆窝
Saphenous opening

阔筋膜
Fascia lata

股神经前皮支
Anterior cutaneous branches of
femoral nerve

腓肠外侧皮神经
Branches of lateral sural
cutaneous nerve

小腿筋膜
Crural fascia

腓浅神经
Superficial fibular nerve

小隐静脉
Small saphenous vein

跖背静脉
Dorsal metatarsal veins

趾背静脉和趾背神经
Dorsal digital nerves and veins

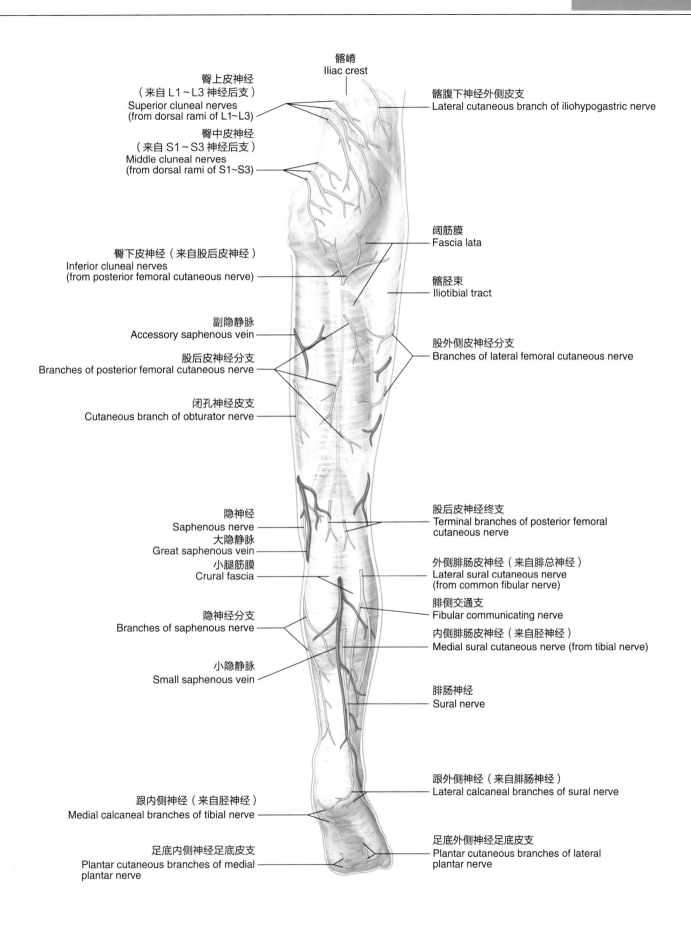

髂嵴
Iliac crest

臀上皮神经
（来自 L1~L3 神经后支）
Superior cluneal nerves
(from dorsal rami of L1~L3)

臀中皮神经
（来自 S1~S3 神经后支）
Middle cluneal nerves
(from dorsal rami of S1~S3)

臀下皮神经（来自股后皮神经）
Inferior cluneal nerves
(from posterior femoral cutaneous nerve)

副隐静脉
Accessory saphenous vein

股后皮神经分支
Branches of posterior femoral cutaneous nerve

闭孔神经皮支
Cutaneous branch of obturator nerve

隐神经
Saphenous nerve

大隐静脉
Great saphenous vein

小腿筋膜
Crural fascia

隐神经分支
Branches of saphenous nerve

小隐静脉
Small saphenous vein

跟内侧神经（来自胫神经）
Medial calcaneal branches of tibial nerve

足底内侧神经足底皮支
Plantar cutaneous branches of medial
plantar nerve

髂腹下神经外侧皮支
Lateral cutaneous branch of iliohypogastric nerve

阔筋膜
Fascia lata

髂胫束
Iliotibial tract

股外侧皮神经分支
Branches of lateral femoral cutaneous nerve

股后皮神经终支
Terminal branches of posterior femoral
cutaneous nerve

外侧腓肠皮神经（来自腓总神经）
Lateral sural cutaneous nerve
(from common fibular nerve)

腓侧交通支
Fibular communicating nerve

内侧腓肠皮神经（来自胫神经）
Medial sural cutaneous nerve (from tibial nerve)

腓肠神经
Sural nerve

跟外侧神经（来自腓肠神经）
Lateral calcaneal branches of sural nerve

足底外侧神经足底皮支
Plantar cutaneous branches of lateral
plantar nerve

图 3-04　　髋骨，外侧面观　Skeleton of the Hip (Os Coxae Bone), Lateral View

A. 骨性标志
Bony features

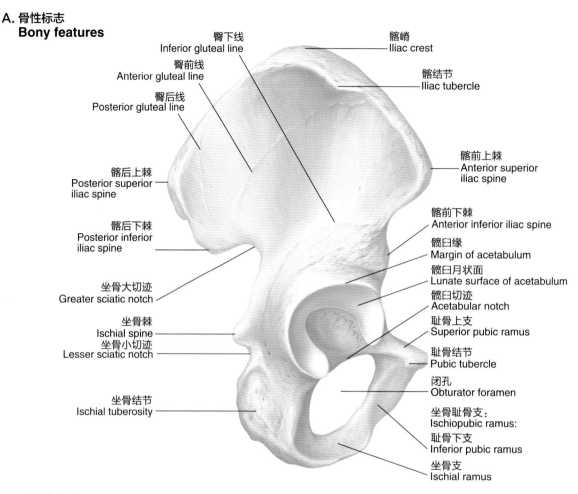

臀下线
Inferior gluteal line

臀前线
Anterior gluteal line

臀后线
Posterior gluteal line

髂嵴
Iliac crest

髂结节
Iliac tubercle

髂前上棘
Anterior superior iliac spine

髂后上棘
Posterior superior iliac spine

髂前下棘
Anterior inferior iliac spine

髂后下棘
Posterior inferior iliac spine

髋臼缘
Margin of acetabulum

坐骨大切迹
Greater sciatic notch

髋臼月状面
Lunate surface of acetabulum

髋臼切迹
Acetabular notch

坐骨棘
Ischial spine

坐骨小切迹
Lesser sciatic notch

耻骨上支
Superior pubic ramus

耻骨结节
Pubic tubercle

闭孔
Obturator foramen

坐骨结节
Ischial tuberosity

坐骨耻骨支：
Ischiopubic ramus:

耻骨下支
Inferior pubic ramus

坐骨支
Ischial ramus

B. 髋骨的组成
Parts of os coxae

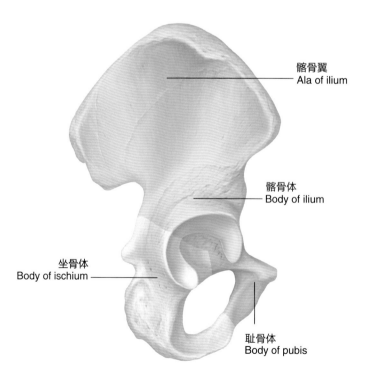

髂骨翼
Ala of ilium

髂骨体
Body of ilium

坐骨体
Body of ischium

耻骨体
Body of pubis

A. 骨性标志
Bony features

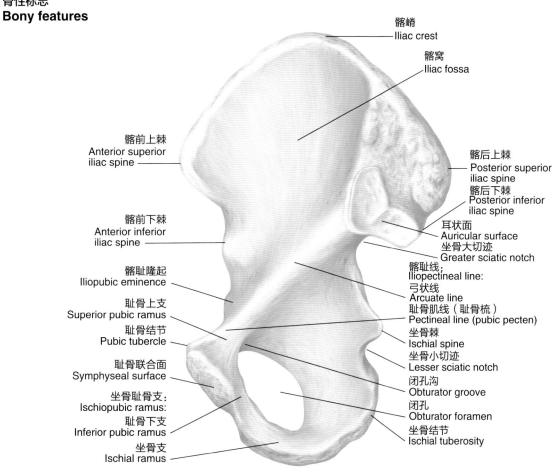

髂嵴
Iliac crest

髂窝
Iliac fossa

髂前上棘
Anterior superior
iliac spine

髂后上棘
Posterior superior
iliac spine

髂后下棘
Posterior inferior
iliac spine

耳状面
Auricular surface

髂前下棘
Anterior inferior
iliac spine

坐骨大切迹
Greater sciatic notch

髂耻隆起
Iliopubic eminence

髂耻线：
Iliopectineal line:

弓状线
Arcuate line

耻骨上支
Superior pubic ramus

耻骨肌线（耻骨梳）
Pectineal line (pubic pecten)

耻骨结节
Pubic tubercle

坐骨棘
Ischial spine

坐骨小切迹
Lesser sciatic notch

耻骨联合面
Symphyseal surface

闭孔沟
Obturator groove

坐骨耻骨支：
Ischiopubic ramus:

闭孔
Obturator foramen

耻骨下支
Inferior pubic ramus

坐骨结节
Ischial tuberosity

坐骨支
Ischial ramus

B. 髋骨部分
Parts of os coxae

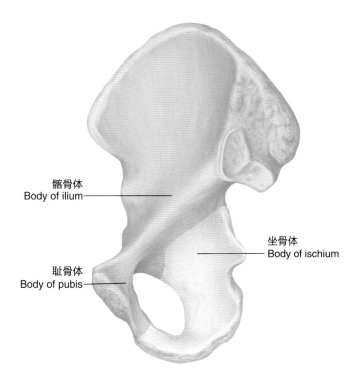

髂骨体
Body of ilium

坐骨体
Body of ischium

耻骨体
Body of pubis

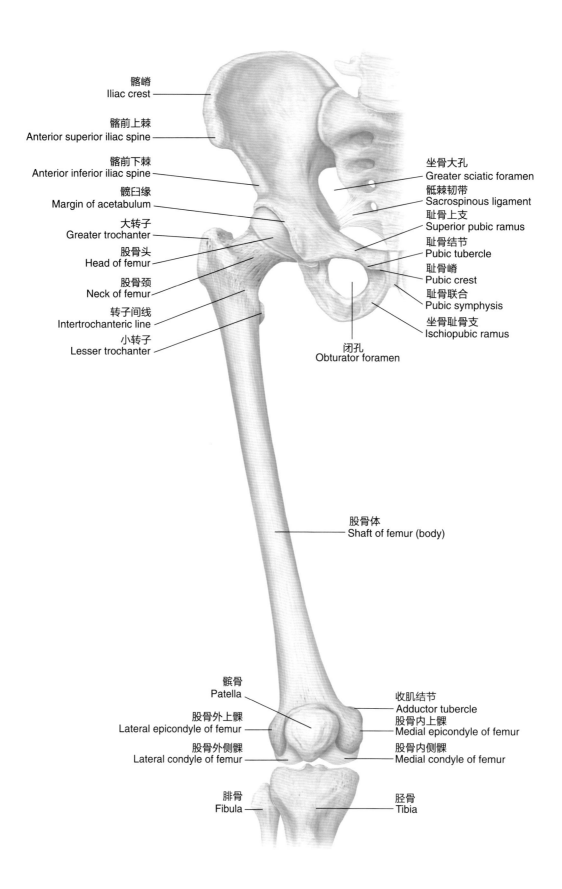

髂嵴
Iliac crest

髂前上棘
Anterior superior iliac spine

髂前下棘
Anterior inferior iliac spine

髋臼缘
Margin of acetabulum

大转子
Greater trochanter

股骨头
Head of femur

股骨颈
Neck of femur

转子间线
Intertrochanteric line

小转子
Lesser trochanter

坐骨大孔
Greater sciatic foramen

骶棘韧带
Sacrospinous ligament

耻骨上支
Superior pubic ramus

耻骨结节
Pubic tubercle

耻骨嵴
Pubic crest

耻骨联合
Pubic symphysis

坐骨耻骨支
Ischiopubic ramus

闭孔
Obturator foramen

股骨体
Shaft of femur (body)

髌骨
Patella

股骨外上髁
Lateral epicondyle of femur

股骨外侧髁
Lateral condyle of femur

腓骨
Fibula

收肌结节
Adductor tubercle

股骨内上髁
Medial epicondyle of femur

股骨内侧髁
Medial condyle of femur

胫骨
Tibia

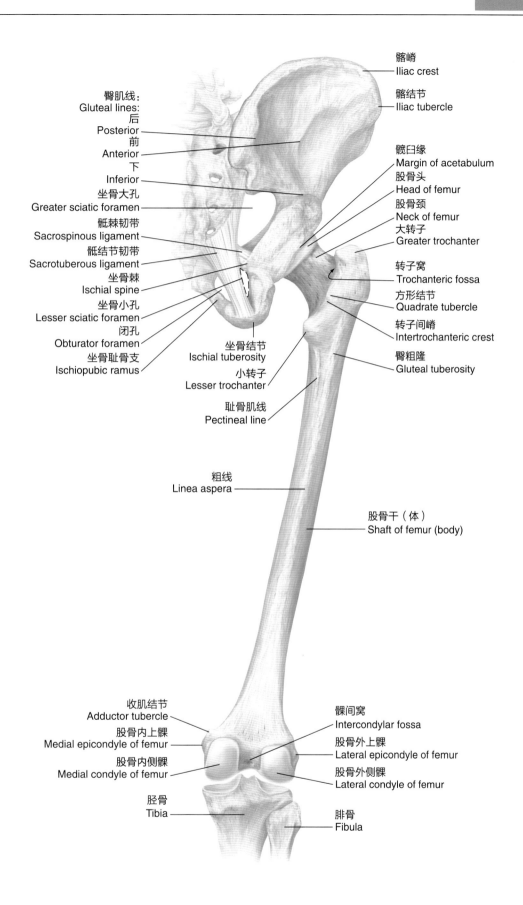

臀肌线：
Gluteal lines:
后
Posterior
前
Anterior
下
Inferior

坐骨大孔
Greater sciatic foramen

骶棘韧带
Sacrospinous ligament

骶结节韧带
Sacrotuberous ligament

坐骨棘
Ischial spine

坐骨小孔
Lesser sciatic foramen

闭孔
Obturator foramen

坐骨耻骨支
Ischiopubic ramus

坐骨结节
Ischial tuberosity

小转子
Lesser trochanter

耻骨肌线
Pectineal line

粗线
Linea aspera

收肌结节
Adductor tubercle

股骨内上髁
Medial epicondyle of femur

股骨内侧髁
Medial condyle of femur

胫骨
Tibia

髂嵴
Iliac crest

髂结节
Iliac tubercle

髋臼缘
Margin of acetabulum

股骨头
Head of femur

股骨颈
Neck of femur

大转子
Greater trochanter

转子窝
Trochanteric fossa

方形结节
Quadrate tubercle

转子间嵴
Intertrochanteric crest

臀粗隆
Gluteal tuberosity

股骨干（体）
Shaft of femur (body)

髁间窝
Intercondylar fossa

股骨外上髁
Lateral epicondyle of femur

股骨外侧髁
Lateral condyle of femur

腓骨
Fibula

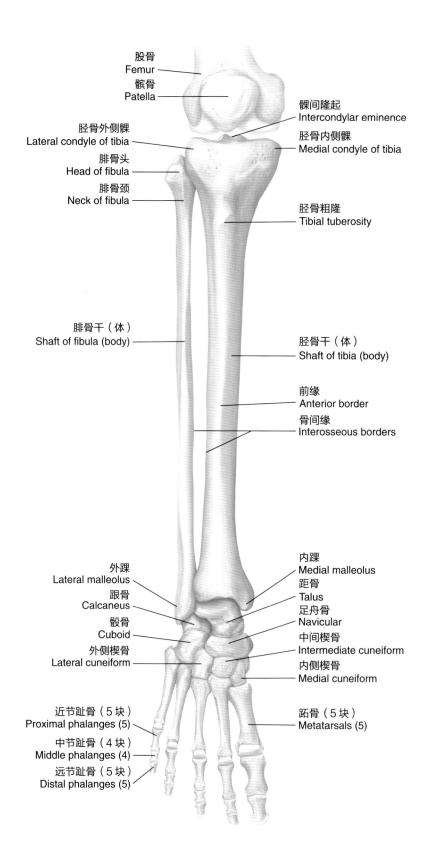

股骨
Femur

髌骨
Patella

髁间隆起
Intercondylar eminence

胫骨外侧髁
Lateral condyle of tibia

胫骨内侧髁
Medial condyle of tibia

腓骨头
Head of fibula

腓骨颈
Neck of fibula

胫骨粗隆
Tibial tuberosity

腓骨干（体）
Shaft of fibula (body)

胫骨干（体）
Shaft of tibia (body)

前缘
Anterior border

骨间缘
Interosseous borders

外踝
Lateral malleolus

内踝
Medial malleolus

距骨
Talus

跟骨
Calcaneus

足舟骨
Navicular

骰骨
Cuboid

中间楔骨
Intermediate cuneiform

外侧楔骨
Lateral cuneiform

内侧楔骨
Medial cuneiform

近节趾骨（5 块）
Proximal phalanges (5)

跖骨（5 块）
Metatarsals (5)

中节趾骨（4 块）
Middle phalanges (4)

远节趾骨（5 块）
Distal phalanges (5)

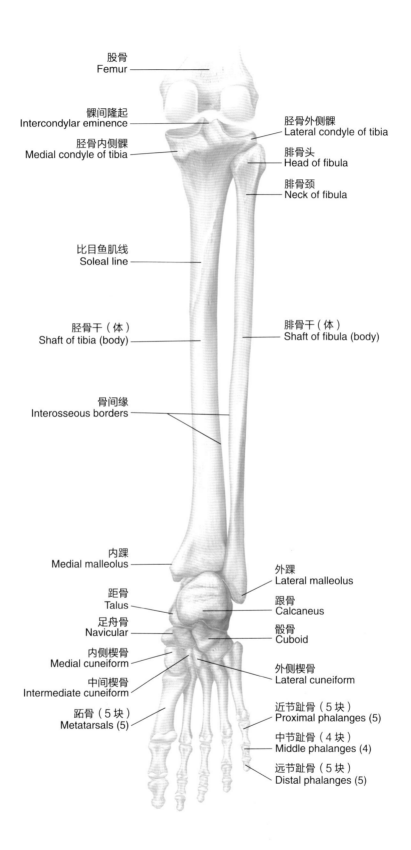

股骨
Femur

髁间隆起
Intercondylar eminence

胫骨外侧髁
Lateral condyle of tibia

胫骨内侧髁
Medial condyle of tibia

腓骨头
Head of fibula

腓骨颈
Neck of fibula

比目鱼肌线
Soleal line

胫骨干（体）
Shaft of tibia (body)

腓骨干（体）
Shaft of fibula (body)

骨间缘
Interosseous borders

内踝
Medial malleolus

外踝
Lateral malleolus

距骨
Talus

跟骨
Calcaneus

足舟骨
Navicular

骰骨
Cuboid

内侧楔骨
Medial cuneiform

外侧楔骨
Lateral cuneiform

中间楔骨
Intermediate cuneiform

跖骨（5 块）
Metatarsals (5)

近节趾骨（5 块）
Proximal phalanges (5)

中节趾骨（4 块）
Middle phalanges (4)

远节趾骨（5 块）
Distal phalanges (5)

图 3-10　下肢的 X 线片　Radiographs of the Lower Limb

A. 髋关节，前面观
Hip joint, anterior view

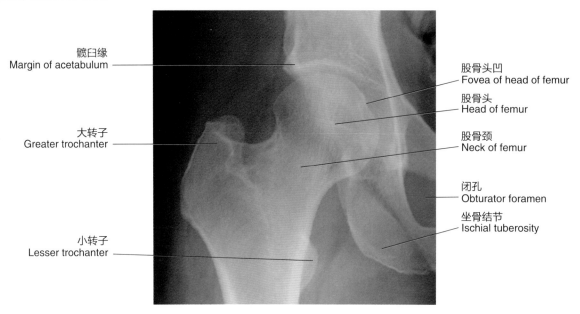

髋臼缘
Margin of acetabulum

大转子
Greater trochanter

小转子
Lesser trochanter

股骨头凹
Fovea of head of femur

股骨头
Head of femur

股骨颈
Neck of femur

闭孔
Obturator foramen

坐骨结节
Ischial tuberosity

B. 膝关节，前面观
Knee joint, anterior view

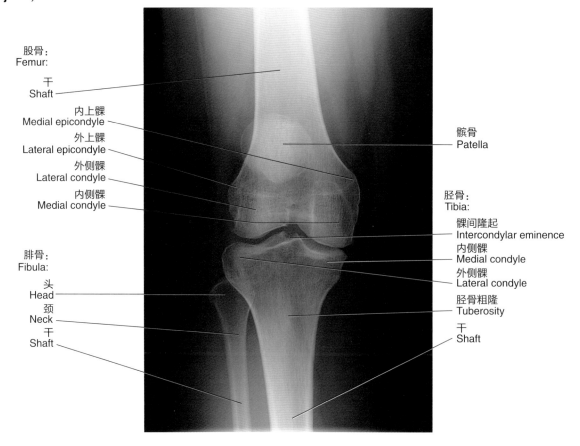

股骨：
Femur:

干
Shaft

内上髁
Medial epicondyle

外上髁
Lateral epicondyle

外侧髁
Lateral condyle

内侧髁
Medial condyle

腓骨：
Fibula:

头
Head

颈
Neck

干
Shaft

髌骨
Patella

胫骨：
Tibia:

髁间隆起
Intercondylar eminence

内侧髁
Medial condyle

外侧髁
Lateral condyle

胫骨粗隆
Tuberosity

干
Shaft

A. 足背面观
Dorsal view

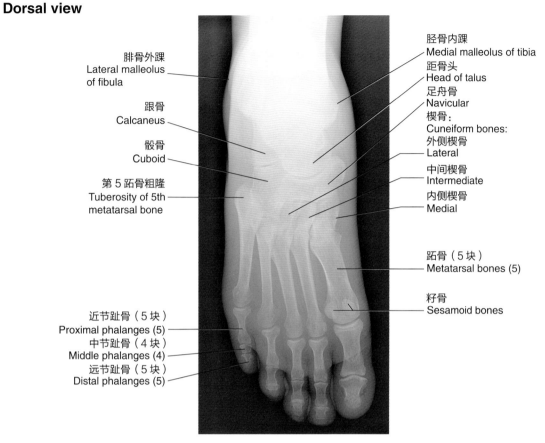

腓骨外踝
Lateral malleolus
of fibula

跟骨
Calcaneus

骰骨
Cuboid

第 5 跖骨粗隆
Tuberosity of 5th
metatarsal bone

近节趾骨（5 块）
Proximal phalanges (5)
中节趾骨（4 块）
Middle phalanges (4)
远节趾骨（5 块）
Distal phalanges (5)

胫骨内踝
Medial malleolus of tibia
距骨头
Head of talus
足舟骨
Navicular
楔骨：
Cuneiform bones:
外侧楔骨
Lateral
中间楔骨
Intermediate
内侧楔骨
Medial

跖骨（5 块）
Metatarsal bones (5)

籽骨
Sesamoid bones

B. 侧面观
Medial view

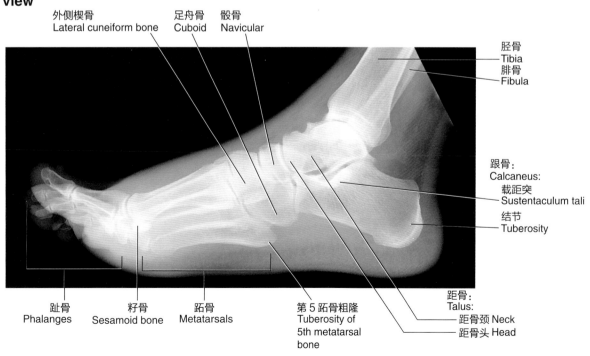

外侧楔骨
Lateral cuneiform bone

足舟骨
Cuboid

骰骨
Navicular

胫骨
Tibia
腓骨
Fibula

跟骨：
Calcaneus:
载距突
Sustentaculum tali
结节
Tuberosity

趾骨
Phalanges

籽骨
Sesamoid bone

跖骨
Metatarsals

第 5 跖骨粗隆
Tuberosity of
5th metatarsal
bone

距骨：
Talus:
距骨颈 Neck
距骨头 Head

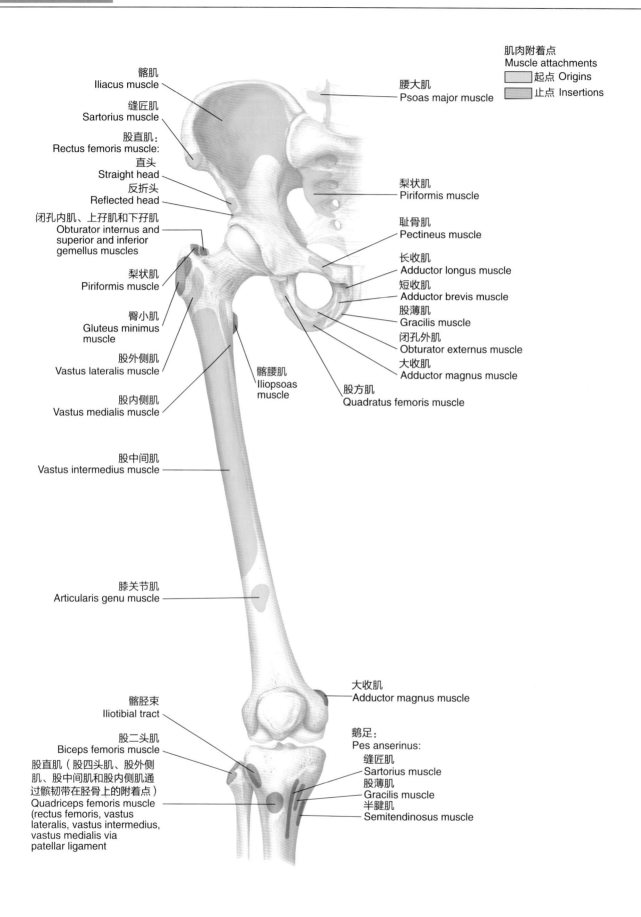

髂肌
Iliacus muscle

缝匠肌
Sartorius muscle

股直肌：
Rectus femoris muscle:

直头
Straight head

反折头
Reflected head

闭孔内肌、上孖肌和下孖肌
Obturator internus and
superior and inferior
gemellus muscles

梨状肌
Piriformis muscle

臀小肌
Gluteus minimus
muscle

股外侧肌
Vastus lateralis muscle

股内侧肌
Vastus medialis muscle

股中间肌
Vastus intermedius muscle

膝关节肌
Articularis genu muscle

髂胫束
Iliotibial tract

股二头肌
Biceps femoris muscle

股直肌（股四头肌、股外侧
肌、股中间肌和股内侧肌通
过髌韧带在胫骨上的附着点）
Quadriceps femoris muscle
(rectus femoris, vastus
lateralis, vastus intermedius,
vastus medialis via
patellar ligament

腰大肌
Psoas major muscle

肌肉附着点
Muscle attachments
起点 Origins
止点 Insertions

梨状肌
Piriformis muscle

耻骨肌
Pectineus muscle

长收肌
Adductor longus muscle

短收肌
Adductor brevis muscle

股薄肌
Gracilis muscle

闭孔外肌
Obturator externus muscle

大收肌
Adductor magnus muscle

股方肌
Quadratus femoris muscle

髂腰肌
Iliopsoas
muscle

大收肌
Adductor magnus muscle

鹅足：
Pes anserinus:
缝匠肌
Sartorius muscle
股薄肌
Gracilis muscle
半腱肌
Semitendinosus muscle

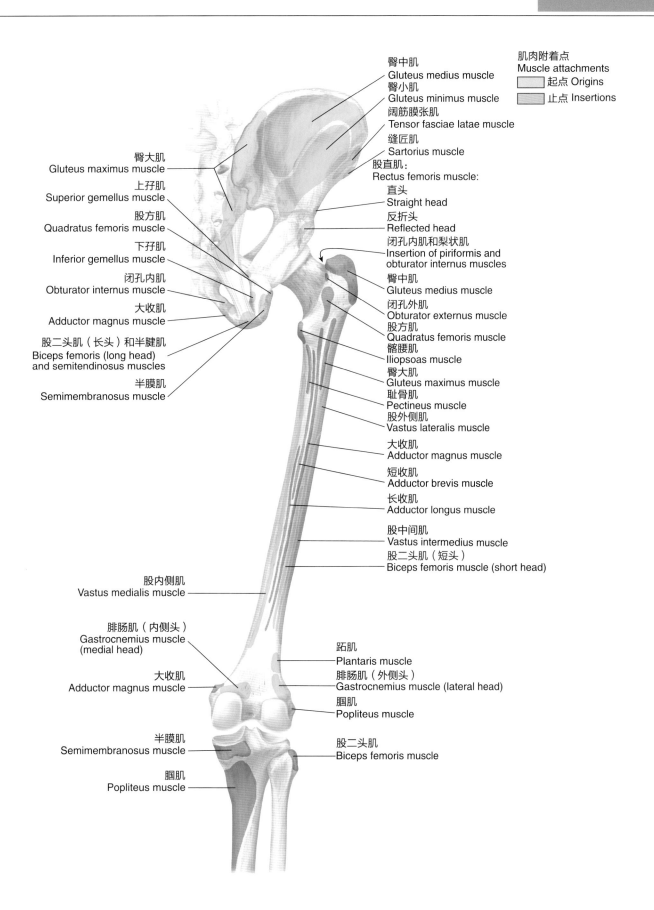

臀中肌
Gluteus medius muscle

臀小肌
Gluteus minimus muscle

阔筋膜张肌
Tensor fasciae latae muscle

缝匠肌
Sartorius muscle

股直肌：
Rectus femoris muscle:

直头
Straight head

反折头
Reflected head

闭孔内肌和梨状肌
Insertion of piriformis and obturator internus muscles

臀中肌
Gluteus medius muscle

闭孔外肌
Obturator externus muscle

股方肌
Quadratus femoris muscle

髂腰肌
Iliopsoas muscle

臀大肌
Gluteus maximus muscle

耻骨肌
Pectineus muscle

股外侧肌
Vastus lateralis muscle

大收肌
Adductor magnus muscle

短收肌
Adductor brevis muscle

长收肌
Adductor longus muscle

股中间肌
Vastus intermedius muscle

股二头肌（短头）
Biceps femoris muscle (short head)

肌肉附着点
Muscle attachments
起点 Origins
止点 Insertions

臀大肌
Gluteus maximus muscle

上孖肌
Superior gemellus muscle

股方肌
Quadratus femoris muscle

下孖肌
Inferior gemellus muscle

闭孔内肌
Obturator internus muscle

大收肌
Adductor magnus muscle

股二头肌（长头）和半腱肌
Biceps femoris (long head) and semitendinosus muscles

半膜肌
Semimembranosus muscle

股内侧肌
Vastus medialis muscle

腓肠肌（内侧头）
Gastrocnemius muscle (medial head)

大收肌
Adductor magnus muscle

半膜肌
Semimembranosus muscle

腘肌
Popliteus muscle

跖肌
Plantaris muscle

腓肠肌（外侧头）
Gastrocnemius muscle (lateral head)

腘肌
Popliteus muscle

股二头肌
Biceps femoris muscle

图 3-14　腰丛　**Lumbar Plexus**

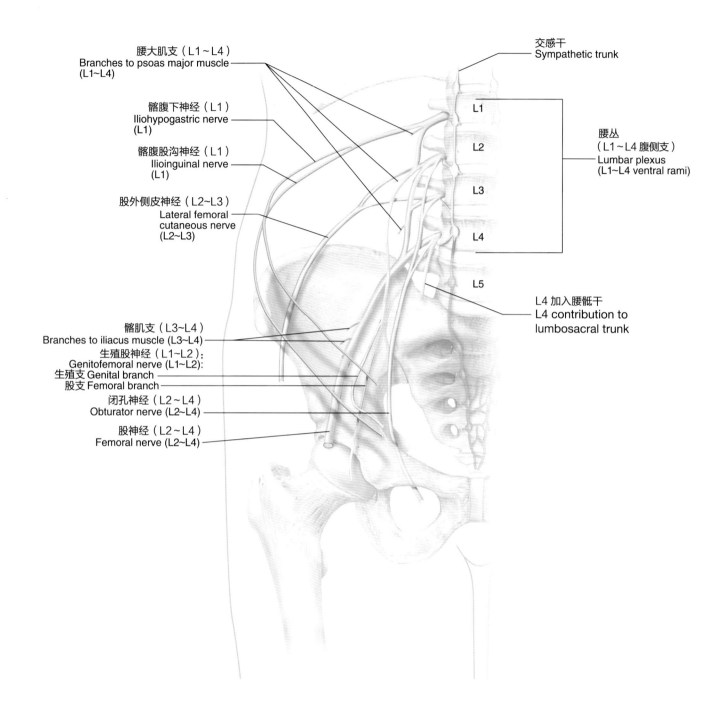

腰大肌支（L1~L4）
Branches to psoas major muscle
(L1~L4)

髂腹下神经（L1）
Iliohypogastric nerve
(L1)

髂腹股沟神经（L1）
Ilioinguinal nerve
(L1)

股外侧皮神经（L2~L3）
Lateral femoral
cutaneous nerve
(L2~L3)

髂肌支（L3~L4）
Branches to iliacus muscle (L3~L4)
生殖股神经（L1~L2）：
Genitofemoral nerve (L1~L2):
生殖支 Genital branch
股支 Femoral branch
闭孔神经（L2~L4）
Obturator nerve (L2~L4)
股神经（L2~L4）
Femoral nerve (L2~L4)

交感干
Sympathetic trunk

L1

L2

L3

L4

腰丛
（L1~L4 腹侧支）
Lumbar plexus
(L1~L4 ventral rami)

L5

L4 加入腰骶干
L4 contribution to
lumbosacral trunk

A. 定位
Orientation

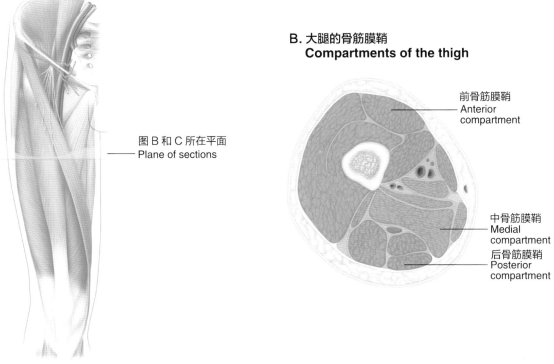

图 B 和 C 所在平面
Plane of sections

B. 大腿的骨筋膜鞘
Compartments of the thigh

前骨筋膜鞘
Anterior compartment

中骨筋膜鞘
Medial compartment

后骨筋膜鞘
Posterior compartment

C. 横断面
Cross section

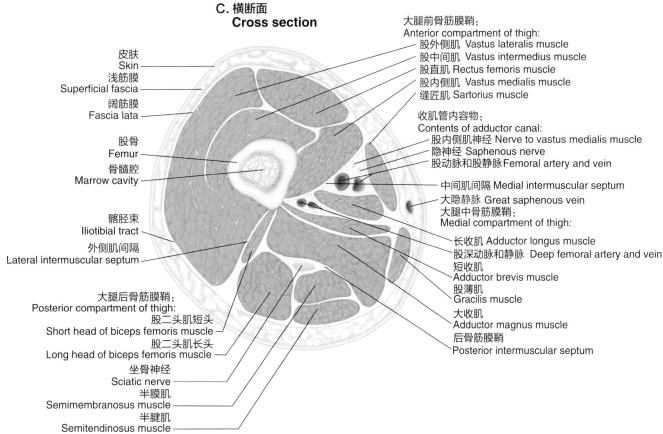

皮肤
Skin

浅筋膜
Superficial fascia

阔筋膜
Fascia lata

股骨
Femur

骨髓腔
Marrow cavity

髂胫束
Iliotibial tract

外侧肌间隔
Lateral intermuscular septum

大腿前骨筋膜鞘:
Anterior compartment of thigh:
股外侧肌 Vastus lateralis muscle
股中间肌 Vastus intermedius muscle
股直肌 Rectus femoris muscle
股内侧肌 Vastus medialis muscle
缝匠肌 Sartorius muscle

收肌管内容物:
Contents of adductor canal:
股内侧肌神经 Nerve to vastus medialis muscle
隐神经 Saphenous nerve
股动脉和股静脉 Femoral artery and vein
中间肌间隔 Medial intermuscular septum
大隐静脉 Great saphenous vein
大腿中骨筋膜鞘:
Medial compartment of thigh:
长收肌 Adductor longus muscle
股深动脉和静脉 Deep femoral artery and vein
短收肌
Adductor brevis muscle
股薄肌
Gracilis muscle
大收肌
Adductor magnus muscle
后骨筋膜鞘
Posterior intermuscular septum

大腿后骨筋膜鞘:
Posterior compartment of thigh:
股二头肌短头
Short head of biceps femoris muscle
股二头肌长头
Long head of biceps femoris muscle
坐骨神经
Sciatic nerve
半膜肌
Semimembranosus muscle
半腱肌
Semitendinosus muscle

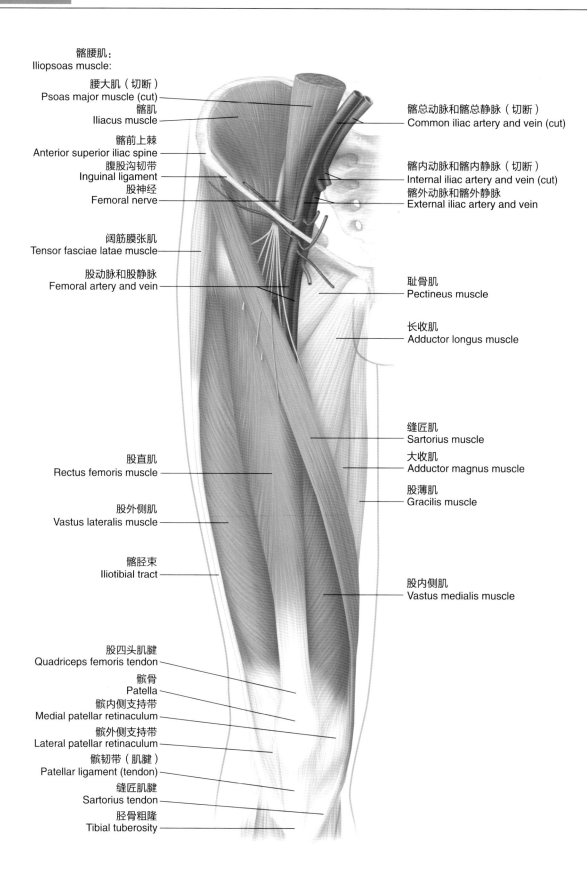

髂腰肌：
Iliopsoas muscle:

腰大肌（切断）
Psoas major muscle (cut)

髂肌
Iliacus muscle

髂前上棘
Anterior superior iliac spine

腹股沟韧带
Inguinal ligament

股神经
Femoral nerve

阔筋膜张肌
Tensor fasciae latae muscle

股动脉和股静脉
Femoral artery and vein

股直肌
Rectus femoris muscle

股外侧肌
Vastus lateralis muscle

髂胫束
Iliotibial tract

股四头肌腱
Quadriceps femoris tendon

髌骨
Patella

髌内侧支持带
Medial patellar retinaculum

髌外侧支持带
Lateral patellar retinaculum

髌韧带（肌腱）
Patellar ligament (tendon)

缝匠肌腱
Sartorius tendon

胫骨粗隆
Tibial tuberosity

髂总动脉和髂总静脉（切断）
Common iliac artery and vein (cut)

髂内动脉和髂内静脉（切断）
Internal iliac artery and vein (cut)

髂外动脉和髂外静脉
External iliac artery and vein

耻骨肌
Pectineus muscle

长收肌
Adductor longus muscle

缝匠肌
Sartorius muscle

大收肌
Adductor magnus muscle

股薄肌
Gracilis muscle

股内侧肌
Vastus medialis muscle

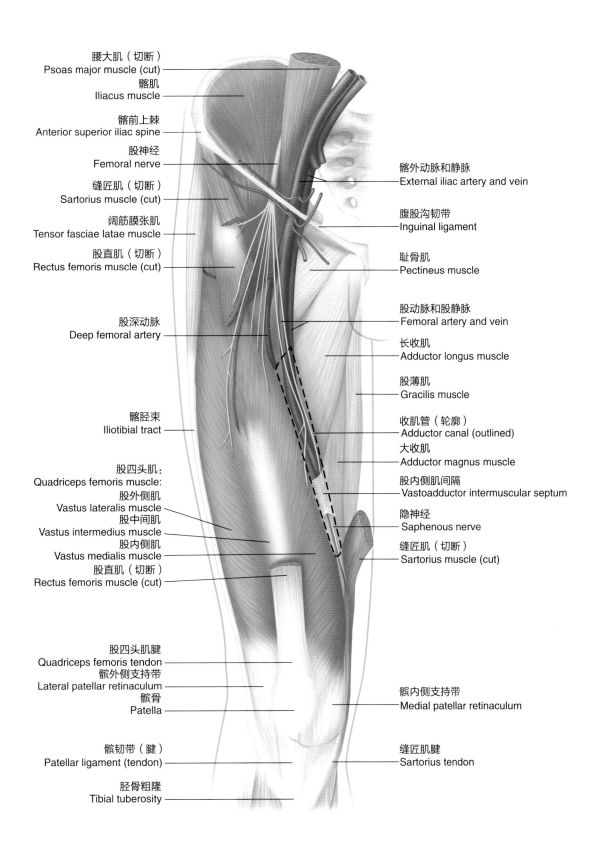

腰大肌（切断）
Psoas major muscle (cut)

髂肌
Iliacus muscle

髂前上棘
Anterior superior iliac spine

股神经
Femoral nerve

缝匠肌（切断）
Sartorius muscle (cut)

阔筋膜张肌
Tensor fasciae latae muscle

股直肌（切断）
Rectus femoris muscle (cut)

股深动脉
Deep femoral artery

髂胫束
Iliotibial tract

股四头肌：
Quadriceps femoris muscle:

股外侧肌
Vastus lateralis muscle

股中间肌
Vastus intermedius muscle

股内侧肌
Vastus medialis muscle

股直肌（切断）
Rectus femoris muscle (cut)

股四头肌腱
Quadriceps femoris tendon

髌外侧支持带
Lateral patellar retinaculum

髌骨
Patella

髌韧带（腱）
Patellar ligament (tendon)

胫骨粗隆
Tibial tuberosity

髂外动脉和静脉
External iliac artery and vein

腹股沟韧带
Inguinal ligament

耻骨肌
Pectineus muscle

股动脉和股静脉
Femoral artery and vein

长收肌
Adductor longus muscle

股薄肌
Gracilis muscle

收肌管（轮廓）
Adductor canal (outlined)

大收肌
Adductor magnus muscle

股内侧肌间隔
Vastoadductor intermuscular septum

隐神经
Saphenous nerve

缝匠肌（切断）
Sartorius muscle (cut)

髌内侧支持带
Medial patellar retinaculum

缝匠肌腱
Sartorius tendon

图 3-18   股三角 Femoral Triangle

A. 前面观
Anterior view

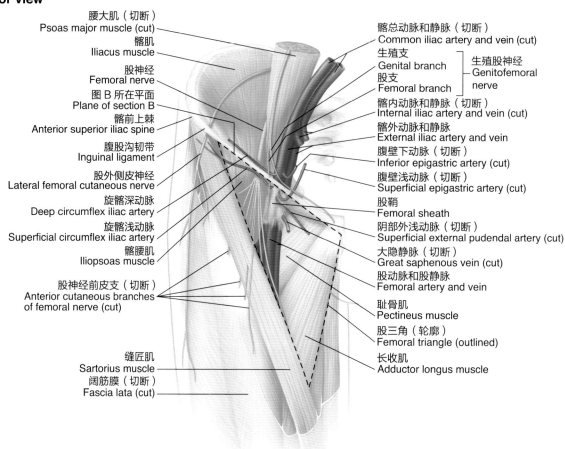

腰大肌（切断）
Psoas major muscle (cut)

髂肌
Iliacus muscle

股神经
Femoral nerve

图 B 所在平面
Plane of section B

髂前上棘
Anterior superior iliac spine

腹股沟韧带
Inguinal ligament

股外侧皮神经
Lateral femoral cutaneous nerve

旋髂深动脉
Deep circumflex iliac artery

旋髂浅动脉
Superficial circumflex iliac artery

髂腰肌
Iliopsoas muscle

股神经前皮支（切断）
Anterior cutaneous branches
of femoral nerve (cut)

缝匠肌
Sartorius muscle

阔筋膜（切断）
Fascia lata (cut)

髂总动脉和静脉（切断）
Common iliac artery and vein (cut)

生殖支
Genital branch
股支
Femoral branch
生殖股神经
Genitofemoral nerve

髂内动脉和静脉（切断）
Internal iliac artery and vein (cut)

髂外动脉和静脉
External iliac artery and vein

腹壁下动脉（切断）
Inferior epigastric artery (cut)

腹壁浅动脉（切断）
Superficial epigastric artery (cut)

股鞘
Femoral sheath

阴部外浅动脉（切断）
Superficial external pudendal artery (cut)

大隐静脉（切断）
Great saphenous vein (cut)

股动脉和股静脉
Femoral artery and vein

耻骨肌
Pectineus muscle

股三角（轮廓）
Femoral triangle (outlined)

长收肌
Adductor longus muscle

B. 经股鞘断面
Section through the femoral sheath

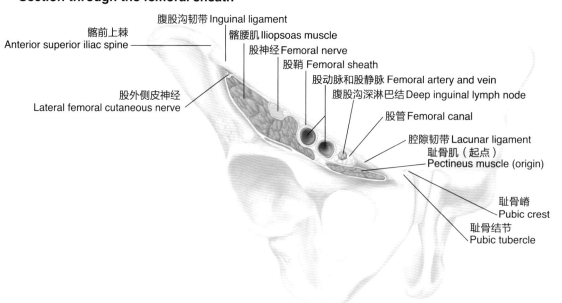

髂前上棘
Anterior superior iliac spine

腹股沟韧带 Inguinal ligament

髂腰肌 Iliopsoas muscle

股神经 Femoral nerve

股鞘 Femoral sheath

股动脉和股静脉 Femoral artery and vein

腹股沟深淋巴结 Deep inguinal lymph node

股外侧皮神经
Lateral femoral cutaneous nerve

股管 Femoral canal

腔隙韧带 Lacunar ligament
耻骨肌（起点）
Pectineus muscle (origin)

耻骨嵴
Pubic crest

耻骨结节
Pubic tubercle

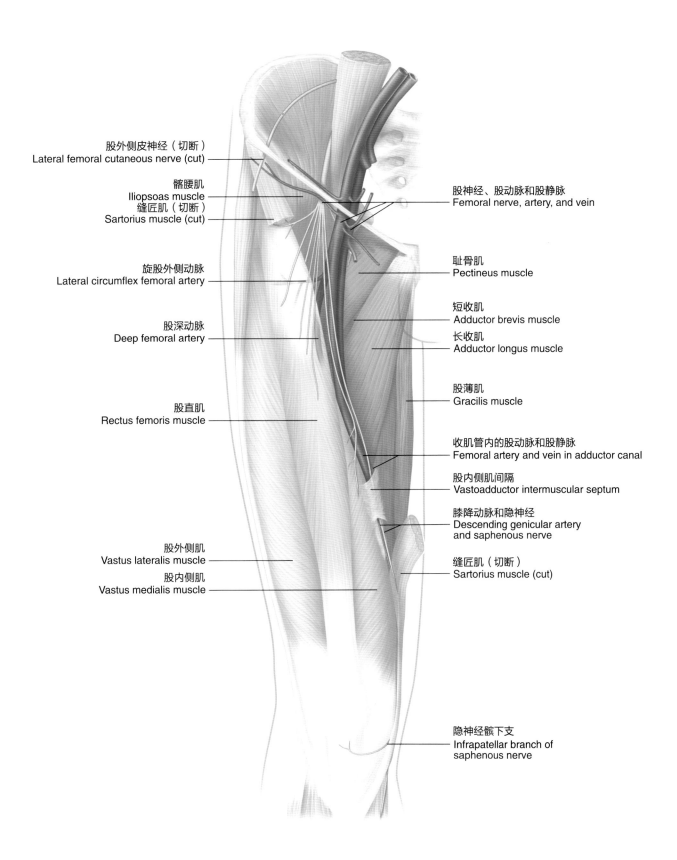

股外侧皮神经（切断）
Lateral femoral cutaneous nerve (cut)

髂腰肌
Iliopsoas muscle
缝匠肌（切断）
Sartorius muscle (cut)

旋股外侧动脉
Lateral circumflex femoral artery

股深动脉
Deep femoral artery

股直肌
Rectus femoris muscle

股外侧肌
Vastus lateralis muscle
股内侧肌
Vastus medialis muscle

股神经、股动脉和股静脉
Femoral nerve, artery, and vein

耻骨肌
Pectineus muscle

短收肌
Adductor brevis muscle
长收肌
Adductor longus muscle

股薄肌
Gracilis muscle

收肌管内的股动脉和股静脉
Femoral artery and vein in adductor canal

股内侧肌间隔
Vastoadductor intermuscular septum

膝降动脉和隐神经
Descending genicular artery
and saphenous nerve

缝匠肌（切断）
Sartorius muscle (cut)

隐神经髌下支
Infrapatellar branch of
saphenous nerve

图 3-20

股内侧区肌群，中层解剖
Muscles of the Medial Thigh, Intermediate Dissection

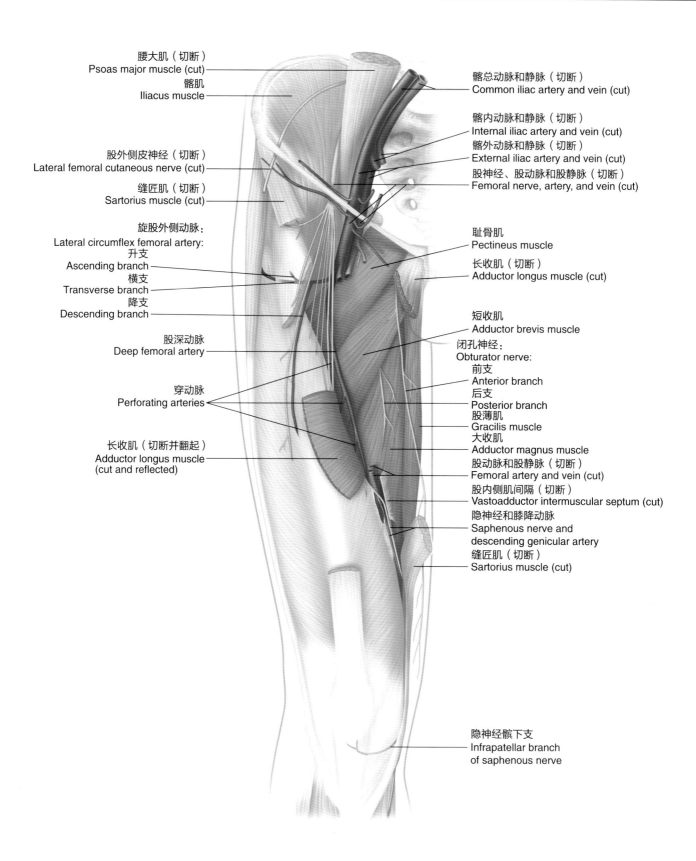

腰大肌（切断）
Psoas major muscle (cut)

髂肌
Iliacus muscle

股外侧皮神经（切断）
Lateral femoral cutaneous nerve (cut)

缝匠肌（切断）
Sartorius muscle (cut)

旋股外侧动脉：
Lateral circumflex femoral artery:
升支
Ascending branch
横支
Transverse branch
降支
Descending branch

股深动脉
Deep femoral artery

穿动脉
Perforating arteries

长收肌（切断并翻起）
Adductor longus muscle
(cut and reflected)

髂总动脉和静脉（切断）
Common iliac artery and vein (cut)

髂内动脉和静脉（切断）
Internal iliac artery and vein (cut)
髂外动脉和静脉（切断）
External iliac artery and vein (cut)
股神经、股动脉和股静脉（切断）
Femoral nerve, artery, and vein (cut)

耻骨肌
Pectineus muscle
长收肌（切断）
Adductor longus muscle (cut)

短收肌
Adductor brevis muscle
闭孔神经：
Obturator nerve:
前支
Anterior branch
后支
Posterior branch
股薄肌
Gracilis muscle
大收肌
Adductor magnus muscle
股动脉和股静脉（切断）
Femoral artery and vein (cut)
股内侧肌间隔（切断）
Vastoadductor intermuscular septum (cut)
隐神经和膝降动脉
Saphenous nerve and
descending genicular artery
缝匠肌（切断）
Sartorius muscle (cut)

隐神经髌下支
Infrapatellar branch
of saphenous nerve

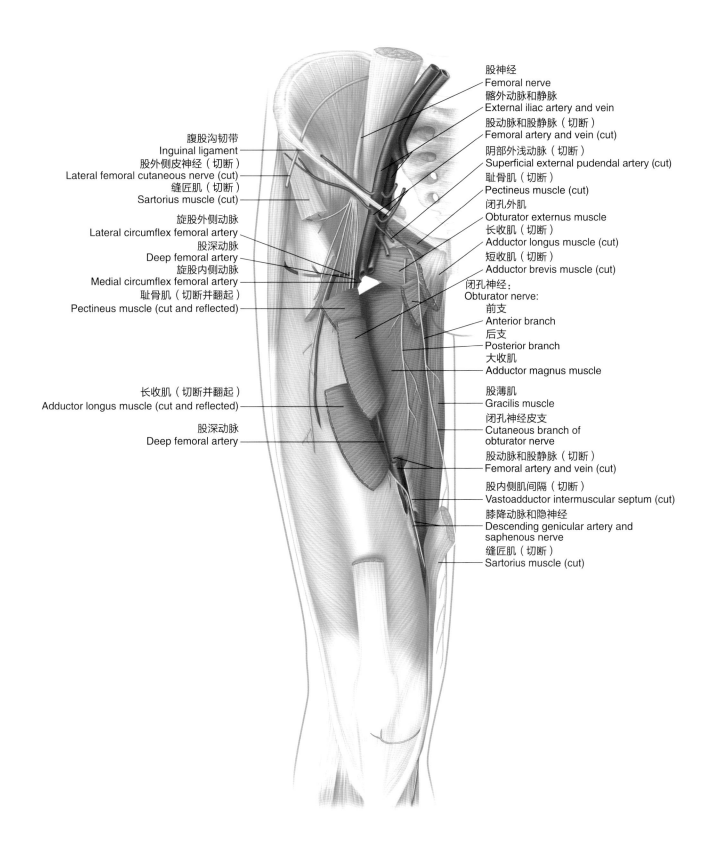

腹股沟韧带
Inguinal ligament
股外侧皮神经（切断）
Lateral femoral cutaneous nerve (cut)
缝匠肌（切断）
Sartorius muscle (cut)

旋股外侧动脉
Lateral circumflex femoral artery
股深动脉
Deep femoral artery
旋股内侧动脉
Medial circumflex femoral artery
耻骨肌（切断并翻起）
Pectineus muscle (cut and reflected)

长收肌（切断并翻起）
Adductor longus muscle (cut and reflected)

股深动脉
Deep femoral artery

股神经
Femoral nerve
髂外动脉和静脉
External iliac artery and vein
股动脉和股静脉（切断）
Femoral artery and vein (cut)
阴部外浅动脉（切断）
Superficial external pudendal artery (cut)
耻骨肌（切断）
Pectineus muscle (cut)
闭孔外肌
Obturator externus muscle
长收肌（切断）
Adductor longus muscle (cut)
短收肌（切断）
Adductor brevis muscle (cut)

闭孔神经：
Obturator nerve:
前支
Anterior branch
后支
Posterior branch
大收肌
Adductor magnus muscle
股薄肌
Gracilis muscle
闭孔神经皮支
Cutaneous branch of obturator nerve
股动脉和股静脉（切断）
Femoral artery and vein (cut)
股内侧肌间隔（切断）
Vastoadductor intermuscular septum (cut)
膝降动脉和隐神经
Descending genicular artery and saphenous nerve
缝匠肌（切断）
Sartorius muscle (cut)

图 3-22

股前内侧区的动脉，浅层解剖
Arteries of the Anterior and Medial Thigh, Superficial Dissection

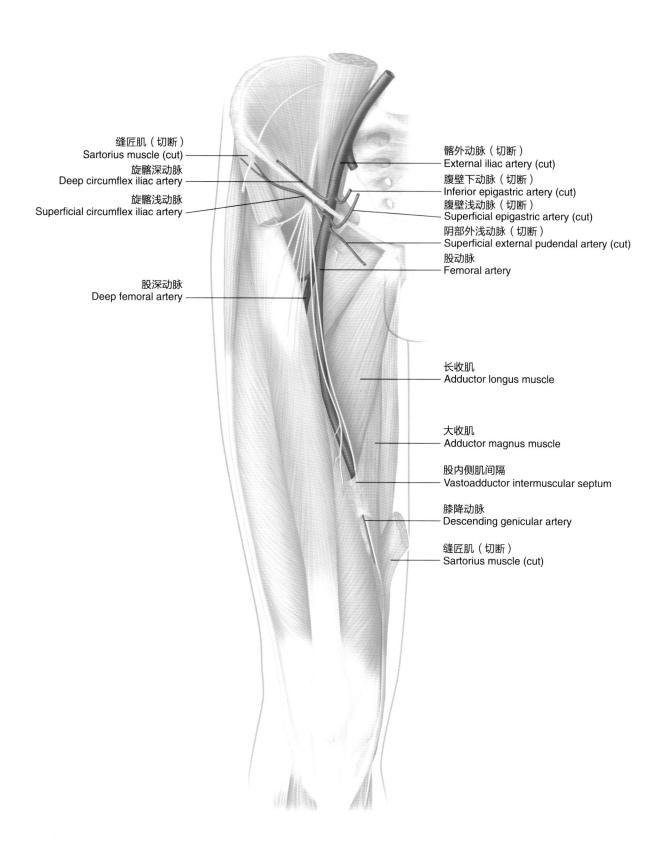

缝匠肌（切断）
Sartorius muscle (cut)

旋髂深动脉
Deep circumflex iliac artery

旋髂浅动脉
Superficial circumflex iliac artery

股深动脉
Deep femoral artery

髂外动脉（切断）
External iliac artery (cut)

腹壁下动脉（切断）
Inferior epigastric artery (cut)

腹壁浅动脉（切断）
Superficial epigastric artery (cut)

阴部外浅动脉（切断）
Superficial external pudendal artery (cut)

股动脉
Femoral artery

长收肌
Adductor longus muscle

大收肌
Adductor magnus muscle

股内侧肌间隔
Vastoadductor intermuscular septum

膝降动脉
Descending genicular artery

缝匠肌（切断）
Sartorius muscle (cut)

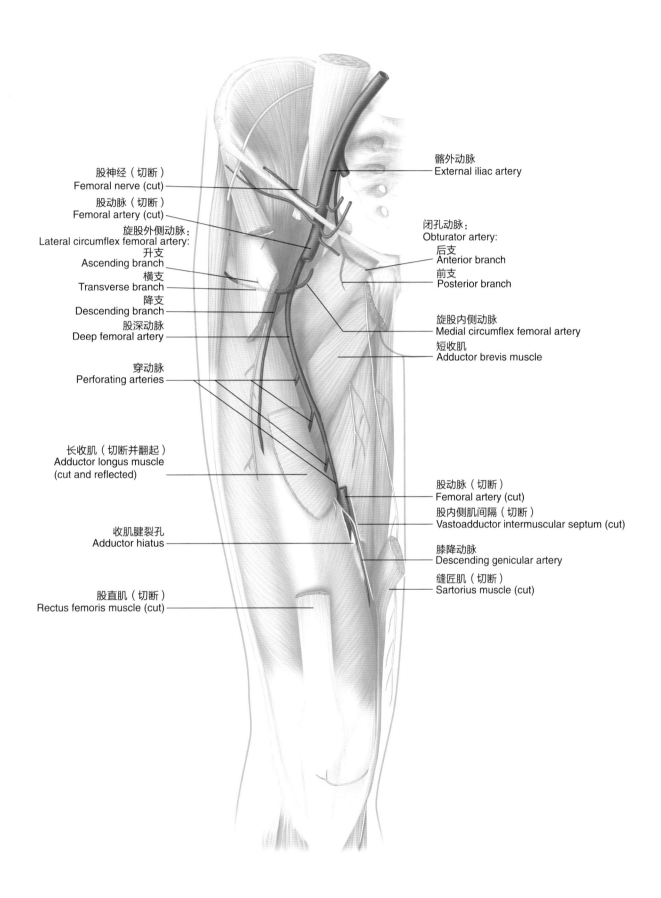

股神经（切断）
Femoral nerve (cut)

股动脉（切断）
Femoral artery (cut)

旋股外侧动脉：
Lateral circumflex femoral artery:
升支
Ascending branch
横支
Transverse branch
降支
Descending branch
股深动脉
Deep femoral artery

穿动脉
Perforating arteries

长收肌（切断并翻起）
Adductor longus muscle
(cut and reflected)

收肌腱裂孔
Adductor hiatus

股直肌（切断）
Rectus femoris muscle (cut)

髂外动脉
External iliac artery

闭孔动脉：
Obturator artery:
后支
Anterior branch
前支
Posterior branch

旋股内侧动脉
Medial circumflex femoral artery
短收肌
Adductor brevis muscle

股动脉（切断）
Femoral artery (cut)
股内侧肌间隔（切断）
Vastoadductor intermuscular septum (cut)
膝降动脉
Descending genicular artery
缝匠肌（切断）
Sartorius muscle (cut)

图 3-24　　**股前内侧区的神经　Nerves of the Anterior and Medial Thigh**

A. 浅层解剖
Superficial dissection

B. 深层解剖
Deep dissection

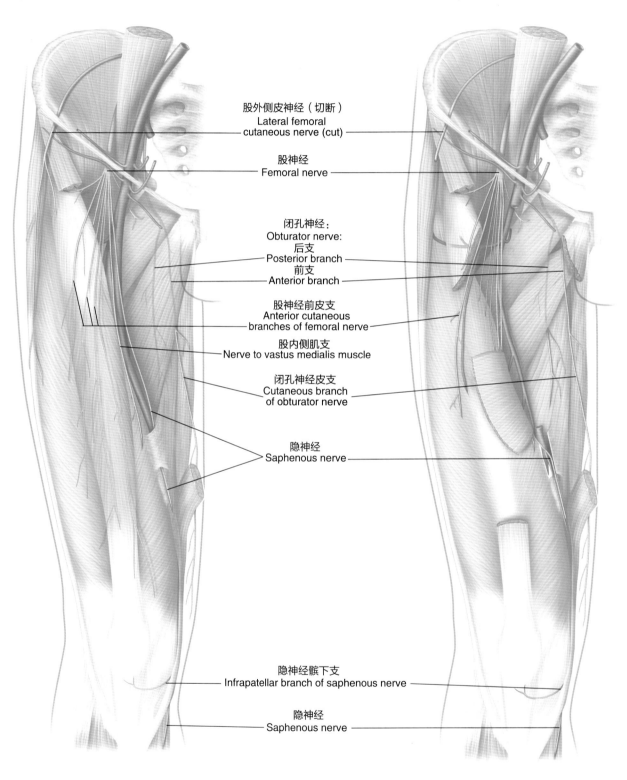

股外侧皮神经（切断）
Lateral femoral
cutaneous nerve (cut)

股神经
Femoral nerve

闭孔神经：
Obturator nerve:
后支
Posterior branch
前支
Anterior branch

股神经前皮支
Anterior cutaneous
branches of femoral nerve

股内侧肌支
Nerve to vastus medialis muscle

闭孔神经皮支
Cutaneous branch
of obturator nerve

隐神经
Saphenous nerve

隐神经髌下支
Infrapatellar branch of saphenous nerve

隐神经
Saphenous nerve

A. 前面观
Anterior view

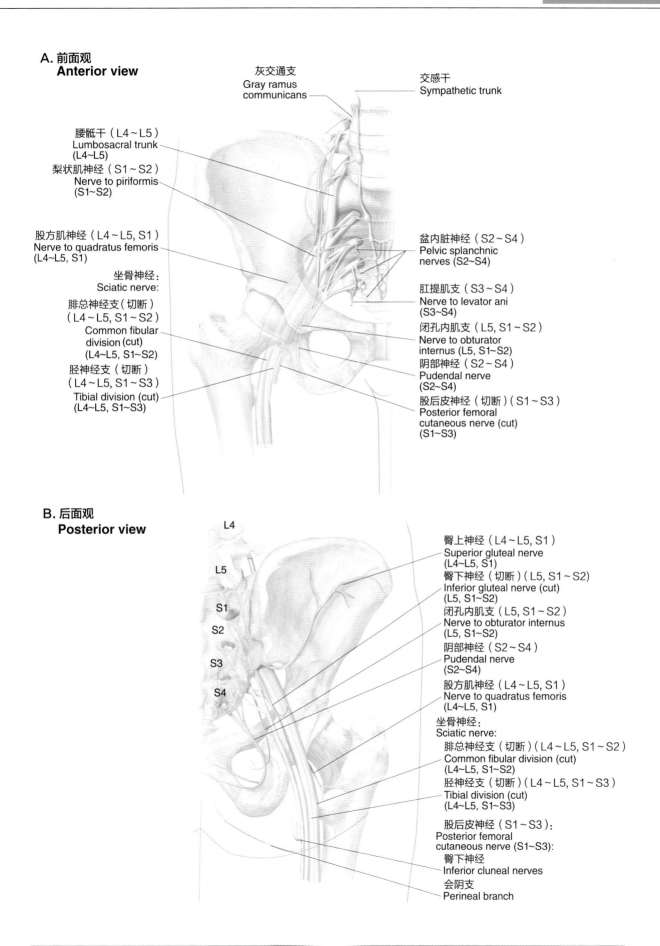

灰交通支
Gray ramus
communicans

交感干
Sympathetic trunk

腰骶干（L4~L5）
Lumbosacral trunk
(L4~L5)

梨状肌神经（S1~S2）
Nerve to piriformis
(S1~S2)

股方肌神经（L4~L5, S1）
Nerve to quadratus femoris
(L4~L5, S1)

坐骨神经：
Sciatic nerve:

腓总神经支（切断）
（L4~L5, S1~S2）
Common fibular
division (cut)
(L4~L5, S1~S2)

胫神经支（切断）
（L4~L5, S1~S3）
Tibial division (cut)
(L4~L5, S1~S3)

盆内脏神经（S2~S4）
Pelvic splanchnic
nerves (S2~S4)

肛提肌支（S3~S4）
Nerve to levator ani
(S3~S4)

闭孔内肌支（L5, S1~S2）
Nerve to obturator
internus (L5, S1~S2)

阴部神经（S2~S4）
Pudendal nerve
(S2~S4)

股后皮神经（切断）（S1~S3）
Posterior femoral
cutaneous nerve (cut)
(S1~S3)

B. 后面观
Posterior view

L4

L5

S1

S2

S3

S4

臀上神经（L4~L5, S1）
Superior gluteal nerve
(L4~L5, S1)

臀下神经（切断）（L5, S1~S2）
Inferior gluteal nerve (cut)
(L5, S1~S2)

闭孔内肌支（L5, S1~S2）
Nerve to obturator internus
(L5, S1~S2)

阴部神经（S2~S4）
Pudendal nerve
(S2~S4)

股方肌神经（L4~L5, S1）
Nerve to quadratus femoris
(L4~L5, S1)

坐骨神经：
Sciatic nerve:

腓总神经支（切断）（L4~L5, S1~S2）
Common fibular division (cut)
(L4~L5, S1~S2)

胫神经支（切断）（L4~L5, S1~S3）
Tibial division (cut)
(L4~L5, S1~S3)

股后皮神经（S1~S3）：
Posterior femoral
cutaneous nerve (S1~S3):

臀下神经
Inferior cluneal nerves

会阴支
Perineal branch

图 3-26　　臀部肌群　Muscles of the Gluteal Region

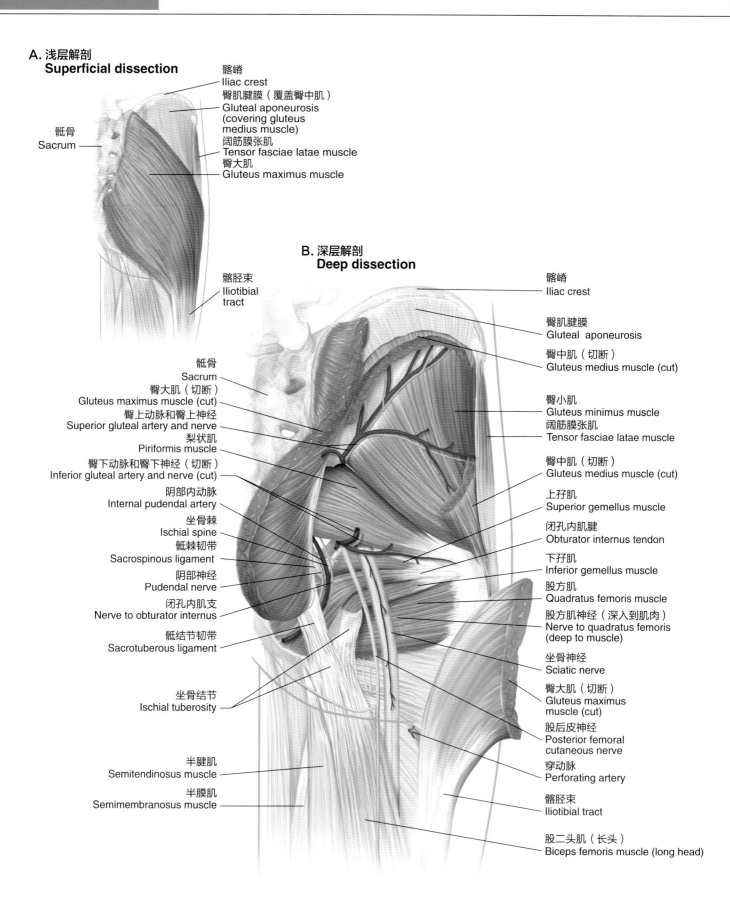

A. 浅层解剖
Superficial dissection

髂嵴
Iliac crest

臀肌腱膜（覆盖臀中肌）
Gluteal aponeurosis (covering gluteus medius muscle)

阔筋膜张肌
Tensor fasciae latae muscle

臀大肌
Gluteus maximus muscle

骶骨
Sacrum

髂胫束
Iliotibial tract

B. 深层解剖
Deep dissection

骶骨
Sacrum

臀大肌（切断）
Gluteus maximus muscle (cut)

臀上动脉和臀上神经
Superior gluteal artery and nerve

梨状肌
Piriformis muscle

臀下动脉和臀下神经（切断）
Inferior gluteal artery and nerve (cut)

阴部内动脉
Internal pudendal artery

坐骨棘
Ischial spine

骶棘韧带
Sacrospinous ligament

阴部神经
Pudendal nerve

闭孔内肌支
Nerve to obturator internus

骶结节韧带
Sacrotuberous ligament

坐骨结节
Ischial tuberosity

半腱肌
Semitendinosus muscle

半膜肌
Semimembranosus muscle

髂嵴
Iliac crest

臀肌腱膜
Gluteal aponeurosis

臀中肌（切断）
Gluteus medius muscle (cut)

臀小肌
Gluteus minimus muscle

阔筋膜张肌
Tensor fasciae latae muscle

臀中肌（切断）
Gluteus medius muscle (cut)

上孖肌
Superior gemellus muscle

闭孔内肌腱
Obturator internus tendon

下孖肌
Inferior gemellus muscle

股方肌
Quadratus femoris muscle

股方肌神经（深入到肌肉）
Nerve to quadratus femoris (deep to muscle)

坐骨神经
Sciatic nerve

臀大肌（切断）
Gluteus maximus muscle (cut)

股后皮神经
Posterior femoral cutaneous nerve

穿动脉
Perforating artery

髂胫束
Iliotibial tract

股二头肌（长头）
Biceps femoris muscle (long head)

A. 动脉
Arteries

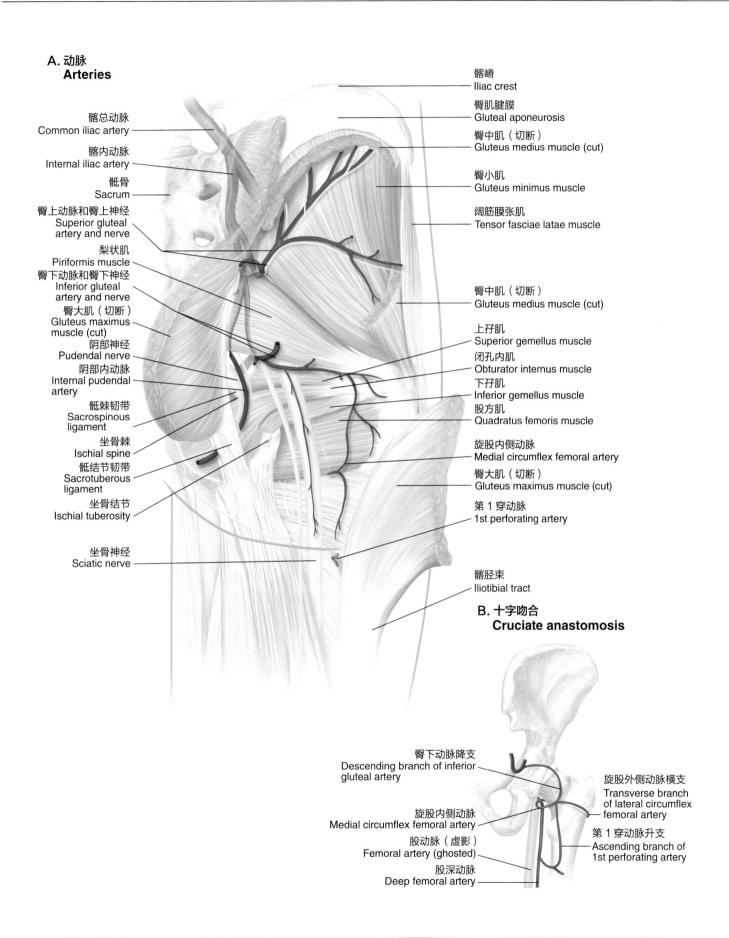

髂嵴
Iliac crest

臀肌腱膜
Gluteal aponeurosis

臀中肌（切断）
Gluteus medius muscle (cut)

臀小肌
Gluteus minimus muscle

阔筋膜张肌
Tensor fasciae latae muscle

臀中肌（切断）
Gluteus medius muscle (cut)

上孖肌
Superior gemellus muscle

闭孔内肌
Obturator internus muscle

下孖肌
Inferior gemellus muscle

股方肌
Quadratus femoris muscle

旋股内侧动脉
Medial circumflex femoral artery

臀大肌（切断）
Gluteus maximus muscle (cut)

第 1 穿动脉
1st perforating artery

髂胫束
Iliotibial tract

髂总动脉
Common iliac artery

髂内动脉
Internal iliac artery

骶骨
Sacrum

臀上动脉和臀上神经
Superior gluteal artery and nerve

梨状肌
Piriformis muscle

臀下动脉和臀下神经
Inferior gluteal artery and nerve

臀大肌（切断）
Gluteus maximus muscle (cut)

阴部神经
Pudendal nerve

阴部内动脉
Internal pudendal artery

骶棘韧带
Sacrospinous ligament

坐骨棘
Ischial spine

骶结节韧带
Sacrotuberous ligament

坐骨结节
Ischial tuberosity

坐骨神经
Sciatic nerve

B. 十字吻合
Cruciate anastomosis

臀下动脉降支
Descending branch of inferior gluteal artery

旋股外侧动脉横支
Transverse branch of lateral circumflex femoral artery

旋股内侧动脉
Medial circumflex femoral artery

第 1 穿动脉升支
Ascending branch of 1st perforating artery

股动脉（虚影）
Femoral artery (ghosted)

股深动脉
Deep femoral artery

图 3-28 　臀部的神经　Nerves of the Gluteal Region

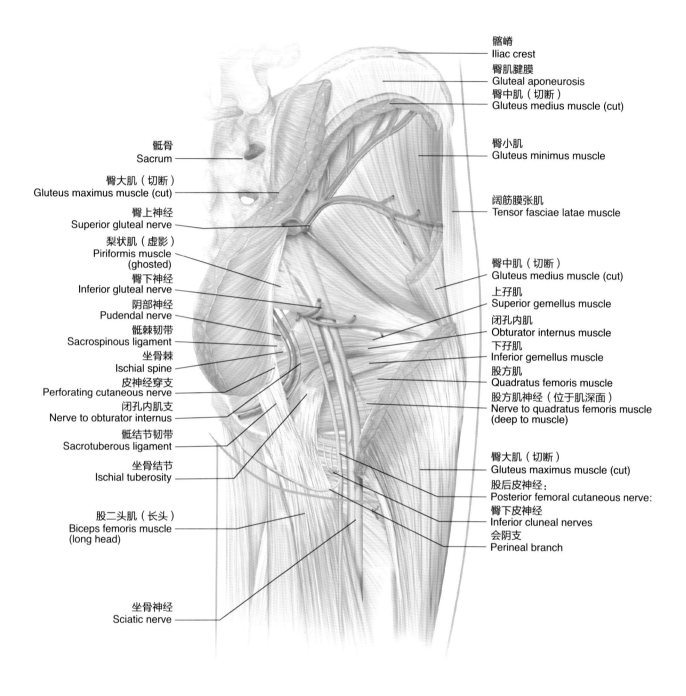

髂嵴
Iliac crest

臀肌腱膜
Gluteal aponeurosis

臀中肌（切断）
Gluteus medius muscle (cut)

臀小肌
Gluteus minimus muscle

阔筋膜张肌
Tensor fasciae latae muscle

臀中肌（切断）
Gluteus medius muscle (cut)

上孖肌
Superior gemellus muscle

闭孔内肌
Obturator internus muscle

下孖肌
Inferior gemellus muscle

股方肌
Quadratus femoris muscle

股方肌神经（位于肌深面）
Nerve to quadratus femoris muscle
(deep to muscle)

臀大肌（切断）
Gluteus maximus muscle (cut)

股后皮神经：
Posterior femoral cutaneous nerve:

臀下皮神经
Inferior cluneal nerves

会阴支
Perineal branch

骶骨
Sacrum

臀大肌（切断）
Gluteus maximus muscle (cut)

臀上神经
Superior gluteal nerve

梨状肌（虚影）
Piriformis muscle
(ghosted)

臀下神经
Inferior gluteal nerve

阴部神经
Pudendal nerve

骶棘韧带
Sacrospinous ligament

坐骨棘
Ischial spine

皮神经穿支
Perforating cutaneous nerve

闭孔内肌支
Nerve to obturator internus

骶结节韧带
Sacrotuberous ligament

坐骨结节
Ischial tuberosity

股二头肌（长头）
Biceps femoris muscle
(long head)

坐骨神经
Sciatic nerve

A. 浅层解剖
Superficial dissection

B. 深层解剖
Deep dissection

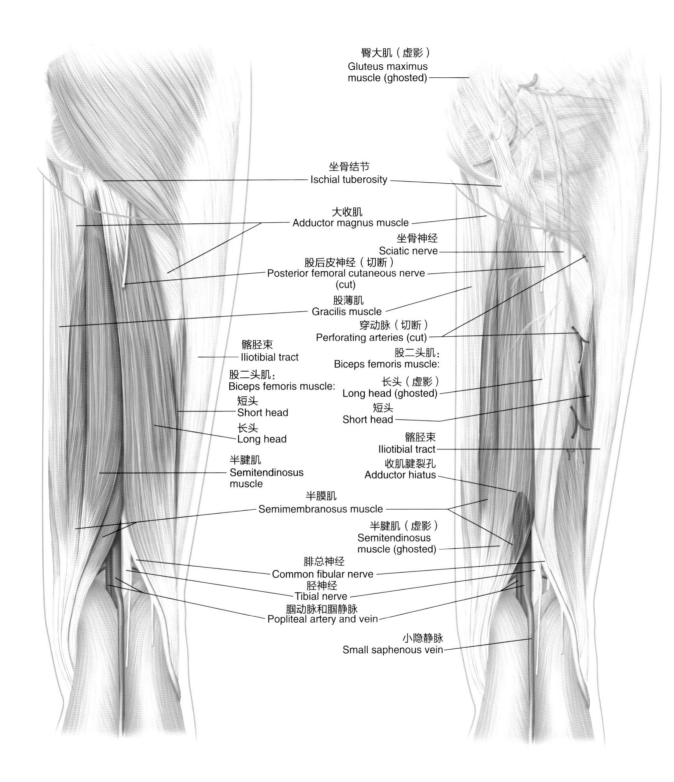

臀大肌（虚影）
Gluteus maximus
muscle (ghosted)

坐骨结节
Ischial tuberosity

大收肌
Adductor magnus muscle

坐骨神经
Sciatic nerve

股后皮神经（切断）
Posterior femoral cutaneous nerve
(cut)

股薄肌
Gracilis muscle

穿动脉（切断）
Perforating arteries (cut)

股二头肌：
Biceps femoris muscle:

髂胫束
Iliotibial tract

股二头肌：
Biceps femoris muscle:

长头（虚影）
Long head (ghosted)

短头
Short head

短头
Short head

长头
Long head

髂胫束
Iliotibial tract

半腱肌
Semitendinosus
muscle

收肌腱裂孔
Adductor hiatus

半膜肌
Semimembranosus muscle

半腱肌（虚影）
Semitendinosus
muscle (ghosted)

腓总神经
Common fibular nerve

胫神经
Tibial nerve

腘动脉和腘静脉
Popliteal artery and vein

小隐静脉
Small saphenous vein

图 3-30　下肢远端的肌肉附着点　Muscle Attachments of the Distal Lower Limb

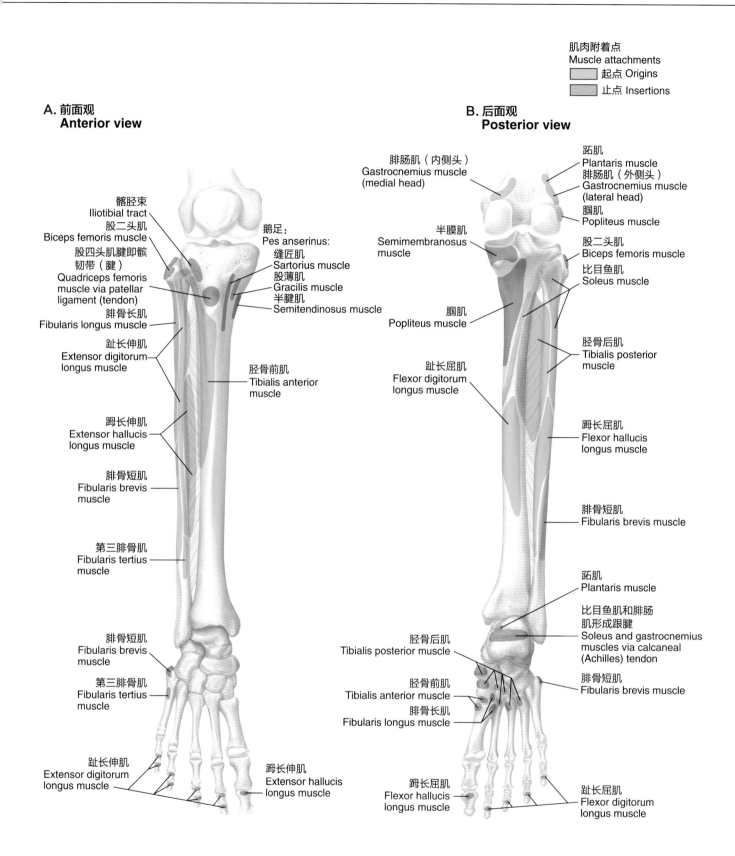

肌肉附着点
Muscle attachments
起点 Origins
止点 Insertions

A. 前面观
Anterior view

髂胫束
Iliotibial tract
股二头肌
Biceps femoris muscle
股四头肌腱即髌
韧带（腱）
Quadriceps femoris
muscle via patellar
ligament (tendon)
腓骨长肌
Fibularis longus muscle
趾长伸肌
Extensor digitorum
longus muscle
𧿹长伸肌
Extensor hallucis
longus muscle
腓骨短肌
Fibularis brevis
muscle
第三腓骨肌
Fibularis tertius
muscle
腓骨短肌
Fibularis brevis
muscle
第三腓骨肌
Fibularis tertius
muscle
趾长伸肌
Extensor digitorum
longus muscle

鹅足：
Pes anserinus:
缝匠肌
Sartorius muscle
股薄肌
Gracilis muscle
半腱肌
Semitendinosus muscle

胫骨前肌
Tibialis anterior
muscle

𧿹长伸肌
Extensor hallucis
longus muscle

B. 后面观
Posterior view

腓肠肌（内侧头）
Gastrocnemius muscle
(medial head)
半膜肌
Semimembranosus
muscle
腘肌
Popliteus muscle
趾长屈肌
Flexor digitorum
longus muscle

跖肌
Plantaris muscle
腓肠肌（外侧头）
Gastrocnemius muscle
(lateral head)
腘肌
Popliteus muscle
股二头肌
Biceps femoris muscle
比目鱼肌
Soleus muscle
胫骨后肌
Tibialis posterior
muscle
𧿹长屈肌
Flexor hallucis
longus muscle
腓骨短肌
Fibularis brevis muscle

跖肌
Plantaris muscle
比目鱼肌和腓肠
肌形成跟腱
Soleus and gastrocnemius
muscles via calcaneal
(Achilles) tendon
腓骨短肌
Fibularis brevis muscle

胫骨后肌
Tibialis posterior muscle
胫骨前肌
Tibialis anterior muscle
腓骨长肌
Fibularis longus muscle

𧿹长屈肌
Flexor hallucis
longus muscle
趾长屈肌
Flexor digitorum
longus muscle

注：足固有肌附着点没有显示
Note: Attachments of intrinsic muscles of foot not shown

A. 浅层解剖
Superficial dissection

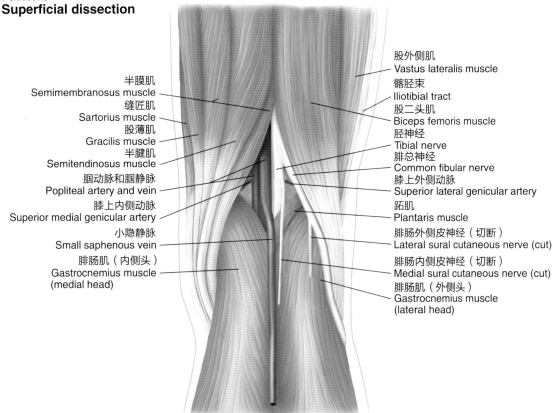

半膜肌
Semimembranosus muscle

缝匠肌
Sartorius muscle

股薄肌
Gracilis muscle

半腱肌
Semitendinosus muscle

腘动脉和腘静脉
Popliteal artery and vein

膝上内侧动脉
Superior medial genicular artery

小隐静脉
Small saphenous vein

腓肠肌（内侧头）
Gastrocnemius muscle
(medial head)

股外侧肌
Vastus lateralis muscle

髂胫束
Iliotibial tract

股二头肌
Biceps femoris muscle

胫神经
Tibial nerve

腓总神经
Common fibular nerve

膝上外侧动脉
Superior lateral genicular artery

跖肌
Plantaris muscle

腓肠外侧皮神经（切断）
Lateral sural cutaneous nerve (cut)

腓肠内侧皮神经（切断）
Medial sural cutaneous nerve (cut)

腓肠肌（外侧头）
Gastrocnemius muscle
(lateral head)

B. 深层解剖
Deep dissection

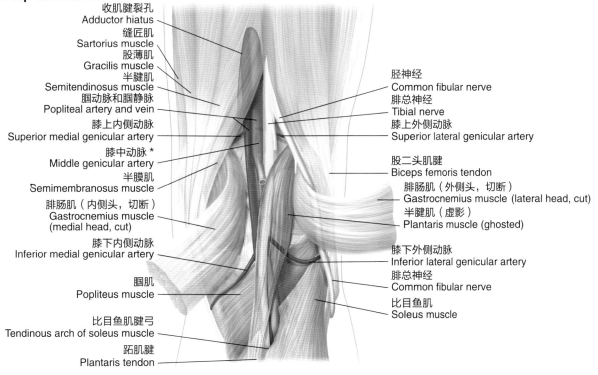

收肌腱裂孔
Adductor hiatus

缝匠肌
Sartorius muscle

股薄肌
Gracilis muscle

半腱肌
Semitendinosus muscle

腘动脉和腘静脉
Popliteal artery and vein

膝上内侧动脉
Superior medial genicular artery

膝中动脉 *
Middle genicular artery

半膜肌
Semimembranosus muscle

腓肠肌（内侧头，切断）
Gastrocnemius muscle
(medial head, cut)

膝下内侧动脉
Inferior medial genicular artery

腘肌
Popliteus muscle

比目鱼肌腱弓
Tendinous arch of soleus muscle

跖肌腱
Plantaris tendon

胫神经
Common fibular nerve

腓总神经
Tibial nerve

膝上外侧动脉
Superior lateral genicular artery

股二头肌腱
Biceps femoris tendon

腓肠肌（外侧头，切断）
Gastrocnemius muscle (lateral head, cut)

半腱肌（虚影）
Plantaris muscle (ghosted)

膝下外侧动脉
Inferior lateral genicular artery

腓总神经
Common fibular nerve

比目鱼肌
Soleus muscle

* 译者注：为腘静脉虚影下的动脉

图 3-32　小腿的骨筋膜鞘　Compartmental Organization of the Leg

A. 定位
Orientation

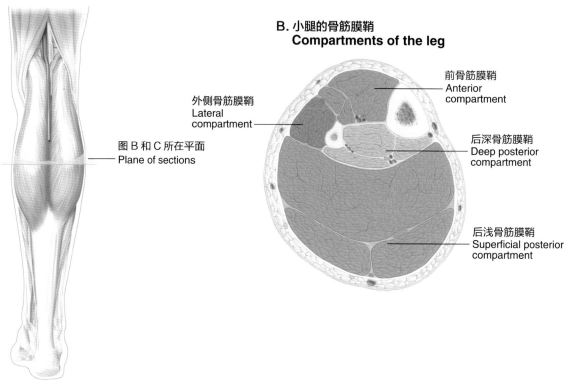

图 B 和 C 所在平面
Plane of sections

B. 小腿的骨筋膜鞘
Compartments of the leg

外侧骨筋膜鞘
Lateral
compartment

前骨筋膜鞘
Anterior
compartment

后深骨筋膜鞘
Deep posterior
compartment

后浅骨筋膜鞘
Superficial posterior
compartment

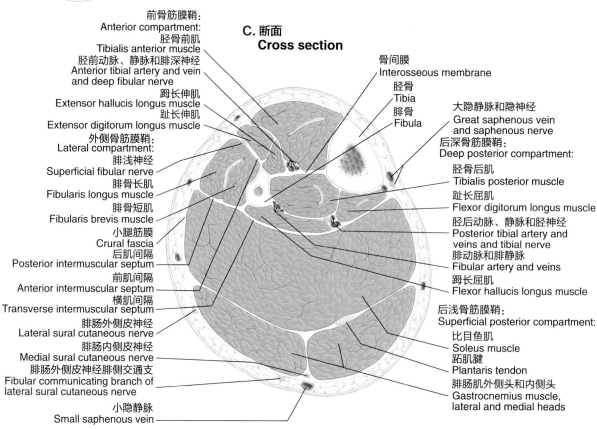

前骨筋膜鞘：
Anterior compartment:
胫骨前肌
Tibialis anterior muscle
胫前动脉、静脉和腓深神经
Anterior tibial artery and vein
and deep fibular nerve
踇长伸肌
Extensor hallucis longus muscle
趾长伸肌
Extensor digitorum longus muscle
外侧骨筋膜鞘：
Lateral compartment:
腓浅神经
Superficial fibular nerve
腓骨长肌
Fibularis longus muscle
腓骨短肌
Fibularis brevis muscle
小腿筋膜
Crural fascia
后肌间隔
Posterior intermuscular septum
前肌间隔
Anterior intermuscular septum
横肌间隔
Transverse intermuscular septum
腓肠外侧皮神经
Lateral sural cutaneous nerve
腓肠内侧皮神经
Medial sural cutaneous nerve
腓肠外侧皮神经腓侧交通支
Fibular communicating branch of
lateral sural cutaneous nerve
小隐静脉
Small saphenous vein

C. 断面
Cross section

骨间膜
Interosseous membrane
胫骨
Tibia
腓骨
Fibula
大隐静脉和隐神经
Great saphenous vein
and saphenous nerve
后深骨筋膜鞘：
Deep posterior compartment:
胫骨后肌
Tibialis posterior muscle
趾长屈肌
Flexor digitorum longus muscle
胫后动脉、静脉和胫神经
Posterior tibial artery and
veins and tibial nerve
腓动脉和腓静脉
Fibular artery and veins
踇长屈肌
Flexor hallucis longus muscle
后浅骨筋膜鞘：
Superficial posterior compartment:
比目鱼肌
Soleus muscle
跖肌腱
Plantaris tendon
腓肠肌外侧头和内侧头
Gastrocnemius muscle,
lateral and medial heads

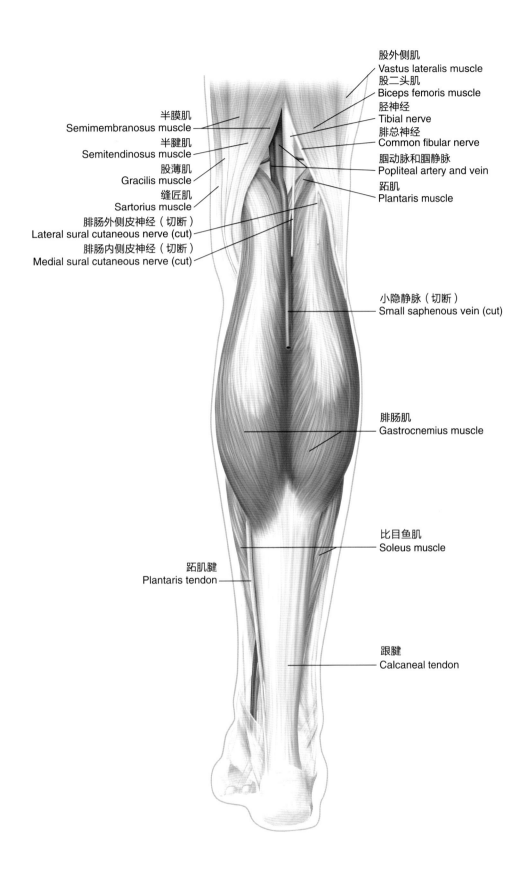

股外侧肌
Vastus lateralis muscle

股二头肌
Biceps femoris muscle

胫神经
Tibial nerve

腓总神经
Common fibular nerve

腘动脉和腘静脉
Popliteal artery and vein

跖肌
Plantaris muscle

半膜肌
Semimembranosus muscle

半腱肌
Semitendinosus muscle

股薄肌
Gracilis muscle

缝匠肌
Sartorius muscle

腓肠外侧皮神经（切断）
Lateral sural cutaneous nerve (cut)

腓肠内侧皮神经（切断）
Medial sural cutaneous nerve (cut)

小隐静脉（切断）
Small saphenous vein (cut)

腓肠肌
Gastrocnemius muscle

比目鱼肌
Soleus muscle

跖肌腱
Plantaris tendon

跟腱
Calcaneal tendon

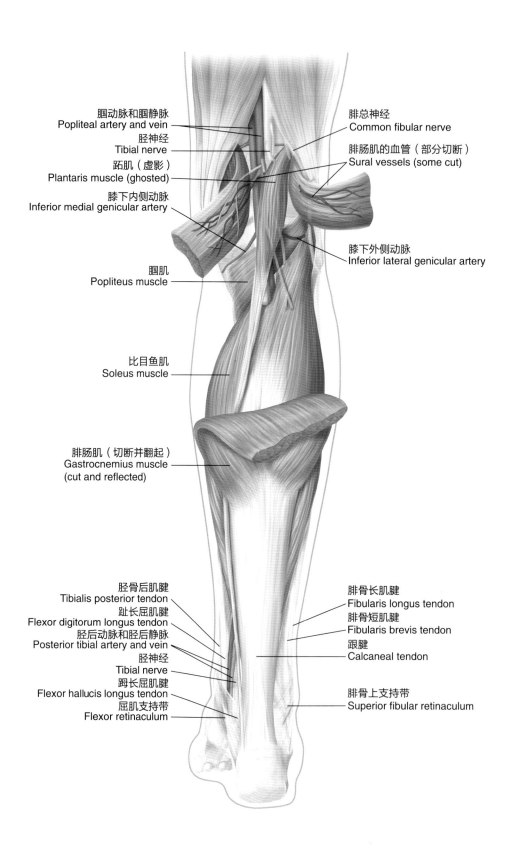

腘动脉和腘静脉
Popliteal artery and vein

胫神经
Tibial nerve

跖肌（虚影）
Plantaris muscle (ghosted)

膝下内侧动脉
Inferior medial genicular artery

腘肌
Popliteus muscle

比目鱼肌
Soleus muscle

腓肠肌（切断并翻起）
Gastrocnemius muscle
(cut and reflected)

腓总神经
Common fibular nerve

腓肠肌的血管（部分切断）
Sural vessels (some cut)

膝下外侧动脉
Inferior lateral genicular artery

胫骨后肌腱
Tibialis posterior tendon

趾长屈肌腱
Flexor digitorum longus tendon

胫后动脉和胫后静脉
Posterior tibial artery and vein

胫神经
Tibial nerve

蹞长屈肌腱
Flexor hallucis longus tendon

屈肌支持带
Flexor retinaculum

腓骨长肌腱
Fibularis longus tendon

腓骨短肌腱
Fibularis brevis tendon

跟腱
Calcaneal tendon

腓骨上支持带
Superior fibular retinaculum

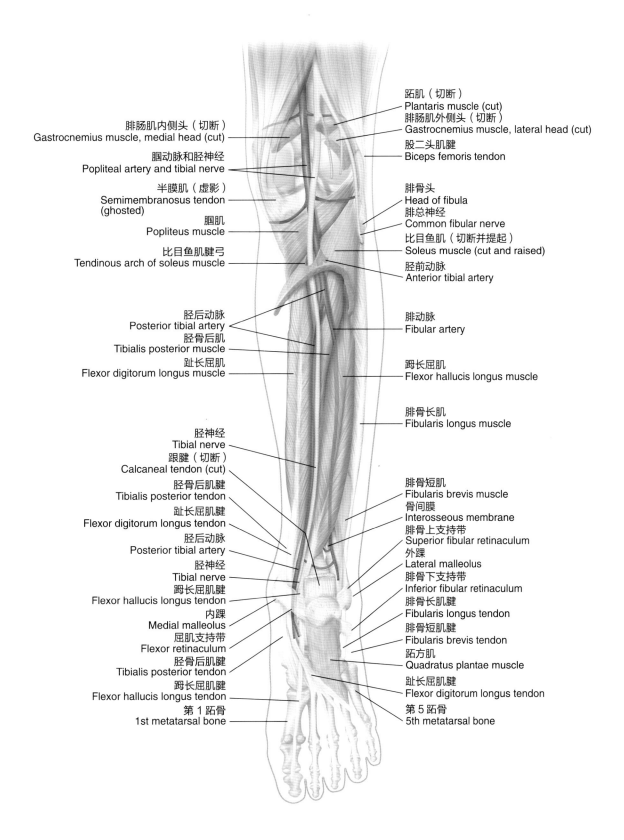

腓肠肌内侧头（切断）
Gastrocnemius muscle, medial head (cut)

腘动脉和胫神经
Popliteal artery and tibial nerve

半膜肌（虚影）
Semimembranosus tendon (ghosted)

腘肌
Popliteus muscle

比目鱼肌腱弓
Tendinous arch of soleus muscle

胫后动脉
Posterior tibial artery

胫骨后肌
Tibialis posterior muscle

趾长屈肌
Flexor digitorum longus muscle

胫神经
Tibial nerve

跟腱（切断）
Calcaneal tendon (cut)

胫骨后肌腱
Tibialis posterior tendon

趾长屈肌腱
Flexor digitorum longus tendon

胫后动脉
Posterior tibial artery

胫神经
Tibial nerve

跛长屈肌腱
Flexor hallucis longus tendon

内踝
Medial malleolus

屈肌支持带
Flexor retinaculum

胫骨后肌腱
Tibialis posterior tendon

跛长屈肌腱
Flexor hallucis longus tendon

第 1 跖骨
1st metatarsal bone

跖肌（切断）
Plantaris muscle (cut)

腓肠肌外侧头（切断）
Gastrocnemius muscle, lateral head (cut)

股二头肌腱
Biceps femoris tendon

腓骨头
Head of fibula

腓总神经
Common fibular nerve

比目鱼肌（切断并提起）
Soleus muscle (cut and raised)

胫前动脉
Anterior tibial artery

腓动脉
Fibular artery

跛长屈肌
Flexor hallucis longus muscle

腓骨长肌
Fibularis longus muscle

腓骨短肌
Fibularis brevis muscle

骨间膜
Interosseous membrane

腓骨上支持带
Superior fibular retinaculum

外踝
Lateral malleolus

腓骨下支持带
Inferior fibular retinaculum

腓骨长肌腱
Fibularis longus tendon

腓骨短肌腱
Fibularis brevis tendon

跖方肌
Quadratus plantae muscle

趾长屈肌腱
Flexor digitorum longus tendon

第 5 跖骨
5th metatarsal bone

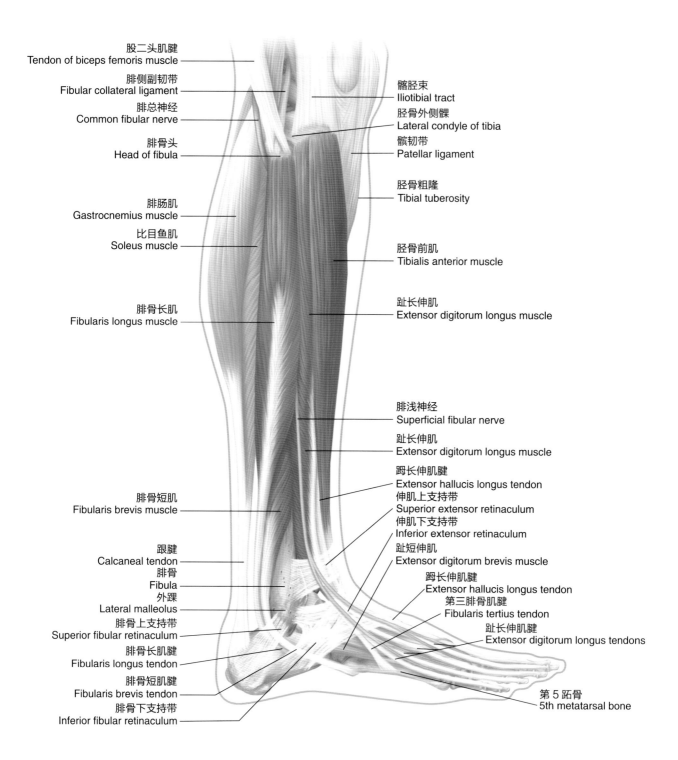

股二头肌腱
Tendon of biceps femoris muscle

腓侧副韧带
Fibular collateral ligament

腓总神经
Common fibular nerve

腓骨头
Head of fibula

腓肠肌
Gastrocnemius muscle

比目鱼肌
Soleus muscle

腓骨长肌
Fibularis longus muscle

腓骨短肌
Fibularis brevis muscle

跟腱
Calcaneal tendon

腓骨
Fibula

外踝
Lateral malleolus

腓骨上支持带
Superior fibular retinaculum

腓骨长肌腱
Fibularis longus tendon

腓骨短肌腱
Fibularis brevis tendon

腓骨下支持带
Inferior fibular retinaculum

髂胫束
Iliotibial tract

胫骨外侧髁
Lateral condyle of tibia

髌韧带
Patellar ligament

胫骨粗隆
Tibial tuberosity

胫骨前肌
Tibialis anterior muscle

趾长伸肌
Extensor digitorum longus muscle

腓浅神经
Superficial fibular nerve

趾长伸肌
Extensor digitorum longus muscle

踇长伸肌腱
Extensor hallucis longus tendon

伸肌上支持带
Superior extensor retinaculum

伸肌下支持带
Inferior extensor retinaculum

趾短伸肌
Extensor digitorum brevis muscle

踇长伸肌腱
Extensor hallucis longus tendon

第三腓骨肌腱
Fibularis tertius tendon

趾长伸肌腱
Extensor digitorum longus tendons

第 5 跖骨
5th metatarsal bone

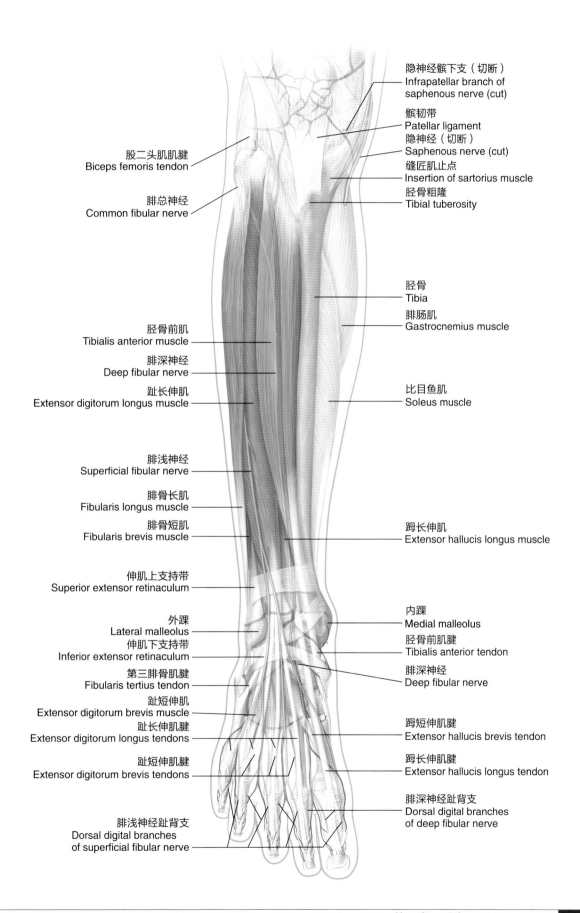

隐神经髌下支（切断）
Infrapatellar branch of
saphenous nerve (cut)

髌韧带
Patellar ligament
隐神经（切断）
Saphenous nerve (cut)

缝匠肌止点
Insertion of sartorius muscle

胫骨粗隆
Tibial tuberosity

股二头肌肌腱
Biceps femoris tendon

腓总神经
Common fibular nerve

胫骨
Tibia

腓肠肌
Gastrocnemius muscle

胫骨前肌
Tibialis anterior muscle

腓深神经
Deep fibular nerve

趾长伸肌
Extensor digitorum longus muscle

比目鱼肌
Soleus muscle

腓浅神经
Superficial fibular nerve

腓骨长肌
Fibularis longus muscle

腓骨短肌
Fibularis brevis muscle

踇长伸肌
Extensor hallucis longus muscle

伸肌上支持带
Superior extensor retinaculum

外踝
Lateral malleolus
伸肌下支持带
Inferior extensor retinaculum

内踝
Medial malleolus

胫骨前肌腱
Tibialis anterior tendon

腓深神经
Deep fibular nerve

第三腓骨肌腱
Fibularis tertius tendon

趾短伸肌
Extensor digitorum brevis muscle
趾长伸肌腱
Extensor digitorum longus tendons

踇短伸肌腱
Extensor hallucis brevis tendon

趾短伸肌腱
Extensor digitorum brevis tendons

踇长伸肌腱
Extensor hallucis longus tendon

腓深神经趾背支
Dorsal digital branches
of deep fibular nerve

腓浅神经趾背支
Dorsal digital branches
of superficial fibular nerve

图 3-38　小腿的动脉　Arteries of the Leg

A. 后面观
Posterior view

B. 前面观
Anterior view

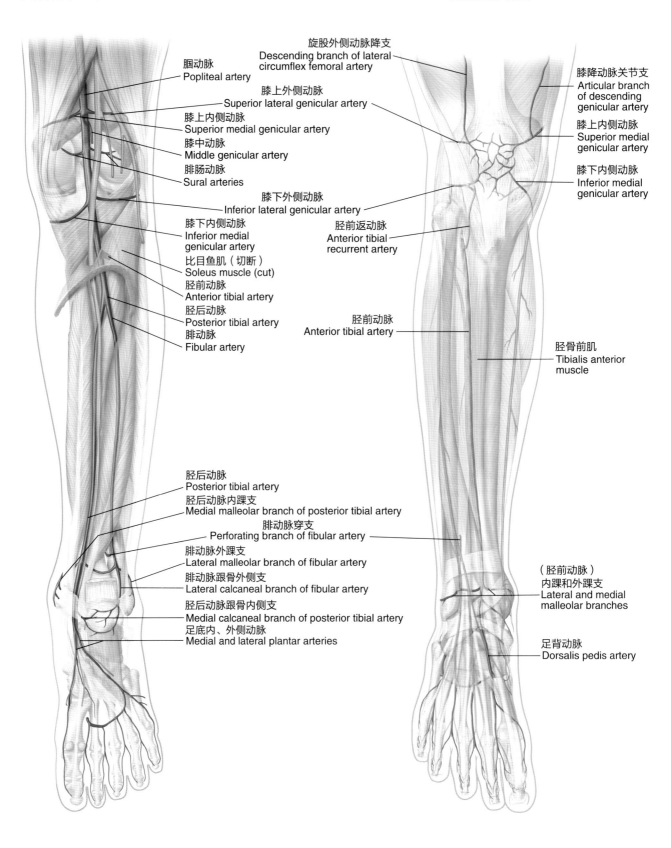

旋股外侧动脉降支
Descending branch of lateral
circumflex femoral artery

腘动脉
Popliteal artery

膝上外侧动脉
Superior lateral genicular artery

膝上内侧动脉
Superior medial genicular artery

膝中动脉
Middle genicular artery

腓肠动脉
Sural arteries

膝下外侧动脉
Inferior lateral genicular artery

膝下内侧动脉
Inferior medial
genicular artery

比目鱼肌（切断）
Soleus muscle (cut)

胫前动脉
Anterior tibial artery

胫后动脉
Posterior tibial artery

腓动脉
Fibular artery

膝降动脉关节支
Articular branch
of descending
genicular artery

膝上内侧动脉
Superior medial
genicular artery

膝下内侧动脉
Inferior medial
genicular artery

胫前返动脉
Anterior tibial
recurrent artery

胫前动脉
Anterior tibial artery

胫骨前肌
Tibialis anterior
muscle

胫后动脉
Posterior tibial artery

胫后动脉内踝支
Medial malleolar branch of posterior tibial artery

腓动脉穿支
Perforating branch of fibular artery

腓动脉外踝支
Lateral malleolar branch of fibular artery

腓动脉跟骨外侧支
Lateral calcaneal branch of fibular artery

胫后动脉跟骨内侧支
Medial calcaneal branch of posterior tibial artery

足底内、外侧动脉
Medial and lateral plantar arteries

（胫前动脉）
内踝和外踝支
Lateral and medial
malleolar branches

足背动脉
Dorsalis pedis artery

A. 后面观
Posterior view

B. 前面观
Anterior view

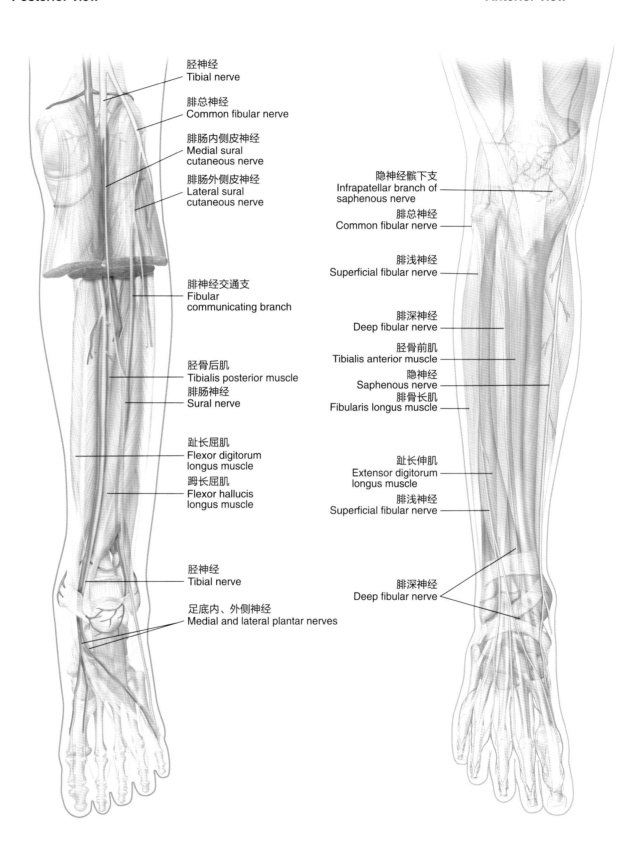

胫神经
Tibial nerve

腓总神经
Common fibular nerve

腓肠内侧皮神经
Medial sural
cutaneous nerve

腓肠外侧皮神经
Lateral sural
cutaneous nerve

腓神经交通支
Fibular
communicating branch

胫骨后肌
Tibialis posterior muscle

腓肠神经
Sural nerve

趾长屈肌
Flexor digitorum
longus muscle

踇长屈肌
Flexor hallucis
longus muscle

胫神经
Tibial nerve

足底内、外侧神经
Medial and lateral plantar nerves

隐神经髌下支
Infrapatellar branch of
saphenous nerve

腓总神经
Common fibular nerve

腓浅神经
Superficial fibular nerve

腓深神经
Deep fibular nerve

胫骨前肌
Tibialis anterior muscle

隐神经
Saphenous nerve

腓骨长肌
Fibularis longus muscle

趾长伸肌
Extensor digitorum
longus muscle

腓浅神经
Superficial fibular nerve

腓深神经
Deep fibular nerve

图 3-40 足骨 **Skeleton of the Foot**

A. 背面观
Dorsal view

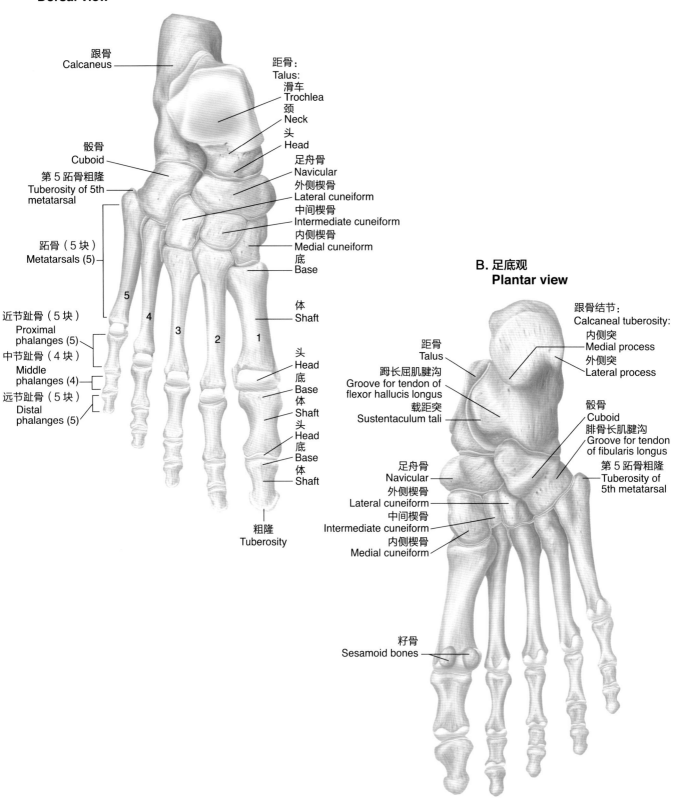

跟骨
Calcaneus

距骨：
Talus:
　滑车
　Trochlea
　颈
　Neck
　头
　Head

骰骨
Cuboid

足舟骨
Navicular

第 5 跖骨粗隆
Tuberosity of 5th
metatarsal

外侧楔骨
Lateral cuneiform

中间楔骨
Intermediate cuneiform

内侧楔骨
Medial cuneiform

跖骨（5 块）
Metatarsals (5)

底
Base

体
Shaft

B. 足底观
Plantar view

近节趾骨（5 块）
Proximal
phalanges (5)

中节趾骨（4 块）
Middle
phalanges (4)

远节趾骨（5 块）
Distal
phalanges (5)

头
Head

底
Base

体
Shaft

头
Head

底
Base

体
Shaft

粗隆
Tuberosity

距骨
Talus

跟骨结节：
Calcaneal tuberosity:
　内侧突
　Medial process
　外侧突
　Lateral process

蹰长屈肌腱沟
Groove for tendon of
flexor hallucis longus

载距突
Sustentaculum tali

骰骨
Cuboid

腓骨长肌腱沟
Groove for tendon
of fibularis longus

第 5 跖骨粗隆
Tuberosity of
5th metatarsal

足舟骨
Navicular

外侧楔骨
Lateral cuneiform

中间楔骨
Intermediate cuneiform

内侧楔骨
Medial cuneiform

籽骨
Sesamoid bones

A. 内侧面观
Medial view

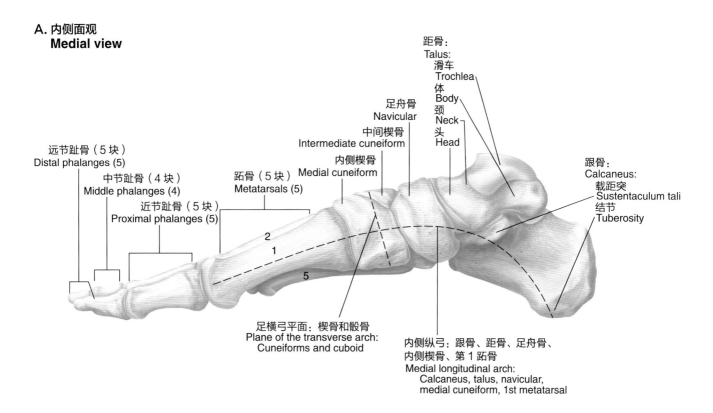

距骨：
Talus:
滑车
Trochlea
体
Body
颈
Neck
头
Head

足舟骨
Navicular

中间楔骨
Intermediate cuneiform

内侧楔骨
Medial cuneiform

跟骨：
Calcaneus:
载距突
Sustentaculum tali
结节
Tuberosity

远节趾骨（5 块）
Distal phalanges (5)

中节趾骨（4 块）
Middle phalanges (4)

近节趾骨（5 块）
Proximal phalanges (5)

跖骨（5 块）
Metatarsals (5)

2
1
5

足横弓平面：楔骨和骰骨
Plane of the transverse arch:
Cuneiforms and cuboid

内侧纵弓：跟骨、距骨、足舟骨、
内侧楔骨、第 1 跖骨
Medial longitudinal arch:
Calcaneus, talus, navicular,
medial cuneiform, 1st metatarsal

B. 外侧面观
Lateral view

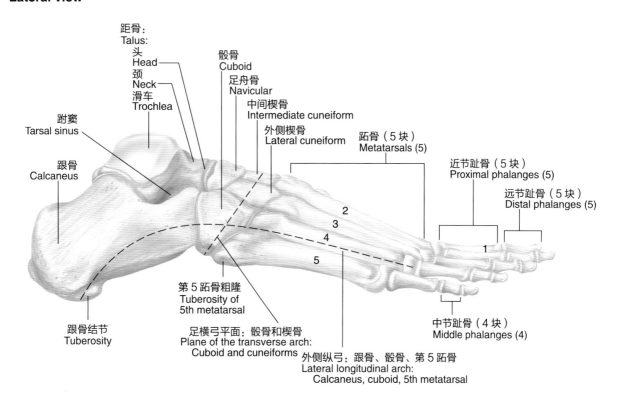

距骨：
Talus:
头
Head
颈
Neck
滑车
Trochlea

骰骨
Cuboid

足舟骨
Navicular

中间楔骨
Intermediate cuneiform

外侧楔骨
Lateral cuneiform

跗窦
Tarsal sinus

跟骨
Calcaneus

跖骨（5 块）
Metatarsals (5)

近节趾骨（5 块）
Proximal phalanges (5)

远节趾骨（5 块）
Distal phalanges (5)

2
3
4
5
1

第 5 跖骨粗隆
Tuberosity of
5th metatarsal

跟骨结节
Tuberosity

足横弓平面：骰骨和楔骨
Plane of the transverse arch:
Cuboid and cuneiforms

中节趾骨（4 块）
Middle phalanges (4)

外侧纵弓：跟骨、骰骨、第 5 跖骨
Lateral longitudinal arch:
Calcaneus, cuboid, 5th metatarsal

图 3-42　足肌群附着点，足背观　**Muscle Attachments of the Foot, Dorsal Surface**

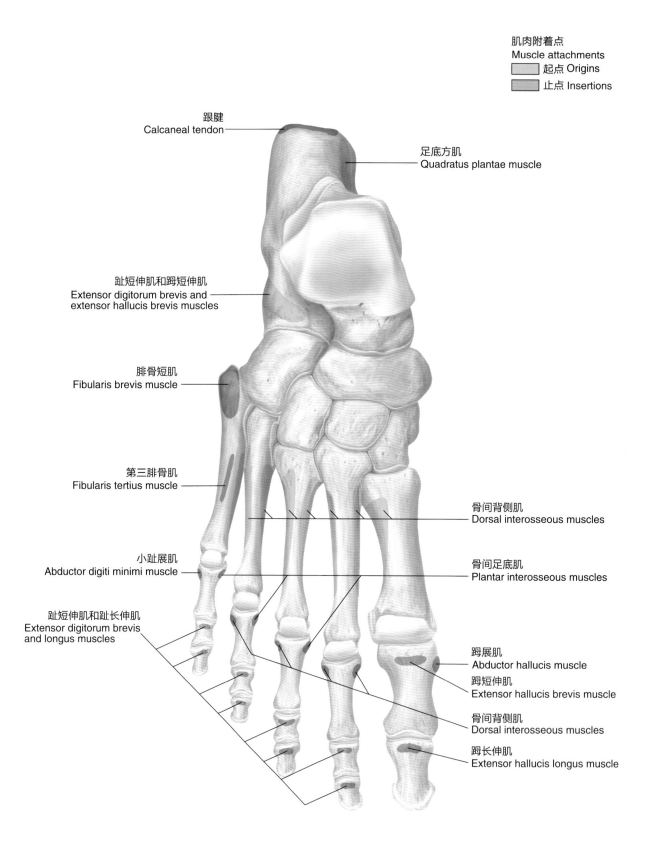

肌肉附着点
Muscle attachments
起点 Origins
止点 Insertions

跟腱
Calcaneal tendon

足底方肌
Quadratus plantae muscle

趾短伸肌和踇短伸肌
Extensor digitorum brevis and extensor hallucis brevis muscles

腓骨短肌
Fibularis brevis muscle

第三腓骨肌
Fibularis tertius muscle

骨间背侧肌
Dorsal interosseous muscles

小趾展肌
Abductor digiti minimi muscle

骨间足底肌
Plantar interosseous muscles

趾短伸肌和趾长伸肌
Extensor digitorum brevis and longus muscles

踇展肌
Abductor hallucis muscle

踇短伸肌
Extensor hallucis brevis muscle

骨间背侧肌
Dorsal interosseous muscles

踇长伸肌
Extensor hallucis longus muscle

肌肉附着点
Muscle attachments

□ 起点 Origins

■ 止点 Insertions

展肌
Abductor hallucis muscle

趾短屈肌
Flexor digitorum brevis muscle

小趾展肌
Abductor digiti minimi muscle

足底方肌
Quadratus plantae muscle

胫骨后肌
Tibialis posterior muscle

腓骨长肌
Fibularis longus muscle

胫骨前肌
Tibialis anterior muscle

踇短屈肌
Flexor hallucis brevis muscle

踇展肌和短屈肌外侧头
Adductor hallucis muscle and lateral head of flexor hallucis brevis muscle

踇展肌和短屈肌内侧头
Abductor hallucis muscle and medial head of flexor hallucis brevis muscle

踇长屈肌
Flexor hallucis longus muscle

小趾短屈肌
Flexor digiti minimi brevis muscle

踇短屈肌
Flexor hallucis brevis muscle

踇展肌（斜头）
Adductor hallucis muscle (oblique head)

骨间足底肌
Plantar interosseous muscles

小趾展肌和小趾短屈肌
Abductor digiti minimi and flexor digiti minimi brevis muscles

骨间足底肌
Plantar interosseous muscles

趾短屈肌
Flexor digitorum brevis muscle

趾长屈肌
Flexor digitorum longus muscle

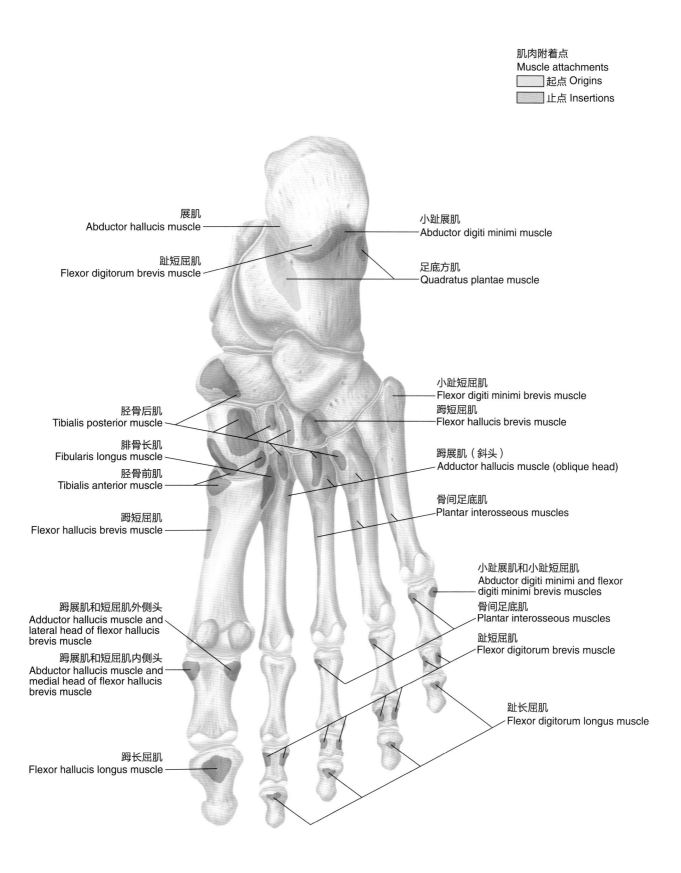

图 3-44

足背皮神经和浅静脉
Cutaneous Nerves and Superficial Veins of the Dorsum of the Foot

A. 解剖
Dissection

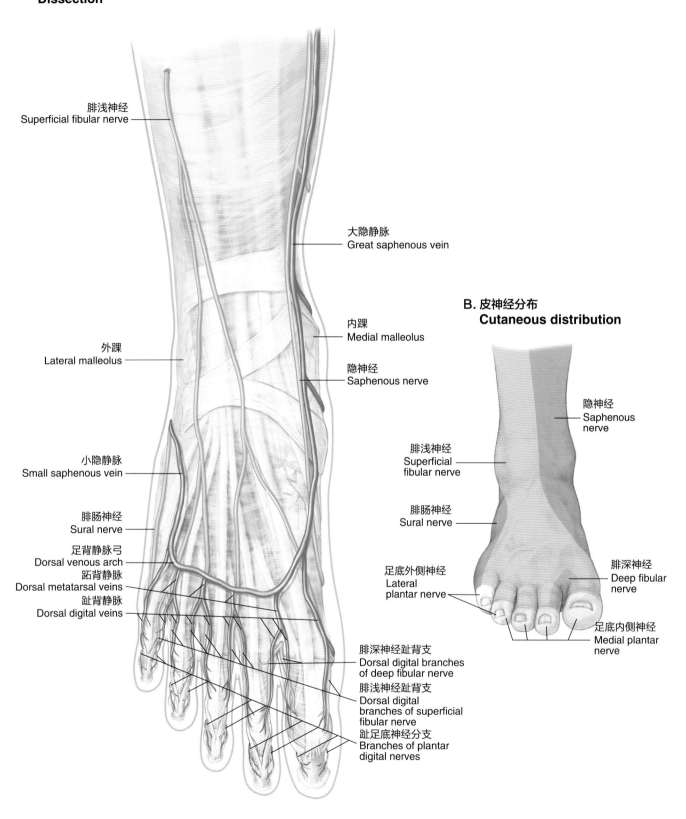

腓浅神经
Superficial fibular nerve

大隐静脉
Great saphenous vein

内踝
Medial malleolus

外踝
Lateral malleolus

隐神经
Saphenous nerve

小隐静脉
Small saphenous vein

腓肠神经
Sural nerve

足背静脉弓
Dorsal venous arch

跖背静脉
Dorsal metatarsal veins

趾背静脉
Dorsal digital veins

腓深神经趾背支
Dorsal digital branches
of deep fibular nerve

腓浅神经趾背支
Dorsal digital
branches of superficial
fibular nerve

趾足底神经分支
Branches of plantar
digital nerves

B. 皮神经分布
Cutaneous distribution

隐神经
Saphenous
nerve

腓浅神经
Superficial
fibular nerve

腓肠神经
Sural nerve

足底外侧神经
Lateral
plantar nerve

腓深神经
Deep fibular
nerve

足底内侧神经
Medial plantar
nerve

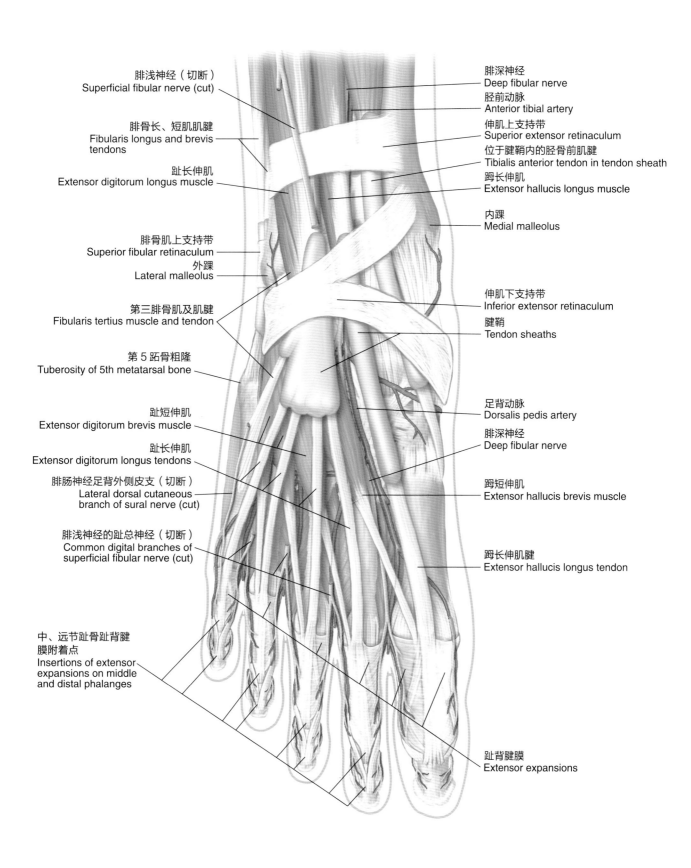

腓浅神经（切断）
Superficial fibular nerve (cut)

腓骨长、短肌肌腱
Fibularis longus and brevis tendons

趾长伸肌
Extensor digitorum longus muscle

腓骨肌上支持带
Superior fibular retinaculum

外踝
Lateral malleolus

第三腓骨肌及肌腱
Fibularis tertius muscle and tendon

第 5 跖骨粗隆
Tuberosity of 5th metatarsal bone

趾短伸肌
Extensor digitorum brevis muscle

趾长伸肌
Extensor digitorum longus tendons

腓肠神经足背外侧皮支（切断）
Lateral dorsal cutaneous branch of sural nerve (cut)

腓浅神经的趾总神经（切断）
Common digital branches of superficial fibular nerve (cut)

中、远节趾骨趾背腱膜附着点
Insertions of extensor expansions on middle and distal phalanges

腓深神经
Deep fibular nerve

胫前动脉
Anterior tibial artery

伸肌上支持带
Superior extensor retinaculum

位于腱鞘内的胫骨前肌腱
Tibialis anterior tendon in tendon sheath

踇长伸肌
Extensor hallucis longus muscle

内踝
Medial malleolus

伸肌下支持带
Inferior extensor retinaculum

腱鞘
Tendon sheaths

足背动脉
Dorsalis pedis artery

腓深神经
Deep fibular nerve

踇短伸肌
Extensor hallucis brevis muscle

踇长伸肌腱
Extensor hallucis longus tendon

趾背腱膜
Extensor expansions

图 3-46　足背，深层解剖　Dorsum of the Foot, Deep Dissection

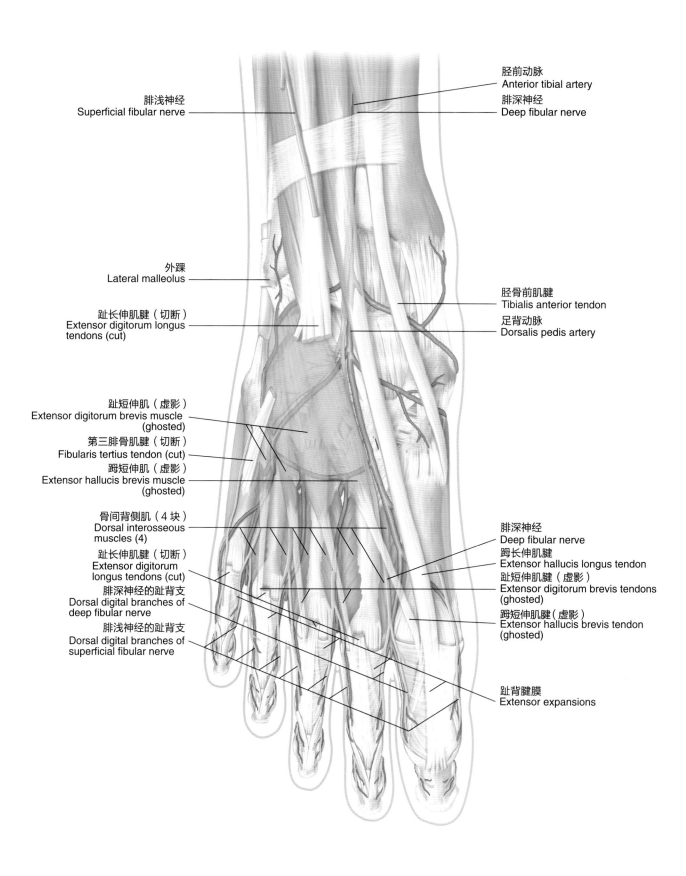

腓浅神经
Superficial fibular nerve

胫前动脉
Anterior tibial artery

腓深神经
Deep fibular nerve

外踝
Lateral malleolus

胫骨前肌腱
Tibialis anterior tendon

足背动脉
Dorsalis pedis artery

趾长伸肌腱（切断）
Extensor digitorum longus
tendons (cut)

趾短伸肌（虚影）
Extensor digitorum brevis muscle
(ghosted)

第三腓骨肌腱（切断）
Fibularis tertius tendon (cut)

踇短伸肌（虚影）
Extensor hallucis brevis muscle
(ghosted)

骨间背侧肌（4 块）
Dorsal interosseous
muscles (4)

趾长伸肌腱（切断）
Extensor digitorum
longus tendons (cut)

腓深神经的趾背支
Dorsal digital branches of
deep fibular nerve

腓浅神经的趾背支
Dorsal digital branches of
superficial fibular nerve

腓深神经
Deep fibular nerve

踇长伸肌腱
Extensor hallucis longus tendon

趾短伸肌腱（虚影）
Extensor digitorum brevis tendons
(ghosted)

踇短伸肌腱（虚影）
Extensor hallucis brevis tendon
(ghosted)

趾背腱膜
Extensor expansions

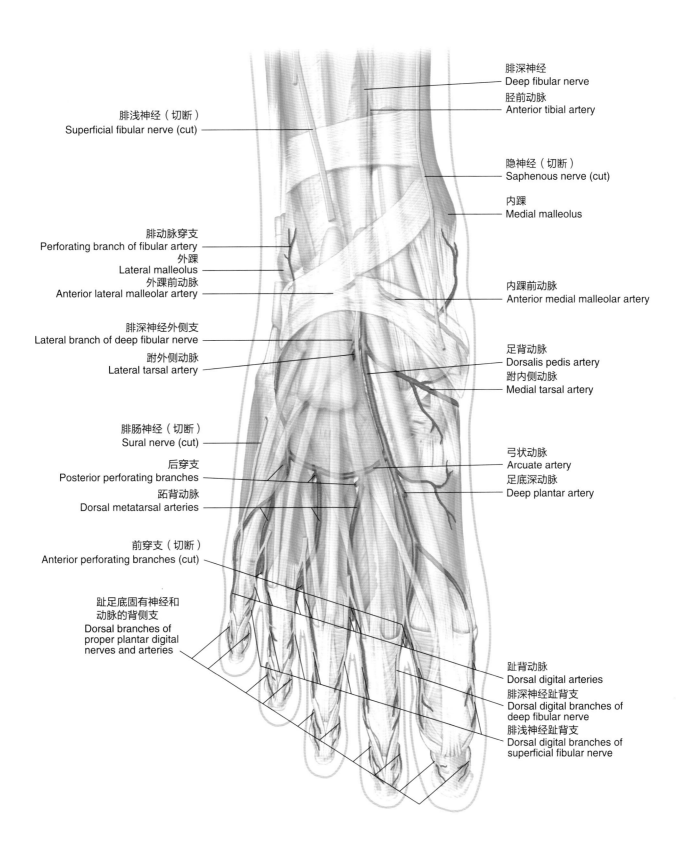

腓深神经
Deep fibular nerve

胫前动脉
Anterior tibial artery

腓浅神经（切断）
Superficial fibular nerve (cut)

隐神经（切断）
Saphenous nerve (cut)

内踝
Medial malleolus

腓动脉穿支
Perforating branch of fibular artery

外踝
Lateral malleolus

外踝前动脉
Anterior lateral malleolar artery

内踝前动脉
Anterior medial malleolar artery

腓深神经外侧支
Lateral branch of deep fibular nerve

跗外侧动脉
Lateral tarsal artery

足背动脉
Dorsalis pedis artery

跗内侧动脉
Medial tarsal artery

腓肠神经（切断）
Sural nerve (cut)

后穿支
Posterior perforating branches

弓状动脉
Arcuate artery

足底深动脉
Deep plantar artery

跖背动脉
Dorsal metatarsal arteries

前穿支（切断）
Anterior perforating branches (cut)

趾足底固有神经和
动脉的背侧支
Dorsal branches of
proper plantar digital
nerves and arteries

趾背动脉
Dorsal digital arteries

腓深神经趾背支
Dorsal digital branches of
deep fibular nerve

腓浅神经趾背支
Dorsal digital branches of
superficial fibular nerve

图 3-48　足底的皮神经 Cutaneous Nerves of the Sole of the Foot

A. 解剖
Dissection

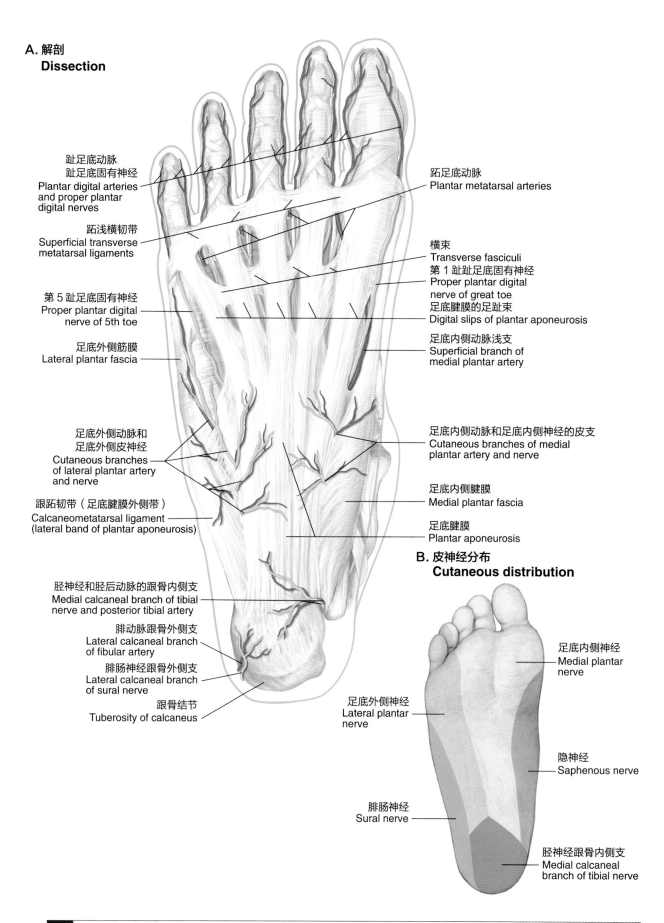

趾足底动脉
趾足底固有神经
Plantar digital arteries
and proper plantar
digital nerves

跖浅横韧带
Superficial transverse
metatarsal ligaments

第 5 趾趾足底固有神经
Proper plantar digital
nerve of 5th toe

足底外侧筋膜
Lateral plantar fascia

足底外侧动脉和
足底外侧皮神经
Cutaneous branches
of lateral plantar artery
and nerve

跟跖韧带（足底腱膜外侧带）
Calcaneometatarsal ligament
(lateral band of plantar aponeurosis)

胫神经和胫后动脉的跟骨内侧支
Medial calcaneal branch of tibial
nerve and posterior tibial artery

腓动脉跟骨外侧支
Lateral calcaneal branch
of fibular artery

腓肠神经跟骨外侧支
Lateral calcaneal branch
of sural nerve

跟骨结节
Tuberosity of calcaneus

跖足底动脉
Plantar metatarsal arteries

横束
Transverse fasciculi
第 1 趾趾足底固有神经
Proper plantar digital
nerve of great toe
足底腱膜的足趾束
Digital slips of plantar aponeurosis

足底内侧动脉浅支
Superficial branch of
medial plantar artery

足底内侧动脉和足底内侧神经的皮支
Cutaneous branches of medial
plantar artery and nerve

足底内侧腱膜
Medial plantar fascia

足底腱膜
Plantar aponeurosis

B. 皮神经分布
Cutaneous distribution

足底内侧神经
Medial plantar
nerve

足底外侧神经
Lateral plantar
nerve

隐神经
Saphenous nerve

腓肠神经
Sural nerve

胫神经跟骨内侧支
Medial calcaneal
branch of tibial nerve

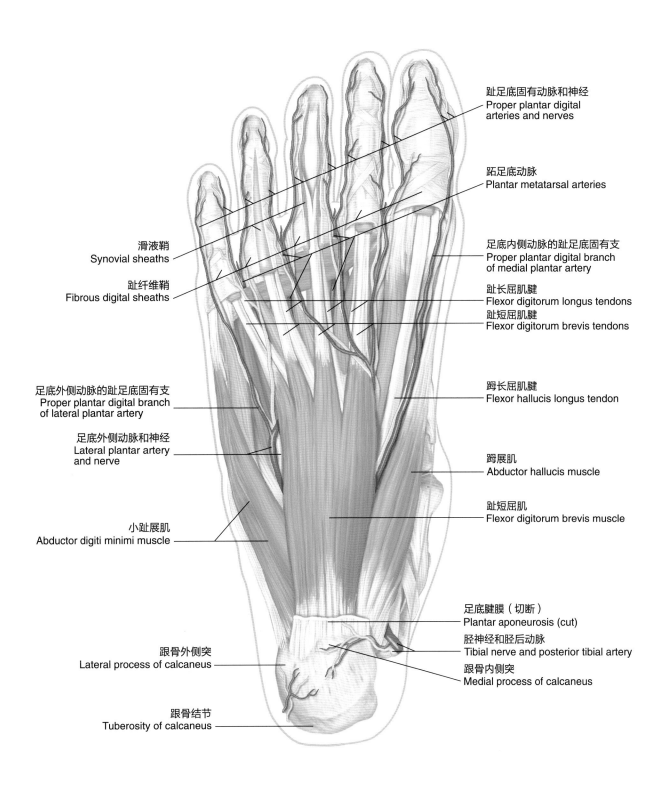

趾足底固有动脉和神经
Proper plantar digital arteries and nerves

跖足底动脉
Plantar metatarsal arteries

滑液鞘
Synovial sheaths

趾纤维鞘
Fibrous digital sheaths

足底内侧动脉的趾足底固有支
Proper plantar digital branch of medial plantar artery

趾长屈肌腱
Flexor digitorum longus tendons

趾短屈肌腱
Flexor digitorum brevis tendons

足底外侧动脉的趾足底固有支
Proper plantar digital branch of lateral plantar artery

足底外侧动脉和神经
Lateral plantar artery and nerve

小趾展肌
Abductor digiti minimi muscle

𬌗长屈肌腱
Flexor hallucis longus tendon

𬌗展肌
Abductor hallucis muscle

趾短屈肌
Flexor digitorum brevis muscle

足底腱膜（切断）
Plantar aponeurosis (cut)

胫神经和胫后动脉
Tibial nerve and posterior tibial artery

跟骨内侧突
Medial process of calcaneus

跟骨外侧突
Lateral process of calcaneus

跟骨结节
Tuberosity of calcaneus

图 3-50   足底肌，第二层   Muscles of the Sole of the Foot, Second Layer

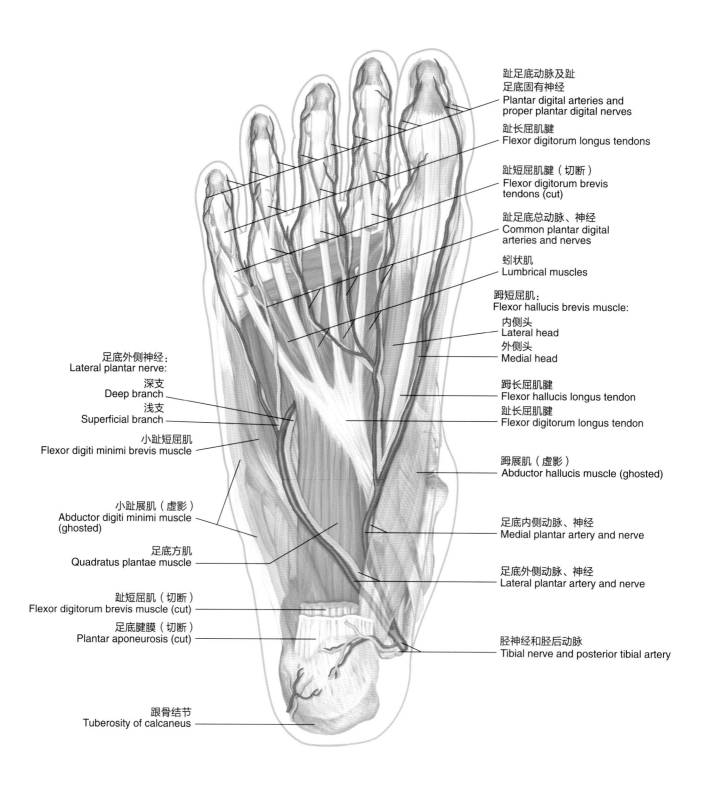

趾足底动脉及趾
足底固有神经
Plantar digital arteries and
proper plantar digital nerves

趾长屈肌腱
Flexor digitorum longus tendons

趾短屈肌腱（切断）
Flexor digitorum brevis
tendons (cut)

趾足底总动脉、神经
Common plantar digital
arteries and nerves

蚓状肌
Lumbrical muscles

踇短屈肌：
Flexor hallucis brevis muscle:

内侧头
Lateral head

外侧头
Medial head

踇长屈肌腱
Flexor hallucis longus tendon

趾长屈肌腱
Flexor digitorum longus tendon

踇展肌（虚影）
Abductor hallucis muscle (ghosted)

足底内侧动脉、神经
Medial plantar artery and nerve

足底外侧动脉、神经
Lateral plantar artery and nerve

胫神经和胫后动脉
Tibial nerve and posterior tibial artery

足底外侧神经：
Lateral plantar nerve:

深支
Deep branch

浅支
Superficial branch

小趾短屈肌
Flexor digiti minimi brevis muscle

小趾展肌（虚影）
Abductor digiti minimi muscle
(ghosted)

足底方肌
Quadratus plantae muscle

趾短屈肌（切断）
Flexor digitorum brevis muscle (cut)

足底腱膜（切断）
Plantar aponeurosis (cut)

跟骨结节
Tuberosity of calcaneus

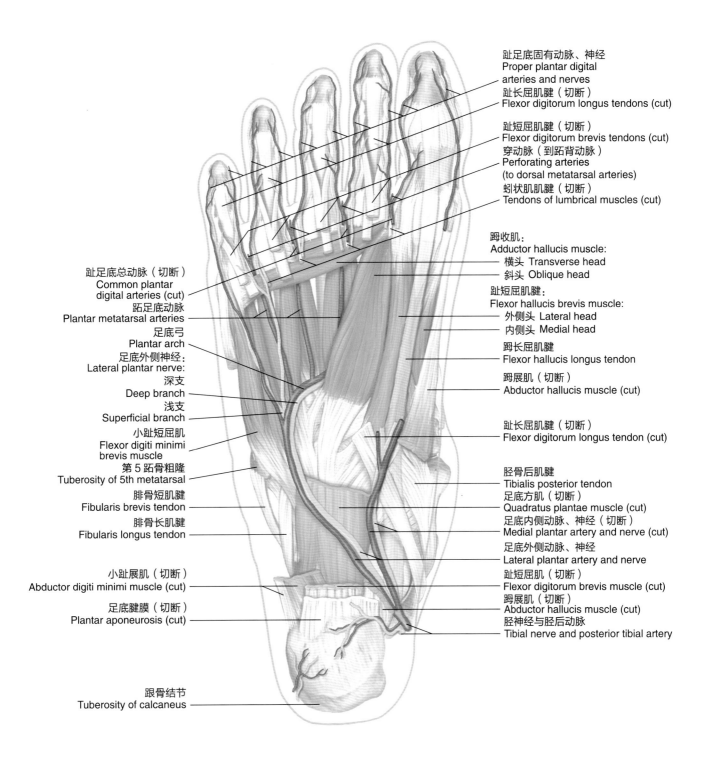

趾足底固有动脉、神经
Proper plantar digital
arteries and nerves

趾长屈肌腱（切断）
Flexor digitorum longus tendons (cut)

趾短屈肌腱（切断）
Flexor digitorum brevis tendons (cut)

穿动脉（到跖背动脉）
Perforating arteries
(to dorsal metatarsal arteries)

蚓状肌肌腱（切断）
Tendons of lumbrical muscles (cut)

踇收肌：
Adductor hallucis muscle:
横头 Transverse head
斜头 Oblique head

趾短屈肌腱：
Flexor hallucis brevis muscle:
外侧头 Lateral head
内侧头 Medial head

踇长屈肌腱
Flexor hallucis longus tendon

踇展肌（切断）
Abductor hallucis muscle (cut)

趾长屈肌腱（切断）
Flexor digitorum longus tendon (cut)

胫骨后肌腱
Tibialis posterior tendon

足底方肌（切断）
Quadratus plantae muscle (cut)

足底内侧动脉、神经（切断）
Medial plantar artery and nerve (cut)

足底外侧动脉、神经
Lateral plantar artery and nerve

趾短屈肌（切断）
Flexor digitorum brevis muscle (cut)

踇展肌（切断）
Abductor hallucis muscle (cut)

胫神经与胫后动脉
Tibial nerve and posterior tibial artery

趾足底总动脉（切断）
Common plantar
digital arteries (cut)

跖足底动脉
Plantar metatarsal arteries

足底弓
Plantar arch

足底外侧神经：
Lateral plantar nerve:
深支
Deep branch
浅支
Superficial branch

小趾短屈肌
Flexor digiti minimi
brevis muscle

第 5 跖骨粗隆
Tuberosity of 5th metatarsal

腓骨短肌腱
Fibularis brevis tendon

腓骨长肌腱
Fibularis longus tendon

小趾展肌（切断）
Abductor digiti minimi muscle (cut)

足底腱膜（切断）
Plantar aponeurosis (cut)

跟骨结节
Tuberosity of calcaneus

图 3-52　足底肌，第四层　Muscles of the Sole of the Foot, Fourth Layer

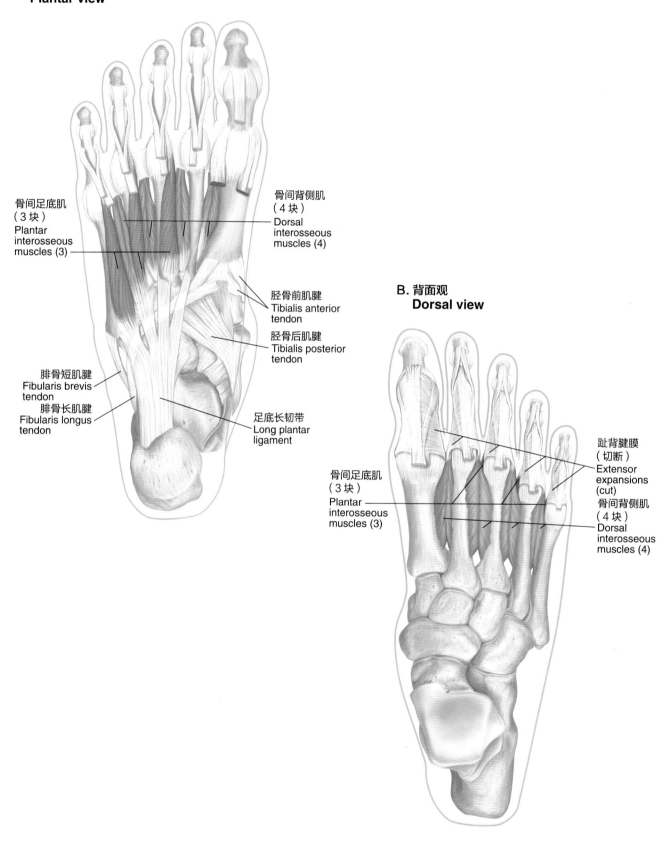

A. 足底观
Plantar view

骨间足底肌
（3 块）
Plantar
interosseous
muscles (3)

骨间背侧肌
（4 块）
Dorsal
interosseous
muscles (4)

胫骨前肌腱
Tibialis anterior
tendon

B. 背面观
Dorsal view

胫骨后肌腱
Tibialis posterior
tendon

腓骨短肌腱
Fibularis brevis
tendon

腓骨长肌腱
Fibularis longus
tendon

足底长韧带
Long plantar
ligament

趾背腱膜
（切断）
Extensor
expansions
(cut)

骨间背侧肌
（4 块）
Dorsal
interosseous
muscles (4)

骨间足底肌
（3 块）
Plantar
interosseous
muscles (3)

A. 动脉
Arteries

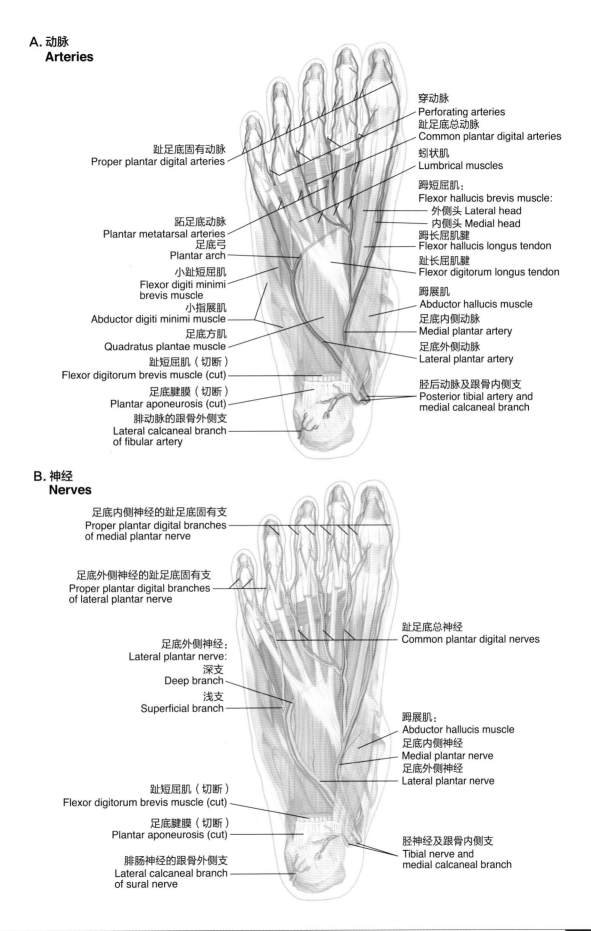

穿动脉
Perforating arteries

趾足底总动脉
Common plantar digital arteries

蚓状肌
Lumbrical muscles

姆短屈肌：
Flexor hallucis brevis muscle:
　外侧头 Lateral head
　内侧头 Medial head

姆长屈肌腱
Flexor hallucis longus tendon

趾长屈肌腱
Flexor digitorum longus tendon

姆展肌
Abductor hallucis muscle

足底内侧动脉
Medial plantar artery

足底外侧动脉
Lateral plantar artery

胫后动脉及跟骨内侧支
Posterior tibial artery and medial calcaneal branch

趾足底固有动脉
Proper plantar digital arteries

跖足底动脉
Plantar metatarsal arteries

足底弓
Plantar arch

小趾短屈肌
Flexor digiti minimi brevis muscle

小指展肌
Abductor digiti minimi muscle

足底方肌
Quadratus plantae muscle

趾短屈肌（切断）
Flexor digitorum brevis muscle (cut)

足底腱膜（切断）
Plantar aponeurosis (cut)

腓动脉的跟骨外侧支
Lateral calcaneal branch of fibular artery

B. 神经
Nerves

足底内侧神经的趾足底固有支
Proper plantar digital branches of medial plantar nerve

足底外侧神经的趾足底固有支
Proper plantar digital branches of lateral plantar nerve

趾足底总神经
Common plantar digital nerves

足底外侧神经：
Lateral plantar nerve:
深支
Deep branch
浅支
Superficial branch

姆展肌：
Abductor hallucis muscle
足底内侧神经
Medial plantar nerve
足底外侧神经
Lateral plantar nerve

趾短屈肌（切断）
Flexor digitorum brevis muscle (cut)

足底腱膜（切断）
Plantar aponeurosis (cut)

腓肠神经的跟骨外侧支
Lateral calcaneal branch of sural nerve

胫神经及跟骨内侧支
Tibial nerve and medial calcaneal branch

图 3-54　髋关节，外部形态　Hip Joint, External Features

A. 前面观
Anterior view

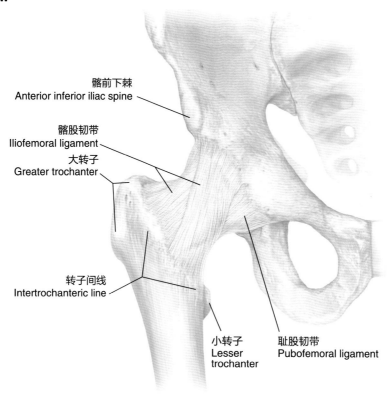

髂前下棘
Anterior inferior iliac spine

髂股韧带
Iliofemoral ligament

大转子
Greater trochanter

转子间线
Intertrochanteric line

小转子
Lesser
trochanter

耻股韧带
Pubofemoral ligament

B. 后面观
Posterior view

髂股韧带
Iliofemoral ligament

坐股韧带
Ischiofemoral ligament

大转子
Greater trochanter

转子间嵴
Intertrochanteric crest

小转子
Lesser trochanter

坐骨棘
Ischial spine

坐骨结节
Ischial tuberosity

A. 外侧面观（打开关节）
Lateral view, joint opened

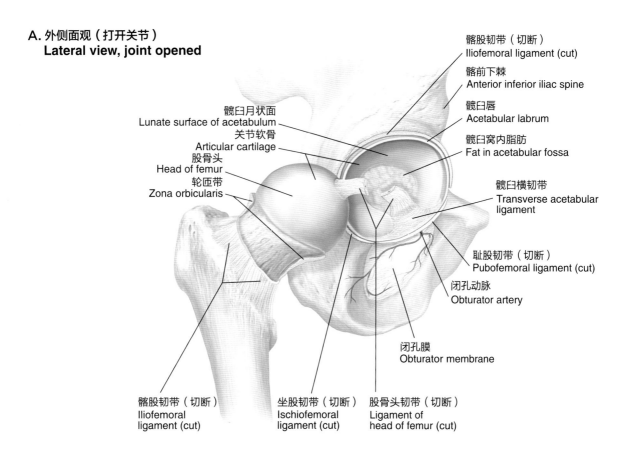

髂股韧带（切断）
Iliofemoral ligament (cut)

髂前下棘
Anterior inferior iliac spine

髋臼唇
Acetabular labrum

髋臼窝内脂肪
Fat in acetabular fossa

髋臼月状面
Lunate surface of acetabulum

关节软骨
Articular cartilage

股骨头
Head of femur

轮匝带
Zona orbicularis

髋臼横韧带
Transverse acetabular ligament

耻股韧带（切断）
Pubofemoral ligament (cut)

闭孔动脉
Obturator artery

闭孔膜
Obturator membrane

髂股韧带（切断）
Iliofemoral ligament (cut)

坐股韧带（切断）
Ischiofemoral ligament (cut)

股骨头韧带（切断）
Ligament of head of femur (cut)

B. 血供
Blood supply

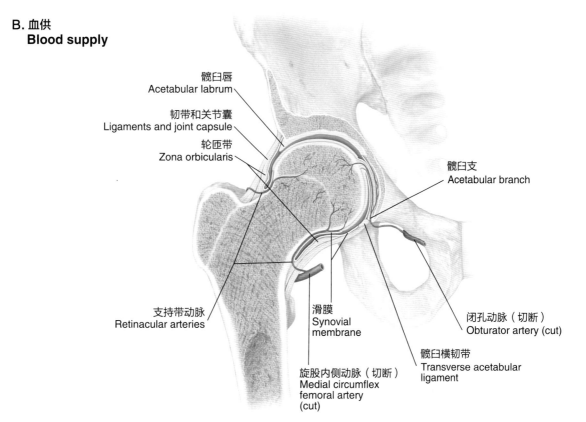

髋臼唇
Acetabular labrum

韧带和关节囊
Ligaments and joint capsule

轮匝带
Zona orbicularis

髋臼支
Acetabular branch

支持带动脉
Retinacular arteries

滑膜
Synovial membrane

旋股内侧动脉（切断）
Medial circumflex femoral artery (cut)

髋臼横韧带
Transverse acetabular ligament

闭孔动脉（切断）
Obturator artery (cut)

图 3-56   膝关节，前面观和后面观   Knee Joint, Anterior and Posterior Views

A. 右膝，前面观
Right knee, anterior view

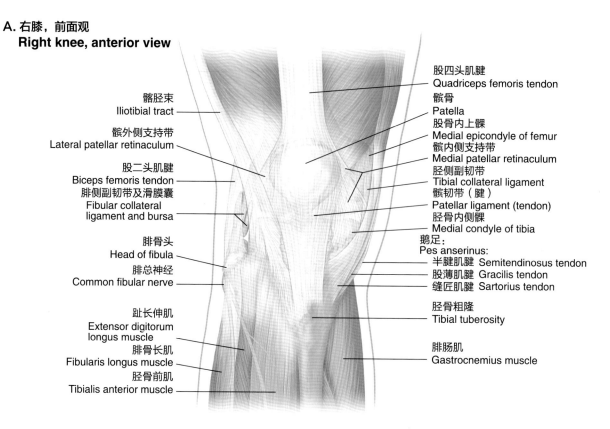

髂胫束
Iliotibial tract

髌外侧支持带
Lateral patellar retinaculum

股二头肌腱
Biceps femoris tendon

腓侧副韧带及滑膜囊
Fibular collateral
ligament and bursa

腓骨头
Head of fibula

腓总神经
Common fibular nerve

趾长伸肌
Extensor digitorum
longus muscle

腓骨长肌
Fibularis longus muscle

胫骨前肌
Tibialis anterior muscle

股四头肌腱
Quadriceps femoris tendon

髌骨
Patella

股骨内上髁
Medial epicondyle of femur

髌内侧支持带
Medial patellar retinaculum

胫侧副韧带
Tibial collateral ligament

髌韧带（腱）
Patellar ligament (tendon)

胫骨内侧髁
Medial condyle of tibia

鹅足：
Pes anserinus:

半腱肌腱 Semitendinosus tendon

股薄肌腱 Gracilis tendon

缝匠肌腱 Sartorius tendon

胫骨粗隆
Tibial tuberosity

腓肠肌
Gastrocnemius muscle

B. 右膝，后面观
Right knee, posterior view

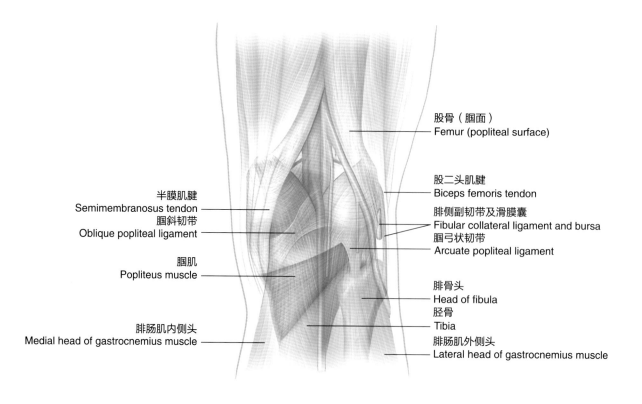

半膜肌腱
Semimembranosus tendon

腘斜韧带
Oblique popliteal ligament

腘肌
Popliteus muscle

腓肠肌内侧头
Medial head of gastrocnemius muscle

股骨（腘面）
Femur (popliteal surface)

股二头肌腱
Biceps femoris tendon

腓侧副韧带及滑膜囊
Fibular collateral ligament and bursa

腘弓状韧带
Arcuate popliteal ligament

腓骨头
Head of fibula

胫骨
Tibia

腓肠肌外侧头
Lateral head of gastrocnemius muscle

A. 右膝，内侧面观
Right knee, medial view

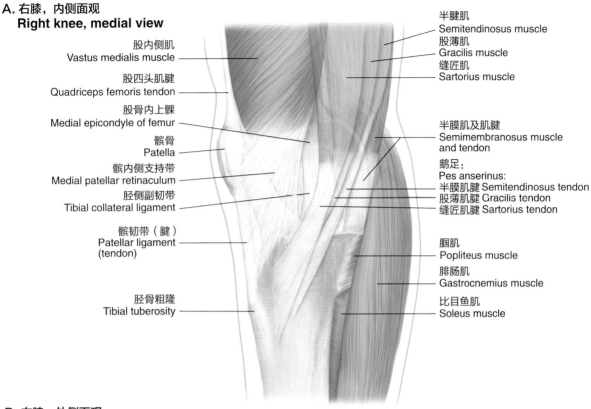

股内侧肌
Vastus medialis muscle

股四头肌腱
Quadriceps femoris tendon

股骨内上髁
Medial epicondyle of femur

髌骨
Patella

髌内侧支持带
Medial patellar retinaculum

胫侧副韧带
Tibial collateral ligament

髌韧带（腱）
Patellar ligament
(tendon)

胫骨粗隆
Tibial tuberosity

半腱肌
Semitendinosus muscle

股薄肌
Gracilis muscle

缝匠肌
Sartorius muscle

半膜肌及肌腱
Semimembranosus muscle
and tendon

鹅足：
Pes anserinus:
半膜肌腱 Semitendinosus tendon
股薄肌腱 Gracilis tendon
缝匠肌腱 Sartorius tendon

腘肌
Popliteus muscle

腓肠肌
Gastrocnemius muscle

比目鱼肌
Soleus muscle

B. 右膝，外侧面观
Right knee, lateral view

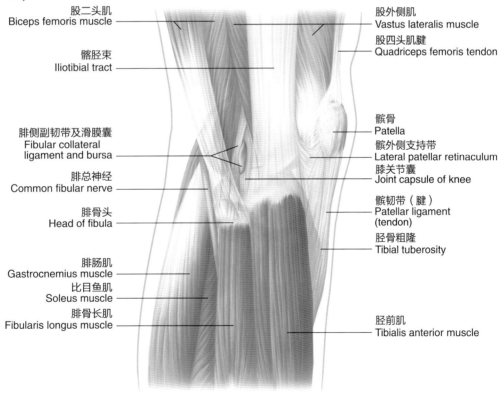

股二头肌
Biceps femoris muscle

髂胫束
Iliotibial tract

腓侧副韧带及滑膜囊
Fibular collateral
ligament and bursa

腓总神经
Common fibular nerve

腓骨头
Head of fibula

腓肠肌
Gastrocnemius muscle

比目鱼肌
Soleus muscle

腓骨长肌
Fibularis longus muscle

股外侧肌
Vastus lateralis muscle

股四头肌腱
Quadriceps femoris tendon

髌骨
Patella

髌外侧支持带
Lateral patellar retinaculum

膝关节囊
Joint capsule of knee

髌韧带（腱）
Patellar ligament
(tendon)

胫骨粗隆
Tibial tuberosity

胫前肌
Tibialis anterior muscle

图 3-58　膝关节，内面观　Knee Joint, Internal View

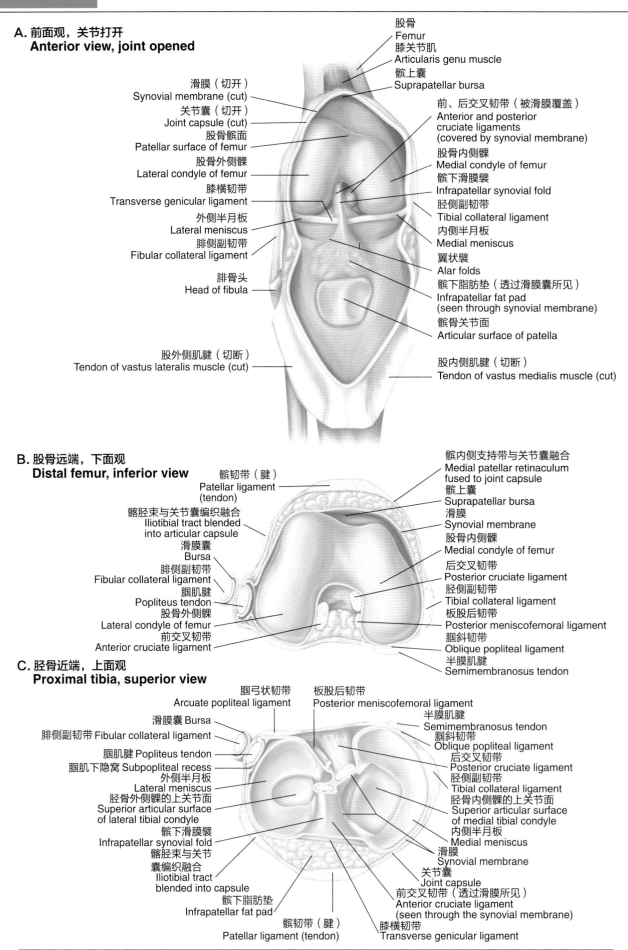

A. 前面观，关节打开
Anterior view, joint opened

股骨
Femur

膝关节肌
Articularis genu muscle

髌上囊
Suprapatellar bursa

滑膜（切开）
Synovial membrane (cut)

关节囊（切开）
Joint capsule (cut)

股骨髌面
Patellar surface of femur

股骨外侧髁
Lateral condyle of femur

膝横韧带
Transverse genicular ligament

外侧半月板
Lateral meniscus

腓侧副韧带
Fibular collateral ligament

腓骨头
Head of fibula

股外侧肌腱（切断）
Tendon of vastus lateralis muscle (cut)

前、后交叉韧带（被滑膜覆盖）
Anterior and posterior
cruciate ligaments
(covered by synovial membrane)

股骨内侧髁
Medial condyle of femur

髌下滑膜襞
Infrapatellar synovial fold

胫侧副韧带
Tibial collateral ligament

内侧半月板
Medial meniscus

翼状襞
Alar folds

髌下脂肪垫（透过滑膜囊所见）
Infrapatellar fat pad
(seen through synovial membrane)

髌骨关节面
Articular surface of patella

股内侧肌腱（切断）
Tendon of vastus medialis muscle (cut)

B. 股骨远端，下面观
Distal femur, inferior view

髌韧带（腱）
Patellar ligament
(tendon)

髂胫束与关节囊编织融合
Iliotibial tract blended
into articular capsule

滑膜囊
Bursa

腓侧副韧带
Fibular collateral ligament

腘肌腱
Popliteus tendon

股骨外侧髁
Lateral condyle of femur

前交叉韧带
Anterior cruciate ligament

髌内侧支持带与关节囊融合
Medial patellar retinaculum
fused to joint capsule

髌上囊
Suprapatellar bursa

滑膜
Synovial membrane

股骨内侧髁
Medial condyle of femur

后交叉韧带
Posterior cruciate ligament

胫侧副韧带
Tibial collateral ligament

板股后韧带
Posterior meniscofemoral ligament

腘斜韧带
Oblique popliteal ligament

半膜肌腱
Semimembranosus tendon

C. 胫骨近端，上面观
Proximal tibia, superior view

腘弓状韧带
Arcuate popliteal ligament

滑膜囊 Bursa

腓侧副韧带 Fibular collateral ligament

腘肌腱 Popliteus tendon

腘肌下隐窝 Subpopliteal recess

外侧半月板
Lateral meniscus

胫骨外侧髁的上关节面
Superior articular surface
of lateral tibial condyle

髌下滑膜襞
Infrapatellar synovial fold

髂胫束与关节囊编织融合
Iliotibial tract
blended into capsule

髌下脂肪垫
Infrapatellar fat pad

髌韧带（腱）
Patellar ligament (tendon)

板股后韧带
Posterior meniscofemoral ligament

半膜肌腱
Semimembranosus tendon

腘斜韧带
Oblique popliteal ligament

后交叉韧带
Posterior cruciate ligament

胫侧副韧带
Tibial collateral ligament

胫骨内侧髁的上关节面
Superior articular surface
of medial tibial condyle

内侧半月板
Medial meniscus

滑膜
Synovial membrane

关节囊
Joint capsule

前交叉韧带（透过滑膜所见）
Anterior cruciate ligament
(seen through the synovial membrane)

膝横韧带
Transverse genicular ligament

A. 韧带，前面观
Ligaments, anterior view

B. 韧带，后面观
Ligaments, posterior view

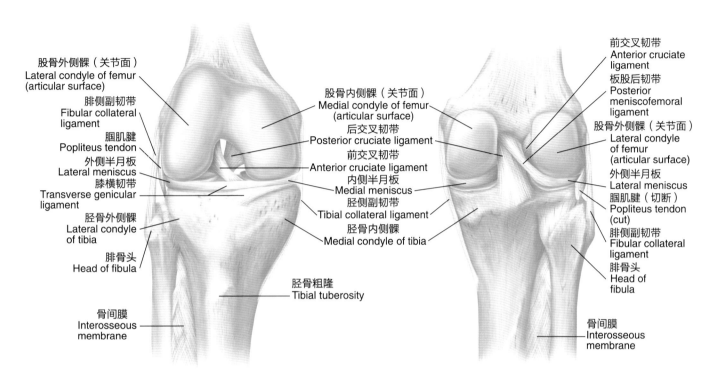

股骨外侧髁（关节面）
Lateral condyle of femur (articular surface)

腓侧副韧带
Fibular collateral ligament

腘肌腱
Popliteus tendon

外侧半月板
Lateral meniscus

膝横韧带
Transverse genicular ligament

胫骨外侧髁
Lateral condyle of tibia

腓骨头
Head of fibula

骨间膜
Interosseous membrane

股骨内侧髁（关节面）
Medial condyle of femur (articular surface)

后交叉韧带
Posterior cruciate ligament

前交叉韧带
Anterior cruciate ligament

内侧半月板
Medial meniscus

胫骨副韧带
Tibial collateral ligament

胫骨内侧髁
Medial condyle of tibia

胫骨粗隆
Tibial tuberosity

前交叉韧带
Anterior cruciate ligament

板股后韧带
Posterior meniscofemoral ligament

股骨外侧髁（关节面）
Lateral condyle of femur (articular surface)

外侧半月板
Lateral meniscus

腘肌腱（切断）
Popliteus tendon (cut)

腓侧副韧带
Fibular collateral ligament

腓骨头
Head of fibula

骨间膜
Interosseous membrane

C. 膝关节伸直时的交叉韧带，外侧面观
Cruciate ligaments, lateral view, knee extended

D. 膝关节屈曲时的交叉韧带，外侧面观
Cruciate ligaments, lateral view, knee flexed

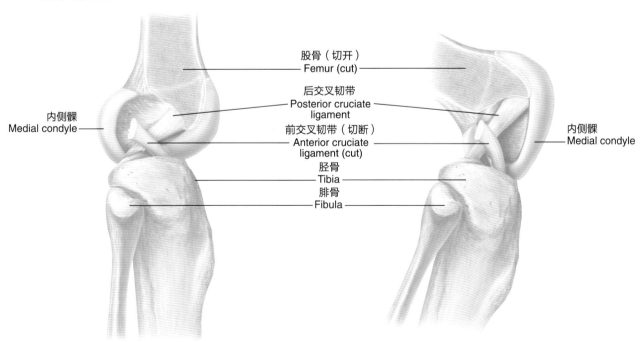

内侧髁
Medial condyle

股骨（切开）
Femur (cut)

后交叉韧带
Posterior cruciate ligament

前交叉韧带（切断）
Anterior cruciate ligament (cut)

胫骨
Tibia

腓骨
Fibula

内侧髁
Medial condyle

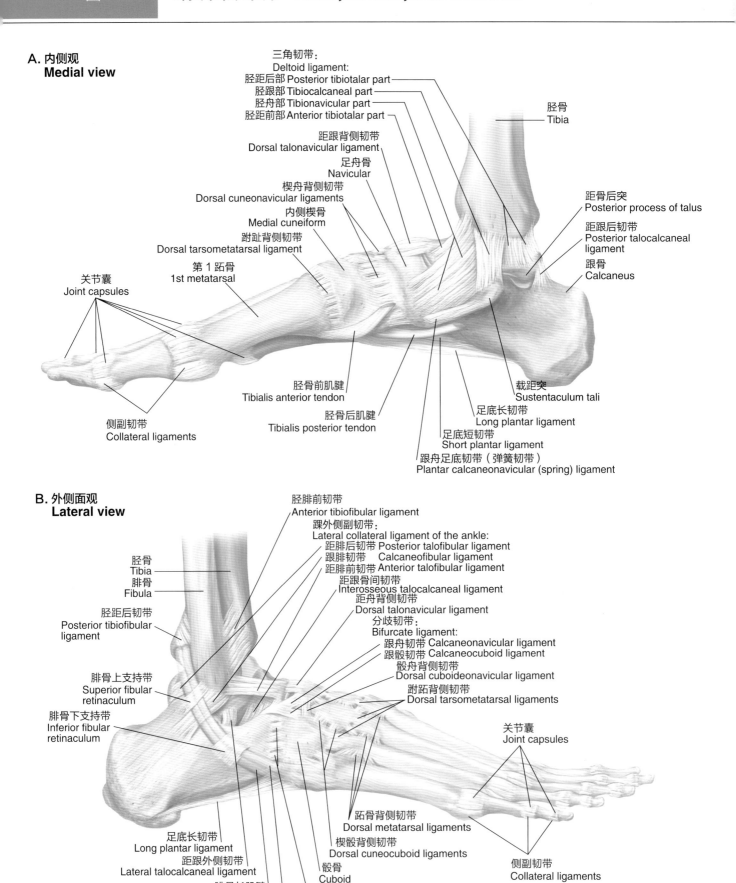

A. 内侧观
Medial view

三角韧带：
Deltoid ligament:
胫距后部 Posterior tibiotalar part
胫跟部 Tibiocalcaneal part
胫舟部 Tibionavicular part
胫距前部 Anterior tibiotalar part

距跟背侧韧带
Dorsal talonavicular ligament

足舟骨
Navicular

楔舟背侧韧带
Dorsal cuneonavicular ligaments

内侧楔骨
Medial cuneiform

跗趾背侧韧带
Dorsal tarsometatarsal ligament

第 1 跖骨
1st metatarsal

关节囊
Joint capsules

侧副韧带
Collateral ligaments

胫骨
Tibia

距骨后突
Posterior process of talus

距跟后韧带
Posterior talocalcaneal ligament

跟骨
Calcaneus

载距突
Sustentaculum tali

足底长韧带
Long plantar ligament

足底短韧带
Short plantar ligament

跟舟足底韧带（弹簧韧带）
Plantar calcaneonavicular (spring) ligament

胫骨前肌腱
Tibialis anterior tendon

胫骨后肌腱
Tibialis posterior tendon

B. 外侧面观
Lateral view

胫腓前韧带
Anterior tibiofibular ligament

踝外侧副韧带：
Lateral collateral ligament of the ankle:
距腓后韧带 Posterior talofibular ligament
跟腓韧带 Calcaneofibular ligament
距腓前韧带 Anterior talofibular ligament

距跟骨间韧带
Interosseous talocalcaneal ligament

距舟背侧韧带
Dorsal talonavicular ligament

分歧韧带：
Bifurcate ligament:
跟舟韧带 Calcaneonavicular ligament
跟骰韧带 Calcaneocuboid ligament

骰舟背侧韧带
Dorsal cuboideonavicular ligament

跗跖背侧韧带
Dorsal tarsometatarsal ligaments

胫骨
Tibia
腓骨
Fibula

胫距后韧带
Posterior tibiofibular ligament

腓骨上支持带
Superior fibular retinaculum

腓骨下支持带
Inferior fibular retinaculum

关节囊
Joint capsules

侧副韧带
Collateral ligaments

跖骨背侧韧带
Dorsal metatarsal ligaments

楔骰背侧韧带
Dorsal cuneocuboid ligaments

骰骨
Cuboid

跟骰背侧韧带
Dorsal calcaneocuboid ligaments

足底长韧带
Long plantar ligament

距跟外侧韧带
Lateral talocalcaneal ligament

腓骨长肌腱
Fibularis longus tendon

腓骨短肌腱
Fibularis brevis tendon

A. 足底观
Plantar view

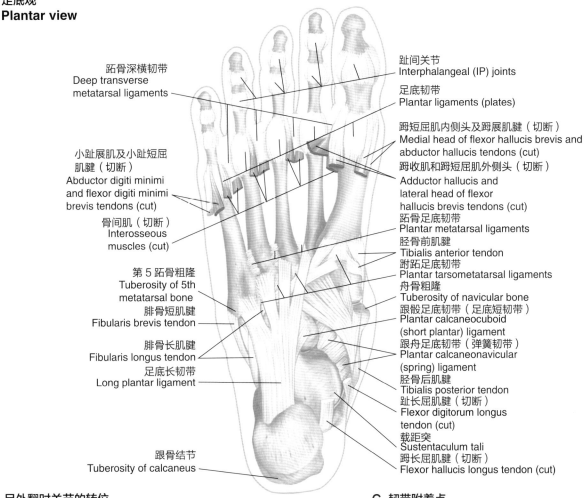

跖骨深横韧带
Deep transverse
metatarsal ligaments

小趾展肌及小趾短屈
肌腱（切断）
Abductor digiti minimi
and flexor digiti minimi
brevis tendons (cut)

骨间肌（切断）
Interosseous
muscles (cut)

第 5 跖骨粗隆
Tuberosity of 5th
metatarsal bone

腓骨短肌腱
Fibularis brevis tendon

腓骨长肌腱
Fibularis longus tendon

足底长韧带
Long plantar ligament

跟骨结节
Tuberosity of calcaneus

趾间关节
Interphalangeal (IP) joints

足底韧带
Plantar ligaments (plates)

蹈短屈肌内侧头及蹈展肌腱（切断）
Medial head of flexor hallucis brevis and
abductor hallucis tendons (cut)

蹈收肌和蹈短屈肌外侧头（切断）
Adductor hallucis and
lateral head of flexor
hallucis brevis tendons (cut)

跖骨足底韧带
Plantar metatarsal ligaments

胫骨前肌腱
Tibialis anterior tendon

跗跖足底韧带
Plantar tarsometatarsal ligaments

舟骨粗隆
Tuberosity of navicular bone

跟骰足底韧带（足底短韧带）
Plantar calcaneocuboid
(short plantar) ligament

跟舟足底韧带（弹簧韧带）
Plantar calcaneonavicular
(spring) ligament

胫骨后肌腱
Tibialis posterior tendon

趾长屈肌腱（切断）
Flexor digitorum longus
tendon (cut)

载距突
Sustentaculum tali

蹈长屈肌腱（切断）
Flexor hallucis longus tendon (cut)

B. 足外翻时关节的转位
Joints of inversion and eversion

C. 韧带附着点
Ligament attachments

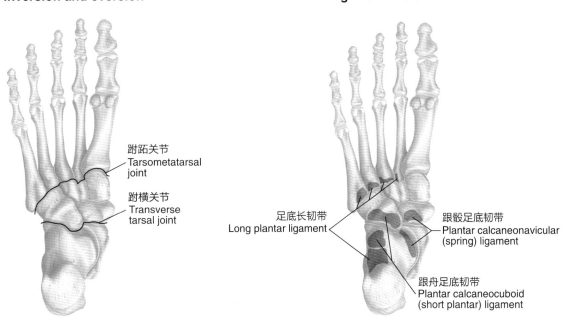

跗跖关节
Tarsometatarsal
joint

跗横关节
Transverse
tarsal joint

足底长韧带
Long plantar ligament

跟骰足底韧带
Plantar calcaneonavicular
(spring) ligament

跟舟足底韧带
Plantar calcaneocuboid
(short plantar) ligament

图 3-62　下肢动脉　Arteries of the Lower Limb

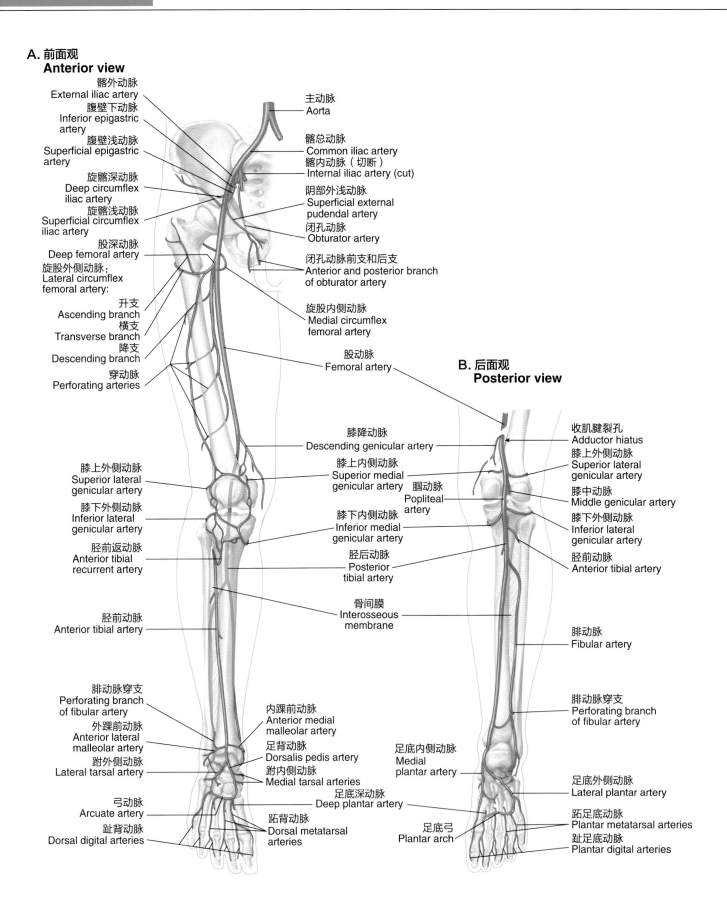

A. 前面观
Anterior view

髂外动脉
External iliac artery

腹壁下动脉
Inferior epigastric artery

腹壁浅动脉
Superficial epigastric artery

旋髂深动脉
Deep circumflex iliac artery

旋髂浅动脉
Superficial circumflex iliac artery

股深动脉
Deep femoral artery

旋股外侧动脉：
Lateral circumflex femoral artery:

升支
Ascending branch

横支
Transverse branch

降支
Descending branch

穿动脉
Perforating arteries

主动脉
Aorta

髂总动脉
Common iliac artery

髂内动脉（切断）
Internal iliac artery (cut)

阴部外浅动脉
Superficial external pudendal artery

闭孔动脉
Obturator artery

闭孔动脉前支和后支
Anterior and posterior branch of obturator artery

旋股内侧动脉
Medial circumflex femoral artery

股动脉
Femoral artery

B. 后面观
Posterior view

膝降动脉
Descending genicular artery

膝上内侧动脉
Superior medial genicular artery

膝下内侧动脉
Inferior medial genicular artery

胫后动脉
Posterior tibial artery

骨间膜
Interosseous membrane

收肌腱裂孔
Adductor hiatus

膝上外侧动脉
Superior lateral genicular artery

膝中动脉
Middle genicular artery

膝下外侧动脉
Inferior lateral genicular artery

胫前动脉
Anterior tibial artery

腘动脉
Popliteal artery

腓动脉
Fibular artery

腓动脉穿支
Perforating branch of fibular artery

膝上外侧动脉
Superior lateral genicular artery

膝下外侧动脉
Inferior lateral genicular artery

胫前返动脉
Anterior tibial recurrent artery

胫前动脉
Anterior tibial artery

腓动脉穿支
Perforating branch of fibular artery

外踝前动脉
Anterior lateral malleolar artery

跗外侧动脉
Lateral tarsal artery

弓动脉
Arcuate artery

趾背动脉
Dorsal digital arteries

内踝前动脉
Anterior medial malleolar artery

足背动脉
Dorsalis pedis artery

跗内侧动脉
Medial tarsal arteries

足底深动脉
Deep plantar artery

跖背动脉
Dorsal metatarsal arteries

足底内侧动脉
Medial plantar artery

足底外侧动脉
Lateral plantar artery

跖足底动脉
Plantar metatarsal arteries

趾足底动脉
Plantar digital arteries

足底弓
Plantar arch

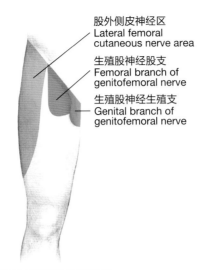

股外侧皮神经区
Lateral femoral
cutaneous nerve area

生殖股神经股支
Femoral branch of
genitofemoral nerve

生殖股神经生殖支
Genital branch of
genitofemoral nerve

A. 股外侧皮神经和生殖股神经
**Lateral femoral cutaneous
and genitofemoral nerves**

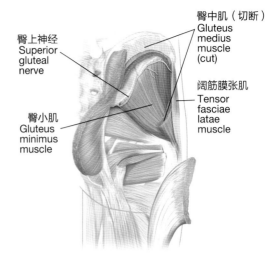

臀上神经
Superior
gluteal
nerve

臀中肌（切断）
Gluteus
medius
muscle
(cut)

阔筋膜张肌
Tensor
fasciae
latae
muscle

臀小肌
Gluteus
minimus
muscle

B. 臀上神经
Superior gluteal nerve

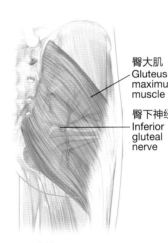

臀大肌
Gluteus
maximus
muscle

臀下神经
Inferior
gluteal
nerve

C. 臀下神经
Inferior gluteal nerve

闭孔内神经
Nerve to
obturator
internus

上孖肌
Superior
gemellus
muscle

闭孔内肌
Obturator
internus
muscle

D. 闭孔内肌神经
Nerve to obturator internus

股方肌神经
Nerve to
quadratus
femoris

下孖肌
Inferior
gemellus
muscle

股方肌
Quadratus
femoris
muscle

E. 股方肌神经
Nerve to quadratus femoris

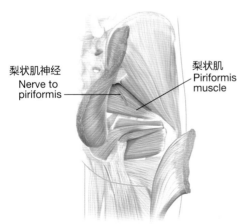

梨状肌神经
Nerve to
piriformis

梨状肌
Piriformis
muscle

F. 梨状肌神经
Nerve to piriformis

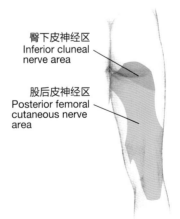

臀下皮神经区
Inferior cluneal
nerve area

股后皮神经区
Posterior femoral
cutaneous nerve
area

G. 股后皮区
Posterior femoral cutaneous

图 3-64   股神经 Femoral Nerve

A. 前面观
Anterior view

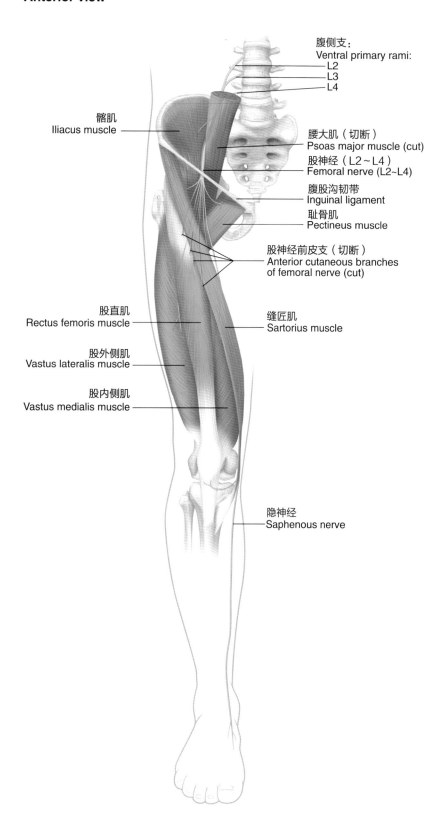

腹侧支：
Ventral primary rami:
— L2
— L3
— L4

髂肌
Iliacus muscle

腰大肌（切断）
Psoas major muscle (cut)

股神经（L2~L4）
Femoral nerve (L2~L4)

腹股沟韧带
Inguinal ligament

耻骨肌
Pectineus muscle

股神经前皮支（切断）
Anterior cutaneous branches
of femoral nerve (cut)

股直肌
Rectus femoris muscle

缝匠肌
Sartorius muscle

股外侧肌
Vastus lateralis muscle

股内侧肌
Vastus medialis muscle

隐神经
Saphenous nerve

B. 皮神经分布，前面观
Cutaneous distribution,
anterior view

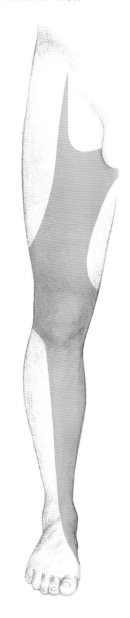

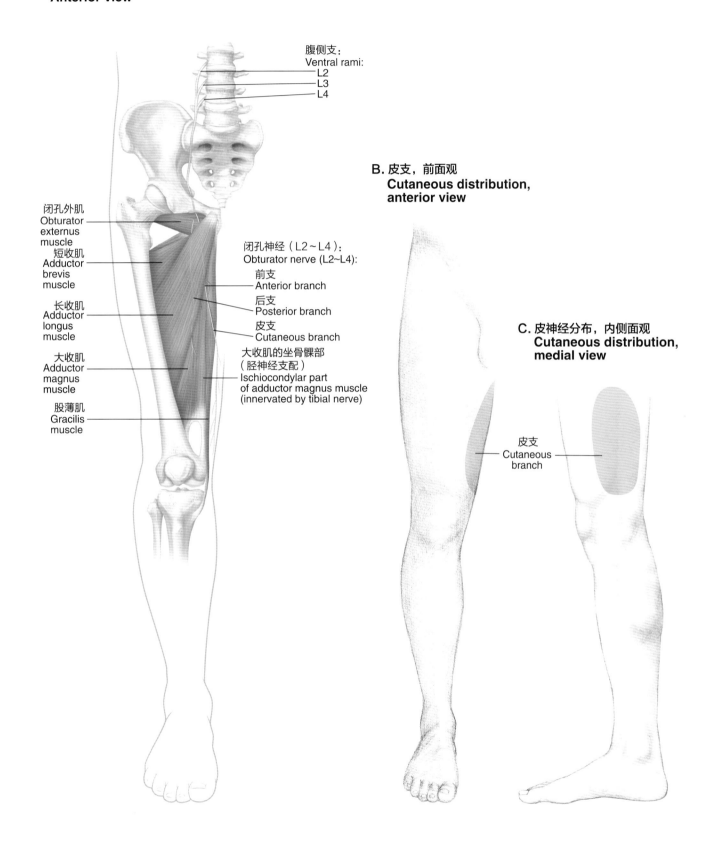

A. 前面观
Anterior view

腹侧支：
Ventral rami:
- L2
- L3
- L4

闭孔外肌
Obturator
externus
muscle

短收肌
Adductor
brevis
muscle

长收肌
Adductor
longus
muscle

大收肌
Adductor
magnus
muscle

股薄肌
Gracilis
muscle

闭孔神经（L2~L4）：
Obturator nerve (L2~L4):

前支
Anterior branch

后支
Posterior branch

皮支
Cutaneous branch

大收肌的坐骨髁部
（胫神经支配）
Ischiocondylar part
of adductor magnus muscle
(innervated by tibial nerve)

B. 皮支，前面观
**Cutaneous distribution,
anterior view**

C. 皮神经分布，内侧面观
**Cutaneous distribution,
medial view**

皮支
Cutaneous
branch

图 3-66　腓总神经　Common Fibular Nerve

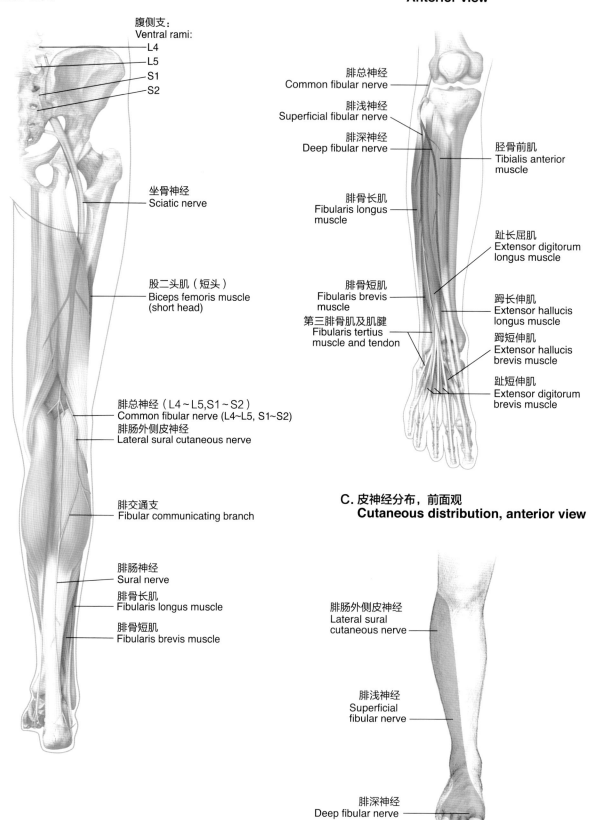

A. 后面观
Posterior view

腹侧支：
Ventral rami:
- L4
- L5
- S1
- S2

坐骨神经
Sciatic nerve

股二头肌（短头）
Biceps femoris muscle
(short head)

腓总神经（L4~L5,S1~S2）
Common fibular nerve (L4~L5, S1~S2)
腓肠外侧皮神经
Lateral sural cutaneous nerve

腓交通支
Fibular communicating branch

腓肠神经
Sural nerve
腓骨长肌
Fibularis longus muscle
腓骨短肌
Fibularis brevis muscle

B. 前面观
Anterior view

腓总神经
Common fibular nerve
腓浅神经
Superficial fibular nerve
腓深神经
Deep fibular nerve
胫骨前肌
Tibialis anterior muscle
腓骨长肌
Fibularis longus muscle
趾长屈肌
Extensor digitorum longus muscle
腓骨短肌
Fibularis brevis muscle
𧿹长伸肌
Extensor hallucis longus muscle
第三腓骨肌及肌腱
Fibularis tertius muscle and tendon
𧿹短伸肌
Extensor hallucis brevis muscle
趾短伸肌
Extensor digitorum brevis muscle

C. 皮神经分布，前面观
Cutaneous distribution, anterior view

腓肠外侧皮神经
Lateral sural cutaneous nerve

腓浅神经
Superficial fibular nerve

腓深神经
Deep fibular nerve

A. 浅层
Superficial view

B. 深层
Deep view

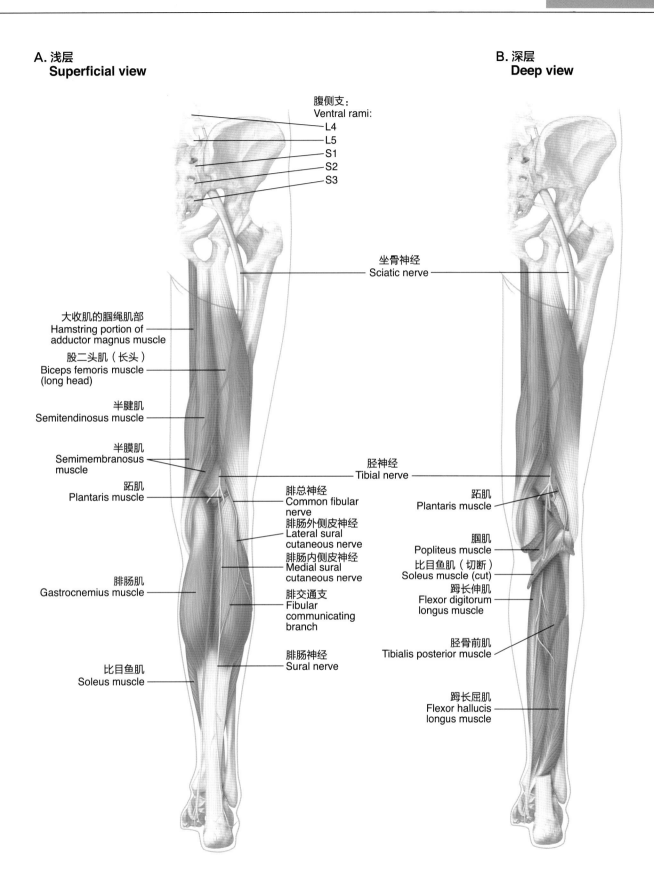

腹侧支：
Ventral rami:
L4
L5
S1
S2
S3

坐骨神经
Sciatic nerve

大收肌的腘绳肌部
Hamstring portion of adductor magnus muscle

股二头肌（长头）
Biceps femoris muscle (long head)

半腱肌
Semitendinosus muscle

半膜肌
Semimembranosus muscle

跖肌
Plantaris muscle

胫神经
Tibial nerve

腓总神经
Common fibular nerve

腓肠外侧皮神经
Lateral sural cutaneous nerve

腓肠内侧皮神经
Medial sural cutaneous nerve

腓肠肌
Gastrocnemius muscle

腓交通支
Fibular communicating branch

比目鱼肌
Soleus muscle

腓肠神经
Sural nerve

跖肌
Plantaris muscle

腘肌
Popliteus muscle

比目鱼肌（切断）
Soleus muscle (cut)

趾长伸肌
Flexor digitorum longus muscle

胫骨前肌
Tibialis posterior muscle

蹬长屈肌
Flexor hallucis longus muscle

图 3-68

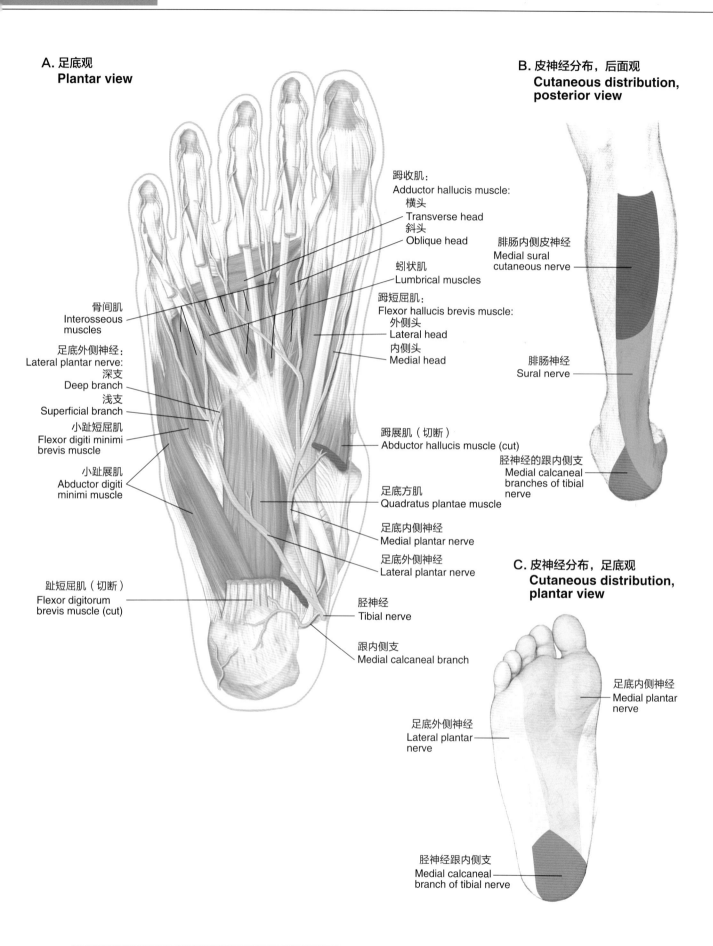

A. 足底观
Plantar view

B. 皮神经分布，后面观
Cutaneous distribution, posterior view

C. 皮神经分布，足底观
Cutaneous distribution, plantar view

蹬收肌：
Adductor hallucis muscle:
横头
Transverse head
斜头
Oblique head

蚓状肌
Lumbrical muscles

蹬短屈肌：
Flexor hallucis brevis muscle:
外侧头
Lateral head
内侧头
Medial head

骨间肌
Interosseous muscles

足底外侧神经：
Lateral plantar nerve:
深支
Deep branch
浅支
Superficial branch

小趾短屈肌
Flexor digiti minimi brevis muscle

小趾展肌
Abductor digiti minimi muscle

趾短屈肌（切断）
Flexor digitorum brevis muscle (cut)

蹬展肌（切断）
Abductor hallucis muscle (cut)

足底方肌
Quadratus plantae muscle

足底内侧神经
Medial plantar nerve

足底外侧神经
Lateral plantar nerve

胫神经
Tibial nerve

跟内侧支
Medial calcaneal branch

腓肠内侧皮神经
Medial sural cutaneous nerve

腓肠神经
Sural nerve

胫神经的跟内侧支
Medial calcaneal branches of tibial nerve

足底内侧神经
Medial plantar nerve

足底外侧神经
Lateral plantar nerve

胫神经跟内侧支
Medial calcaneal branch of tibial nerve

A. 前面观
Anterior view

B. 后面观
Posterior view

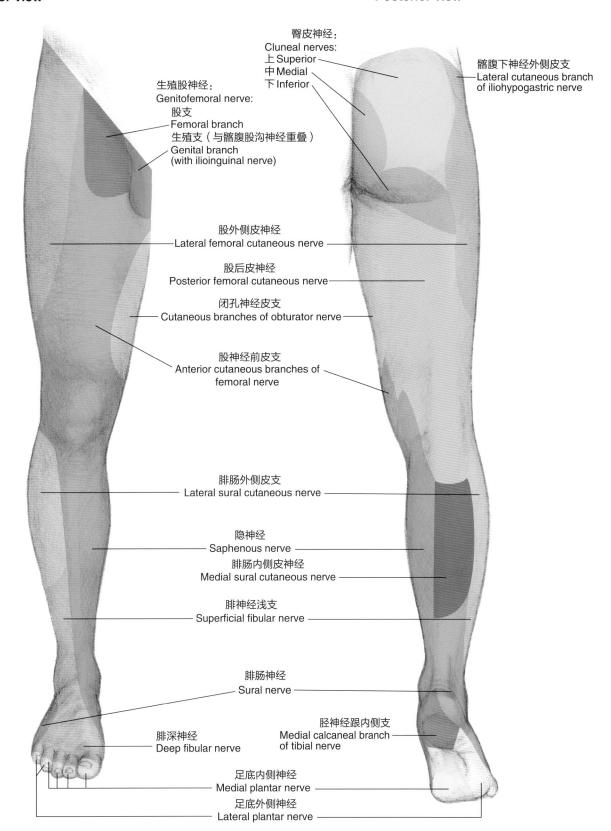

臀皮神经：
Cluneal nerves:
上 Superior
中 Medial
下 Inferior

生殖股神经：
Genitofemoral nerve:
股支
Femoral branch
生殖支（与髂腹股沟神经重叠）
Genital branch
(with ilioinguinal nerve)

髂腹下神经外侧皮支
Lateral cutaneous branch
of iliohypogastric nerve

股外侧皮神经
Lateral femoral cutaneous nerve

股后皮神经
Posterior femoral cutaneous nerve

闭孔神经皮支
Cutaneous branches of obturator nerve

股神经前皮支
Anterior cutaneous branches of
femoral nerve

腓肠外侧皮支
Lateral sural cutaneous nerve

隐神经
Saphenous nerve

腓肠内侧皮神经
Medial sural cutaneous nerve

腓神经浅支
Superficial fibular nerve

腓肠神经
Sural nerve

腓深神经
Deep fibular nerve

胫神经跟内侧支
Medial calcaneal branch
of tibial nerve

足底内侧神经
Medial plantar nerve

足底外侧神经
Lateral plantar nerve

图 3-70　　**下肢皮区　Dermatomes of the Lower Limb**

A. 前面观
Anterior view

B. 后面观
Posterior view

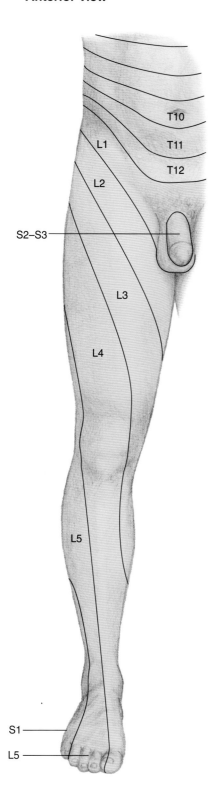

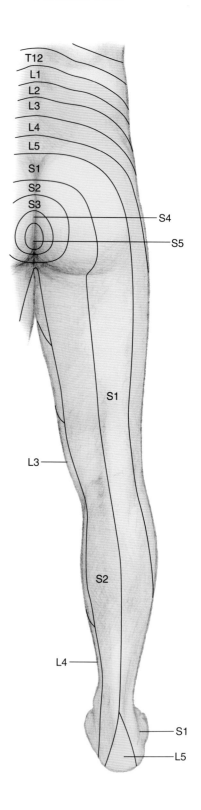

A. 前面观
Anterior view

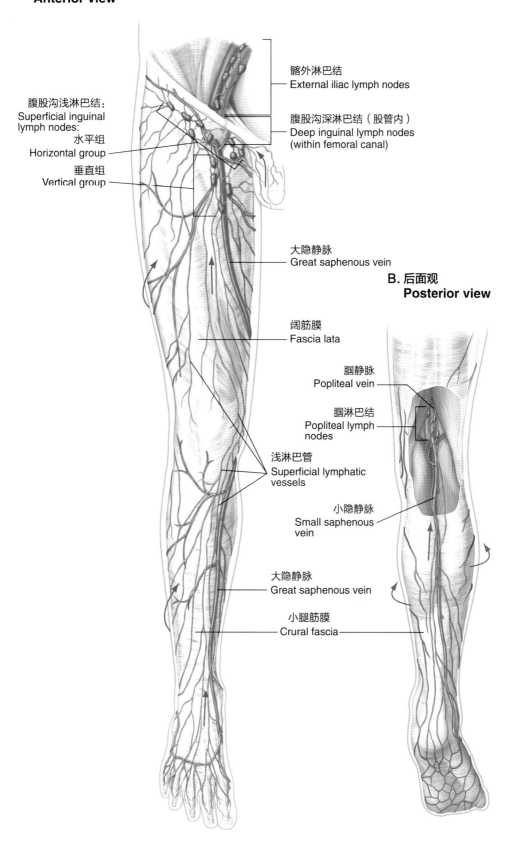

髂外淋巴结
External iliac lymph nodes

腹股沟深淋巴结（股管内）
Deep inguinal lymph nodes
(within femoral canal)

腹股沟浅淋巴结：
Superficial inguinal
lymph nodes:

水平组
Horizontal group

垂直组
Vertical group

大隐静脉
Great saphenous vein

B. 后面观
Posterior view

阔筋膜
Fascia lata

腘静脉
Popliteal vein

腘淋巴结
Popliteal lymph
nodes

浅淋巴管
Superficial lymphatic
vessels

小隐静脉
Small saphenous
vein

大隐静脉
Great saphenous vein

小腿筋膜
Crural fascia

下肢肌						
名称	**起点**	**止点**	**主要作用**	**神经支配**	**动脉**	**注释**
髂腰肌（图3-16）	髂肌（起自髂窝）和腰大肌（起自腰椎）组成	股骨小转子	屈大腿，屈曲和侧弯腰椎	L2~L4脊神经前支和来自股神经的分支	髂腰动脉和旋髂深动脉	
缝匠肌（图3-16）	髂前上棘	胫骨内侧面（鹅足）	屈曲、外展和外旋大腿；屈小腿	股神经	股动脉、旋股外侧动脉和膝降动脉	
股四头肌（图3-16）	4块肌组成：股直肌、股外侧肌、股中间肌和股内侧肌	通过髌韧带止于胫骨粗隆	伸膝关节；股直肌屈大腿	股神经	股动脉、旋股外侧动脉	
股直肌（图3-16）	直头：髂前下棘；反折头：髋臼上缘上方	髌骨和胫骨粗隆（借髌韧带）	伸小腿、屈大腿	股神经	股动脉、旋股外侧动脉	股直肌是股四头肌的一部分
股外侧肌（图3-16）	外内侧肌间隔、粗线外侧唇和臀肌粗隆	髌骨和髌外侧支持带	伸小腿	股神经	股动脉、旋股外侧动脉	股外侧肌是股四头肌的一部分
股内侧肌（图3-16）	内侧肌间隔、粗线内侧唇	髌骨和髌内侧支持带	伸小腿	股神经	股动脉、旋股外侧动脉	股内侧肌是股四头肌的一部分
股中间肌（图3-16）	股骨前面和外侧面	髌骨	伸小腿	股神经	股动脉、旋股外侧动脉	股中间肌是股四头肌的一部分
耻骨肌（图3-16）	耻骨梳	股骨的耻骨肌线	内收、屈曲和内旋大腿	股神经，偶尔有闭孔神经前支	旋股内侧动脉	
股薄肌（图3-16）	耻骨联合和耻骨下支	胫骨内侧面（鹅足）	内收大腿，屈小腿，屈曲和内旋大腿	闭孔神经前支	闭孔动脉和股深动脉	鹅足是股薄肌、缝匠肌和半腱肌的共同止点
长收肌（图3-19）	耻骨上支内侧部	股骨粗线	内收、屈曲和内旋股骨	闭孔神经前支	闭孔动脉和股深动脉	
短收肌（图3-20和图3-21）	耻骨下支	耻骨肌线和粗线（耻骨肌和长收肌深面）	内收、屈曲和内旋股骨	闭孔神经前支	闭孔动脉和股深动脉	闭孔神经前支和后支位于短收肌的前面和后面
大收肌（图3-21）	坐骨耻骨支和坐骨结节	股骨粗线，坐骨部收肌结节	内收、屈曲和内旋股骨后伸股骨（坐骨部）	闭孔神经后支和胫神经（坐骨部）	闭孔动脉和股深动脉	大收肌的坐骨部在胚胎起源和功能上属于腘绳肌，因此受胫神经支配
闭孔外肌	闭孔膜外面（表面）和耻骨上、下支	股骨转子窝	外旋大腿	闭孔神经	闭孔动脉	闭孔外肌腱经股骨颈下方止于其止点
臀大肌（图3-26）	臀后线，骶骨和尾骨后面，骶结节韧带	上部肌束：髂胫束；最下部肌束：股骨的臀肌粗隆	后伸大腿和躯干，外旋股骨	臀下神经	臀下动脉和臀上动脉浅支	
臀中肌（图3-26）	髂骨的臀前线和臀后线之间	股骨大转子	外展和内旋大腿 后伸大腿和躯干，外旋股骨	臀上神经 臀下神经	臀上动脉深支 臀下动脉和臀上动脉浅支	

下肢肌						
名称	起点	止点	主要作用	神经支配	动脉	注释
臀小肌 （图3-26）	髂骨的臀前线以下	股骨大转子前缘	外展、内旋（前部肌束）和外旋（后部肌束）髋关节 屈曲、外展和内旋大腿	臀上神经	臀上动脉深支	
阔筋膜张肌 （图3-17）	髂嵴前部，髂前上棘	髂胫束	屈曲、外展和内旋大腿	臀上神经	臀上动脉深支	
梨状肌 （图3-26）	骶骨前面	股骨大转子上缘	外旋和外展大腿	S1~S2 前支	骶外侧动脉、臀上动脉、臀下动脉	梨状肌离开骨盆穿过坐骨大孔
闭孔内肌 （图3-26 和图3-28）	闭孔周缘和闭孔膜内面	大转子、转子窝内面	外旋和外展大腿	闭孔内肌神经（L5，S1~S2）	闭孔动脉，臀下动脉	闭孔内肌穿坐骨小孔离开盆腔
上孖肌 （图3-26 和图3-28）	坐骨棘	闭孔内肌腱	外旋股骨	闭孔内肌神经	臀下动脉	
下孖肌 （图3-26 和图3-28）	坐骨结节	闭孔内肌腱	外旋股骨	股方肌神经	臀下动脉	
股方肌 （图3-26 和图3-28）	坐骨结节外侧缘	转子间嵴下方的股方肌线	外旋股骨	股方肌神经	臀下动脉	股方肌神经也支配下孖肌
股二头肌 （图3-29）	长头：坐骨结节；短头：粗线外侧唇	腓骨头和胫骨外侧髁	后伸大腿，屈小腿	长头 胫神经 短头 腓总神经	股深动脉穿支	
半腱肌 （图3-29）	坐骨结节内下面（与股二头肌共腱）	胫骨内侧面（鹅足）	后伸大腿，屈小腿	胫神经	股深动脉穿支	鹅足是股薄肌、缝匠肌和半腱肌的共同止点
半膜肌 （图3-29）	坐骨结节上外侧面	胫骨内侧髁	后伸大腿，屈小腿	胫神经	股深动脉穿支	
腓肠肌 （图3-33）	股骨；内侧头：股骨内侧髁上方；外侧头：股骨外侧髁上方	借跟腱止于跟骨背面	屈小腿，跖屈足	胫神经	腘动脉的膝关节支和腓肠肌支	腓肠肌和比目鱼肌的跟腱是全身最粗大强大的肌腱
跖肌 （图3-34）	股骨外侧髁上方（腓肠肌外侧头上方）	跟骨背内侧和跟腱	屈小腿，跖屈足	胫神经	腘动脉的膝关节支和腓肠肌支	
比目鱼肌 （图3-34）	腓骨头后面和腓骨干上部，胫骨的比目鱼肌线	借跟腱止于跟骨背面	跖屈足	胫神经	腘动脉的膝下内侧动脉和腓肠肌支	比目鱼肌和腓肠肌的两个头有时称为小腿三头肌
腘肌 （图3-31）	股骨外侧髁（借一条圆韧带）	胫骨后面的比目鱼肌线	屈曲和内旋小腿（伴足跖屈外旋大腿）	胫神经	腘动脉的膝关节支	腘肌解锁膝关节启动小腿屈曲

续表

下肢肌						
名称	起点	止点	主要作用	神经支配	动脉	注释
跗长屈肌（图 3-35）	腓骨下 2/3 的后面	跗趾远节趾骨底	屈跗趾跖趾关节和近侧趾间关节，跖屈足	胫神经	腓动脉	长屈肌对于正常步态的"离地"部分非常重要
趾长屈肌（图 3-35）	胫骨后面的内侧半	第 2~5 趾的远节趾骨底	屈第 2~5 趾的跖趾关节、近侧趾间关节和远侧趾间关节，跖屈足	胫神经	胫后动脉	小腿的趾长屈肌相当于上肢的指深屈肌
胫骨后肌（图 3-35）	骨间膜、腓骨后内侧面、胫骨后外侧面	足舟骨结节和内侧楔骨，第 2~4 跖骨	跖屈足和足内翻	胫神经	胫后动脉	同时作为胫骨前肌的拮抗肌（背屈 / 跖屈）和协同肌（内翻）
跗展肌（图 3-49）	跟骨结节内侧	跗趾近节趾骨底的内侧	外展跗趾；去跗趾关节	足底内侧神经	足底内侧和外侧动脉	
跗收肌（图 3-51）	斜头：第 2~4 跖骨底；横头：第 3~5 跖骨底	跗趾近节趾骨底外侧	内收跗趾（拉跗趾靠近足中线，即第 2 趾）	足底外侧神经深支	足底外侧动脉	
跗短屈肌（图 3-49 和图 3-51）	骰骨、外侧楔骨、第 1 跖骨内侧	内侧肌腹：跗趾近节趾骨内侧；外侧肌腹：近节趾骨外侧	去跗趾跖趾关节	足底内侧神经（外侧肌腹偶尔接受足底外侧神经的支配）	足底内侧和外侧动脉	每个止点的肌腱都含有一块籽骨
趾短屈肌（图 3-49）	跟骨结节、足底腱膜、肌间隔	分叉让趾长屈肌腱通过后止于第 2~5 趾中节趾骨底	屈跖趾关节和第 2~5 趾近侧趾骨间关节	足底内侧神经	足底内侧动脉	
腓骨长肌（图 3-36 和图 3-37）	腓骨上 2/3 外侧面	在足固有肌深面穿过足底止于内侧楔骨和第 1 跖骨底	跖屈和外翻足	腓浅神经	腓动脉	位于腓骨短肌浅面
腓骨短肌（图 3-36 和图 3-37）	腓骨下 1/3 外侧面	第 5 趾骨粗隆底	跖屈和外翻足	腓浅神经	腓动脉	
胫骨前肌（图 3-37）	胫骨外侧髁和胫骨外上面	内侧楔骨内面和第 1 跖骨	背屈和内翻足	腓深神经	胫前动脉	同时作为胫骨后肌的拮抗肌和协同肌
跗长伸肌（图 3-37）	腓骨前面中间 1/2 和骨间膜	跗指远节趾骨底	伸跗趾的跖趾关节和趾间关节	腓深神经	胫前动脉	
跗短伸肌（图 3-45）	跟骨上外侧面	跗趾近节趾骨底背侧	伸跗趾	腓深神经	胫前动脉	常被认为是趾短伸肌最内侧部

下肢肌						
名称	起点	止点	主要作用	神经支配	动脉	注释
趾长伸肌（图3-37）	胫骨外侧髁、腓骨前面、骨间膜外侧部	借趾背腱膜止于外侧4个足趾的背面（中央束止于中节趾骨底，外侧束止于远节趾骨底）	伸外侧4个足趾的跖趾关节、近侧和远侧趾间关节	腓深神经	胫前动脉	
趾短伸肌（图3-45）	跟骨外上面	第2~4趾的趾背腱膜（止于姆趾的是姆短伸肌）	伸第2~4趾	腓深神经	足背动脉	
第三腓骨肌（图3-37和图3-45）	腓骨远端前面	第5跖骨体背面	背屈和外翻足	腓深神经	胫前动脉	第三腓骨肌位于小腿前骨筋膜鞘，而不是外侧骨筋膜鞘（内有腓骨长肌和腓骨短肌）
足底方肌（图3-50）	跟骨前部和跖长韧带	趾长屈肌腱	辅助趾长屈肌屈足趾	足底外侧神经	足底外侧动脉	
足的骨间背侧肌（图3-46、图3-51和图3-52）	4块肌，起自相邻的跖骨体	第2趾近节趾骨底（两侧）和第3、4趾近节趾骨底（外侧）	外展第2~4趾（运动足趾远离中线，中线定义为第2足趾），屈这些足趾的跖趾关节并伸趾间关节	足底外侧神经深支	弓状动脉；足底深动脉	记住背侧肌外展和足底肌内收是以第2趾为标志，可以帮助你记忆骨间肌的附着点
足的骨间足底肌（图3-46、图3-51和图3-52）	第3~5跖骨底内侧	第3~5趾近节趾骨底和趾背腱膜	内收第3~5趾（运动足趾向定义为中线的第2趾靠拢），屈第3~5趾跖趾关节并伸趾间关节	足底外侧神经深支	足底动脉弓；跖底动脉	记住背侧肌外展和足底肌内收是以第2趾为标志，可以帮助你记忆骨间肌的附着点

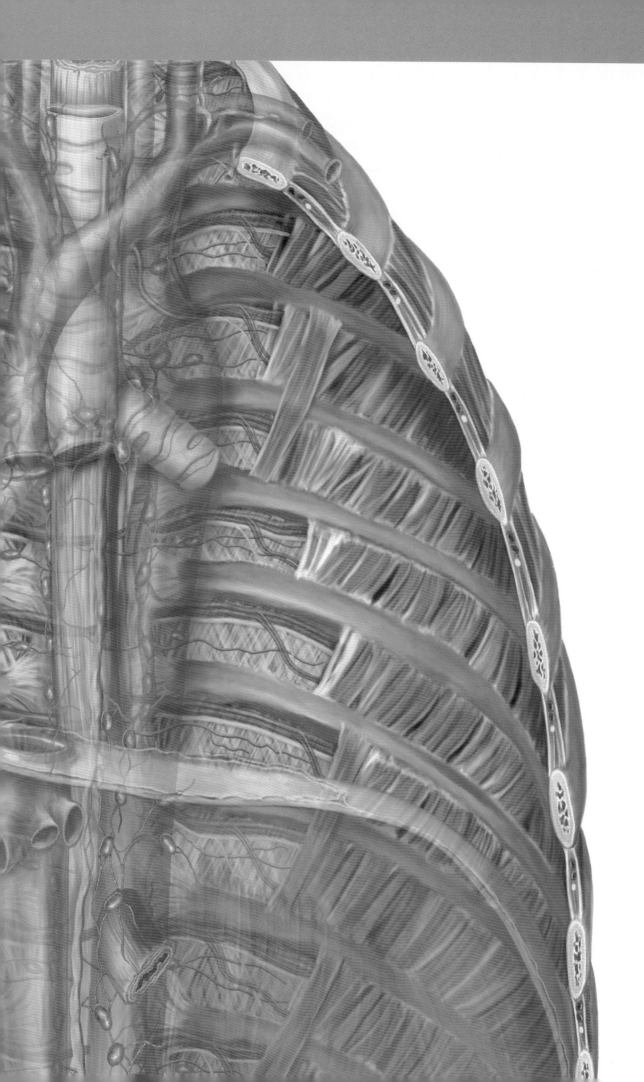

第四章 | 胸部

CHAPTER 4 | **The Thorax**

A. 前面观
Anterior view

可触及的骨性结构
Palpable bony structures

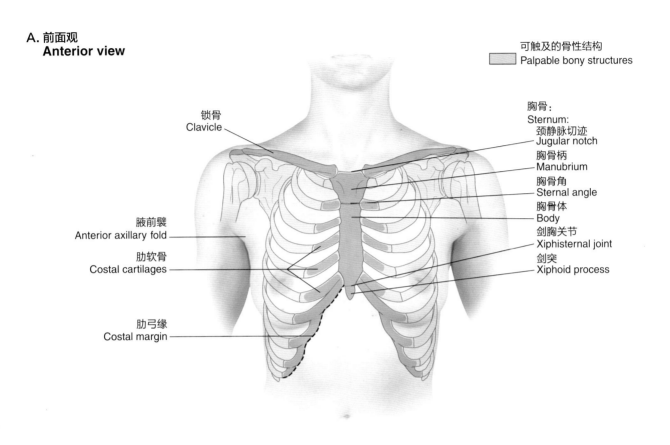

锁骨
Clavicle

胸骨：
Sternum:

颈静脉切迹
Jugular notch

胸骨柄
Manubrium

胸骨角
Sternal angle

胸骨体
Body

剑胸关节
Xiphisternal joint

剑突
Xiphoid process

腋前襞
Anterior axillary fold

肋软骨
Costal cartilages

肋弓缘
Costal margin

B. 标志，前面观
Landmarks, anterior view

C. 标志，侧面观
Landmarks, lateral view

D. 标志，后面观
Landmarks, posterior view

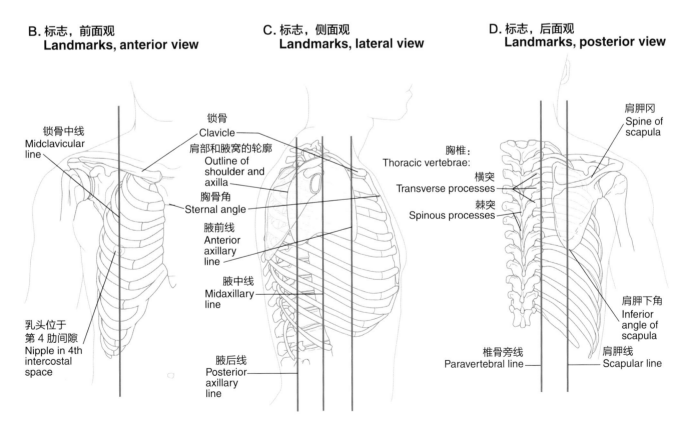

锁骨中线
Midclavicular line

锁骨
Clavicle

肩部和腋窝的轮廓
Outline of shoulder and axilla

胸骨角
Sternal angle

腋前线
Anterior axillary line

腋中线
Midaxillary line

乳头位于第 4 肋间隙
Nipple in 4th intercostal space

腋后线
Posterior axillary line

胸椎：
Thoracic vertebrae:

横突
Transverse processes

棘突
Spinous processes

肩胛冈
Spine of scapula

肩胛下角
Inferior angle of scapula

肩胛线
Scapular line

椎骨旁线
Paravertebral line

图 4-02

胸部的皮神经和浅表血管
Cutaneous Nerves and Superficial Vessels of the Thorax

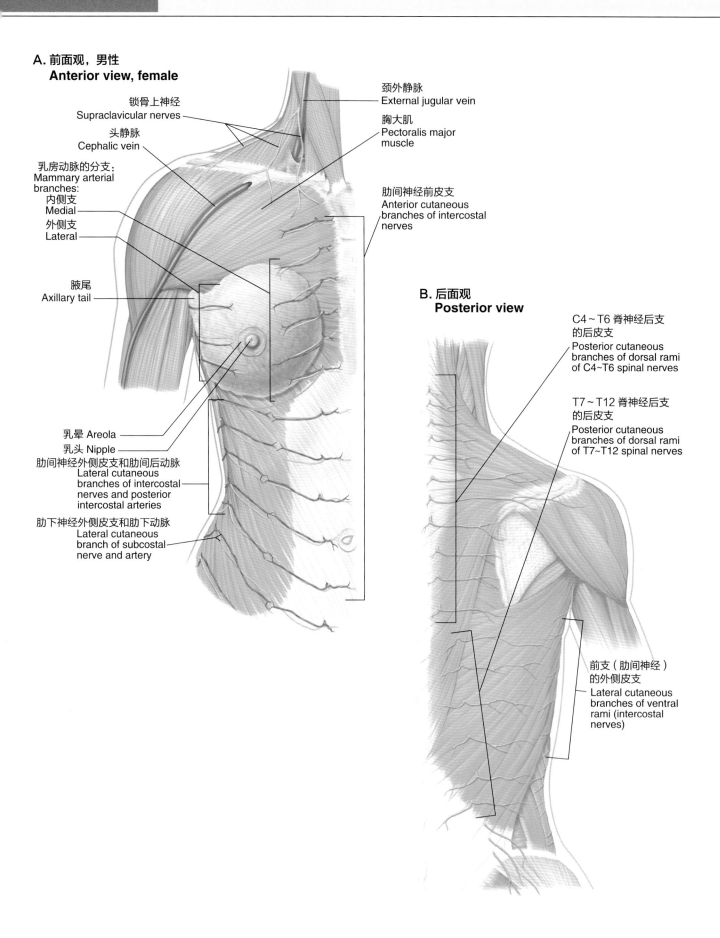

A. 前面观，男性
Anterior view, female

锁骨上神经
Supraclavicular nerves

头静脉
Cephalic vein

乳房动脉的分支：
Mammary arterial
branches:
内侧支
Medial
外侧支
Lateral

腋尾
Axillary tail

乳晕 Areola
乳头 Nipple
肋间神经外侧皮支和肋间后动脉
Lateral cutaneous
branches of intercostal
nerves and posterior
intercostal arteries

肋下神经外侧皮支和肋下动脉
Lateral cutaneous
branch of subcostal
nerve and artery

颈外静脉
External jugular vein

胸大肌
Pectoralis major
muscle

肋间神经前皮支
Anterior cutaneous
branches of intercostal
nerves

B. 后面观
Posterior view

C4～T6 脊神经后支
的后皮支
Posterior cutaneous
branches of dorsal rami
of C4~T6 spinal nerves

T7～T12 脊神经后支
的后皮支
Posterior cutaneous
branches of dorsal rami
of T7~T12 spinal nerves

前支（肋间神经）
的外侧皮支
Lateral cutaneous
branches of ventral
rami (intercostal
nerves)

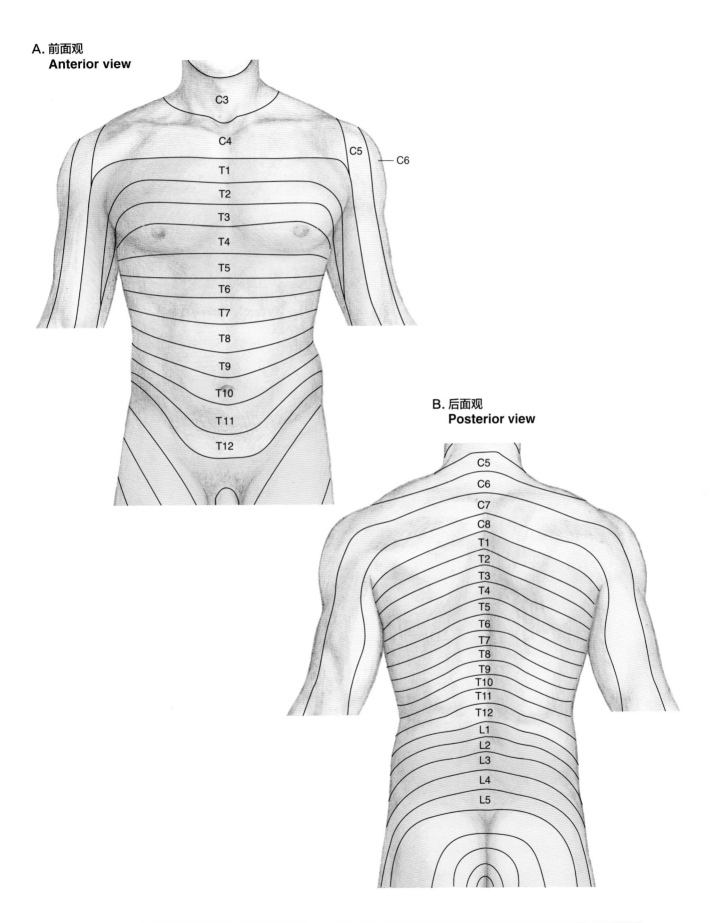

A. 前面观
Anterior view

C3

C4

C5　— C6

T1

T2

T3

T4

T5

T6

T7

T8

T9

T10

T11

T12

B. 后面观
Posterior view

C5

C6

C7

C8

T1

T2

T3

T4

T5

T6

T7

T8

T9

T10

T11

T12

L1

L2

L3

L4

L5

图 4-04　胸壁的骨骼　Skeleton of the Thoracic Wall

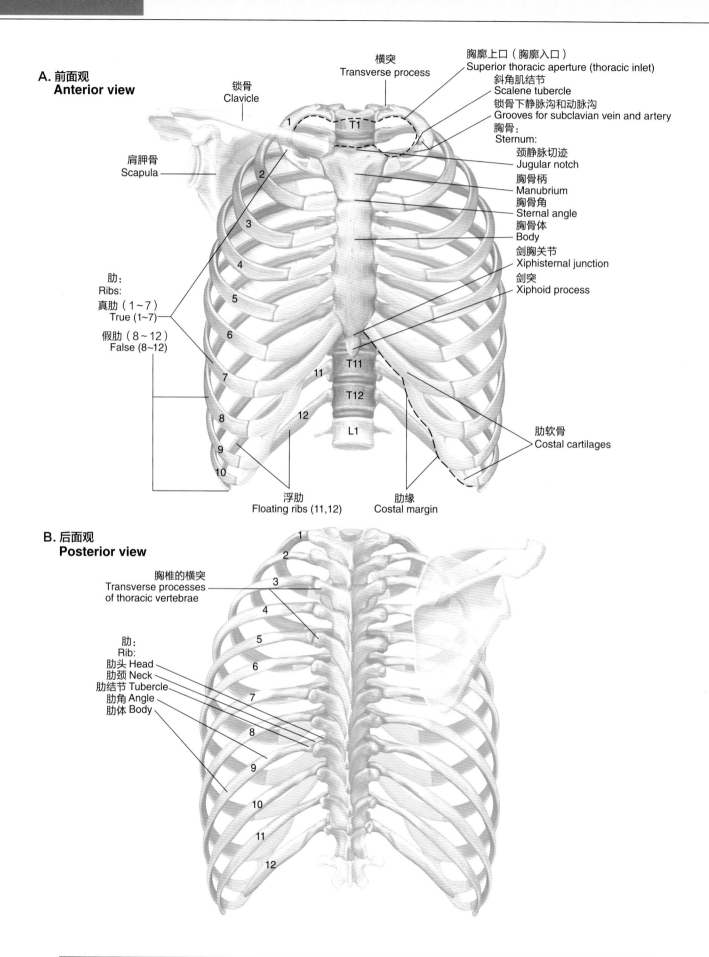

A. 前面观
Anterior view

横突
Transverse process

胸廓上口（胸廓入口）
Superior thoracic aperture (thoracic inlet)
斜角肌结节
Scalene tubercle
锁骨下静脉沟和动脉沟
Grooves for subclavian vein and artery
胸骨：
Sternum:
颈静脉切迹
Jugular notch
胸骨柄
Manubrium
胸骨角
Sternal angle
胸骨体
Body
剑胸关节
Xiphisternal junction
剑突
Xiphoid process

锁骨
Clavicle

肩胛骨
Scapula

肋：
Ribs:
真肋（1~7）
True (1~7)

假肋（8~12）
False (8~12)

肋软骨
Costal cartilages

浮肋
Floating ribs (11,12)

肋缘
Costal margin

B. 后面观
Posterior view

胸椎的横突
Transverse processes
of thoracic vertebrae

肋：
Rib:
肋头 Head
肋颈 Neck
肋结节 Tubercle
肋角 Angle
肋体 Body

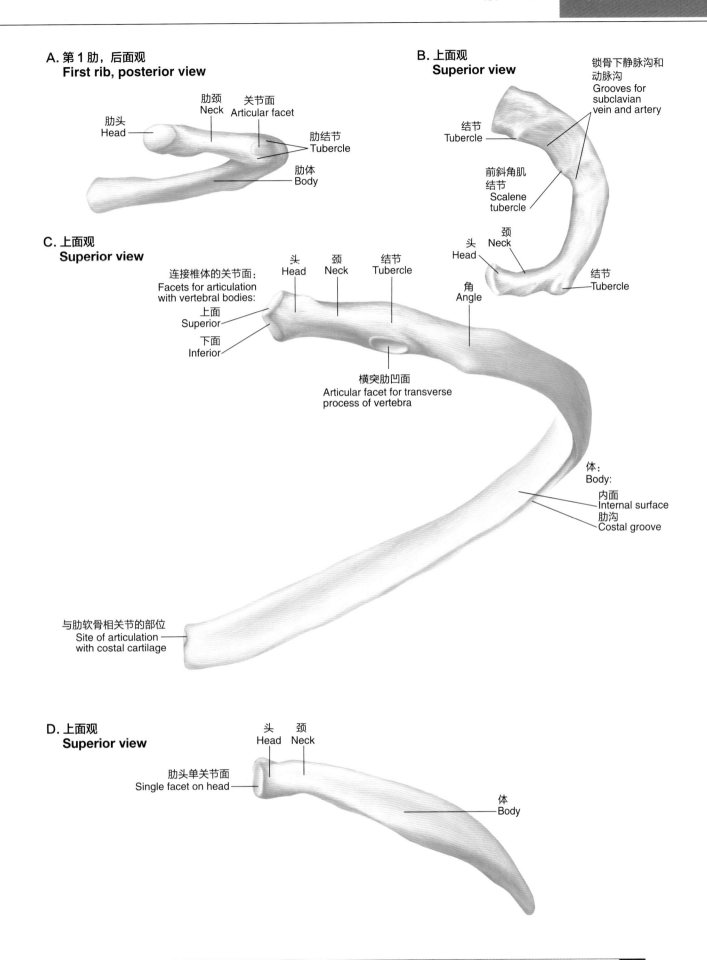

A. 第 1 肋，后面观
First rib, posterior view

肋头
Head

肋颈
Neck

关节面
Articular facet

肋结节
Tubercle

肋体
Body

B. 上面观
Superior view

锁骨下静脉沟和动脉沟
Grooves for subclavian vein and artery

结节
Tubercle

前斜角肌结节
Scalene tubercle

头
Head

颈
Neck

结节
Tubercle

C. 上面观
Superior view

连接椎体的关节面：
Facets for articulation with vertebral bodies:

上面
Superior

下面
Inferior

头
Head

颈
Neck

结节
Tubercle

角
Angle

横突肋凹面
Articular facet for transverse process of vertebra

体：
Body:

内面
Internal surface

肋沟
Costal groove

与肋软骨相关节的部位
Site of articulation with costal cartilage

D. 上面观
Superior view

头
Head

颈
Neck

肋头单关节面
Single facet on head

体
Body

图 4-06　　肋椎关节　Costovertebral and Sternocostal Articulations

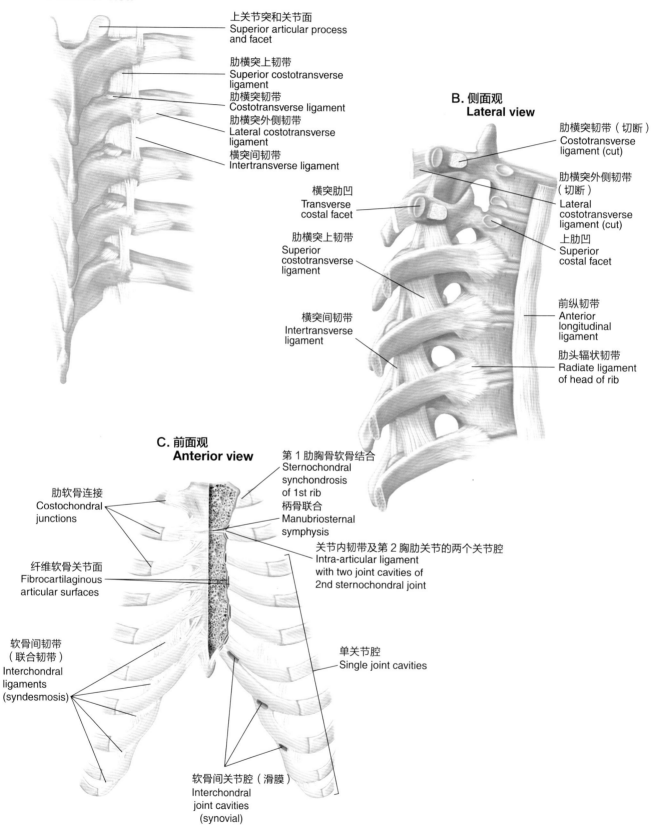

A. 后面观
Posterior view

上关节突和关节面
Superior articular process and facet

肋横突上韧带
Superior costotransverse ligament

肋横突韧带
Costotransverse ligament

肋横突外侧韧带
Lateral costotransverse ligament

横突间韧带
Intertransverse ligament

横突肋凹
Transverse costal facet

肋横突上韧带
Superior costotransverse ligament

横突间韧带
Intertransverse ligament

B. 侧面观
Lateral view

肋横突韧带（切断）
Costotransverse ligament (cut)

肋横突外侧韧带（切断）
Lateral costotransverse ligament (cut)

上肋凹
Superior costal facet

前纵韧带
Anterior longitudinal ligament

肋头辐状韧带
Radiate ligament of head of rib

C. 前面观
Anterior view

肋软骨连接
Costochondral junctions

纤维软骨关节面
Fibrocartilaginous articular surfaces

软骨间韧带
（联合韧带）
Interchondral ligaments (syndesmosis)

第 1 肋胸骨软骨结合
Sternochondral synchondrosis of 1st rib

柄骨联合
Manubriosternal symphysis

关节内韧带及第 2 胸肋关节的两个关节腔
Intra-articular ligament with two joint cavities of 2nd sternochondral joint

单关节腔
Single joint cavities

软骨间关节腔（滑膜）
Interchondral joint cavities (synovial)

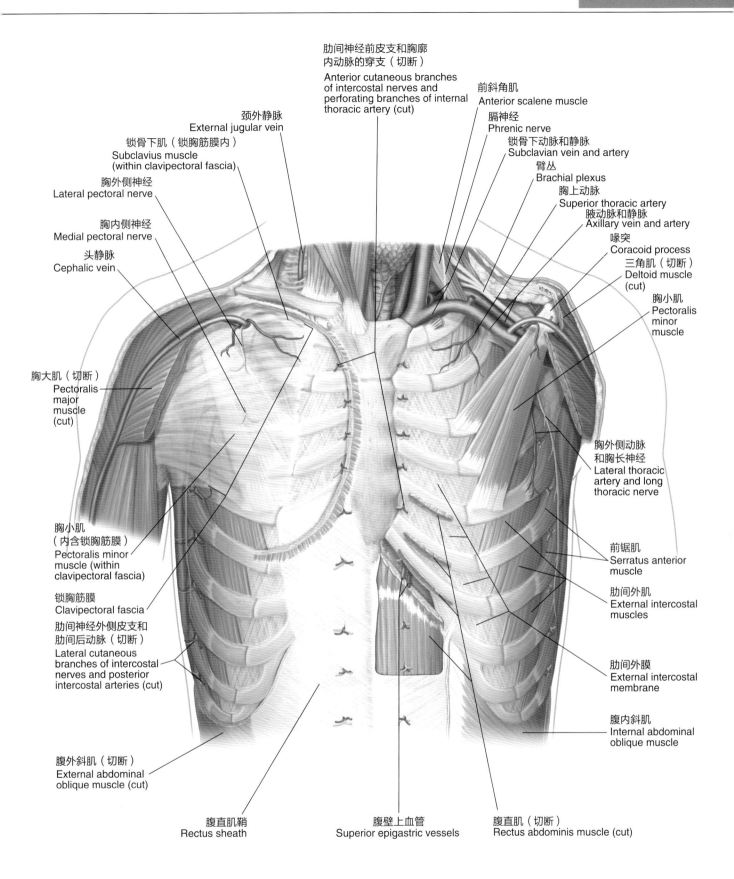

肋间神经前皮支和胸廓
内动脉的穿支（切断）
Anterior cutaneous branches
of intercostal nerves and
perforating branches of internal
thoracic artery (cut)

前斜角肌
Anterior scalene muscle

膈神经
Phrenic nerve

锁骨下动脉和静脉
Subclavian vein and artery

臂丛
Brachial plexus

胸上动脉
Superior thoracic artery

腋动脉和静脉
Axillary vein and artery

喙突
Coracoid process

三角肌（切断）
Deltoid muscle
(cut)

胸小肌
Pectoralis
minor
muscle

颈外静脉
External jugular vein

锁骨下肌（锁胸筋膜内）
Subclavius muscle
(within clavipectoral fascia)

胸外侧神经
Lateral pectoral nerve

胸内侧神经
Medial pectoral nerve

头静脉
Cephalic vein

胸大肌（切断）
Pectoralis
major
muscle
(cut)

胸外侧动脉
和胸长神经
Lateral thoracic
artery and long
thoracic nerve

胸小肌
（内含锁胸筋膜）
Pectoralis minor
muscle (within
clavipectoral fascia)

锁胸筋膜
Clavipectoral fascia

肋间神经外侧皮支和
肋间后动脉（切断）
Lateral cutaneous
branches of intercostal
nerves and posterior
intercostal arteries (cut)

前锯肌
Serratus anterior
muscle

肋间外肌
External intercostal
muscles

肋间外膜
External intercostal
membrane

腹内斜肌
Internal abdominal
oblique muscle

腹外斜肌（切断）
External abdominal
oblique muscle (cut)

腹直肌鞘
Rectus sheath

腹壁上血管
Superior epigastric vessels

腹直肌（切断）
Rectus abdominis muscle (cut)

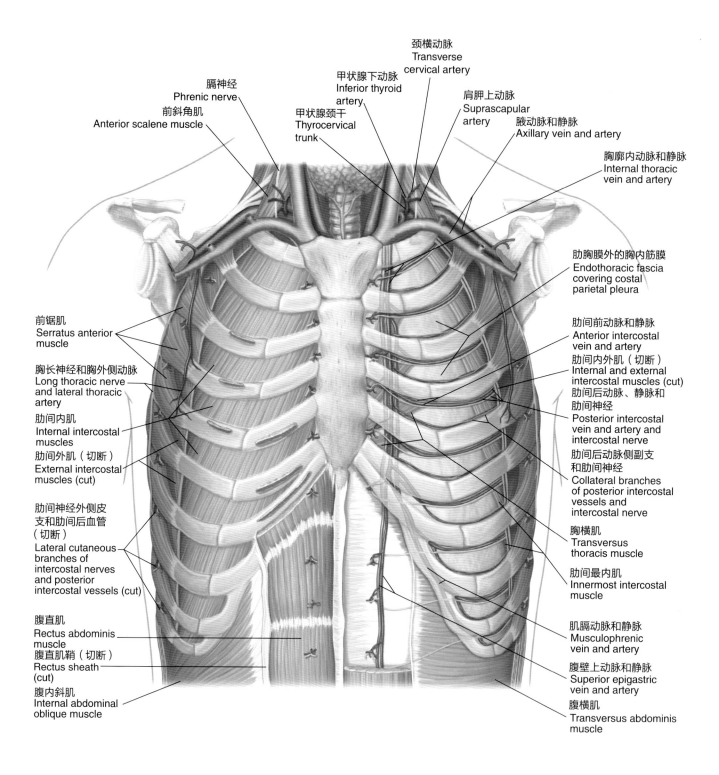

膈神经
Phrenic nerve

前斜角肌
Anterior scalene muscle

甲状腺颈干
Thyrocervical trunk

甲状腺下动脉
Inferior thyroid artery

颈横动脉
Transverse cervical artery

肩胛上动脉
Suprascapular artery

腋动脉和静脉
Axillary vein and artery

胸廓内动脉和静脉
Internal thoracic vein and artery

肋胸膜外的胸内筋膜
Endothoracic fascia covering costal parietal pleura

前锯肌
Serratus anterior muscle

胸长神经和胸外侧动脉
Long thoracic nerve and lateral thoracic artery

肋间内肌
Internal intercostal muscles

肋间外肌（切断）
External intercostal muscles (cut)

肋间神经外侧皮支和肋间后血管（切断）
Lateral cutaneous branches of intercostal nerves and posterior intercostal vessels (cut)

腹直肌
Rectus abdominis muscle

腹直肌鞘（切断）
Rectus sheath (cut)

腹内斜肌
Internal abdominal oblique muscle

肋间前动脉和静脉
Anterior intercostal vein and artery

肋间内外肌（切断）
Internal and external intercostal muscles (cut)

肋间后动脉、静脉和肋间神经
Posterior intercostal vein and artery and intercostal nerve

肋间后动脉侧副支和肋间神经
Collateral branches of posterior intercostal vessels and intercostal nerve

胸横肌
Transversus thoracis muscle

肋间最内肌
Innermost intercostal muscle

肌膈动脉和静脉
Musculophrenic vein and artery

腹壁上动脉和静脉
Superior epigastric vein and artery

腹横肌
Transversus abdominis muscle

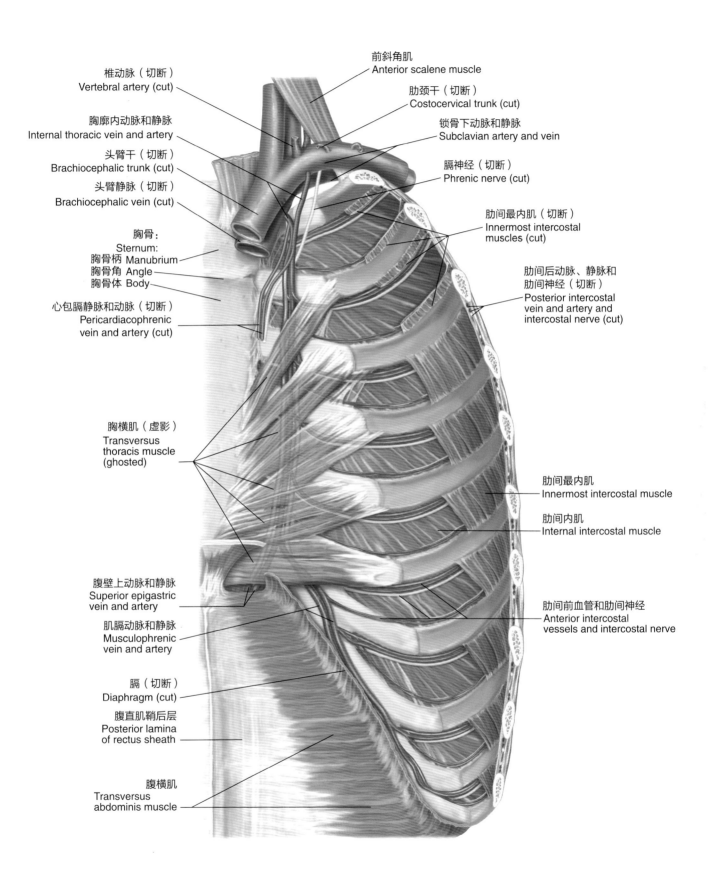

椎动脉（切断）
Vertebral artery (cut)

前斜角肌
Anterior scalene muscle

肋颈干（切断）
Costocervical trunk (cut)

胸廓内动脉和静脉
Internal thoracic vein and artery

锁骨下动脉和静脉
Subclavian artery and vein

头臂干（切断）
Brachiocephalic trunk (cut)

膈神经（切断）
Phrenic nerve (cut)

头臂静脉（切断）
Brachiocephalic vein (cut)

肋间最内肌（切断）
Innermost intercostal muscles (cut)

胸骨：
Sternum:
胸骨柄 Manubrium
胸骨角 Angle
胸骨体 Body

肋间后动脉、静脉和肋间神经（切断）
Posterior intercostal vein and artery and intercostal nerve (cut)

心包膈静脉和动脉（切断）
Pericardiacophrenic vein and artery (cut)

胸横肌（虚影）
Transversus thoracis muscle (ghosted)

肋间最内肌
Innermost intercostal muscle

肋间内肌
Internal intercostal muscle

腹壁上动脉和静脉
Superior epigastric vein and artery

肌膈动脉和静脉
Musculophrenic vein and artery

肋间前血管和肋间神经
Anterior intercostal vessels and intercostal nerve

膈（切断）
Diaphragm (cut)

腹直肌鞘后层
Posterior lamina of rectus sheath

腹横肌
Transversus abdominis muscle

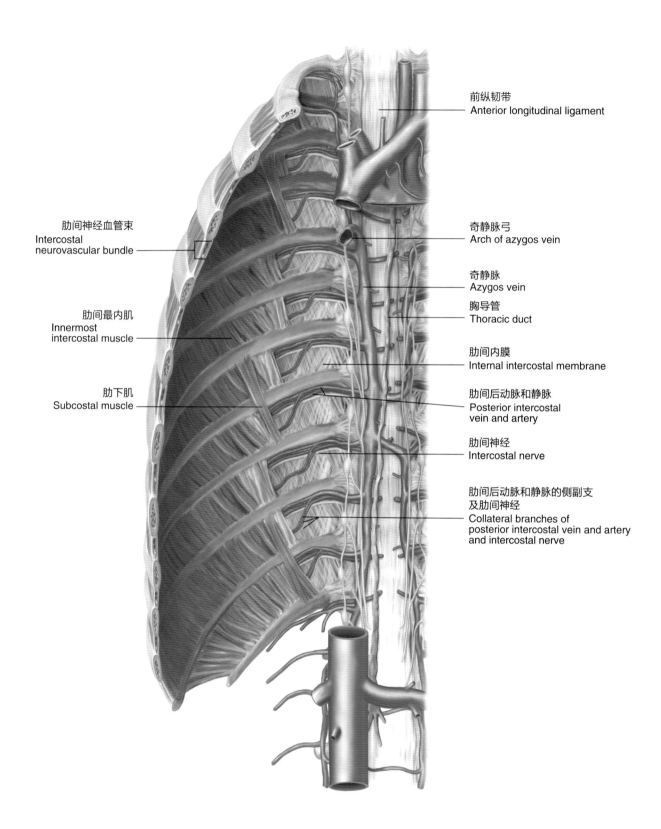

前纵韧带
Anterior longitudinal ligament

肋间神经血管束
Intercostal
neurovascular bundle

肋间最内肌
Innermost
intercostal muscle

肋下肌
Subcostal muscle

奇静脉弓
Arch of azygos vein

奇静脉
Azygos vein

胸导管
Thoracic duct

肋间内膜
Internal intercostal membrane

肋间后动脉和静脉
Posterior intercostal
vein and artery

肋间神经
Intercostal nerve

肋间后动脉和静脉的侧副支
及肋间神经
Collateral branches of
posterior intercostal vein and artery
and intercostal nerve

胸后壁肌，除去胸膜内面观
Muscles of the Posterior Thoracic Wall, Internal View with Pleura Removed

A. 定位
Orientation

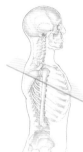

图 B 所在平面
Plane of section B

B. 经第 4 肋间隙的斜断面
Oblique section through 4th intercostal space

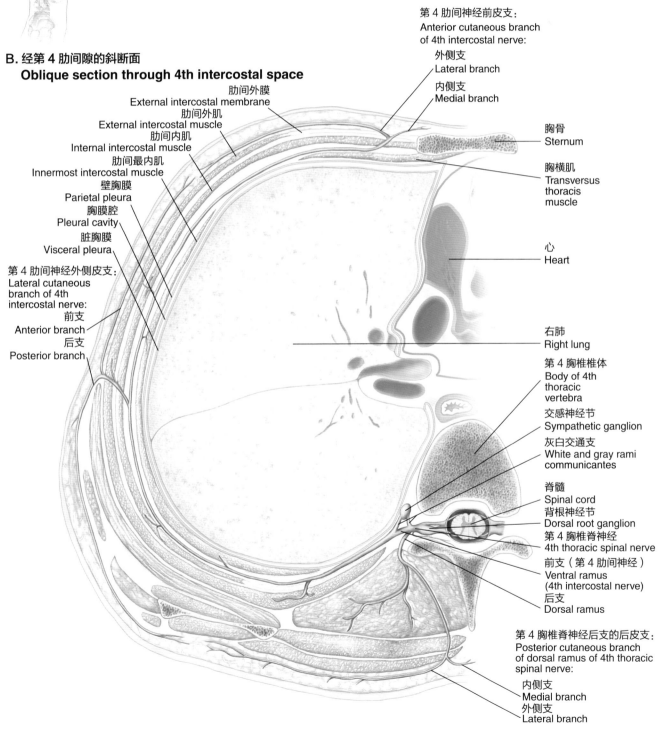

第 4 肋间神经前皮支：
Anterior cutaneous branch
of 4th intercostal nerve:
外侧支
Lateral branch
内侧支
Medial branch

肋间外膜
External intercostal membrane
肋间外肌
External intercostal muscle
肋间内肌
Internal intercostal muscle
肋间最内肌
Innermost intercostal muscle
壁胸膜
Parietal pleura
胸膜腔
Pleural cavity
脏胸膜
Visceral pleura

胸骨
Sternum

胸横肌
Transversus
thoracis
muscle

心
Heart

第 4 肋间神经外侧皮支：
Lateral cutaneous
branch of 4th
intercostal nerve:
前支
Anterior branch
后支
Posterior branch

右肺
Right lung

第 4 胸椎椎体
Body of 4th
thoracic
vertebra
交感神经节
Sympathetic ganglion
灰白交通支
White and gray rami
communicantes
脊髓
Spinal cord
背根神经节
Dorsal root ganglion
第 4 胸椎脊神经
4th thoracic spinal nerve
前支（第 4 肋间神经）
Ventral ramus
(4th intercostal nerve)
后支
Dorsal ramus

第 4 胸椎脊神经后支的后皮支：
Posterior cutaneous branch
of dorsal ramus of 4th thoracic
spinal nerve:
内侧支
Medial branch
外侧支
Lateral branch

图 4-12　第 10 肋间神经的分布　Pattern of the 10th Intercostal Nerve

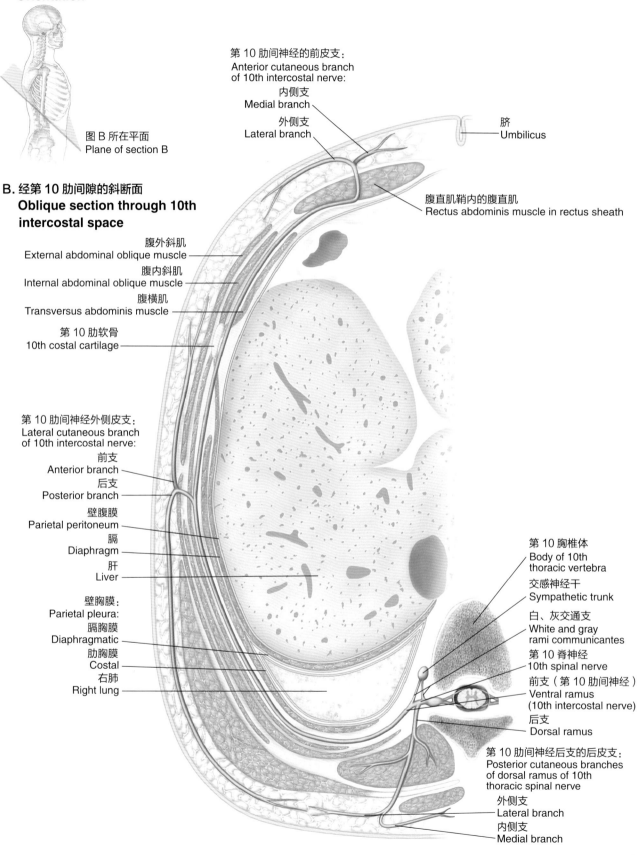

A. 定位
Orientation

图 B 所在平面
Plane of section B

B. 经第 10 肋间隙的斜断面
Oblique section through 10th intercostal space

第 10 肋间神经的前皮支：
Anterior cutaneous branch
of 10th intercostal nerve:

内侧支
Medial branch

外侧支
Lateral branch

脐
Umbilicus

腹直肌鞘内的腹直肌
Rectus abdominis muscle in rectus sheath

腹外斜肌
External abdominal oblique muscle

腹内斜肌
Internal abdominal oblique muscle

腹横肌
Transversus abdominis muscle

第 10 肋软骨
10th costal cartilage

第 10 肋间神经外侧皮支：
Lateral cutaneous branch
of 10th intercostal nerve:

前支
Anterior branch

后支
Posterior branch

壁腹膜
Parietal peritoneum

膈
Diaphragm

肝
Liver

壁胸膜：
Parietal pleura:

膈胸膜
Diaphragmatic

肋胸膜
Costal

右肺
Right lung

第 10 胸椎体
Body of 10th
thoracic vertebra

交感神经干
Sympathetic trunk

白、灰交通支
White and gray
rami communicantes

第 10 脊神经
10th spinal nerve

前支（第 10 肋间神经）
Ventral ramus
(10th intercostal nerve)

后支
Dorsal ramus

第 10 肋间神经后支的后皮支：
Posterior cutaneous branches
of dorsal ramus of 10th
thoracic spinal nerve

外侧支
Lateral branch

内侧支
Medial branch

A. 前面观
Anterior view

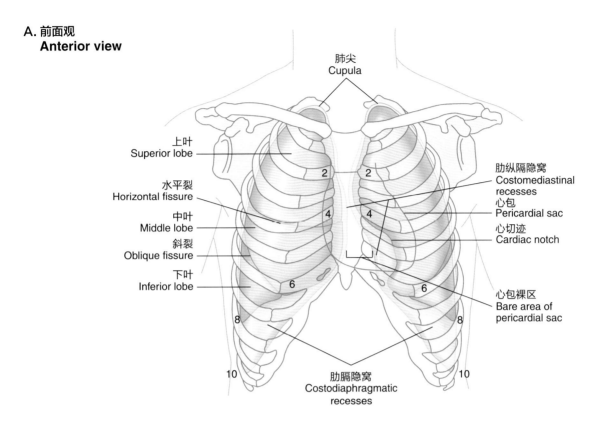

肺尖
Cupula

上叶
Superior lobe

水平裂
Horizontal fissure

中叶
Middle lobe

斜裂
Oblique fissure

下叶
Inferior lobe

肋纵隔隐窝
Costomediastinal
recesses

心包
Pericardial sac

心切迹
Cardiac notch

心包裸区
Bare area of
pericardial sac

肋膈隐窝
Costodiaphragmatic
recesses

B. 后面观
Posterior view

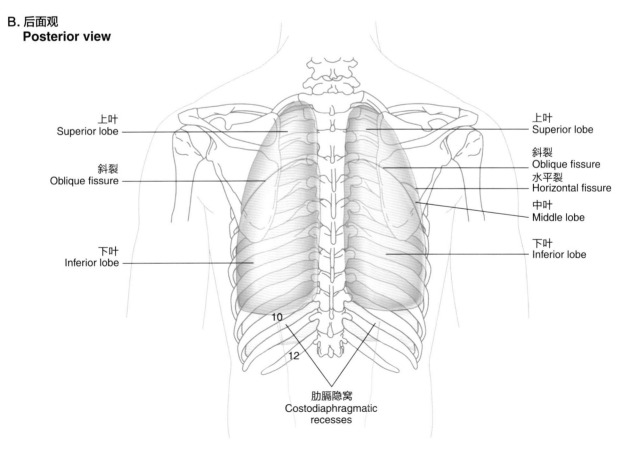

上叶
Superior lobe

斜裂
Oblique fissure

下叶
Inferior lobe

上叶
Superior lobe

斜裂
Oblique fissure

水平裂
Horizontal fissure

中叶
Middle lobe

下叶
Inferior lobe

肋膈隐窝
Costodiaphragmatic
recesses

图 4-14　心和纵隔的体表投影　Surface Projection of the Heart and Mediastinum

A. 心和心瓣膜
Heart and heart valves

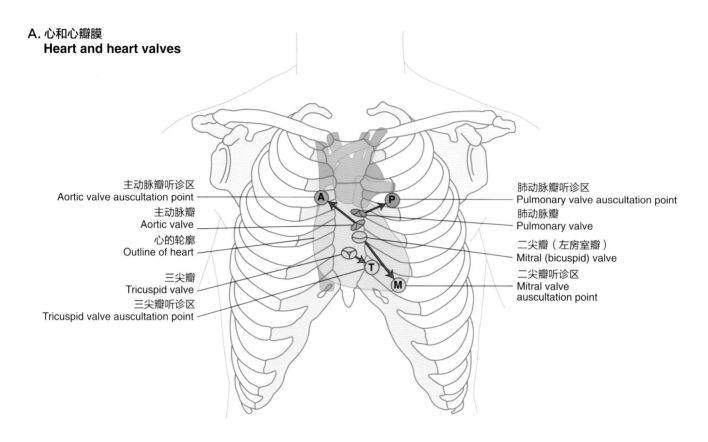

主动脉瓣听诊区
Aortic valve auscultation point

主动脉瓣
Aortic valve

心的轮廓
Outline of heart

三尖瓣
Tricuspid valve

三尖瓣听诊区
Tricuspid valve auscultation point

肺动脉瓣听诊区
Pulmonary valve auscultation point

肺动脉瓣
Pulmonary valve

二尖瓣（左房室瓣）
Mitral (bicuspid) valve

二尖瓣听诊区
Mitral valve
auscultation point

B. 纵隔，前面观
Mediastinum, anterior view

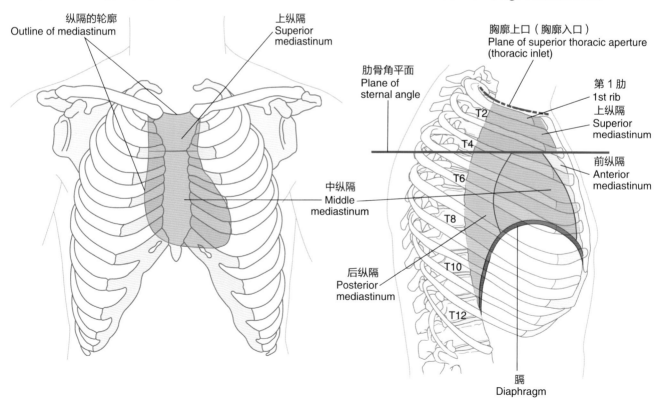

纵隔的轮廓
Outline of mediastinum

上纵隔
Superior
mediastinum

中纵隔
Middle
mediastinum

后纵隔
Posterior
mediastinum

C. 纵隔，右侧面观
Mediastinum, right lateral view

肋骨角平面
Plane of
sternal angle

胸廓上口（胸廓入口）
Plane of superior thoracic aperture
(thoracic inlet)

第 1 肋
1st rib

上纵隔
Superior
mediastinum

前纵隔
Anterior
mediastinum

T2

T4

T6

T8

T10

T12

膈
Diaphragm

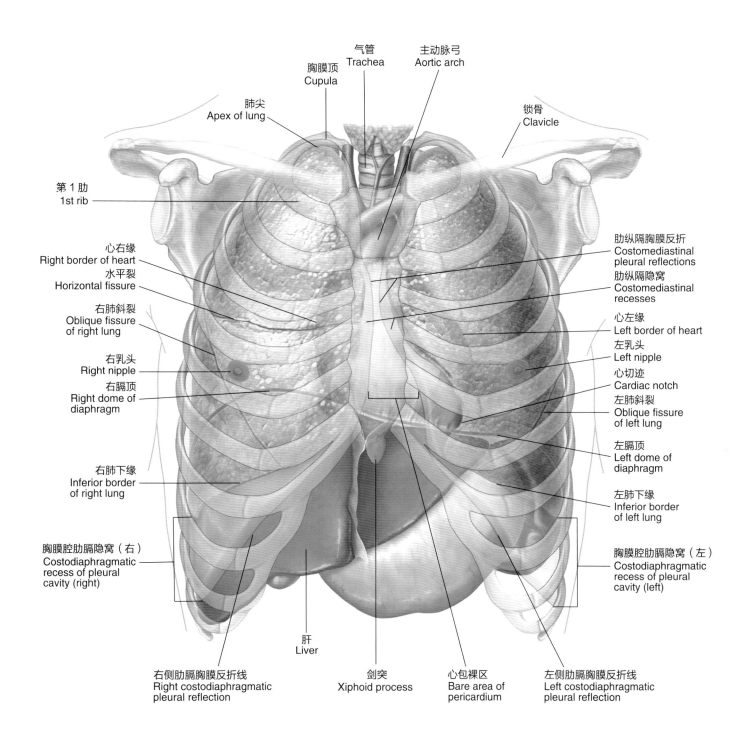

胸膜顶
Cupula

气管
Trachea

主动脉弓
Aortic arch

肺尖
Apex of lung

锁骨
Clavicle

第 1 肋
1st rib

心右缘
Right border of heart

水平裂
Horizontal fissure

右肺斜裂
Oblique fissure
of right lung

右乳头
Right nipple

右膈顶
Right dome of
diaphragm

右肺下缘
Inferior border
of right lung

胸膜腔肋膈隐窝（右）
Costodiaphragmatic
recess of pleural
cavity (right)

肋纵隔胸膜反折
Costomediastinal
pleural reflections

肋纵隔隐窝
Costomediastinal
recesses

心左缘
Left border of heart

左乳头
Left nipple

心切迹
Cardiac notch

左肺斜裂
Oblique fissure
of left lung

左膈顶
Left dome of
diaphragm

左肺下缘
Inferior border
of left lung

胸膜腔肋膈隐窝（左）
Costodiaphragmatic
recess of pleural
cavity (left)

肝
Liver

右侧肋膈胸膜反折线
Right costodiaphragmatic
pleural reflection

剑突
Xiphoid process

心包裸区
Bare area of
pericardium

左侧肋膈胸膜反折线
Left costodiaphragmatic
pleural reflection

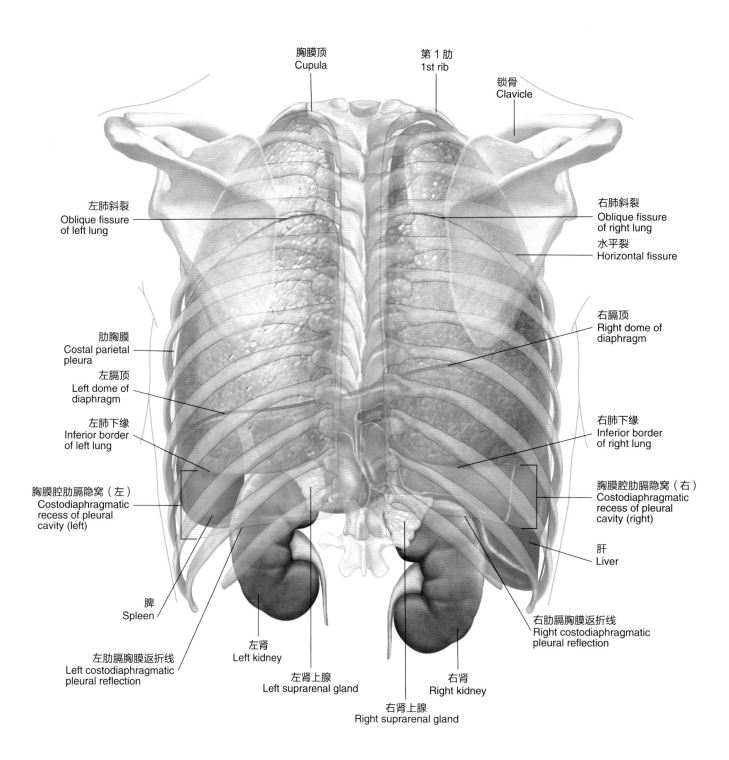

胸膜顶
Cupula

第 1 肋
1st rib

锁骨
Clavicle

左肺斜裂
Oblique fissure
of left lung

右肺斜裂
Oblique fissure
of right lung

水平裂
Horizontal fissure

肋胸膜
Costal parietal
pleura

右膈顶
Right dome of
diaphragm

左膈顶
Left dome of
diaphragm

左肺下缘
Inferior border
of left lung

右肺下缘
Inferior border
of right lung

胸膜腔肋膈隐窝（左）
Costodiaphragmatic
recess of pleural
cavity (left)

胸膜腔肋膈隐窝（右）
Costodiaphragmatic
recess of pleural
cavity (right)

肝
Liver

脾
Spleen

右肋膈胸膜返折线
Right costodiaphragmatic
pleural reflection

左肋膈胸膜返折线
Left costodiaphragmatic
pleural reflection

左肾
Left kidney

左肾上腺
Left suprarenal gland

右肾
Right kidney

右肾上腺
Right suprarenal gland

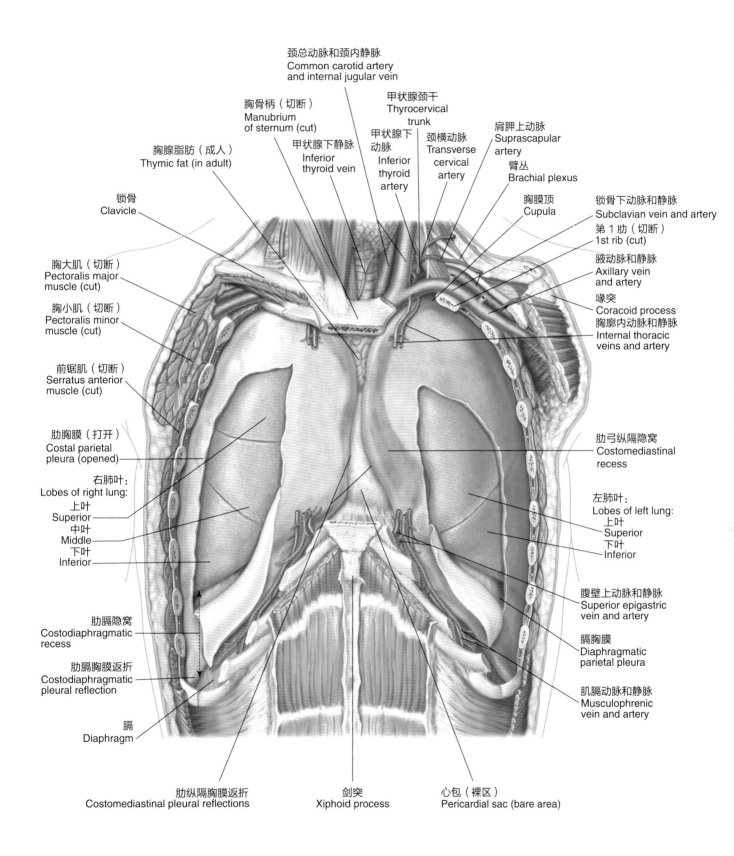

颈总动脉和颈内静脉
Common carotid artery
and internal jugular vein

胸骨柄（切断）
Manubrium
of sternum (cut)

甲状腺颈干
Thyrocervical
trunk

甲状腺下静脉
Inferior
thyroid vein

甲状腺下动脉
Inferior
thyroid
artery

颈横动脉
Transverse
cervical
artery

肩胛上动脉
Suprascapular
artery

臂丛
Brachial plexus

胸膜顶
Cupula

锁骨下动脉和静脉
Subclavian vein and artery

第 1 肋（切断）
1st rib (cut)

腋动脉和静脉
Axillary vein
and artery

喙突
Coracoid process

胸廓内动脉和静脉
Internal thoracic
veins and artery

胸腺脂肪（成人）
Thymic fat (in adult)

锁骨
Clavicle

胸大肌（切断）
Pectoralis major
muscle (cut)

胸小肌（切断）
Pectoralis minor
muscle (cut)

前锯肌（切断）
Serratus anterior
muscle (cut)

肋胸膜（打开）
Costal parietal
pleura (opened)

右肺叶：
Lobes of right lung:
上叶
Superior
中叶
Middle
下叶
Inferior

肋膈隐窝
Costodiaphragmatic
recess

肋膈胸膜返折
Costodiaphragmatic
pleural reflection

膈
Diaphragm

肋弓纵隔隐窝
Costomediastinal
recess

左肺叶：
Lobes of left lung:
上叶
Superior
下叶
Inferior

腹壁上动脉和静脉
Superior epigastric
vein and artery

膈胸膜
Diaphragmatic
parietal pleura

肌膈动脉和静脉
Musculophrenic
vein and artery

肋纵隔胸膜返折
Costomediastinal pleural reflections

剑突
Xiphoid process

心包（裸区）
Pericardial sac (bare area)

图 4-18 **胸腔脏器，心包 Thoracic Viscera, Pericardial Sac**

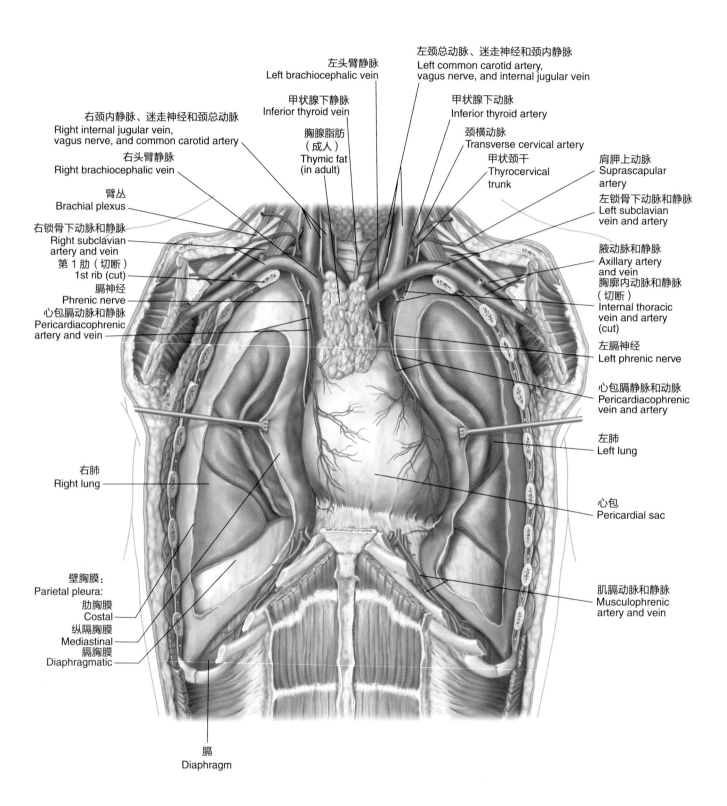

左头臂静脉
Left brachiocephalic vein

左颈总动脉、迷走神经和颈内静脉
Left common carotid artery,
vagus nerve, and internal jugular vein

甲状腺下静脉
Inferior thyroid vein

甲状腺下动脉
Inferior thyroid artery

右颈内静脉、迷走神经和颈总动脉
Right internal jugular vein,
vagus nerve, and common carotid artery

胸腺脂肪
（成人）
Thymic fat
(in adult)

颈横动脉
Transverse cervical artery

右头臂静脉
Right brachiocephalic vein

甲状颈干
Thyrocervical
trunk

肩胛上动脉
Suprascapular
artery

臂丛
Brachial plexus

左锁骨下动脉和静脉
Left subclavian
vein and artery

右锁骨下动脉和静脉
Right subclavian
artery and vein

腋动脉和静脉
Axillary artery
and vein

第 1 肋（切断）
1st rib (cut)

胸廓内动脉和静脉
（切断）
Internal thoracic
vein and artery
(cut)

膈神经
Phrenic nerve

心包膈动脉和静脉
Pericardiacophrenic
artery and vein

左膈神经
Left phrenic nerve

心包膈静脉和动脉
Pericardiacophrenic
vein and artery

左肺
Left lung

右肺
Right lung

心包
Pericardial sac

壁胸膜：
Parietal pleura:
肋胸膜
Costal
纵隔胸膜
Mediastinal
膈胸膜
Diaphragmatic

肌膈动脉和静脉
Musculophrenic
artery and vein

膈
Diaphragm

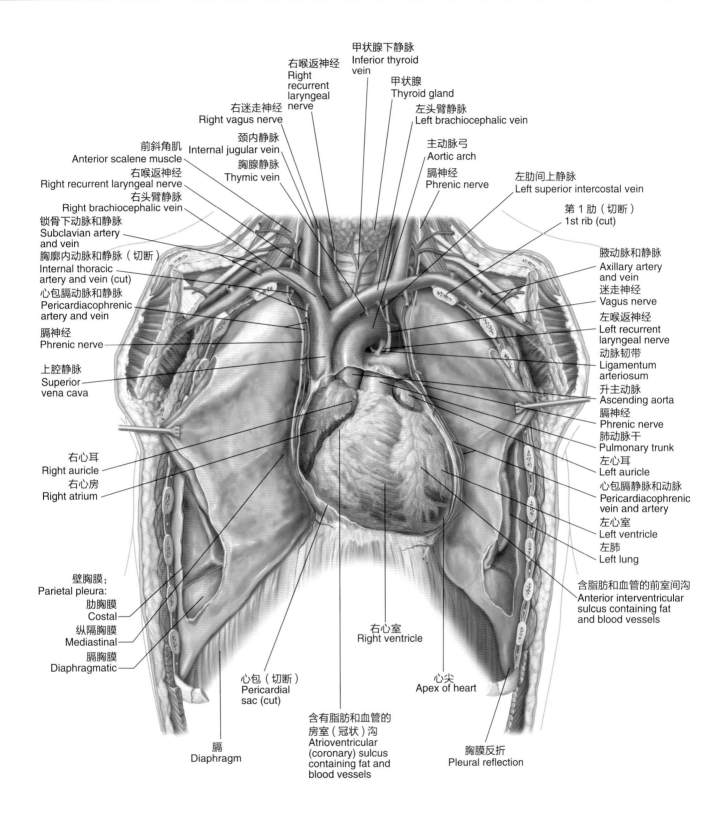

甲状腺下静脉
Inferior thyroid vein

右喉返神经
Right recurrent laryngeal nerve

甲状腺
Thyroid gland

右迷走神经
Right vagus nerve

左头臂静脉
Left brachiocephalic vein

前斜角肌
Anterior scalene muscle

颈内静脉
Internal jugular vein

主动脉弓
Aortic arch

右喉返神经
Right recurrent laryngeal nerve

胸腺静脉
Thymic vein

膈神经
Phrenic nerve

左肋间上静脉
Left superior intercostal vein

右头臂静脉
Right brachiocephalic vein

第 1 肋（切断）
1st rib (cut)

锁骨下动脉和静脉
Subclavian artery and vein

腋动脉和静脉
Axillary artery and vein

胸廓内动脉和静脉（切断）
Internal thoracic artery and vein (cut)

迷走神经
Vagus nerve

心包膈动脉和静脉
Pericardiacophrenic artery and vein

左喉返神经
Left recurrent laryngeal nerve

膈神经
Phrenic nerve

动脉韧带
Ligamentum arteriosum

上腔静脉
Superior vena cava

升主动脉
Ascending aorta

膈神经
Phrenic nerve

肺动脉干
Pulmonary trunk

右心耳
Right auricle

左心耳
Left auricle

右心房
Right atrium

心包膈静脉和动脉
Pericardiacophrenic vein and artery

左心室
Left ventricle

左肺
Left lung

壁胸膜：
Parietal pleura:

肋胸膜
Costal

纵隔胸膜
Mediastinal

膈胸膜
Diaphragmatic

含脂肪和血管的前室间沟
Anterior interventricular sulcus containing fat and blood vessels

右心室
Right ventricle

心包（切断）
Pericardial sac (cut)

心尖
Apex of heart

膈
Diaphragm

含有脂肪和血管的房室（冠状）沟
Atrioventricular (coronary) sulcus containing fat and blood vessels

胸膜反折
Pleural reflection

图 4-20　　**除去心的胸腔脏器　Thoracic Viscera with Heart Removed**

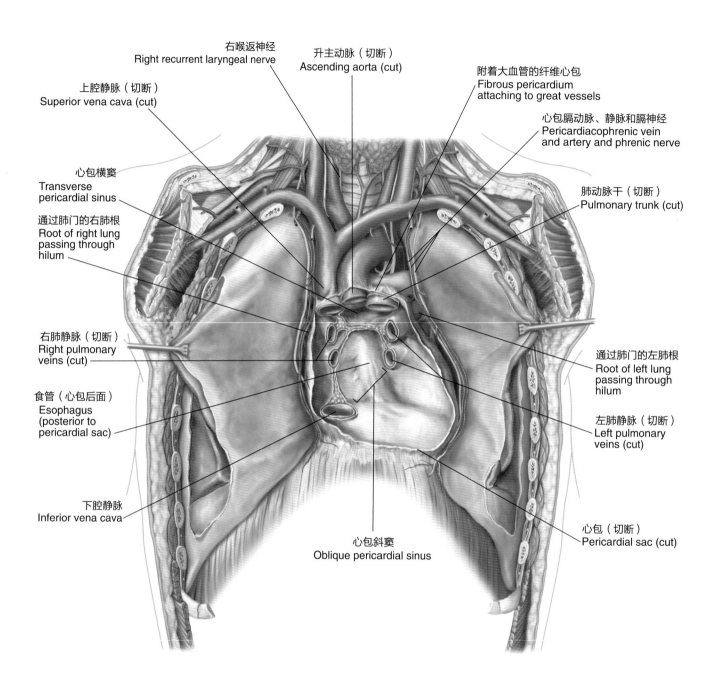

右喉返神经
Right recurrent laryngeal nerve

升主动脉（切断）
Ascending aorta (cut)

上腔静脉（切断）
Superior vena cava (cut)

附着大血管的纤维心包
Fibrous pericardium
attaching to great vessels

心包膈动脉、静脉和膈神经
Pericardiacophrenic vein
and artery and phrenic nerve

心包横窦
Transverse
pericardial sinus

肺动脉干（切断）
Pulmonary trunk (cut)

通过肺门的右肺根
Root of right lung
passing through
hilum

右肺静脉（切断）
Right pulmonary
veins (cut)

通过肺门的左肺根
Root of left lung
passing through
hilum

食管（心包后面）
Esophagus
(posterior to
pericardial sac)

左肺静脉（切断）
Left pulmonary
veins (cut)

下腔静脉
Inferior vena cava

心包（切断）
Pericardial sac (cut)

心包斜窦
Oblique pericardial sinus

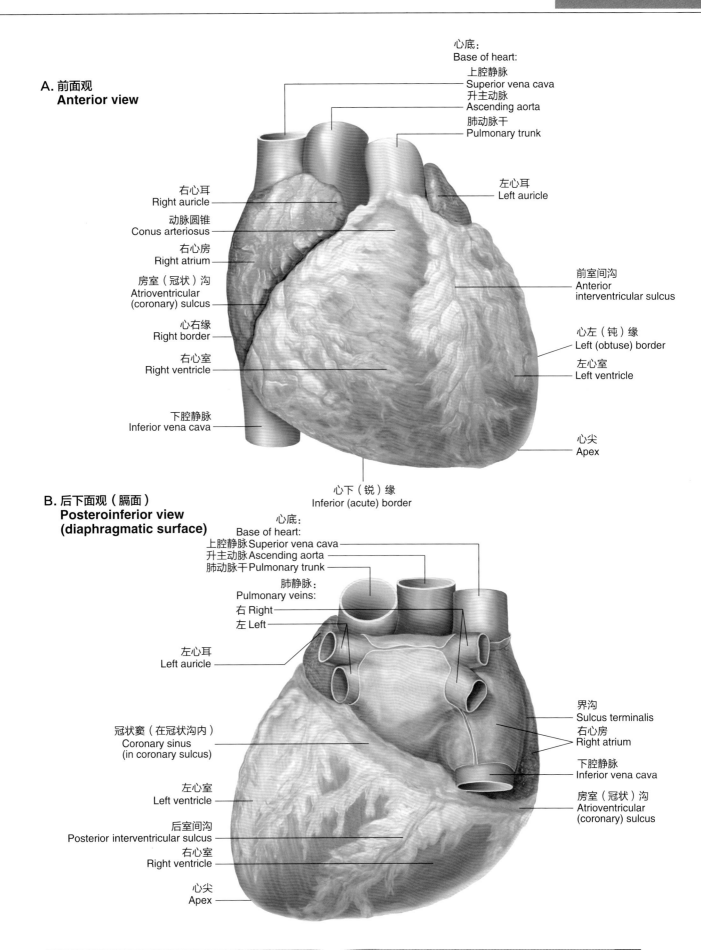

A. 前面观
Anterior view

心底：
Base of heart:

上腔静脉
Superior vena cava
升主动脉
Ascending aorta
肺动脉干
Pulmonary trunk

左心耳
Left auricle

右心耳
Right auricle

动脉圆锥
Conus arteriosus

右心房
Right atrium

房室（冠状）沟
Atrioventricular
(coronary) sulcus

心右缘
Right border

右心室
Right ventricle

下腔静脉
Inferior vena cava

前室间沟
Anterior
interventricular sulcus

心左（钝）缘
Left (obtuse) border

左心室
Left ventricle

心尖
Apex

心下（锐）缘
Inferior (acute) border

B. 后下面观（膈面）
Posteroinferior view
(diaphragmatic surface)

心底：
Base of heart:
上腔静脉 Superior vena cava
升主动脉 Ascending aorta
肺动脉干 Pulmonary trunk
肺静脉：
Pulmonary veins:
右 Right
左 Left

左心耳
Left auricle

冠状窦（在冠状沟内）
Coronary sinus
(in coronary sulcus)

左心室
Left ventricle

后室间沟
Posterior interventricular sulcus

右心室
Right ventricle

心尖
Apex

界沟
Sulcus terminalis
右心房
Right atrium

下腔静脉
Inferior vena cava

房室（冠状）沟
Atrioventricular
(coronary) sulcus

图 4-22　冠状动脉　Coronary Arteries

A. 前面观
Anterior view

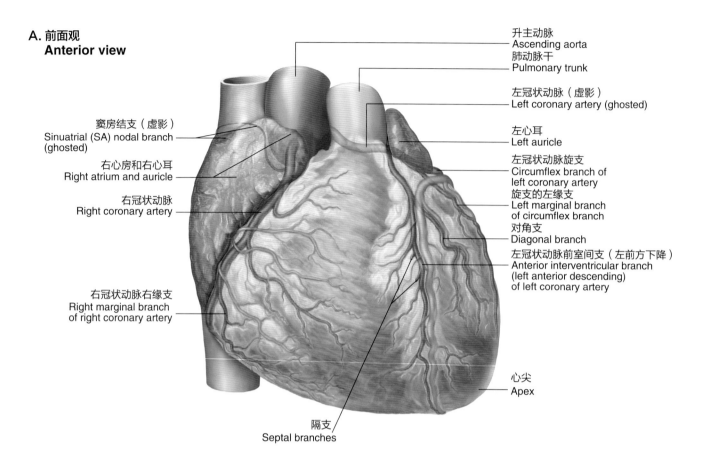

升主动脉
Ascending aorta

肺动脉干
Pulmonary trunk

左冠状动脉（虚影）
Left coronary artery (ghosted)

左心耳
Left auricle

左冠状动脉旋支
Circumflex branch of
left coronary artery

旋支的左缘支
Left marginal branch
of circumflex branch

对角支
Diagonal branch

左冠状动脉前室间支（左前方下降）
Anterior interventricular branch
(left anterior descending)
of left coronary artery

窦房结支（虚影）
Sinuatrial (SA) nodal branch
(ghosted)

右心房和右心耳
Right atrium and auricle

右冠状动脉
Right coronary artery

右冠状动脉右缘支
Right marginal branch
of right coronary artery

心尖
Apex

隔支
Septal branches

B. 后下面观
Posteroinferior view

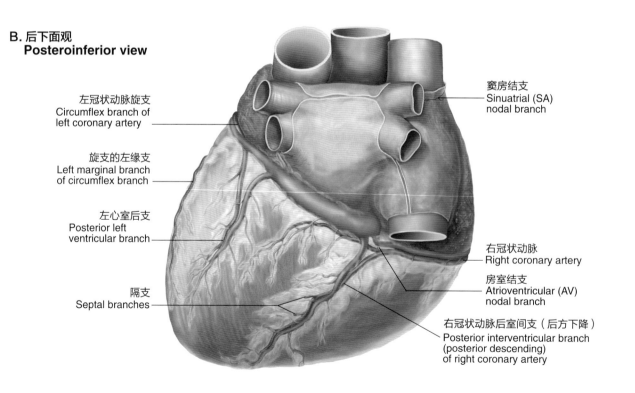

左冠状动脉旋支
Circumflex branch of
left coronary artery

旋支的左缘支
Left marginal branch
of circumflex branch

左心室后支
Posterior left
ventricular branch

隔支
Septal branches

窦房结支
Sinuatrial (SA)
nodal branch

右冠状动脉
Right coronary artery

房室结支
Atrioventricular (AV)
nodal branch

右冠状动脉后室间支（后方下降）
Posterior interventricular branch
(posterior descending)
of right coronary artery

A. 正常动脉模式，前面观
Normal arterial pattern, anterior view

窦房结支（虚影）
Sinuatrial (SA) nodal branch (ghosted)

窦房结的位置
Site of SA node

右冠状动脉
Right coronary artery

右冠状动脉右缘支
Right marginal branch of right coronary artery

升主动脉
Ascending aorta

肺动脉干
Pulmonary trunk

左冠状动脉（虚影）
Left coronary artery (ghosted)

左冠状动脉旋支
Circumflex branch of left coronary artery

左冠状动脉前室间支（左前方下降）
Anterior interventricular branch (left anterior descending) of left coronary artery

对角支
Diagonal branch

旋支的左缘支
Left marginal branch of circumflex branch

心尖
Apex

B. 变异，前面观
Variation, anterior view

窦房结的位置
Site of SA node

窦房结支起于旋支（40%，虚影）
Sinuatrial (SA) nodal branch from circumflex branch (40%, ghosted)

C. 正常动脉分支，后下面观
Normal arterial pattern, posteroinferior view

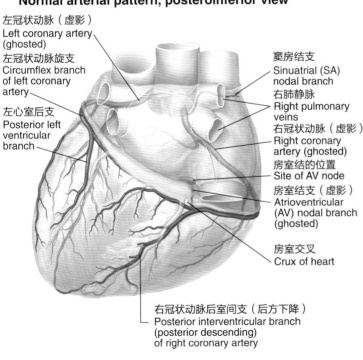

左冠状动脉（虚影）
Left coronary artery (ghosted)

左冠状动脉旋支
Circumflex branch of left coronary artery

左心室后支
Posterior left ventricular branch

窦房结支
Sinuatrial (SA) nodal branch

右肺静脉
Right pulmonary veins

右冠状动脉（虚影）
Right coronary artery (ghosted)

房室结的位置
Site of AV node

房室结支（虚影）
Atrioventricular (AV) nodal branch (ghosted)

房室交叉
Crux of heart

右冠状动脉后室间支（后方下降）
Posterior interventricular branch (posterior descending) of right coronary artery

D. 变异，后下面观
Variation, posteroinferior view

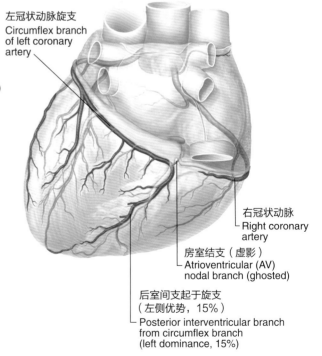

左冠状动脉旋支
Circumflex branch of left coronary artery

右冠状动脉
Right coronary artery

房室结支（虚影）
Atrioventricular (AV) nodal branch (ghosted)

后室间支起于旋支（左侧优势，15%）
Posterior interventricular branch from circumflex branch (left dominance, 15%)

图 4-24　心静脉　Cardiac Veins

A. 前面观
Anterior view

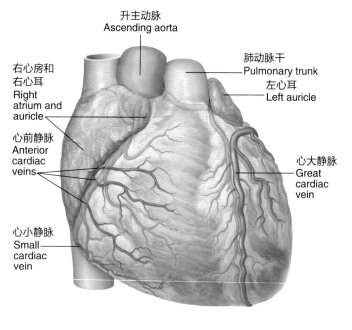

升主动脉
Ascending aorta

肺动脉干
Pulmonary trunk

左心耳
Left auricle

右心房和
右心耳
Right
atrium and
auricle

心前静脉
Anterior
cardiac
veins

心大静脉
Great
cardiac
vein

心小静脉
Small
cardiac
vein

B. 正常静脉模式，前面观
Normal venous pattern, anterior view

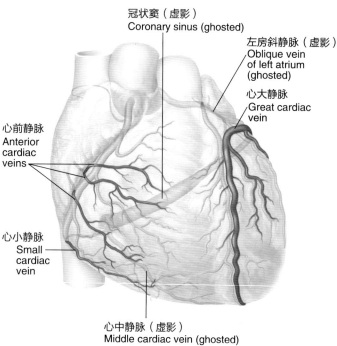

冠状窦（虚影）
Coronary sinus (ghosted)

左房斜静脉（虚影）
Oblique vein
of left atrium
(ghosted)

心大静脉
Great cardiac
vein

心前静脉
Anterior
cardiac
veins

心小静脉
Small
cardiac
vein

心中静脉（虚影）
Middle cardiac vein (ghosted)

C. 后下面观
Posteroinferior view

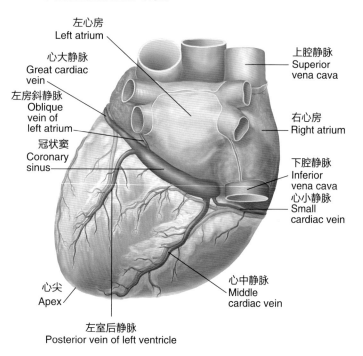

左心房
Left atrium

心大静脉
Great cardiac
vein

上腔静脉
Superior
vena cava

左房斜静脉
Oblique
vein of
left atrium

冠状窦
Coronary
sinus

右心房
Right atrium

下腔静脉
Inferior
vena cava

心小静脉
Small
cardiac vein

心尖
Apex

心中静脉
Middle
cardiac vein

左室后静脉
Posterior vein of left ventricle

D. 正常静脉模式，后下面观
Normal venous pattern, posteroinferior view

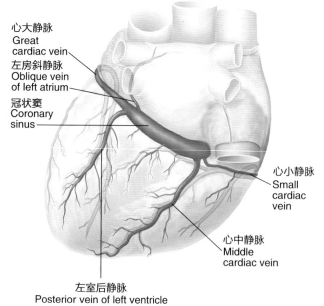

心大静脉
Great
cardiac vein

左房斜静脉
Oblique vein
of left atrium

冠状窦
Coronary
sinus

心小静脉
Small
cardiac
vein

心中静脉
Middle
cardiac vein

左室后静脉
Posterior vein of left ventricle

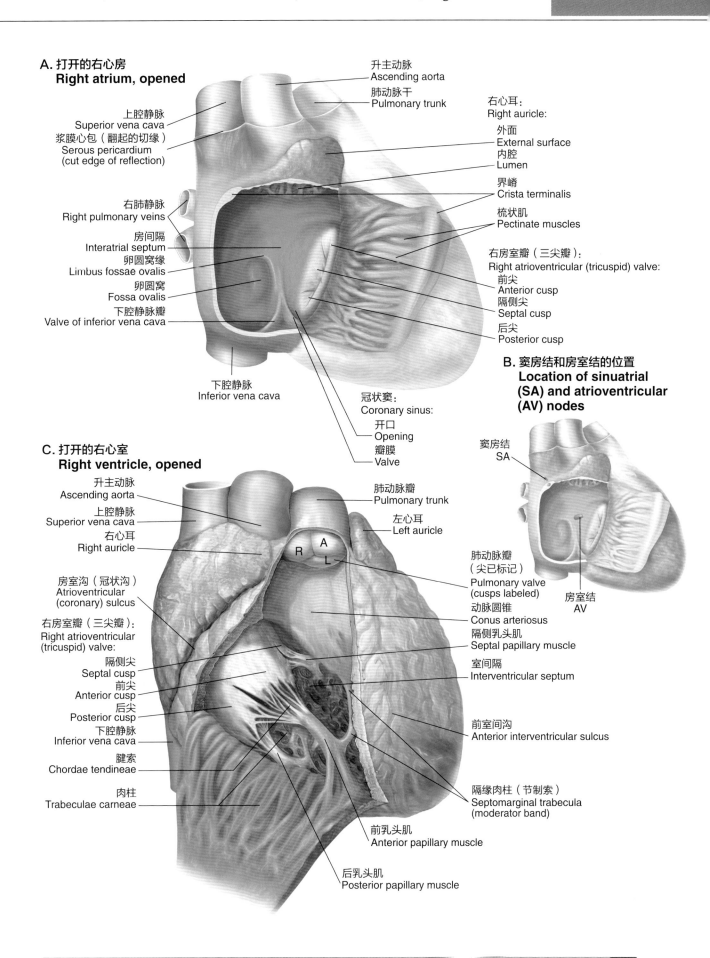

A. 打开的右心房
Right atrium, opened

升主动脉
Ascending aorta

肺动脉干
Pulmonary trunk

上腔静脉
Superior vena cava

浆膜心包（翻起的切缘）
Serous pericardium
(cut edge of reflection)

右肺静脉
Right pulmonary veins

房间隔
Interatrial septum

卵圆窝缘
Limbus fossae ovalis

卵圆窝
Fossa ovalis

下腔静脉瓣
Valve of inferior vena cava

下腔静脉
Inferior vena cava

右心耳：
Right auricle:

外面
External surface

内腔
Lumen

界嵴
Crista terminalis

梳状肌
Pectinate muscles

右房室瓣（三尖瓣）：
Right atrioventricular (tricuspid) valve:

前尖
Anterior cusp

隔侧尖
Septal cusp

后尖
Posterior cusp

冠状窦：
Coronary sinus:

开口
Opening

瓣膜
Valve

B. 窦房结和房室结的位置
Location of sinuatrial (SA) and atrioventricular (AV) nodes

窦房结
SA

肺动脉瓣（尖已标记）
Pulmonary valve (cusps labeled)

房室结
AV

C. 打开的右心室
Right ventricle, opened

升主动脉
Ascending aorta

上腔静脉
Superior vena cava

右心耳
Right auricle

房室沟（冠状沟）
Atrioventricular (coronary) sulcus

右房室瓣（三尖瓣）：
Right atrioventricular (tricuspid) valve:

隔侧尖
Septal cusp

前尖
Anterior cusp

后尖
Posterior cusp

下腔静脉
Inferior vena cava

腱索
Chordae tendineae

肉柱
Trabeculae carneae

肺动脉瓣
Pulmonary trunk

左心耳
Left auricle

R　A　L

肺动脉瓣（尖已标记）
Pulmonary valve (cusps labeled)

动脉圆锥
Conus arteriosus

隔侧乳头肌
Septal papillary muscle

室间隔
Interventricular septum

前室间沟
Anterior interventricular sulcus

隔缘肉柱（节制索）
Septomarginal trabecula (moderator band)

前乳头肌
Anterior papillary muscle

后乳头肌
Posterior papillary muscle

图 4-26　心，内部结构，左心房　Heart, Internal Features, Left Chambers

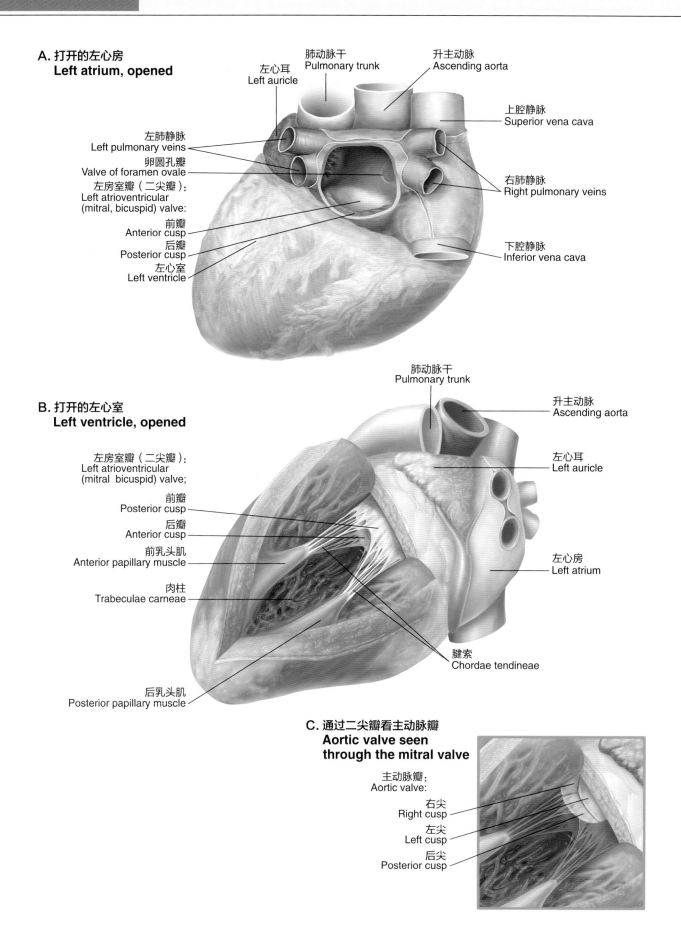

A. 打开的左心房
Left atrium, opened

左心耳
Left auricle

肺动脉干
Pulmonary trunk

升主动脉
Ascending aorta

上腔静脉
Superior vena cava

左肺静脉
Left pulmonary veins

卵圆孔瓣
Valve of foramen ovale

左房室瓣（二尖瓣）：
Left atrioventricular
(mitral, bicuspid) valve:

前瓣
Anterior cusp

后瓣
Posterior cusp

左心室
Left ventricle

右肺静脉
Right pulmonary veins

下腔静脉
Inferior vena cava

B. 打开的左心室
Left ventricle, opened

肺动脉干
Pulmonary trunk

升主动脉
Ascending aorta

左房室瓣（二尖瓣）：
Left atrioventricular
(mitral bicuspid) valve;

前瓣
Posterior cusp

后瓣
Anterior cusp

前乳头肌
Anterior papillary muscle

肉柱
Trabeculae carneae

左心耳
Left auricle

左心房
Left atrium

腱索
Chordae tendineae

后乳头肌
Posterior papillary muscle

C. 通过二尖瓣看主动脉瓣
Aortic valve seen
through the mitral valve

主动脉瓣：
Aortic valve:

右尖
Right cusp

左尖
Left cusp

后尖
Posterior cusp

A. 心的收缩期瓣膜
Valves of Heart in Systole

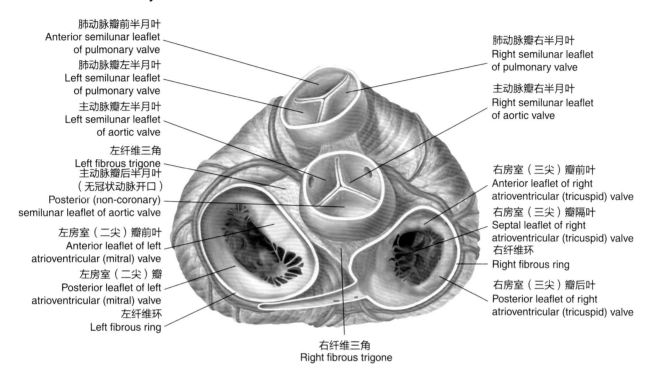

肺动脉瓣前半月叶
Anterior semilunar leaflet
of pulmonary valve

肺动脉瓣左半月叶
Left semilunar leaflet
of pulmonary valve

主动脉瓣左半月叶
Left semilunar leaflet
of aortic valve

左纤维三角
Left fibrous trigone
主动脉瓣后半月叶
（无冠状动脉开口）
Posterior (non-coronary)
semilunar leaflet of aortic valve

左房室（二尖）瓣前叶
Anterior leaflet of left
atrioventricular (mitral) valve

左房室（二尖）瓣
Posterior leaflet of left
atrioventricular (mitral) valve

左纤维环
Left fibrous ring

肺动脉瓣右半月叶
Right semilunar leaflet
of pulmonary valve

主动脉瓣右半月叶
Right semilunar leaflet
of aortic valve

右房室（三尖）瓣前叶
Anterior leaflet of right
atrioventricular (tricuspid) valve

右房室（三尖）瓣隔叶
Septal leaflet of right
atrioventricular (tricuspid) valve
右纤维环
Right fibrous ring

右房室（三尖）瓣后叶
Posterior leaflet of right
atrioventricular (tricuspid) valve

右纤维三角
Right fibrous trigone

B. 收缩期
Systole

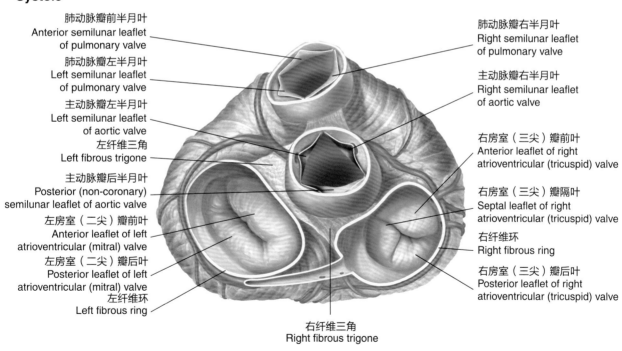

肺动脉瓣前半月叶
Anterior semilunar leaflet
of pulmonary valve

肺动脉瓣左半月叶
Left semilunar leaflet
of pulmonary valve

主动脉瓣左半月叶
Left semilunar leaflet
of aortic valve
左纤维三角
Left fibrous trigone

主动脉瓣后半月叶
Posterior (non-coronary)
semilunar leaflet of aortic valve

左房室（二尖）瓣前叶
Anterior leaflet of left
atrioventricular (mitral) valve
左房室（二尖）瓣后叶
Posterior leaflet of left
atrioventricular (mitral) valve
左纤维环
Left fibrous ring

肺动脉瓣右半月叶
Right semilunar leaflet
of pulmonary valve

主动脉瓣右半月叶
Right semilunar leaflet
of aortic valve

右房室（三尖）瓣前叶
Anterior leaflet of right
atrioventricular (tricuspid) valve

右房室（三尖）瓣隔叶
Septal leaflet of right
atrioventricular (tricuspid) valve

右纤维环
Right fibrous ring

右房室（三尖）瓣后叶
Posterior leaflet of right
atrioventricular (tricuspid) valve

右纤维三角
Right fibrous trigone

图 4-28　心的剖视图　Sectional View of the Heart

A. 图 B 所在平面
Plane of section

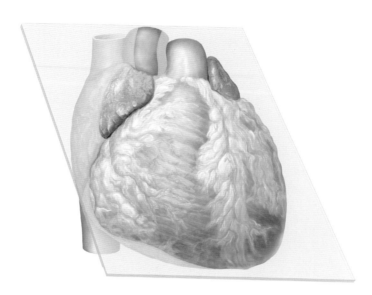

B. 显示心切面的后下部
Section through the heart showing the posteroinferior portion

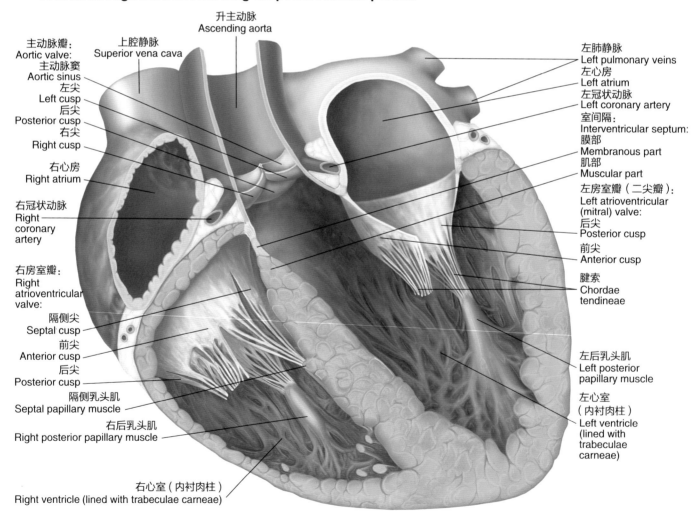

升主动脉
Ascending aorta

主动脉瓣：
Aortic valve:
主动脉窦
Aortic sinus
左尖
Left cusp
后尖
Posterior cusp
右尖
Right cusp

上腔静脉
Superior vena cava

左肺静脉
Left pulmonary veins
左心房
Left atrium
左冠状动脉
Left coronary artery
室间隔：
Interventricular septum:
膜部
Membranous part
肌部
Muscular part

右心房
Right atrium

右冠状动脉
Right
coronary
artery

左房室瓣（二尖瓣）：
Left atrioventricular
(mitral) valve:
后尖
Posterior cusp
前尖
Anterior cusp

右房室瓣：
Right
atrioventricular
valve:

腱索
Chordae
tendineae

隔侧尖
Septal cusp
前尖
Anterior cusp
后尖
Posterior cusp
隔侧乳头肌
Septal papillary muscle
右后乳头肌
Right posterior papillary muscle

左后乳头肌
Left posterior
papillary muscle

左心室
（内衬肉柱）
Left ventricle
(lined with
trabeculae
carneae)

右心室（内衬肉柱）
Right ventricle (lined with trabeculae carneae)

A. 前面观
Anterior view

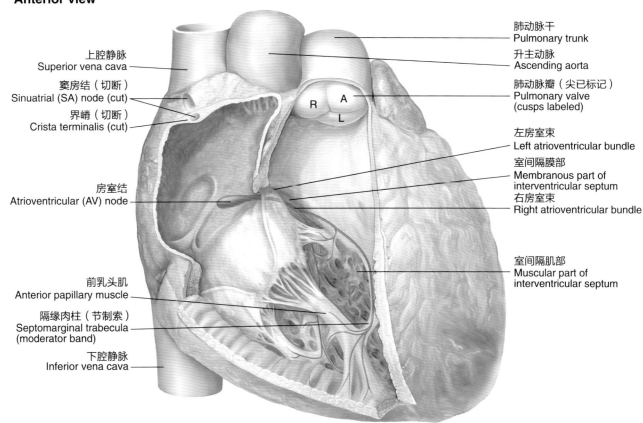

肺动脉干
Pulmonary trunk

升主动脉
Ascending aorta

肺动脉瓣（尖已标记）
Pulmonary valve
(cusps labeled)

左房室束
Left atrioventricular bundle

室间隔膜部
Membranous part of
interventricular septum

右房室束
Right atrioventricular bundle

室间隔肌部
Muscular part of
interventricular septum

上腔静脉
Superior vena cava

窦房结（切断）
Sinuatrial (SA) node (cut)

界嵴（切断）
Crista terminalis (cut)

房室结
Atrioventricular (AV) node

前乳头肌
Anterior papillary muscle

隔缘肉柱（节制索）
Septomarginal trabecula
(moderator band)

下腔静脉
Inferior vena cava

B. 左侧面观
Left lateral view

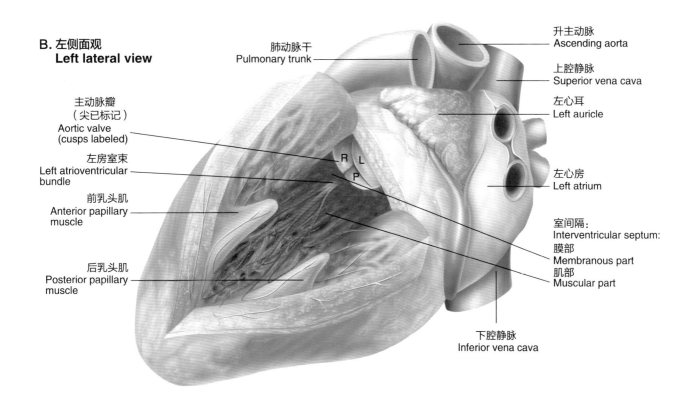

肺动脉干
Pulmonary trunk

升主动脉
Ascending aorta

上腔静脉
Superior vena cava

左心耳
Left auricle

左心房
Left atrium

室间隔：
Interventricular septum:
膜部
Membranous part
肌部
Muscular part

主动脉瓣
（尖已标记）
Aortic valve
(cusps labeled)

左房室束
Left atrioventricular
bundle

前乳头肌
Anterior papillary
muscle

后乳头肌
Posterior papillary
muscle

下腔静脉
Inferior vena cava

图 4-30　胸腔脏器，肺　Thoracic Viscera, Lungs

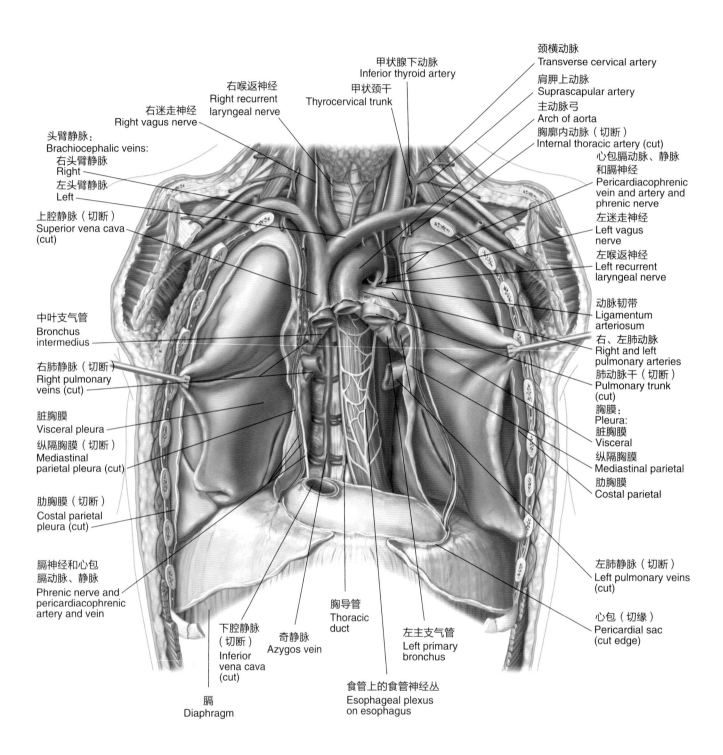

颈横动脉
Transverse cervical artery

肩胛上动脉
Suprascapular artery

主动脉弓
Arch of aorta

胸廓内动脉（切断）
Internal thoracic artery (cut)

心包膈动脉、静脉
和膈神经
Pericardiacophrenic
vein and artery and
phrenic nerve

左迷走神经
Left vagus
nerve

左喉返神经
Left recurrent
laryngeal nerve

动脉韧带
Ligamentum
arteriosum

右、左肺动脉
Right and left
pulmonary arteries

肺动脉干（切断）
Pulmonary trunk
(cut)

胸膜：
Pleura:
脏胸膜
Visceral
纵隔胸膜
Mediastinal parietal
肋胸膜
Costal parietal

左肺静脉（切断）
Left pulmonary veins
(cut)

心包（切缘）
Pericardial sac
(cut edge)

甲状腺下动脉
Inferior thyroid artery

甲状颈干
Thyrocervical trunk

右喉返神经
Right recurrent
laryngeal nerve

右迷走神经
Right vagus nerve

头臂静脉：
Brachiocephalic veins:
右头臂静脉
Right
左头臂静脉
Left

上腔静脉（切断）
Superior vena cava
(cut)

中叶支气管
Bronchus
intermedius

右肺静脉（切断）
Right pulmonary
veins (cut)

脏胸膜
Visceral pleura

纵隔胸膜（切断）
Mediastinal
parietal pleura (cut)

肋胸膜（切断）
Costal parietal
pleura (cut)

膈神经和心包
膈动脉、静脉
Phrenic nerve and
pericardiacophrenic
artery and vein

下腔静脉
（切断）
Inferior
vena cava
(cut)

奇静脉
Azygos vein

膈
Diaphragm

胸导管
Thoracic
duct

左主支气管
Left primary
bronchus

食管上的食管神经丛
Esophageal plexus
on esophagus

A. 右肺
Right lung

B. 左肺
Left lung

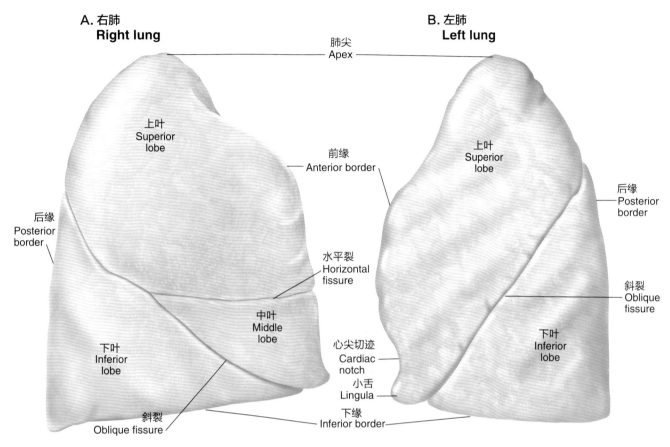

肺尖
Apex

上叶
Superior
lobe

前缘
Anterior border

上叶
Superior
lobe

后缘
Posterior
border

后缘
Posterior
border

水平裂
Horizontal
fissure

斜裂
Oblique
fissure

下叶
Inferior
lobe

中叶
Middle
lobe

心尖切迹
Cardiac
notch

下叶
Inferior
lobe

小舌
Lingula

斜裂
Oblique fissure

下缘
Inferior border

C. 肺的正位片
Radiograph, anterior view

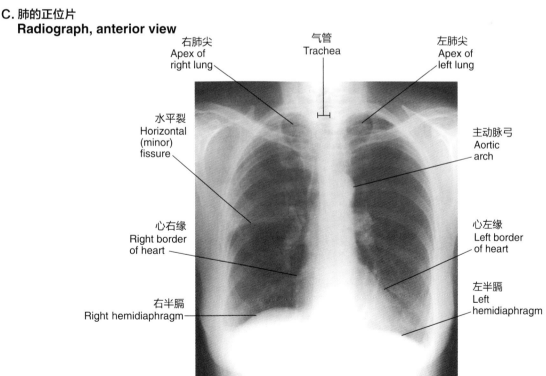

右肺尖
Apex of
right lung

气管
Trachea

左肺尖
Apex of
left lung

水平裂
Horizontal
(minor)
fissure

主动脉弓
Aortic
arch

心右缘
Right border
of heart

心左缘
Left border
of heart

右半膈
Right hemidiaphragm

左半膈
Left
hemidiaphragm

图 4-32　　肺，内面观　Lungs, Medial View

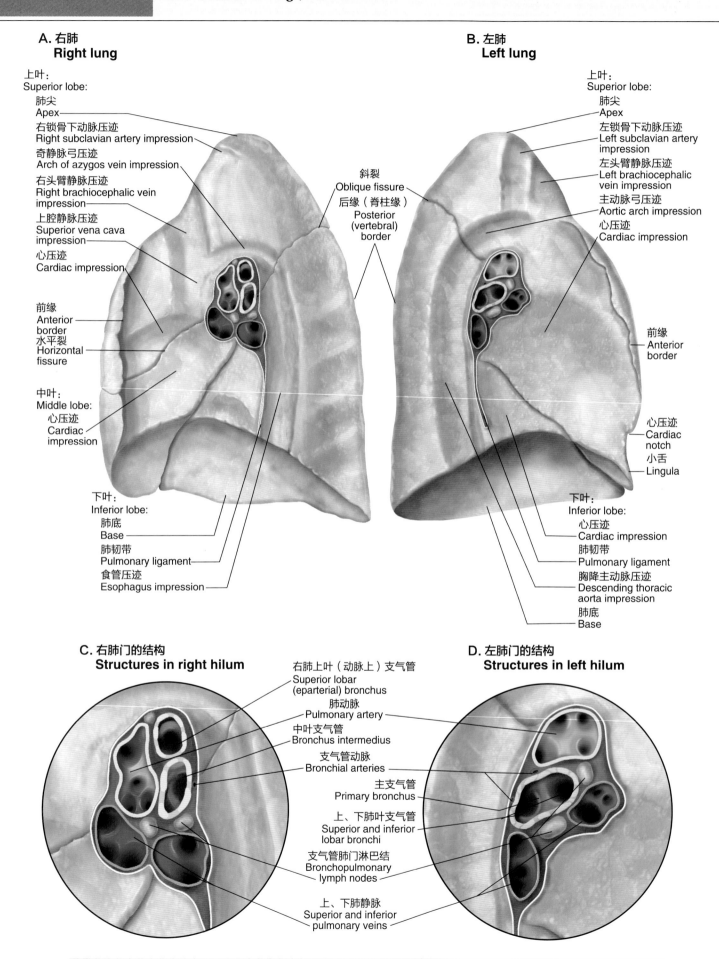

A. 右肺
Right lung

上叶：
Superior lobe:

肺尖
Apex

右锁骨下动脉压迹
Right subclavian artery impression

奇静脉弓压迹
Arch of azygos vein impression

右头臂静脉压迹
Right brachiocephalic vein impression

上腔静脉压迹
Superior vena cava impression

心压迹
Cardiac impression

前缘
Anterior border

水平裂
Horizontal fissure

中叶：
Middle lobe:

心压迹
Cardiac impression

下叶：
Inferior lobe:

肺底
Base

肺韧带
Pulmonary ligament

食管压迹
Esophagus impression

斜裂
Oblique fissure

后缘（脊柱缘）
Posterior (vertebral) border

B. 左肺
Left lung

上叶：
Superior lobe:

肺尖
Apex

左锁骨下动脉压迹
Left subclavian artery impression

左头臂静脉压迹
Left brachiocephalic vein impression

主动脉弓压迹
Aortic arch impression

心压迹
Cardiac impression

前缘
Anterior border

心压迹
Cardiac notch

小舌
Lingula

下叶：
Inferior lobe:

心压迹
Cardiac impression

肺韧带
Pulmonary ligament

胸降主动脉压迹
Descending thoracic aorta impression

肺底
Base

C. 右肺门的结构
Structures in right hilum

D. 左肺门的结构
Structures in left hilum

右肺上叶（动脉上）支气管
Superior lobar (eparterial) bronchus

肺动脉
Pulmonary artery

中叶支气管
Bronchus intermedius

支气管动脉
Bronchial arteries

主支气管
Primary bronchus

上、下肺叶支气管
Superior and inferior lobar bronchi

支气管肺门淋巴结
Bronchopulmonary lymph nodes

上、下肺静脉
Superior and inferior pulmonary veins

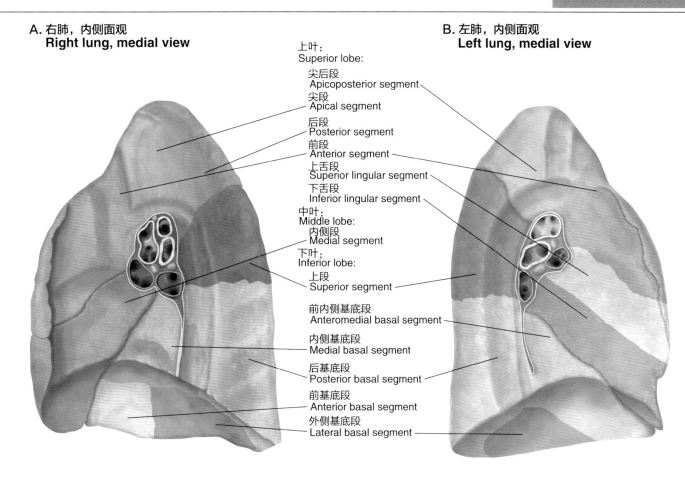

A. 右肺，内侧面观
Right lung, medial view

B. 左肺，内侧面观
Left lung, medial view

上叶：
Superior lobe:

尖后段
Apicoposterior segment

尖段
Apical segment

后段
Posterior segment

前段
Anterior segment

上舌段
Superior lingular segment

下舌段
Inferior lingular segment

中叶：
Middle lobe:

内侧段
Medial segment

下叶：
Inferior lobe:

上段
Superior segment

前内侧基底段
Anteromedial basal segment

内侧基底段
Medial basal segment

后基底段
Posterior basal segment

前基底段
Anterior basal segment

外侧基底段
Lateral basal segment

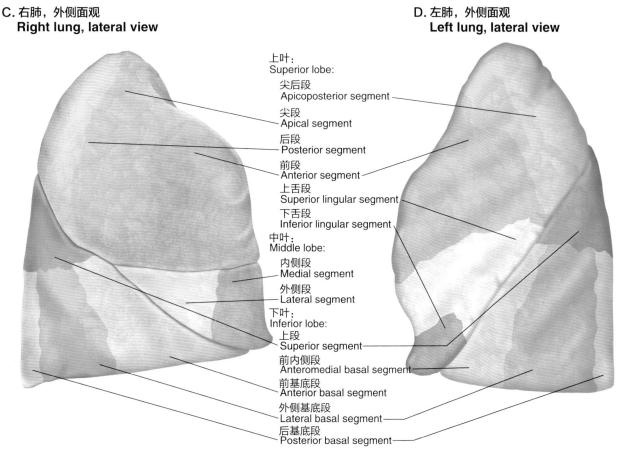

C. 右肺，外侧面观
Right lung, lateral view

D. 左肺，外侧面观
Left lung, lateral view

上叶：
Superior lobe:

尖后段
Apicoposterior segment

尖段
Apical segment

后段
Posterior segment

前段
Anterior segment

上舌段
Superior lingular segment

下舌段
Inferior lingular segment

中叶：
Middle lobe:

内侧段
Medial segment

外侧段
Lateral segment

下叶：
Inferior lobe:

上段
Superior segment

前内侧段
Anteromedial basal segment

前基底段
Anterior basal segment

外侧基底段
Lateral basal segment

后基底段
Posterior basal segment

图 4-34　气管和支气管树　Trachea and Bronchial Tree

A. 前面观
Anterior view

B. 横断面，上面观
Cross section, superior view

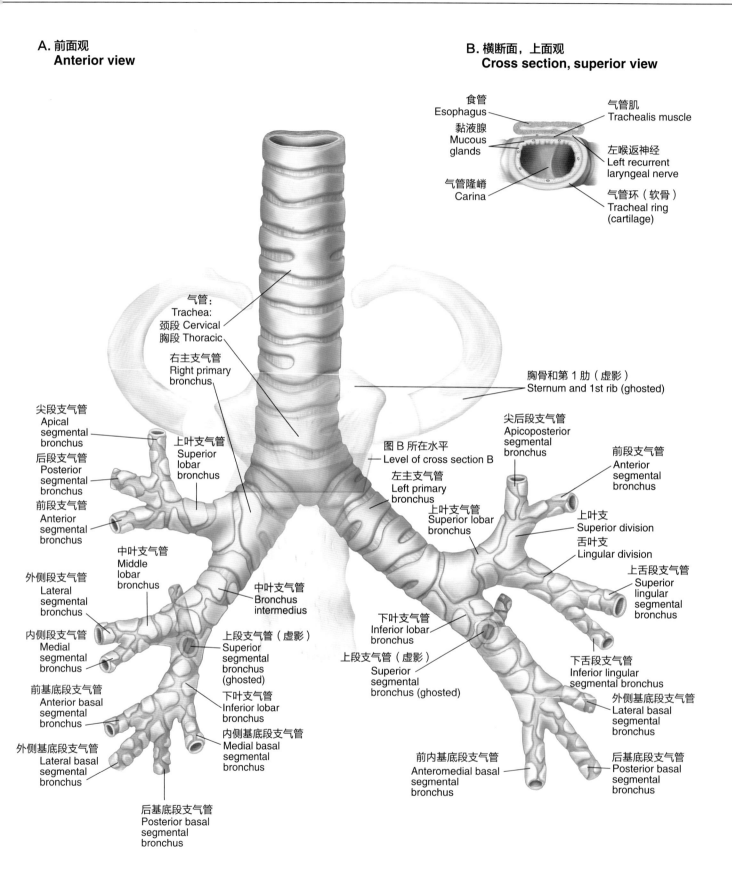

食管
Esophagus

气管肌
Trachealis muscle

黏液腺
Mucous glands

左喉返神经
Left recurrent laryngeal nerve

气管隆嵴
Carina

气管环（软骨）
Tracheal ring (cartilage)

气管：
Trachea:
颈段 Cervical
胸段 Thoracic

右主支气管
Right primary bronchus

胸骨和第 1 肋（虚影）
Sternum and 1st rib (ghosted)

尖段支气管
Apical segmental bronchus

后段支气管
Posterior segmental bronchus

前段支气管
Anterior segmental bronchus

上叶支气管
Superior lobar bronchus

图 B 所在水平
Level of cross section B

左主支气管
Left primary bronchus

上叶支气管
Superior lobar bronchus

尖后段支气管
Apicoposterior segmental bronchus

前段支气管
Anterior segmental bronchus

上叶支
Superior division

舌叶支
Lingular division

上舌段支气管
Superior lingular segmental bronchus

外侧段支气管
Lateral segmental bronchus

中叶支气管
Middle lobar bronchus

中叶支气管
Bronchus intermedius

内侧段支气管
Medial segmental bronchus

上段支气管（虚影）
Superior segmental bronchus (ghosted)

下叶支气管
Inferior lobar bronchus

上段支气管（虚影）
Superior segmental bronchus (ghosted)

下舌段支气管
Inferior lingular segmental bronchus

下叶支气管
Inferior lobar bronchus

外侧基底段支气管
Lateral basal segmental bronchus

前基底段支气管
Anterior basal segmental bronchus

内侧基底段支气管
Medial basal segmental bronchus

后基底段支气管
Posterior basal segmental bronchus

外侧基底段支气管
Lateral basal segmental bronchus

后基底段支气管
Posterior basal segmental bronchus

前内基底段支气管
Anteromedial basal segmental bronchus

A. 肺的血管
Pulmonary vessels

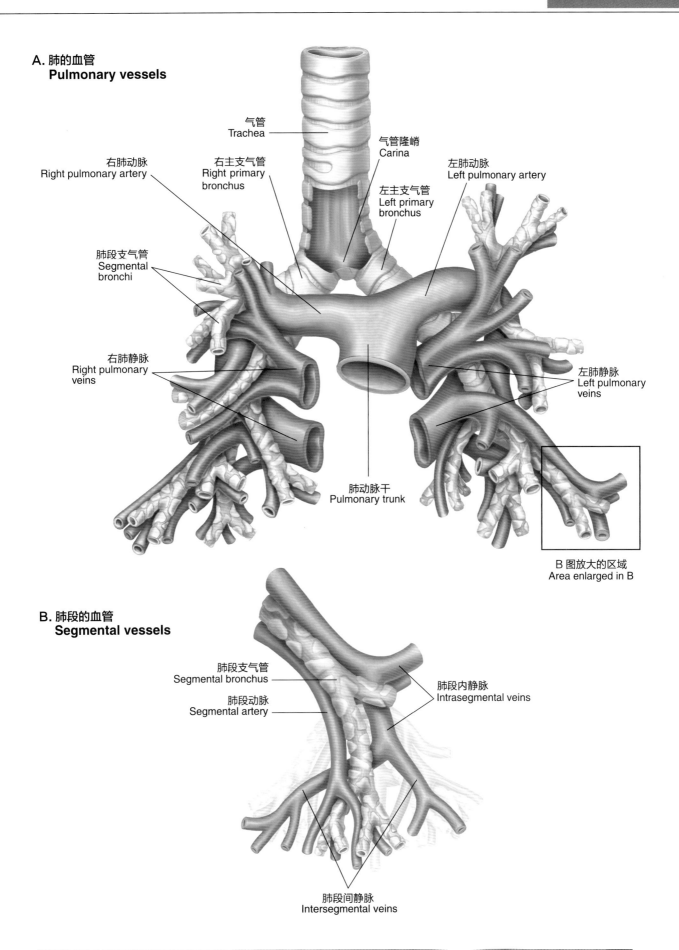

气管
Trachea

气管隆嵴
Carina

右肺动脉
Right pulmonary artery

右主支气管
Right primary bronchus

左主支气管
Left primary bronchus

左肺动脉
Left pulmonary artery

肺段支气管
Segmental bronchi

右肺静脉
Right pulmonary veins

左肺静脉
Left pulmonary veins

肺动脉干
Pulmonary trunk

B 图放大的区域
Area enlarged in B

B. 肺段的血管
Segmental vessels

肺段支气管
Segmental bronchus

肺段动脉
Segmental artery

肺段内静脉
Intrasegmental veins

肺段间静脉
Intersegmental veins

图 4-36　　纵隔，右侧面观　Mediastinum, Right Lateral View

A. 纵隔分部
Parts of the mediastinum

胸骨角平面
Plane of the sternal angle

T2
T4
T6
T8

第 1 肋
1st rib

上纵隔
Superior mediastinum

前纵隔
Anterior mediastinum

中纵隔
Middle mediastinum

后纵隔
Posterior mediastinum

膈
Diaphragm

B. 解剖
Dissection

臂丛（切断）
Brachial plexus (cut)

前斜角肌
Anterior scalene muscle

膈神经
Phrenic nerve

第 1 肋
1st rib

右迷走神经
Right vagus nerve

气管
Trachea

食管
Esophagus

胸内脏神经
Thoracic visceral nerves

右肋间上静脉
Right superior intercostal vein

奇静脉弓
Arch of azygos vein

肋间后血管和神经
Posterior intercostal vessels and intercostal nerve

右主支气管（切断）
Right primary bronchus (cut)

右支气管动脉
Right bronchial artery

右肺动脉（切断）
Right pulmonary artery (cut)

交感神经干
Sympathetic trunk

奇静脉
Azygos vein

加入胸腔脏大神经的分支
Contributions to greater thoracic splanchnic nerve

肋胸膜（切断）
Costal parietal pleura (cut)

右颈总动脉
Right common carotid artery

右颈内静脉
Right internal jugular vein

右锁骨下动脉和静脉（切断）
Right subclavian artery and vein (cut)

右胸廓内血管（切断）
Right internal thoracic vessels (cut)

胸腺脂肪（透过纵隔胸膜）
Thymic fat (seen through mediastinal parietal pleura)

胸骨角
Sternal angle

上腔静脉
Superior vena cava

纵隔胸膜（切断）
Mediastinal parietal pleura (cut)

肋纵隔隐窝
Costomediastinal recess

肋胸膜（切断）
Costal parietal pleura (cut)

膈神经及心包膈血管
Phrenic nerve and pericardiacophrenic vessels

心包
Pericardial sac

下腔静脉
Inferior vena cava

膈
Diaphragm

右肺静脉（切断）
Right pulmonary veins (cut)

食管丛（神经、血管）
Esophageal plexus

肺韧带（切断）
Pulmonary ligament (cut)

A. 纵隔分部
Parts of the mediastinum

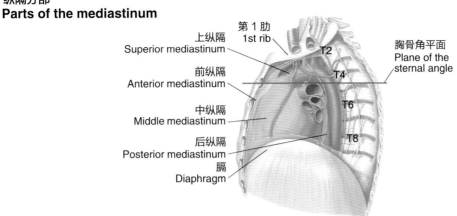

上纵隔
Superior mediastinum

第 1 肋
1st rib

T2

胸骨角平面
Plane of the
sternal angle

前纵隔
Anterior mediastinum

T4

中纵隔
Middle mediastinum

T6

后纵隔
Posterior mediastinum

T8

膈
Diaphragm

B. 解剖
Dissection

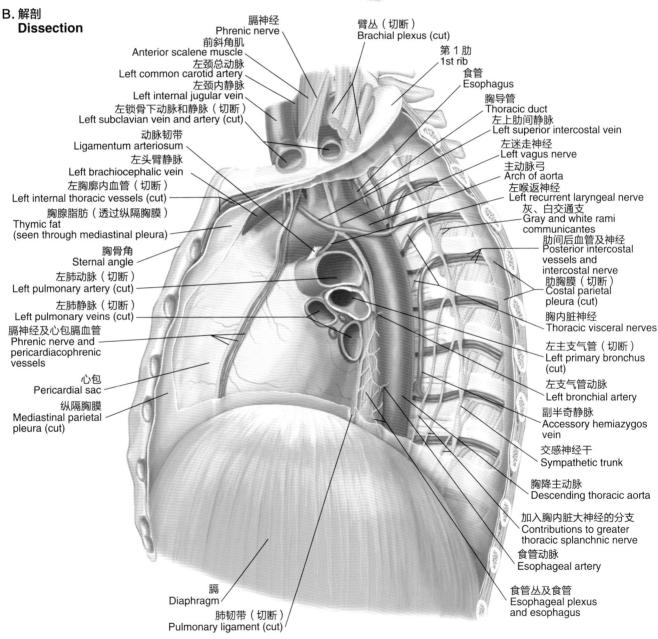

膈神经
Phrenic nerve

前斜角肌
Anterior scalene muscle

左颈总动脉
Left common carotid artery

左颈内静脉
Left internal jugular vein

左锁骨下动脉和静脉（切断）
Left subclavian vein and artery (cut)

动脉韧带
Ligamentum arteriosum

左头臂静脉
Left brachiocephalic vein

左胸廓内血管（切断）
Left internal thoracic vessels (cut)

胸腺脂肪（透过纵隔胸膜）
Thymic fat
(seen through mediastinal pleura)

胸骨角
Sternal angle

左肺动脉（切断）
Left pulmonary artery (cut)

左肺静脉（切断）
Left pulmonary veins (cut)

膈神经及心包膈血管
Phrenic nerve and
pericardiacophrenic
vessels

心包
Pericardial sac

纵隔胸膜
Mediastinal parietal
pleura (cut)

膈
Diaphragm

肺韧带（切断）
Pulmonary ligament (cut)

臂丛（切断）
Brachial plexus (cut)

第 1 肋
1st rib

食管
Esophagus

胸导管
Thoracic duct

左上肋间静脉
Left superior intercostal vein

左迷走神经
Left vagus nerve

主动脉弓
Arch of aorta

左喉返神经
Left recurrent laryngeal nerve

灰、白交通支
Gray and white rami
communicantes

肋间后血管及神经
Posterior intercostal
vessels and
intercostal nerve

肋胸膜（切断）
Costal parietal
pleura (cut)

胸内脏神经
Thoracic visceral nerves

左主支气管（切断）
Left primary bronchus
(cut)

左支气管动脉
Left bronchial artery

副半奇静脉
Accessory hemiazygos
vein

交感神经干
Sympathetic trunk

胸降主动脉
Descending thoracic aorta

加入胸内脏大神经的分支
Contributions to greater
thoracic splanchnic nerve

食管动脉
Esophageal artery

食管丛及食管
Esophageal plexus
and esophagus

A. 纵隔分部
Parts of the mediastinum

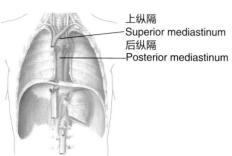

上纵隔
Superior mediastinum
后纵隔
Posterior mediastinum

B. 解剖
Dissection

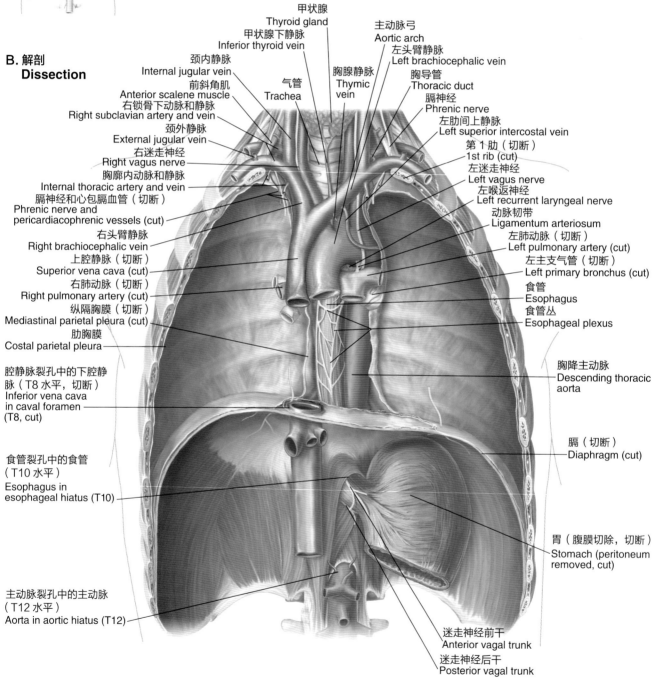

甲状腺
Thyroid gland
甲状腺下静脉
Inferior thyroid vein
颈内静脉
Internal jugular vein
前斜角肌
Anterior scalene muscle
右锁骨下动脉和静脉
Right subclavian artery and vein
颈外静脉
External jugular vein
右迷走神经
Right vagus nerve
胸廓内动脉和静脉
Internal thoracic artery and vein
膈神经和心包膈血管（切断）
Phrenic nerve and
pericardiacophrenic vessels (cut)
右头臂静脉
Right brachiocephalic vein
上腔静脉（切断）
Superior vena cava (cut)
右肺动脉（切断）
Right pulmonary artery (cut)
纵隔胸膜（切断）
Mediastinal parietal pleura (cut)
肋胸膜
Costal parietal pleura

腔静脉裂孔中的下腔静脉（T8 水平，切断）
Inferior vena cava
in caval foramen
(T8, cut)

食管裂孔中的食管
（T10 水平）
Esophagus in
esophageal hiatus (T10)

主动脉裂孔中的主动脉
（T12 水平）
Aorta in aortic hiatus (T12)

气管
Trachea

胸腺静脉
Thymic
vein

主动脉弓
Aortic arch
左头臂静脉
Left brachiocephalic vein
胸导管
Thoracic duct
膈神经
Phrenic nerve
左肋间上静脉
Left superior intercostal vein
第 1 肋（切断）
1st rib (cut)
左迷走神经
Left vagus nerve
左喉返神经
Left recurrent laryngeal nerve
动脉韧带
Ligamentum arteriosum
左肺动脉（切断）
Left pulmonary artery (cut)
左主支气管（切断）
Left primary bronchus (cut)
食管
Esophagus
食管丛
Esophageal plexus

胸降主动脉
Descending thoracic
aorta

膈（切断）
Diaphragm (cut)

胃（腹膜切除，切断）
Stomach (peritoneum
removed, cut)

迷走神经前干
Anterior vagal trunk
迷走神经后干
Posterior vagal trunk

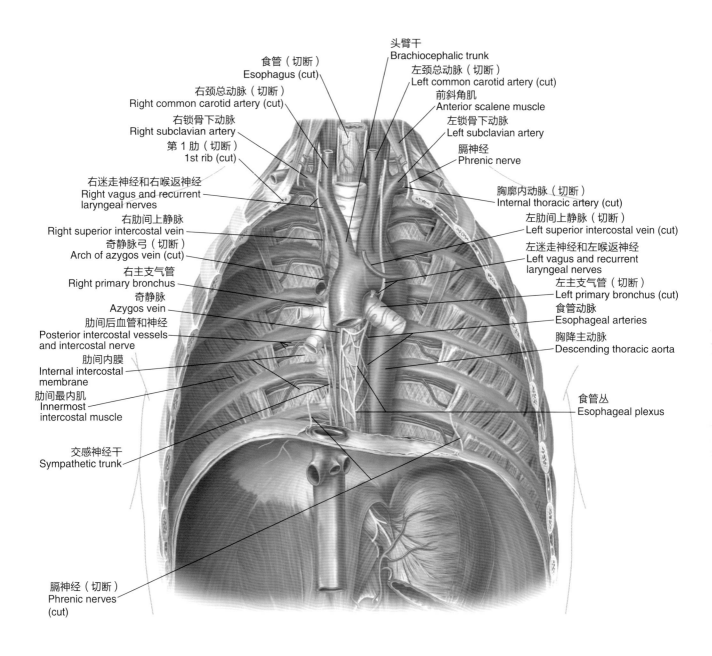

食管（切断）
Esophagus (cut)

头臂干
Brachiocephalic trunk

左颈总动脉（切断）
Left common carotid artery (cut)

右颈总动脉（切断）
Right common carotid artery (cut)

前斜角肌
Anterior scalene muscle

右锁骨下动脉
Right subclavian artery

左锁骨下动脉
Left subclavian artery

第 1 肋（切断）
1st rib (cut)

膈神经
Phrenic nerve

右迷走神经和右喉返神经
Right vagus and recurrent
laryngeal nerves

胸廓内动脉（切断）
Internal thoracic artery (cut)

右肋间上静脉
Right superior intercostal vein

左肋间上静脉（切断）
Left superior intercostal vein (cut)

奇静脉弓（切断）
Arch of azygos vein (cut)

左迷走神经和左喉返神经
Left vagus and recurrent
laryngeal nerves

右主支气管
Right primary bronchus

左主支气管（切断）
Left primary bronchus (cut)

奇静脉
Azygos vein

食管动脉
Esophageal arteries

肋间后血管和神经
Posterior intercostal vessels
and intercostal nerve

胸降主动脉
Descending thoracic aorta

肋间内膜
Internal intercostal
membrane

肋间最内肌
Innermost
intercostal muscle

食管丛
Esophageal plexus

交感神经干
Sympathetic trunk

膈神经（切断）
Phrenic nerves
(cut)

图 4-40　胸后壁的动脉　Arteries of the Posterior Thoracic Wall

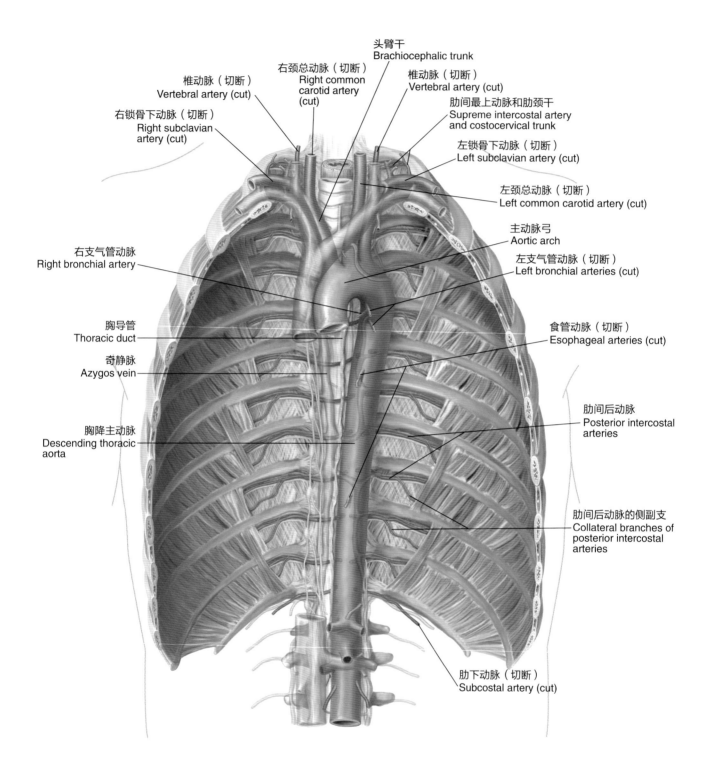

椎动脉（切断）
Vertebral artery (cut)

右颈总动脉（切断）
Right common
carotid artery
(cut)

头臂干
Brachiocephalic trunk

椎动脉（切断）
Vertebral artery (cut)

肋间最上动脉和肋颈干
Supreme intercostal artery
and costocervical trunk

右锁骨下动脉（切断）
Right subclavian
artery (cut)

左锁骨下动脉（切断）
Left subclavian artery (cut)

左颈总动脉（切断）
Left common carotid artery (cut)

主动脉弓
Aortic arch

右支气管动脉
Right bronchial artery

左支气管动脉（切断）
Left bronchial arteries (cut)

胸导管
Thoracic duct

食管动脉（切断）
Esophageal arteries (cut)

奇静脉
Azygos vein

肋间后动脉
Posterior intercostal
arteries

胸降主动脉
Descending thoracic
aorta

肋间后动脉的侧副支
Collateral branches of
posterior intercostal
arteries

肋下动脉（切断）
Subcostal artery (cut)

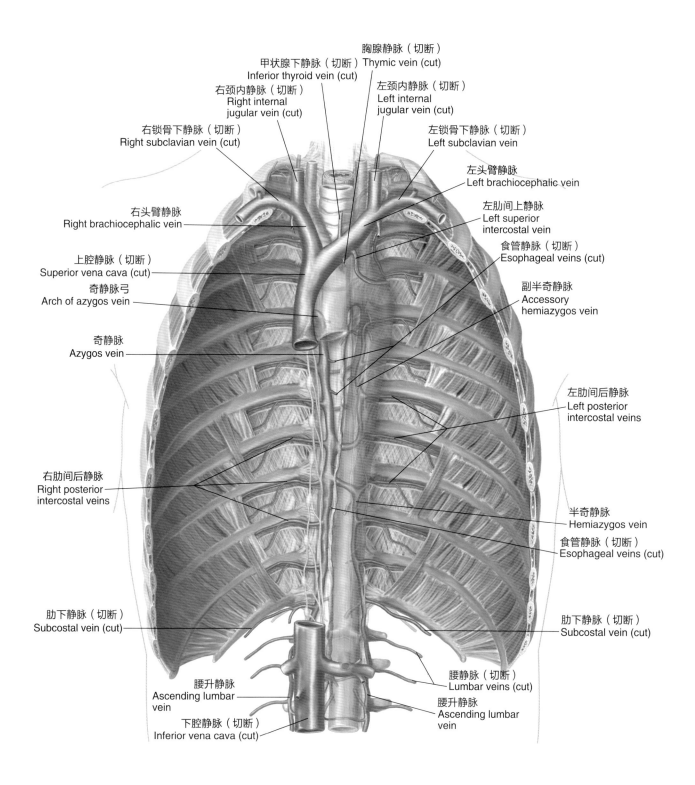

胸腺静脉（切断）
Thymic vein (cut)

甲状腺下静脉（切断）
Inferior thyroid vein (cut)

右颈内静脉（切断）
Right internal
jugular vein (cut)

左颈内静脉（切断）
Left internal
jugular vein (cut)

右锁骨下静脉（切断）
Right subclavian vein (cut)

左锁骨下静脉（切断）
Left subclavian vein

左头臂静脉
Left brachiocephalic vein

右头臂静脉
Right brachiocephalic vein

左肋间上静脉
Left superior
intercostal vein

上腔静脉（切断）
Superior vena cava (cut)

食管静脉（切断）
Esophageal veins (cut)

奇静脉弓
Arch of azygos vein

副半奇静脉
Accessory
hemiazygos vein

奇静脉
Azygos vein

左肋间后静脉
Left posterior
intercostal veins

右肋间后静脉
Right posterior
intercostal veins

半奇静脉
Hemiazygos vein

食管静脉（切断）
Esophageal veins (cut)

肋下静脉（切断）
Subcostal vein (cut)

肋下静脉（切断）
Subcostal vein (cut)

腰升静脉
Ascending lumbar
vein

腰静脉（切断）
Lumbar veins (cut)

腰升静脉
Ascending lumbar
vein

下腔静脉（切断）
Inferior vena cava (cut)

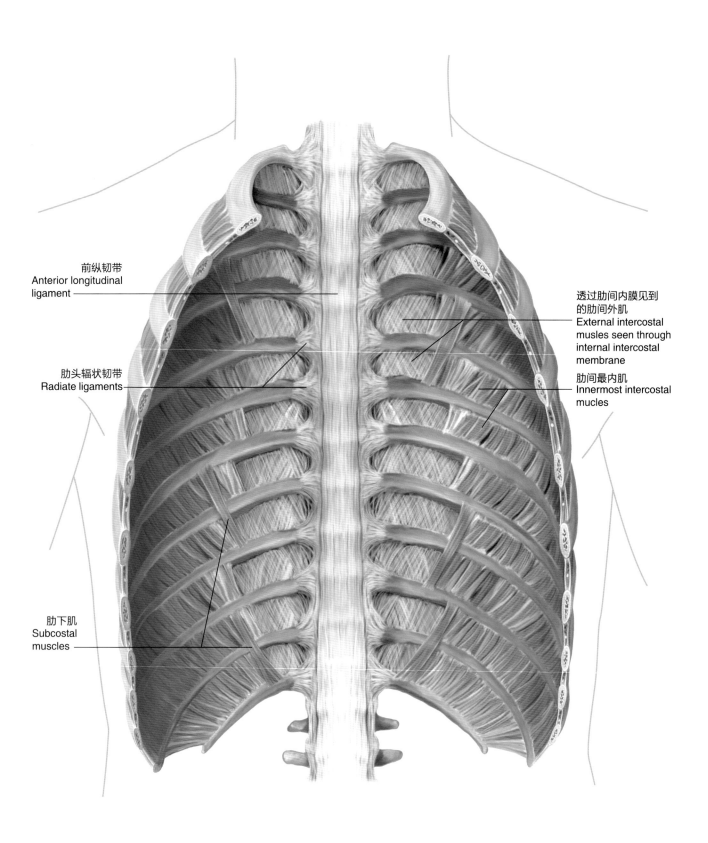

前纵韧带
Anterior longitudinal
ligament

肋头辐状韧带
Radiate ligaments

肋下肌
Subcostal
muscles

透过肋间内膜见到
的肋间外肌
External intercostal
musles seen through
internal intercostal
membrane

肋间最内肌
Innermost intercostal
mucles

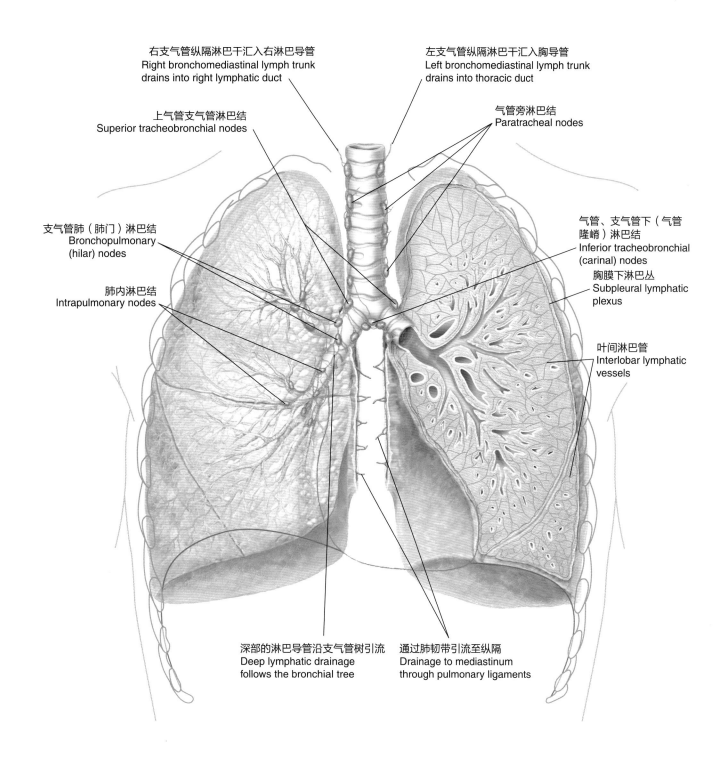

右支气管纵隔淋巴干汇入右淋巴导管
Right bronchomediastinal lymph trunk
drains into right lymphatic duct

左支气管纵隔淋巴干汇入胸导管
Left bronchomediastinal lymph trunk
drains into thoracic duct

上气管支气管淋巴结
Superior tracheobronchial nodes

气管旁淋巴结
Paratracheal nodes

支气管肺（肺门）淋巴结
Bronchopulmonary
(hilar) nodes

气管、支气管下（气管
隆嵴）淋巴结
Inferior tracheobronchial
(carinal) nodes

胸膜下淋巴丛
Subpleural lymphatic
plexus

肺内淋巴结
Intrapulmonary nodes

叶间淋巴管
Interlobar lymphatic
vessels

深部的淋巴导管沿支气管树引流
Deep lymphatic drainage
follows the bronchial tree

通过肺韧带引流至纵隔
Drainage to mediastinum
through pulmonary ligaments

图 4-44　胸前壁的淋巴　Lymphatics of the Anterior Thoracic Wall

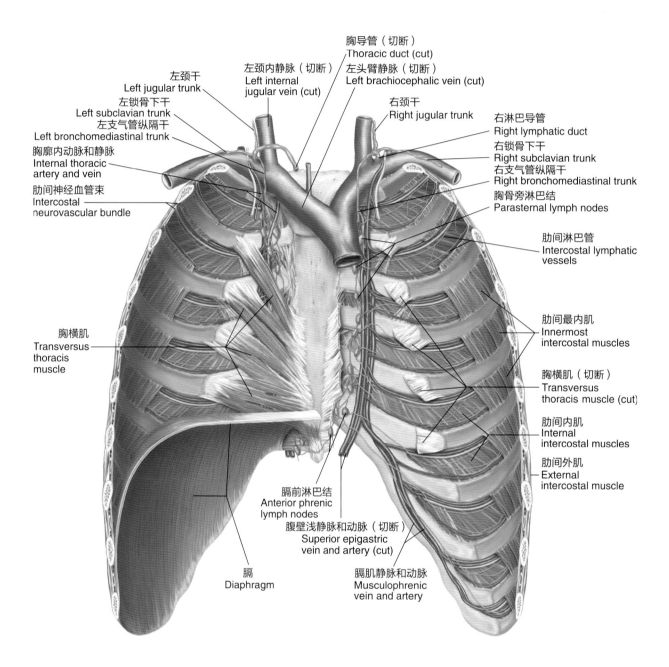

左颈干
Left jugular trunk

左锁骨下干
Left subclavian trunk

左支气管纵隔干
Left bronchomediastinal trunk

胸廓内动脉和静脉
Internal thoracic
artery and vein

肋间神经血管束
Intercostal
neurovascular bundle

左颈内静脉（切断）
Left internal
jugular vein (cut)

胸导管（切断）
Thoracic duct (cut)

左头臂静脉（切断）
Left brachiocephalic vein (cut)

右颈干
Right jugular trunk

右淋巴导管
Right lymphatic duct

右锁骨下干
Right subclavian trunk

右支气管纵隔干
Right bronchomediastinal trunk

胸骨旁淋巴结
Parasternal lymph nodes

肋间淋巴管
Intercostal lymphatic
vessels

胸横肌
Transversus
thoracis
muscle

肋间最内肌
Innermost
intercostal muscles

胸横肌（切断）
Transversus
thoracis muscle (cut)

肋间内肌
Internal
intercostal muscles

肋间外肌
External
intercostal muscle

膈前淋巴结
Anterior phrenic
lymph nodes

腹壁浅静脉和动脉（切断）
Superior epigastric
vein and artery (cut)

膈
Diaphragm

膈肌静脉和动脉
Musculophrenic
vein and artery

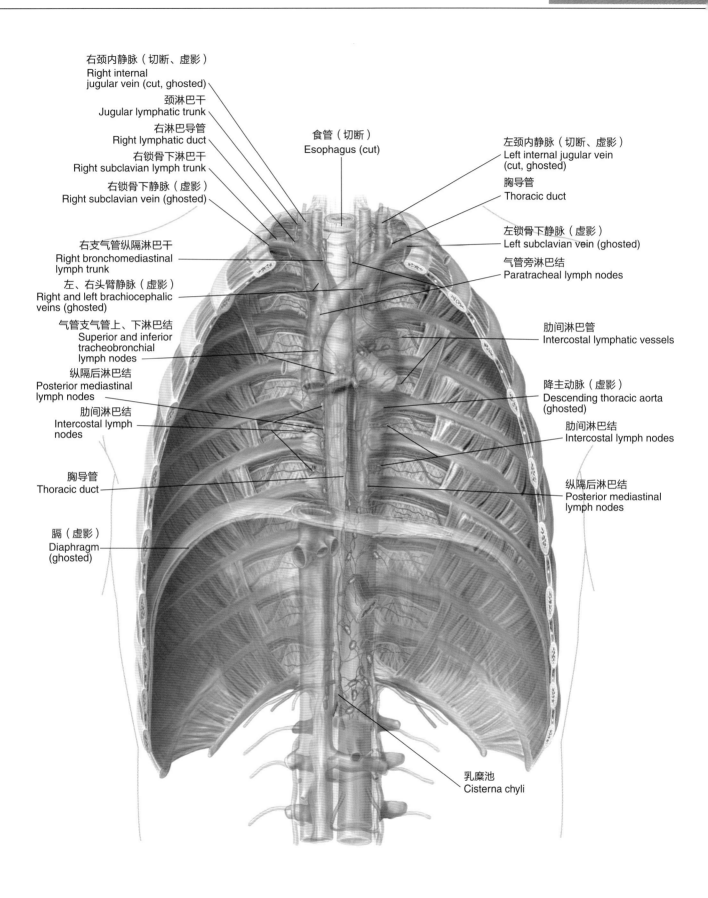

右颈内静脉（切断、虚影）
Right internal
jugular vein (cut, ghosted)

颈淋巴干
Jugular lymphatic trunk

右淋巴导管
Right lymphatic duct

右锁骨下淋巴干
Right subclavian lymph trunk

右锁骨下静脉（虚影）
Right subclavian vein (ghosted)

右支气管纵隔淋巴干
Right bronchomediastinal
lymph trunk

左、右头臂静脉（虚影）
Right and left brachiocephalic
veins (ghosted)

气管支气管上、下淋巴结
Superior and inferior
tracheobronchial
lymph nodes

纵隔后淋巴结
Posterior mediastinal
lymph nodes

肋间淋巴结
Intercostal lymph
nodes

胸导管
Thoracic duct

膈（虚影）
Diaphragm
(ghosted)

食管（切断）
Esophagus (cut)

左颈内静脉（切断、虚影）
Left internal jugular vein
(cut, ghosted)

胸导管
Thoracic duct

左锁骨下静脉（虚影）
Left subclavian vein (ghosted)

气管旁淋巴结
Paratracheal lymph nodes

肋间淋巴管
Intercostal lymphatic vessels

降主动脉（虚影）
Descending thoracic aorta
(ghosted)

肋间淋巴结
Intercostal lymph nodes

纵隔后淋巴结
Posterior mediastinal
lymph nodes

乳糜池
Cisterna chyli

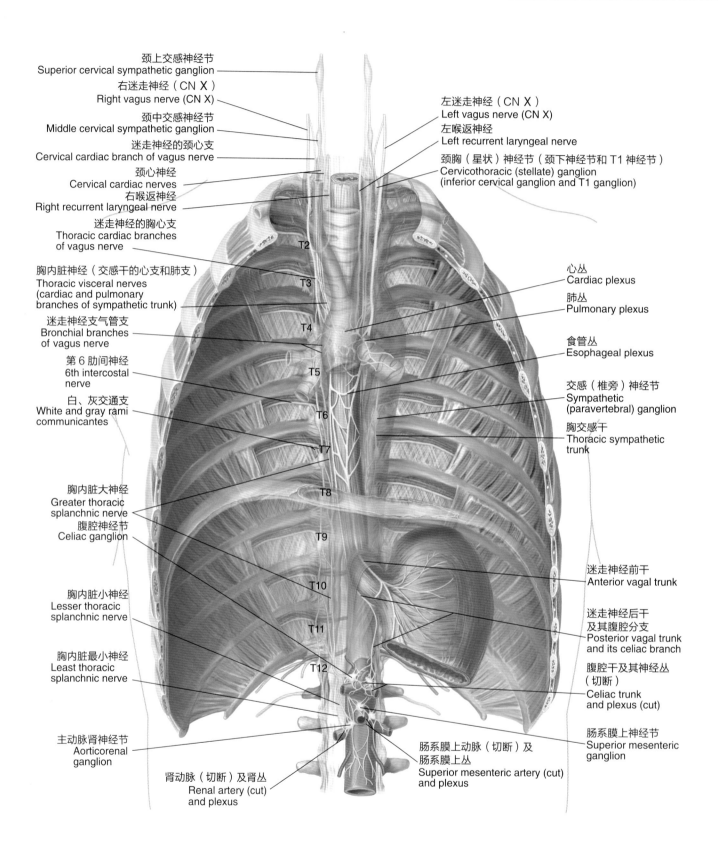

颈上交感神经节
Superior cervical sympathetic ganglion

右迷走神经（CN X）
Right vagus nerve (CN X)

颈中交感神经节
Middle cervical sympathetic ganglion

迷走神经的颈心支
Cervical cardiac branch of vagus nerve

颈心神经
Cervical cardiac nerves

右喉返神经
Right recurrent laryngeal nerve

迷走神经的胸心支
Thoracic cardiac branches
of vagus nerve

胸内脏神经（交感干的心支和肺支）
Thoracic visceral nerves
(cardiac and pulmonary
branches of sympathetic trunk)

迷走神经支气管支
Bronchial branches
of vagus nerve

第 6 肋间神经
6th intercostal
nerve

白、灰交通支
White and gray rami
communicantes

胸内脏大神经
Greater thoracic
splanchnic nerve

腹腔神经节
Celiac ganglion

胸内脏小神经
Lesser thoracic
splanchnic nerve

胸内脏最小神经
Least thoracic
splanchnic nerve

主动脉肾神经节
Aorticorenal
ganglion

肾动脉（切断）及肾丛
Renal artery (cut)
and plexus

左迷走神经（CN X）
Left vagus nerve (CN X)

左喉返神经
Left recurrent laryngeal nerve

颈胸（星状）神经节（颈下神经节和 T1 神经节）
Cervicothoracic (stellate) ganglion
(inferior cervical ganglion and T1 ganglion)

心丛
Cardiac plexus

肺丛
Pulmonary plexus

食管丛
Esophageal plexus

交感（椎旁）神经节
Sympathetic
(paravertebral) ganglion

胸交感干
Thoracic sympathetic
trunk

迷走神经前干
Anterior vagal trunk

迷走神经后干
及其腹腔分支
Posterior vagal trunk
and its celiac branch

腹腔干及其神经丛
（切断）
Celiac trunk
and plexus (cut)

肠系膜上神经节
Superior mesenteric
ganglion

肠系膜上动脉（切断）及
肠系膜上丛
Superior mesenteric artery (cut)
and plexus

T2
T3
T4
T5
T6
T7
T8
T9
T10
T11
T12

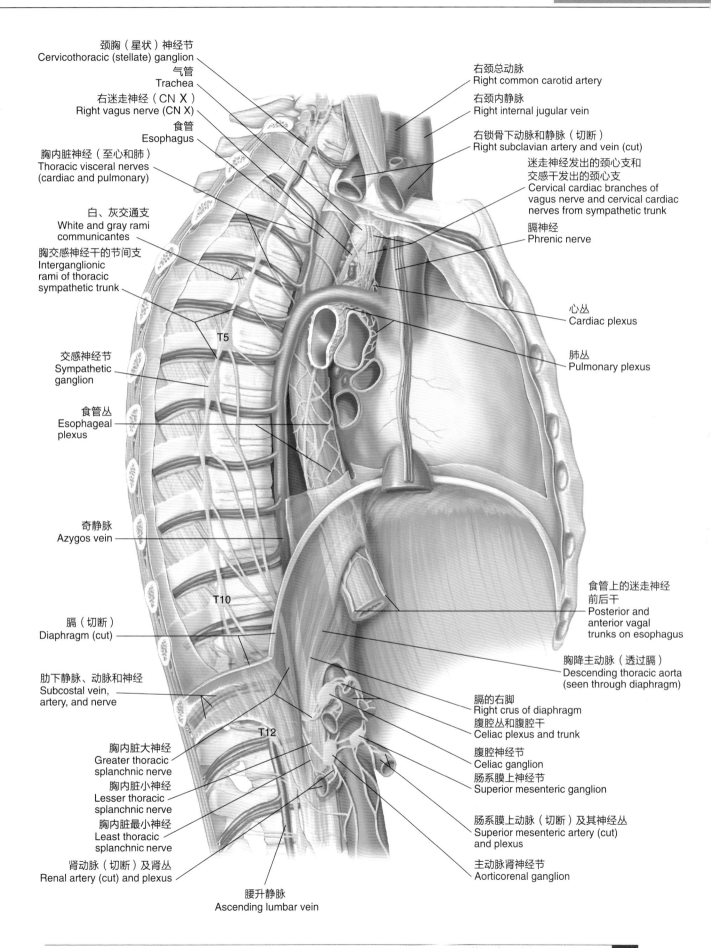

颈胸（星状）神经节
Cervicothoracic (stellate) ganglion

气管
Trachea

右迷走神经（CN X）
Right vagus nerve (CN X)

食管
Esophagus

胸内脏神经（至心和肺）
Thoracic visceral nerves
(cardiac and pulmonary)

白、灰交通支
White and gray rami
communicantes

胸交感神经干的节间支
Interganglionic
rami of thoracic
sympathetic trunk

交感神经节
Sympathetic
ganglion

食管丛
Esophageal
plexus

奇静脉
Azygos vein

膈（切断）
Diaphragm (cut)

肋下静脉、动脉和神经
Subcostal vein,
artery, and nerve

胸内脏大神经
Greater thoracic
splanchnic nerve

胸内脏小神经
Lesser thoracic
splanchnic nerve

胸内脏最小神经
Least thoracic
splanchnic nerve

肾动脉（切断）及肾丛
Renal artery (cut) and plexus

腰升静脉
Ascending lumbar vein

右颈总动脉
Right common carotid artery

右颈内静脉
Right internal jugular vein

右锁骨下动脉和静脉（切断）
Right subclavian artery and vein (cut)

迷走神经发出的颈心支和
交感干发出的颈心支
Cervical cardiac branches of
vagus nerve and cervical cardiac
nerves from sympathetic trunk

膈神经
Phrenic nerve

心丛
Cardiac plexus

肺丛
Pulmonary plexus

食管上的迷走神经
前后干
Posterior and
anterior vagal
trunks on esophagus

胸降主动脉（透过膈）
Descending thoracic aorta
(seen through diaphragm)

膈的右脚
Right crus of diaphragm

腹腔丛和腹腔干
Celiac plexus and trunk

腹腔神经节
Celiac ganglion

肠系膜上神经节
Superior mesenteric ganglion

肠系膜上动脉（切断）及其神经丛
Superior mesenteric artery (cut)
and plexus

主动脉肾神经节
Aorticorenal ganglion

T5

T10

T12

A. 定位
Orientation

B. 横断面
Cross section

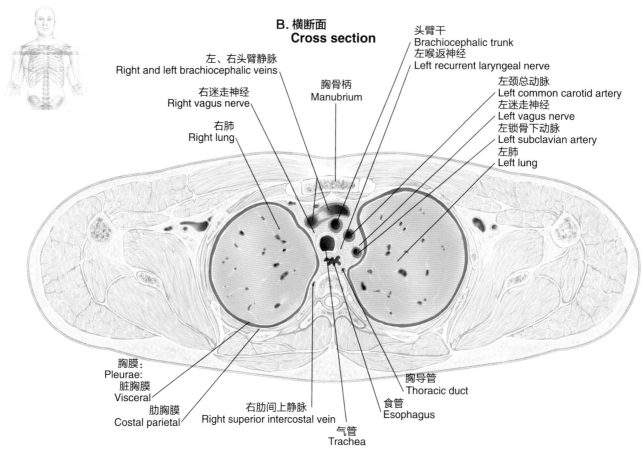

左、右头臂静脉
Right and left brachiocephalic veins

右迷走神经
Right vagus nerve

右肺
Right lung

胸骨柄
Manubrium

头臂干
Brachiocephalic trunk
左喉返神经
Left recurrent laryngeal nerve

左颈总动脉
Left common carotid artery
左迷走神经
Left vagus nerve
左锁骨下动脉
Left subclavian artery
左肺
Left lung

胸膜:
Pleurae:
脏胸膜
Visceral
肋胸膜
Costal parietal

右肋间上静脉
Right superior intercostal vein

气管
Trachea

食管
Esophagus

胸导管
Thoracic duct

C. CT 影像
CT view

右头臂静脉
Right brachiocephalic vein
左头臂静脉
Left brachiocephalic vein

胸骨柄
Manubrium
头臂干
Brachiocephalic trunk

左颈总动脉
Left common carotid artery
左锁骨下动脉
Left subclavian artery

D. CT 影像，肺窗
CT view with lung window

右头臂静脉
Right brachiocephalic vein
左头臂静脉
Left brachiocephalic vein

胸骨柄
Manubrium
头臂干
Brachiocephalic trunk

左颈总动脉
Left common carotid artery
左锁骨下动脉
Left subclavian artery

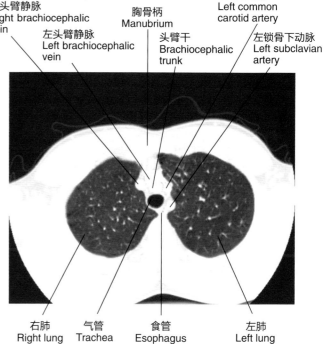

右肺
Right lung
气管
Trachea
食管
Esophagus
左肺
Left lung

右肺
Right lung
气管
Trachea
食管
Esophagus
左肺
Left lung

A. 定位
Orientation

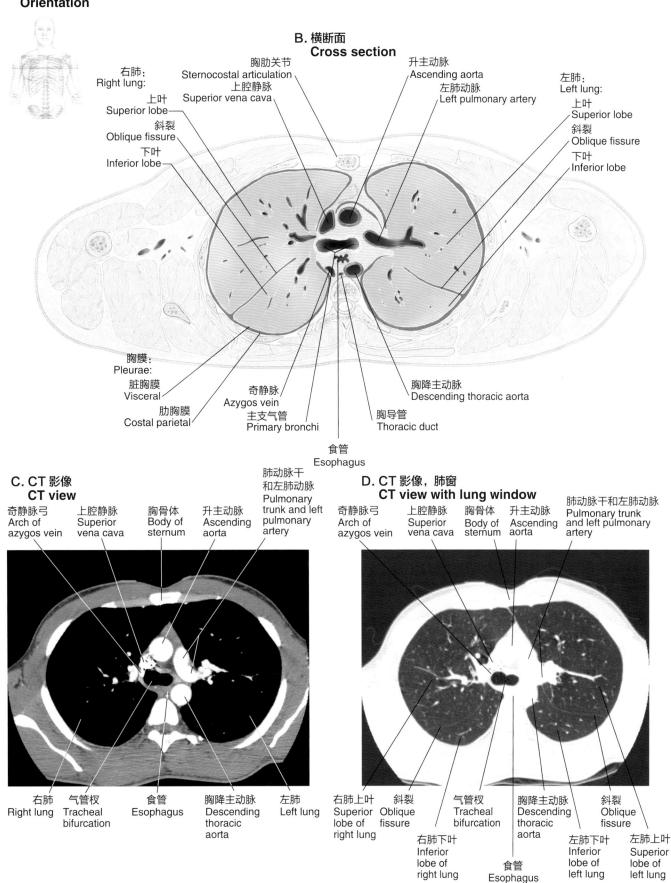

B. 横断面
Cross section

右肺：
Right lung:
上叶
Superior lobe
斜裂
Oblique fissure
下叶
Inferior lobe

胸肋关节
Sternocostal articulation
上腔静脉
Superior vena cava

升主动脉
Ascending aorta
左肺动脉
Left pulmonary artery

左肺：
Left lung:
上叶
Superior lobe
斜裂
Oblique fissure
下叶
Inferior lobe

胸膜：
Pleurae:
脏胸膜
Visceral
肋胸膜
Costal parietal

奇静脉
Azygos vein
主支气管
Primary bronchi

胸降主动脉
Descending thoracic aorta
胸导管
Thoracic duct

食管
Esophagus

C. CT 影像
CT view

奇静脉弓
Arch of
azygos vein
上腔静脉
Superior vena cava
胸骨体
Body of
sternum
升主动脉
Ascending
aorta
肺动脉干
和左肺动脉
Pulmonary
trunk and left
pulmonary
artery

右肺　气管杈
Right lung　Tracheal
bifurcation
食管
Esophagus
胸降主动脉
Descending
thoracic
aorta
左肺
Left lung

D. CT 影像，肺窗
CT view with lung window

奇静脉弓
Arch of
azygos vein
上腔静脉
Superior
vena cava
胸骨体
Body of
sternum
升主动脉
Ascending
aorta
肺动脉干和左肺动脉
Pulmonary trunk
and left pulmonary
artery

右肺上叶
Superior
lobe of
right lung
斜裂
Oblique
fissure
气管杈
Tracheal
bifurcation
胸降主动脉
Descending
thoracic
aorta
斜裂
Oblique
fissure

右肺下叶
Inferior
lobe of
right lung
食管
Esophagus
左肺下叶
Inferior
lobe of
left lung
左肺上叶
Superior
lobe of
left lung

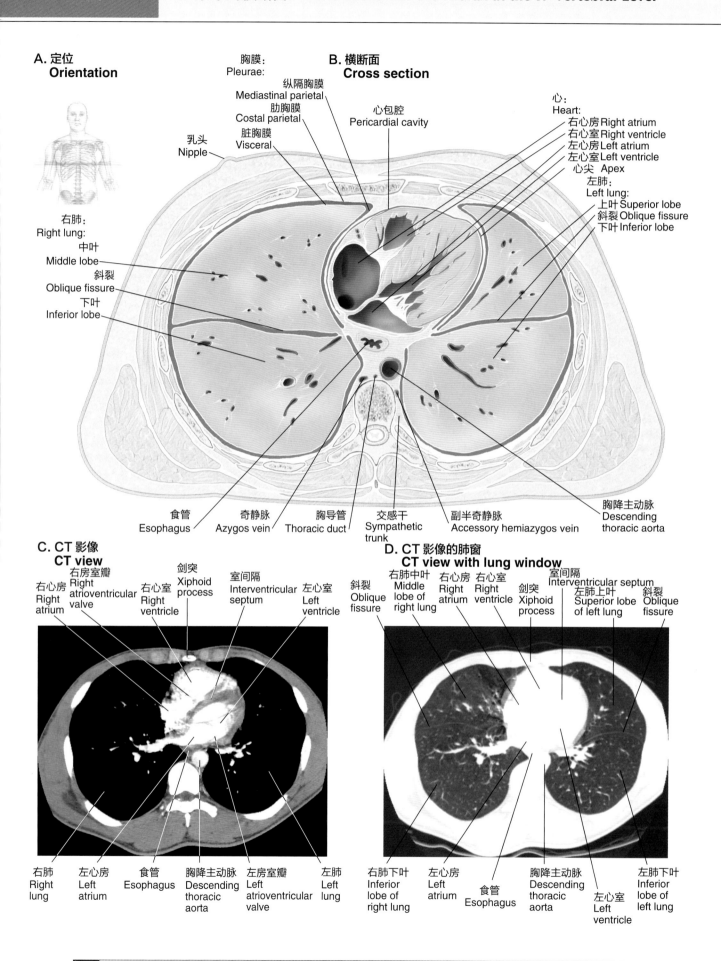

A. 定位
Orientation

胸膜：
Pleurae:

纵隔胸膜
Mediastinal parietal

肋胸膜
Costal parietal

脏胸膜
Visceral

乳头
Nipple

心包腔
Pericardial cavity

B. 横断面
Cross section

心：
Heart:

右心房 Right atrium
右心室 Right ventricle
左心房 Left atrium
左心室 Left ventricle
心尖　Apex

左肺：
Left lung:
上叶 Superior lobe
斜裂 Oblique fissure
下叶 Inferior lobe

右肺：
Right lung:
中叶
Middle lobe
斜裂
Oblique fissure
下叶
Inferior lobe

食管
Esophagus

奇静脉
Azygos vein

胸导管
Thoracic duct

交感干
Sympathetic trunk

副半奇静脉
Accessory hemiazygos vein

胸降主动脉
Descending thoracic aorta

C. CT 影像
CT view

右心房
Right atrium

右房室瓣
Right atrioventricular valve

右心室
Right ventricle

剑突
Xiphoid process

室间隔
Interventricular septum

左心室
Left ventricle

右肺
Right lung

左心房
Left atrium

食管
Esophagus

胸降主动脉
Descending thoracic aorta

左房室瓣
Left atrioventricular valve

左肺
Left lung

D. CT 影像的肺窗
CT view with lung window

斜裂
Oblique fissure

右肺中叶
Middle lobe of right lung

右心房
Right atrium

右心室
Right ventricle

剑突
Xiphoid process

室间隔
Interventricular septum

左肺上叶
Superior lobe of left lung

斜裂
Oblique fissure

右肺下叶
Inferior lobe of right lung

左心房
Left atrium

食管
Esophagus

胸降主动脉
Descending thoracic aorta

左心室
Left ventricle

左肺下叶
Inferior lobe of left lung

胸壁肌						
名称	起点	止点	主要作用	神经支配	动脉	注释
肋间外肌（图4-08）	在一个肋间隙内的肋下缘	下位肋的上缘，肌纤维行向内下	在呼吸过程中维持肋间隙不向外膨出或者向内凹陷	肋间神经（T1~T11）	肋间动脉	共11块；从肋结节伸展至肋骨软骨关节；延续为前方的肋间外膜
肋间内肌（图4-09和图4-10）	肋上缘	上位肋的下缘，肌纤维行向内上方	在呼吸过程中维持肋间隙不向外膨出或者向内凹陷	肋间神经（T1~T11）	肋间动脉	共11块；从胸骨缘伸展至肋角；延续为后方的肋间内膜
肋间最内肌（图4-09和图4-10）	肋上缘	肌纤维向内上方止于上位肋的下缘	在呼吸过程中维持肋间隙不向外膨出或者向内凹陷	肋间神经（T1~T11）	肋间动脉	肋间最内肌与肋间内肌的肌纤维方向一致，唯一的区别是其位于肋间神经血管束的深面
肋下肌（图4-10）	肋角	起点上2~3肋的肋角	压缩肋间隙	肋间神经	肋间动脉	肋下肌、胸横肌和肋间最内肌是最深层的肋间肌
胸横肌（图4-09）	胸骨后面	第2~6肋软骨的内面	用力呼气时压缩胸腔	第2~6肋间神经	胸廓内动脉	胸横肌、肋下肌和肋间最内肌是最深层的肋间肌

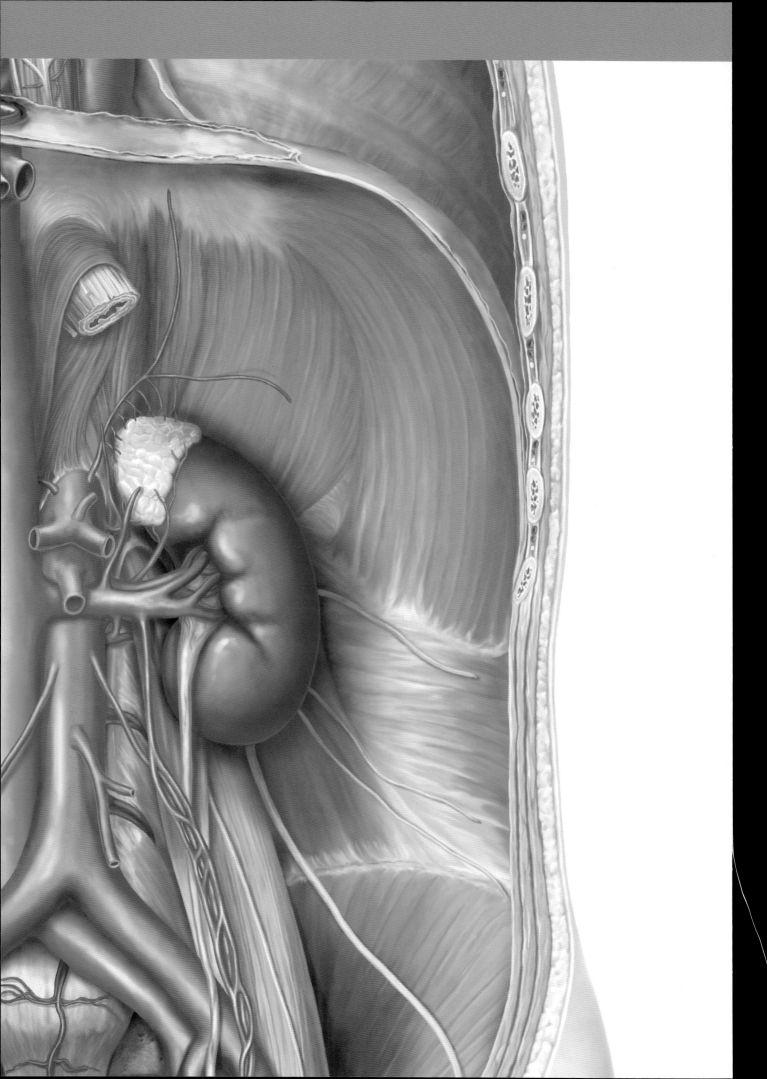

第五章 | 腹部

CHAPTER 5 | **The Abdomen**

A. 可触及的结构
Palpable structures

可触及的骨性结构
Palpable bony structures

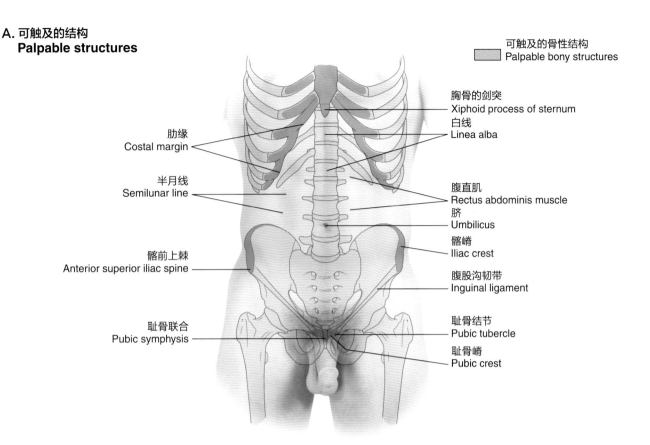

胸骨的剑突
Xiphoid process of sternum

白线
Linea alba

肋缘
Costal margin

腹直肌
Rectus abdominis muscle

脐
Umbilicus

半月线
Semilunar line

髂前上棘
Anterior superior iliac spine

髂嵴
Iliac crest

腹股沟韧带
Inguinal ligament

耻骨联合
Pubic symphysis

耻骨结节
Pubic tubercle

耻骨嵴
Pubic crest

B. 腹部四分法
Abdominal quadrants

C. 腹部分区
Abdominal regions

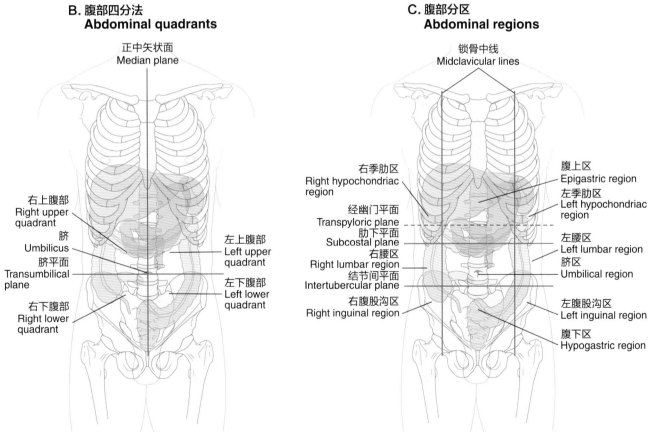

正中矢状面
Median plane

锁骨中线
Midclavicular lines

右上腹部
Right upper quadrant

脐
Umbilicus

脐平面
Transumbilical plane

右下腹部
Right lower quadrant

左上腹部
Left upper quadrant

左下腹部
Left lower quadrant

右季肋区
Right hypochondriac region

经幽门平面
Transpyloric plane

肋下平面
Subcostal plane

右腰区
Right lumbar region

结节间平面
Intertubercular plane

右腹股沟区
Right inguinal region

腹上区
Epigastric region

左季肋区
Left hypochondriac region

左腰区
Left lumbar region

脐区
Umbilical region

左腹股沟区
Left inguinal region

腹下区
Hypogastric region

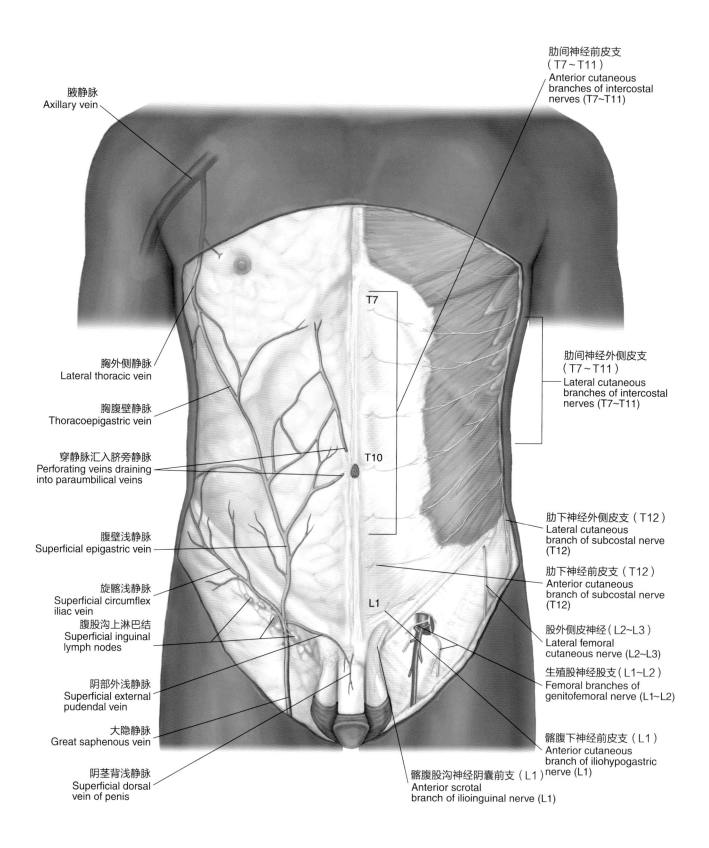

腋静脉
Axillary vein

肋间神经前皮支
（T7~T11）
Anterior cutaneous
branches of intercostal
nerves (T7~T11)

胸外侧静脉
Lateral thoracic vein

肋间神经外侧皮支
（T7~T11）
Lateral cutaneous
branches of intercostal
nerves (T7~T11)

胸腹壁静脉
Thoracoepigastric vein

穿静脉汇入脐旁静脉
Perforating veins draining
into paraumbilical veins

腹壁浅静脉
Superficial epigastric vein

旋髂浅静脉
Superficial circumflex
iliac vein

腹股沟上淋巴结
Superficial inguinal
lymph nodes

阴部外浅静脉
Superficial external
pudendal vein

大隐静脉
Great saphenous vein

阴茎背浅静脉
Superficial dorsal
vein of penis

肋下神经外侧皮支（T12）
Lateral cutaneous
branch of subcostal nerve
(T12)

肋下神经前皮支（T12）
Anterior cutaneous
branch of subcostal nerve
(T12)

股外侧皮神经（L2~L3）
Lateral femoral
cutaneous nerve (L2~L3)

生殖股神经股支（L1~L2）
Femoral branches of
genitofemoral nerve (L1~L2)

髂腹下神经前皮支（L1）
Anterior cutaneous
branch of iliohypogastric
nerve (L1)

髂腹股沟神经阴囊前支（L1）
Anterior scrotal
branch of ilioinguinal nerve (L1)

T7

T10

L1

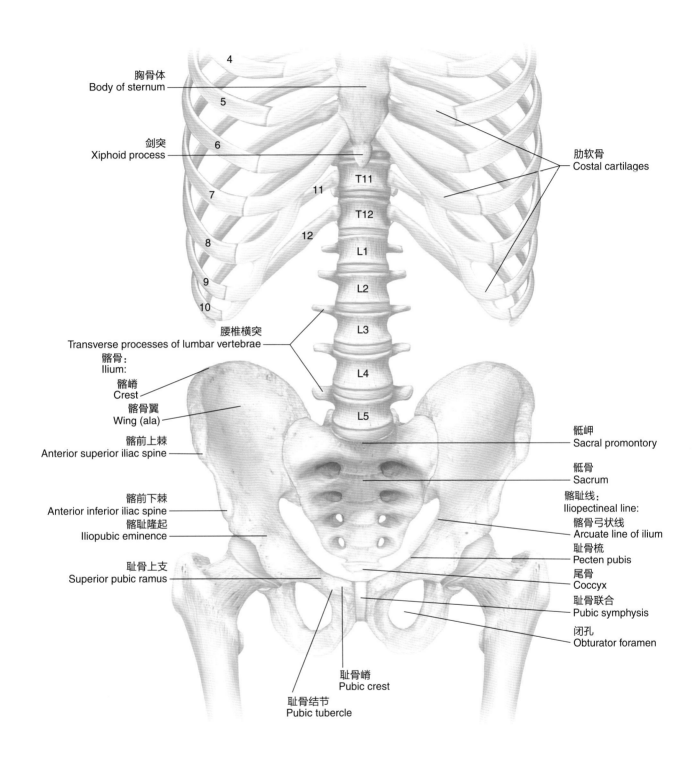

4

胸骨体
Body of sternum

5

剑突
Xiphoid process

6

T11

11

T12

7

12

L1

8

L2

9

L3

10

L4

肋软骨
Costal cartilages

腰椎横突
Transverse processes of lumbar vertebrae

髂骨：
Ilium:

髂嵴
Crest

髂骨翼
Wing (ala)

髂前上棘
Anterior superior iliac spine

髂前下棘
Anterior inferior iliac spine

髂耻隆起
Iliopubic eminence

耻骨上支
Superior pubic ramus

L5

骶岬
Sacral promontory

骶骨
Sacrum

髂耻线：
Iliopectineal line:

髂骨弓状线
Arcuate line of ilium

耻骨梳
Pecten pubis

尾骨
Coccyx

耻骨联合
Pubic symphysis

闭孔
Obturator foramen

耻骨嵴
Pubic crest

耻骨结节
Pubic tubercle

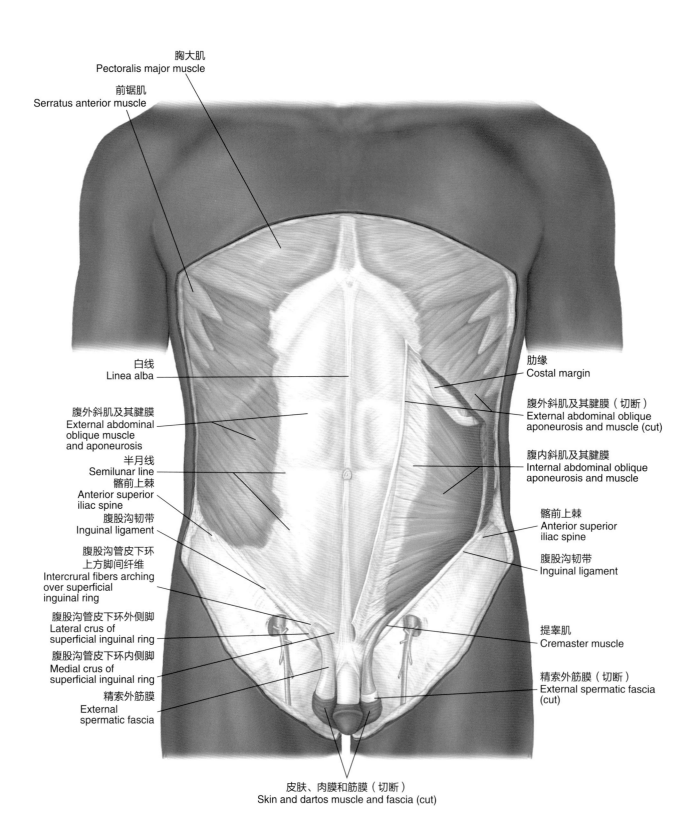

胸大肌
Pectoralis major muscle

前锯肌
Serratus anterior muscle

白线
Linea alba

腹外斜肌及其腱膜
External abdominal
oblique muscle
and aponeurosis

半月线
Semilunar line

髂前上棘
Anterior superior
iliac spine

腹股沟韧带
Inguinal ligament

腹股沟管皮下环
上方脚间纤维
Intercrural fibers arching
over superficial
inguinal ring

腹股沟管皮下环外侧脚
Lateral crus of
superficial inguinal ring

腹股沟管皮下环内侧脚
Medial crus of
superficial inguinal ring

精索外筋膜
External
spermatic fascia

肋缘
Costal margin

腹外斜肌及其腱膜（切断）
External abdominal oblique
aponeurosis and muscle (cut)

腹内斜肌及其腱膜
Internal abdominal oblique
aponeurosis and muscle

髂前上棘
Anterior superior
iliac spine

腹股沟韧带
Inguinal ligament

提睾肌
Cremaster muscle

精索外筋膜（切断）
External spermatic fascia
(cut)

皮肤、肉膜和筋膜（切断）
Skin and dartos muscle and fascia (cut)

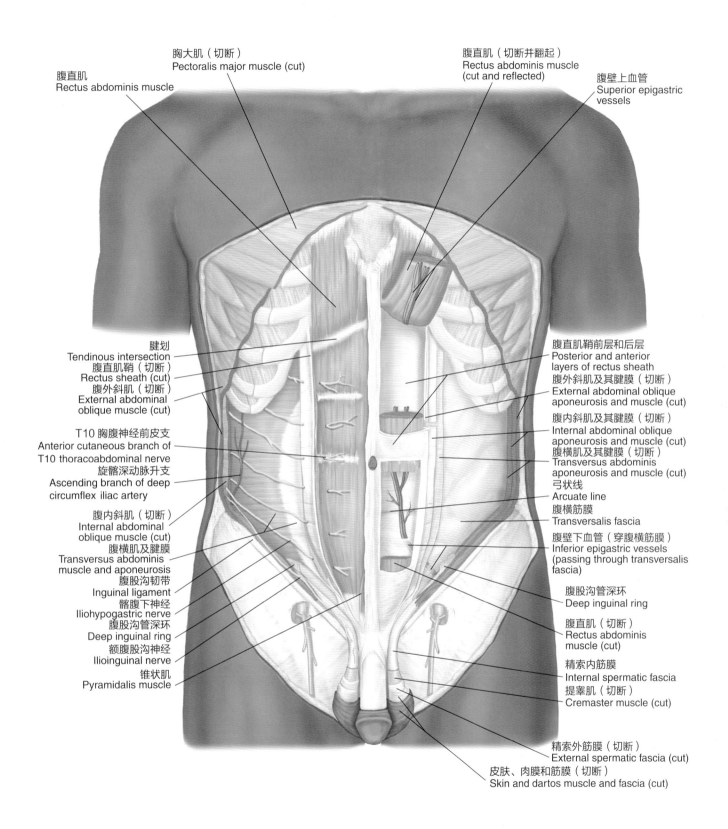

腹直肌（切断）
Pectoralis major muscle (cut)

胸大肌（切断）
Pectoralis major muscle (cut)

腹直肌（切断并翻起）
Rectus abdominis muscle (cut and reflected)

腹壁上血管
Superior epigastric vessels

腹直肌
Rectus abdominis muscle

腱划
Tendinous intersection
腹直肌鞘（切断）
Rectus sheath (cut)
腹外斜肌（切断）
External abdominal oblique muscle (cut)

T10 胸腹神经前皮支
Anterior cutaneous branch of T10 thoracoabdominal nerve
旋髂深动脉升支
Ascending branch of deep circumflex iliac artery

腹内斜肌（切断）
Internal abdominal oblique muscle (cut)
腹横肌及腱膜
Transversus abdominis muscle and aponeurosis
腹股沟韧带
Inguinal ligament
髂腹下神经
Iliohypogastric nerve
腹股沟管深环
Deep inguinal ring
额腹股沟神经
Ilioinguinal nerve
锥状肌
Pyramidalis muscle

腹直肌鞘前层和后层
Posterior and anterior layers of rectus sheath
腹外斜肌及其腱膜（切断）
External abdominal oblique aponeurosis and muscle (cut)
腹内斜肌及其腱膜（切断）
Internal abdominal oblique aponeurosis and muscle (cut)
腹横肌及其腱膜（切断）
Transversus abdominis aponeurosis and muscle (cut)
弓状线
Arcuate line
腹横筋膜
Transversalis fascia
腹壁下血管（穿腹横筋膜）
Inferior epigastric vessels (passing through transversalis fascia)
腹股沟管深环
Deep inguinal ring
腹直肌（切断）
Rectus abdominis muscle (cut)
精索内筋膜
Internal spermatic fascia
提睾肌（切断）
Cremaster muscle (cut)

精索外筋膜（切断）
External spermatic fascia (cut)
皮肤、肉膜和筋膜（切断）
Skin and dartos muscle and fascia (cut)

图 5-06　腹直肌鞘　Rectus Sheath

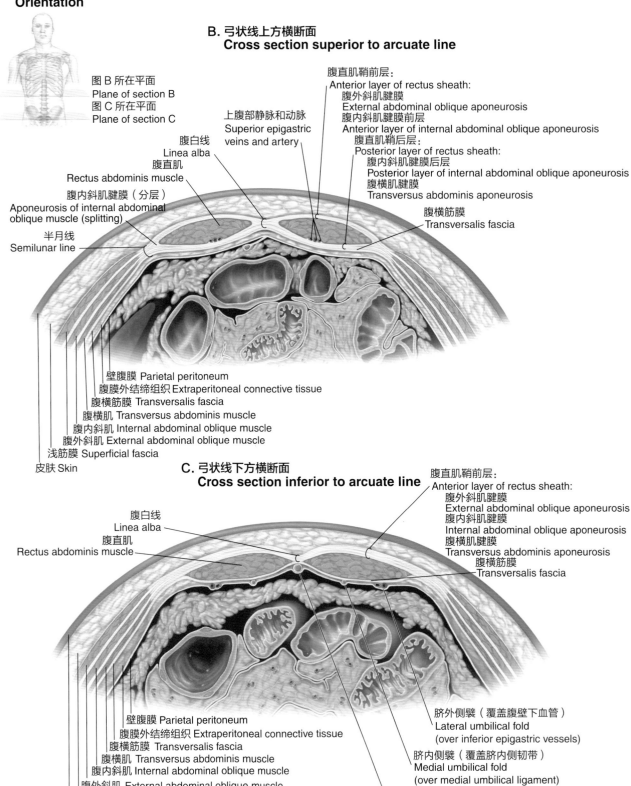

A. 定位
Orientation

图 B 所在平面
Plane of section B
图 C 所在平面
Plane of section C

B. 弓状线上方横断面
Cross section superior to arcuate line

腹白线
Linea alba
腹直肌
Rectus abdominis muscle
腹内斜肌腱膜（分层）
Aponeurosis of internal abdominal
oblique muscle (splitting)
半月线
Semilunar line

上腹部静脉和动脉
Superior epigastric
veins and artery

腹直肌鞘前层：
Anterior layer of rectus sheath:
腹外斜肌腱膜
External abdominal oblique aponeurosis
腹内斜肌腱膜前层
Anterior layer of internal abdominal oblique aponeurosis
腹直肌鞘后层：
Posterior layer of rectus sheath:
腹内斜肌腱膜后层
Posterior layer of internal abdominal oblique aponeurosis
腹横肌腱膜
Transversus abdominis aponeurosis
腹横筋膜
Transversalis fascia

壁腹膜 Parietal peritoneum
腹膜外结缔组织 Extraperitoneal connective tissue
腹横筋膜 Transversalis fascia
腹横肌 Transversus abdominis muscle
腹内斜肌 Internal abdominal oblique muscle
腹外斜肌 External abdominal oblique muscle
浅筋膜 Superficial fascia
皮肤 Skin

C. 弓状线下方横断面
Cross section inferior to arcuate line

腹白线
Linea alba
腹直肌
Rectus abdominis muscle

腹直肌鞘前层：
Anterior layer of rectus sheath:
腹外斜肌腱膜
External abdominal oblique aponeurosis
腹内斜肌腱膜
Internal abdominal oblique aponeurosis
腹横肌腱膜
Transversus abdominis aponeurosis
腹横筋膜
Transversalis fascia

壁腹膜 Parietal peritoneum
腹膜外结缔组织 Extraperitoneal connective tissue
腹横筋膜 Transversalis fascia
腹横肌 Transversus abdominis muscle
腹内斜肌 Internal abdominal oblique muscle
腹外斜肌 External abdominal oblique muscle
浅筋膜 Superficial fascia
皮肤 Skin

脐外侧襞（覆盖腹壁下血管）
Lateral umbilical fold
(over inferior epigastric vessels)
脐内侧襞（覆盖脐内侧韧带）
Medial umbilical fold
(over medial umbilical ligament)
脐正中襞（覆盖脐正中韧带）
Median umbilical fold
(over median umbilical ligament)

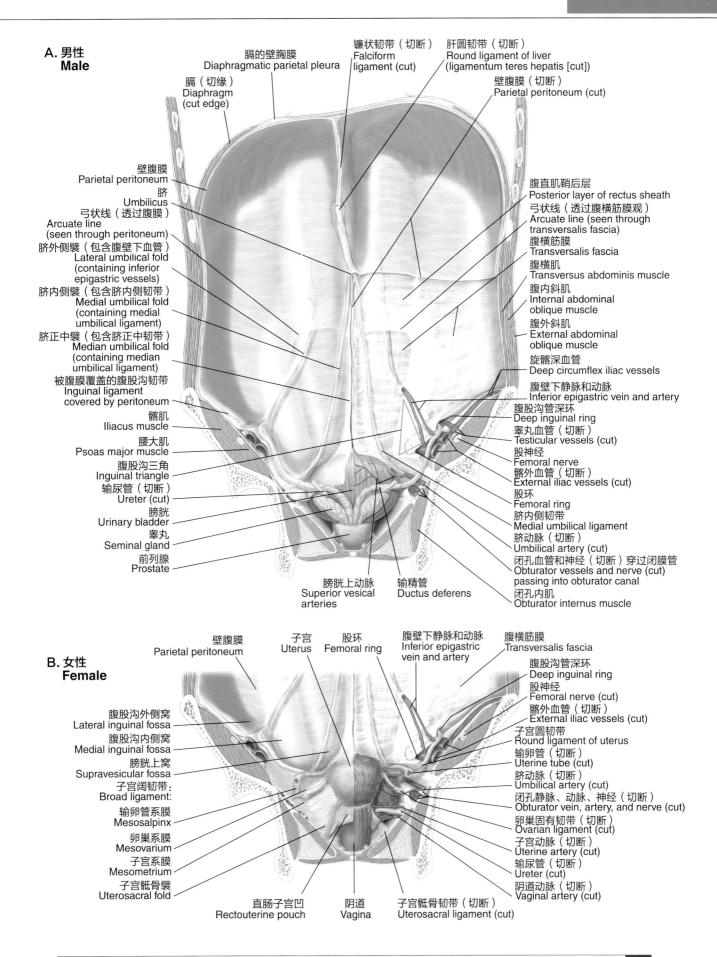

A. 男性
Male

膈的壁胸膜
Diaphragmatic parietal pleura

镰状韧带（切断）
Falciform ligament (cut)

肝圆韧带（切断）
Round ligament of liver
(ligamentum teres hepatis [cut])

膈（切缘）
Diaphragm
(cut edge)

壁腹膜（切断）
Parietal peritoneum (cut)

壁腹膜
Parietal peritoneum

脐
Umbilicus

弓状线（透过腹膜）
Arcuate line
(seen through peritoneum)

脐外侧襞（包含腹壁下血管）
Lateral umbilical fold
(containing inferior
epigastric vessels)

脐内侧襞（包含脐内侧韧带）
Medial umbilical fold
(containing medial
umbilical ligament)

脐正中襞（包含脐正中韧带）
Median umbilical fold
(containing median
umbilical ligament)

被腹膜覆盖的腹股沟韧带
Inguinal ligament
covered by peritoneum

髂肌
Iliacus muscle

腰大肌
Psoas major muscle

腹股沟三角
Inguinal triangle

输尿管（切断）
Ureter (cut)

膀胱
Urinary bladder

睾丸
Seminal gland

前列腺
Prostate

腹直肌鞘后层
Posterior layer of rectus sheath

弓状线（透过腹横筋膜观）
Arcuate line (seen through
transversalis fascia)

腹横筋膜
Transversalis fascia

腹横肌
Transversus abdominis muscle

腹内斜肌
Internal abdominal
oblique muscle

腹外斜肌
External abdominal
oblique muscle

旋髂深血管
Deep circumflex iliac vessels

腹壁下静脉和动脉
Inferior epigastric vein and artery

腹股沟管深环
Deep inguinal ring

睾丸血管（切断）
Testicular vessels (cut)

股神经
Femoral nerve

髂外血管（切断）
External iliac vessels (cut)

股环
Femoral ring

脐内侧韧带
Medial umbilical ligament

脐动脉（切断）
Umbilical artery (cut)

闭孔血管和神经（切断）穿过闭膜管
Obturator vessels and nerve (cut)
passing into obturator canal

闭孔内肌
Obturator internus muscle

膀胱上动脉
Superior vesical arteries

输精管
Ductus deferens

B. 女性
Female

壁腹膜
Parietal peritoneum

子宫
Uterus

股环
Femoral ring

腹壁下静脉和动脉
Inferior epigastric
vein and artery

腹横筋膜
Transversalis fascia

腹股沟管深环
Deep inguinal ring

股神经
Femoral nerve (cut)

髂外血管（切断）
External iliac vessels (cut)

子宫圆韧带
Round ligament of uterus

输卵管（切断）
Uterine tube (cut)

脐动脉（切断）
Umbilical artery (cut)

闭孔静脉、动脉、神经（切断）
Obturator vein, artery, and nerve (cut)

卵巢固有韧带（切断）
Ovarian ligament (cut)

子宫动脉（切断）
Uterine artery (cut)

输尿管（切断）
Ureter (cut)

阴道动脉（切断）
Vaginal artery (cut)

腹股沟外侧窝
Lateral inguinal fossa

腹股沟内侧窝
Medial inguinal fossa

膀胱上窝
Supravesicular fossa

子宫阔韧带：
Broad ligament:

输卵管系膜
Mesosalpinx

卵巢系膜
Mesovarium

子宫系膜
Mesometrium

子宫骶骨襞
Uterosacral fold

直肠子宫凹
Rectouterine pouch

阴道
Vagina

子宫骶骨韧带（切断）
Uterosacral ligament (cut)

图 5-08　　**腹股沟区，浅层　Inguinal Region, Superficial Layer**

A. 女性
Female

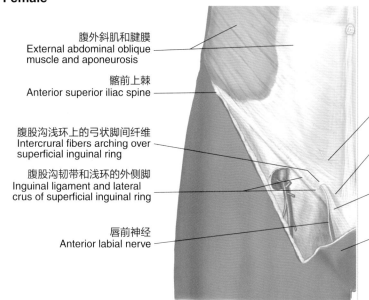

腹外斜肌和腱膜
External abdominal oblique
muscle and aponeurosis

髂前上棘
Anterior superior iliac spine

腹股沟浅环上的弓状脚间纤维
Intercrural fibers arching over
superficial inguinal ring

腹股沟韧带和浅环的外侧脚
Inguinal ligament and lateral
crus of superficial inguinal ring

唇前神经
Anterior labial nerve

髂腹下神经前皮支
Anterior cutaneous branch of iliohypogastric nerve

腹股沟浅环的内侧脚
Medial crus of
superficial inguinal ring

子宫圆韧带
Round ligament of uterus

大阴唇的皮肤、肉膜和筋膜
Skin and dartos muscle and fascia
of labium majus

B. 男性
Male

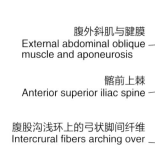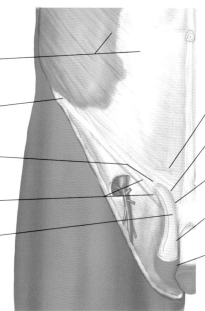

腹外斜肌与腱膜
External abdominal oblique
muscle and aponeurosis

髂前上棘
Anterior superior iliac spine

腹股沟浅环上的弓状脚间纤维
Intercrural fibers arching over
superficial inguinal ring

腹股沟韧带和外侧脚
Inguinal ligament and lateral crus

阴囊前神经
Anterior scrotal nerve

髂腹下神经前皮支
Anterior cutaneous branch of iliohypogastric nerve

腹股沟浅环的内侧脚
Medial crus of
superficial inguinal ring

精索
Spermatic cord

精索外筋膜
External spermatic fascia

皮肤、肉膜和筋膜（切断）
Skin and dartos muscle and fascia (cut)

A. 女性 Female

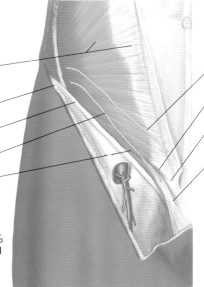

腹内斜肌与腱膜
Internal abdominal oblique
muscle and aponeurosis

髂前上棘
Anterior superior iliac spine

腹股沟韧带
Inguinal ligament

髂腹股沟神经（切断）
Ilioinguinal nerve (cut)*

提睾肌筋膜
Cremaster muscle and fascia

髂腹下神经
Iliohypogastric nerve

腹横筋膜
Transversalis fascia

腹股沟镰（联合腱）
Falx inguinalis (conjoint tendon)

子宫圆韧带
Round ligament of uterus

* 髂腹股沟神经与生殖股神经联合者占 35%
*Ilioinguinal nerve unites with genitofemoral
nerve in 35% of cases

B. 男性 Male

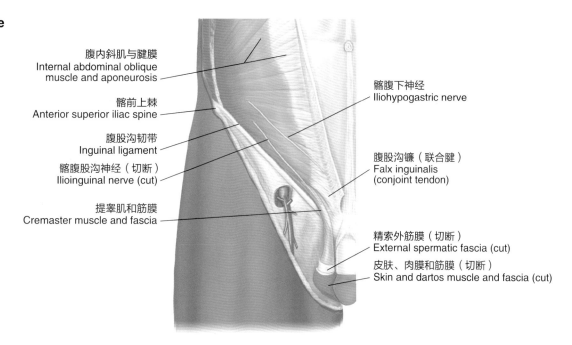

腹内斜肌与腱膜
Internal abdominal oblique
muscle and aponeurosis

髂前上棘
Anterior superior iliac spine

腹股沟韧带
Inguinal ligament

髂腹股沟神经（切断）
Ilioinguinal nerve (cut)

提睾肌和筋膜
Cremaster muscle and fascia

髂腹下神经
Iliohypogastric nerve

腹股沟镰（联合腱）
Falx inguinalis
(conjoint tendon)

精索外筋膜（切断）
External spermatic fascia (cut)

皮肤、肉膜和筋膜（切断）
Skin and dartos muscle and fascia (cut)

图 5-10　腹股沟区，深层　Inguinal Region, Deep Layer

A. 女性
Female

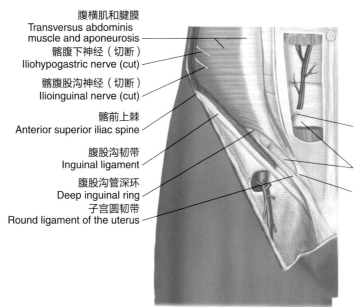

腹横肌和腱膜
Transversus abdominis
muscle and aponeurosis

髂腹下神经（切断）
Iliohypogastric nerve (cut)

髂腹股沟神经（切断）
Ilioinguinal nerve (cut)

髂前上棘
Anterior superior iliac spine

腹股沟韧带
Inguinal ligament

腹股沟管深环
Deep inguinal ring

子宫圆韧带
Round ligament of the uterus

腹壁下血管（穿过腹横筋膜）
Inferior epigastric vessels
(passing through transversalis fascia)

横筋膜
Transversalis fascia

腹股沟镰（联合腱）
Falx inguinalis (conjoint tendon)

B. 男性
Male

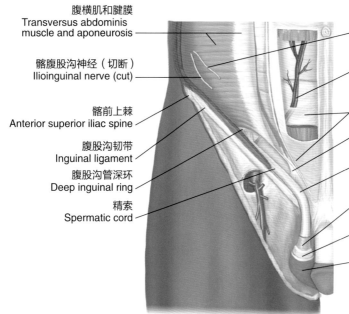

腹横肌和腱膜
Transversus abdominis
muscle and aponeurosis

髂腹股沟神经（切断）
Ilioinguinal nerve (cut)

髂前上棘
Anterior superior iliac spine

腹股沟韧带
Inguinal ligament

腹股沟管深环
Deep inguinal ring

精索
Spermatic cord

髂下腹神经（切断）
Iliohypogastric nerve (cut)

腹壁下血管（穿过腹横筋膜）
Inferior epigastric vessels
(passing through transversalis fascia)

腹横筋膜
Transversalis fascia

腹股沟镰（联合腱）
Falx inguinalis (conjoint tendon)

精索内筋膜
Internal spermatic fascia

提睾肌和筋膜（切断）
Cremasteric muscle and fascia (cut)

精索外筋膜（切断）
External spermatic fascia (cut)

皮肤、肉膜和筋膜（切断）
Skin and dartos muscle and fascia (cut)

A. 女性
Female

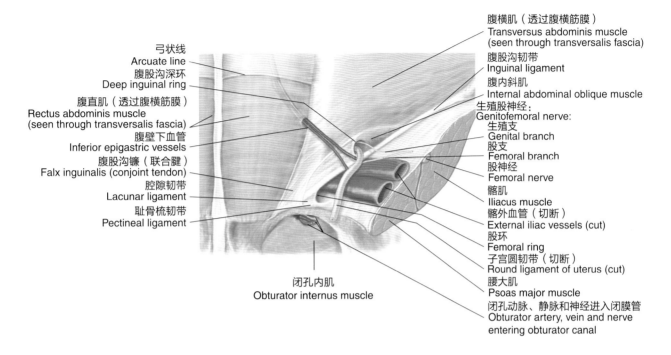

弓状线
Arcuate line
腹股沟深环
Deep inguinal ring

腹直肌（透过腹横筋膜）
Rectus abdominis muscle
(seen through transversalis fascia)
腹壁下血管
Inferior epigastric vessels
腹股沟镰（联合腱）
Falx inguinalis (conjoint tendon)
腔隙韧带
Lacunar ligament
耻骨梳韧带
Pectineal ligament

腹横肌（透过腹横筋膜）
Transversus abdominis muscle
(seen through transversalis fascia)
腹股沟韧带
Inguinal ligament
腹内斜肌
Internal abdominal oblique muscle
生殖股神经：
Genitofemoral nerve:
生殖支
Genital branch
股支
Femoral branch
股神经
Femoral nerve
髂肌
Iliacus muscle
髂外血管（切断）
External iliac vessels (cut)
股环
Femoral ring
子宫圆韧带（切断）
Round ligament of uterus (cut)
腰大肌
Psoas major muscle
闭孔动脉、静脉和神经进入闭膜管
Obturator artery, vein and nerve
entering obturator canal

闭孔内肌
Obturator internus muscle

B. 男性
Male

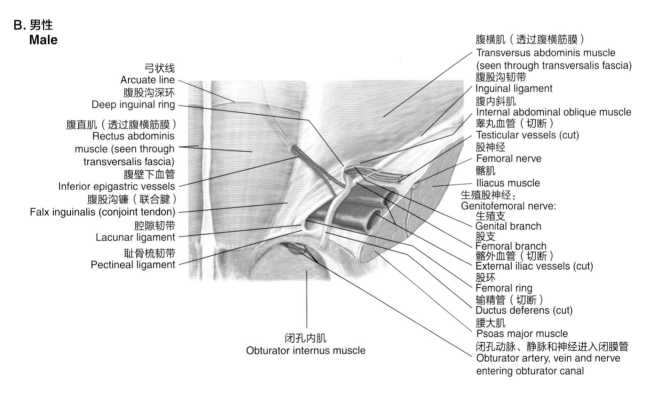

弓状线
Arcuate line
腹股沟深环
Deep inguinal ring

腹直肌（透过腹横筋膜）
Rectus abdominis
muscle (seen through
transversalis fascia)
腹壁下血管
Inferior epigastric vessels
腹股沟镰（联合腱）
Falx inguinalis (conjoint tendon)
腔隙韧带
Lacunar ligament
耻骨梳韧带
Pectineal ligament

腹横肌（透过腹横筋膜）
Transversus abdominis muscle
(seen through transversalis fascia)
腹股沟韧带
Inguinal ligament
腹内斜肌
Internal abdominal oblique muscle
睾丸血管（切断）
Testicular vessels (cut)
股神经
Femoral nerve
髂肌
Iliacus muscle
生殖股神经：
Genitofemoral nerve:
生殖支
Genital branch
股支
Femoral branch
髂外血管（切断）
External iliac vessels (cut)
股环
Femoral ring
输精管（切断）
Ductus deferens (cut)
腰大肌
Psoas major muscle
闭孔动脉、静脉和神经进入闭膜管
Obturator artery, vein and nerve
entering obturator canal

闭孔内肌
Obturator internus muscle

图 5-12　腹股沟区，男性　Inguinal Region, Male

A. 解剖
Dissection

腹外斜肌和腱膜（切断并翻开）
External abdominal oblique muscle and aponeurosis (cut and reflected)

髂前上棘
Anterior superior iliac spine

腹股沟韧带
Inguinal ligament

腹股沟管深环
Deep inguinal ring

腹壁下血管
Inferior epigastric vessels

腹股沟三角内的腹横筋膜
Transversalis fascia within inguinal triangle

提睾肌
Cremaster muscle

腔隙韧带
Lacunar ligament

耻骨梳韧带
Pectineal ligament

腹内斜肌（切断并翻开）
Internal abdominal oblique muscle (cut and reflected)

腹横肌
Transversus abdominis muscle

腹股沟镰
Falx inguinalis

内侧脚
Medial crus

腹股沟管浅环
Superficial inguinal ring

精索
Spermatic cord

外侧脚
Lateral crus

B. 分层便于显示
Layers separated for visibility

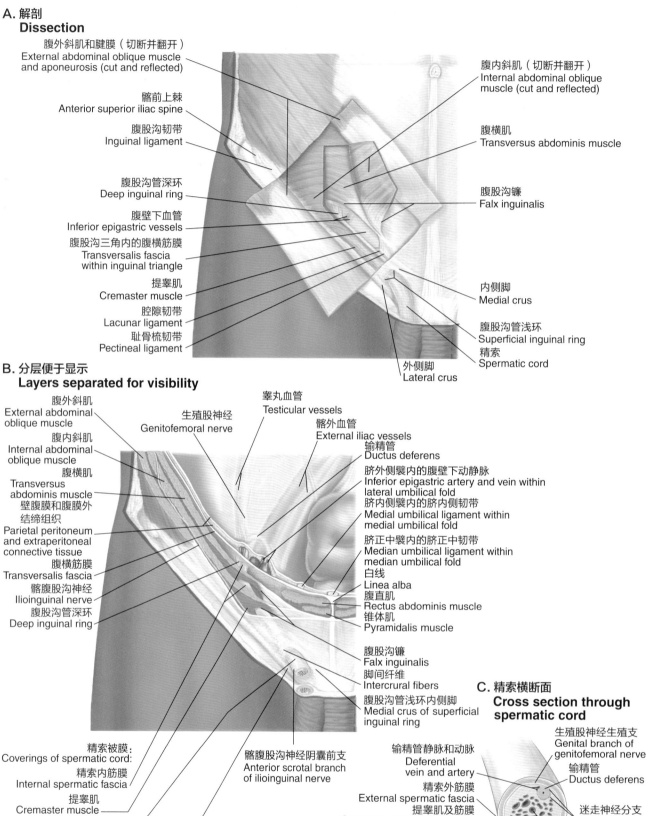

腹外斜肌
External abdominal oblique muscle

腹内斜肌
Internal abdominal oblique muscle

腹横肌
Transversus abdominis muscle

壁腹膜和腹膜外结缔组织
Parietal peritoneum and extraperitoneal connective tissue

腹横筋膜
Transversalis fascia

髂腹股沟神经
Ilioinguinal nerve

腹股沟管深环
Deep inguinal ring

生殖股神经
Genitofemoral nerve

睾丸血管
Testicular vessels

髂外血管
External iliac vessels

输精管
Ductus deferens

脐外侧襞内的腹壁下动静脉
Inferior epigastric artery and vein within lateral umbilical fold

脐内侧襞内的脐内侧韧带
Medial umbilical ligament within medial umbilical fold

脐正中襞内的脐正中韧带
Median umbilical ligament within median umbilical fold

白线
Linea alba

腹直肌
Rectus abdominis muscle

锥体肌
Pyramidalis muscle

腹股沟镰
Falx inguinalis

脚间纤维
Intercrural fibers

腹股沟管浅环内侧脚
Medial crus of superficial inguinal ring

精索被膜：
Coverings of spermatic cord:

精索内筋膜
Internal spermatic fascia

提睾肌
Cremaster muscle

精索外筋膜
External spermatic fascia

腹股沟管浅环外侧脚
Lateral crus of superficial inguinal ring

髂腹股沟神经阴囊前支
Anterior scrotal branch of ilioinguinal nerve

C. 精索横断面
Cross section through spermatic cord

输精管静脉和动脉
Deferential vein and artery

精索外筋膜
External spermatic fascia

提睾肌及筋膜
Cremaster muscle and fascia

精索内筋膜
Internal spermatic fascia

蔓状静脉丛
Pampiniform plexus

生殖股神经生殖支
Genital branch of genitofemoral nerve

输精管
Ductus deferens

迷走神经分支
Branches of vagus nerve

睾丸动脉
Testicular artery

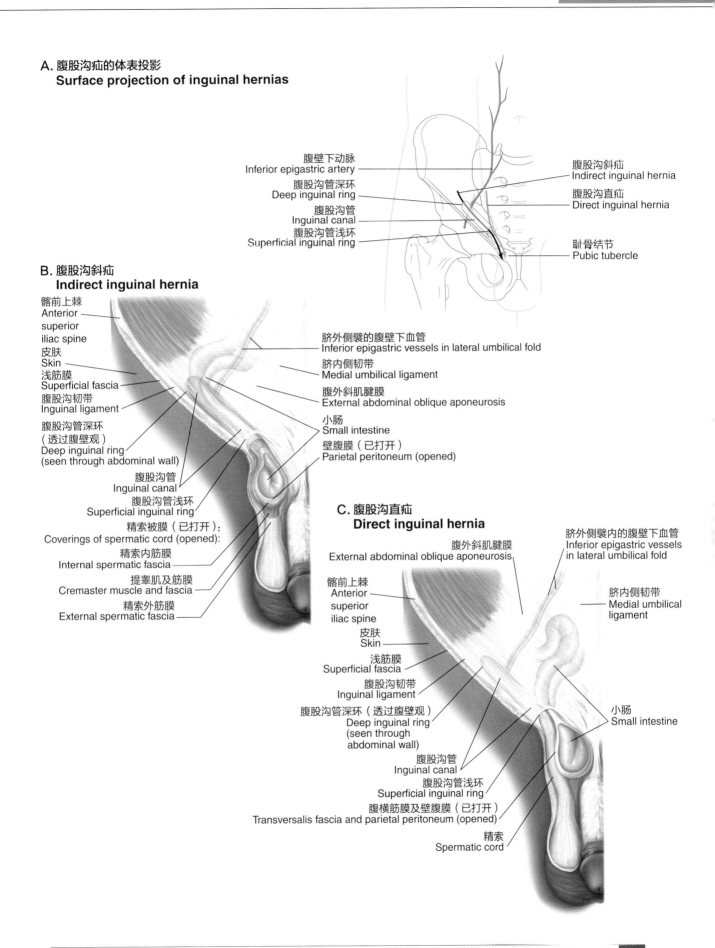

A. 腹股沟疝的体表投影
Surface projection of inguinal hernias

腹壁下动脉
Inferior epigastric artery

腹股沟管深环
Deep inguinal ring

腹股沟管
Inguinal canal

腹股沟管浅环
Superficial inguinal ring

腹股沟斜疝
Indirect inguinal hernia

腹股沟直疝
Direct inguinal hernia

耻骨结节
Pubic tubercle

B. 腹股沟斜疝
Indirect inguinal hernia

髂前上棘
Anterior superior iliac spine

皮肤
Skin

浅筋膜
Superficial fascia

腹股沟韧带
Inguinal ligament

腹股沟管深环
（透过腹壁观）
Deep inguinal ring
(seen through abdominal wall)

腹股沟管
Inguinal canal

腹股沟管浅环
Superficial inguinal ring

精索被膜（已打开）：
Coverings of spermatic cord (opened):

精索内筋膜
Internal spermatic fascia

提睾肌及筋膜
Cremaster muscle and fascia

精索外筋膜
External spermatic fascia

脐外侧襞的腹壁下血管
Inferior epigastric vessels in lateral umbilical fold

脐内侧韧带
Medial umbilical ligament

腹外斜肌腱膜
External abdominal oblique aponeurosis

小肠
Small intestine

壁腹膜（已打开）
Parietal peritoneum (opened)

C. 腹股沟直疝
Direct inguinal hernia

腹外斜肌腱膜
External abdominal oblique aponeurosis

髂前上棘
Anterior superior iliac spine

皮肤
Skin

浅筋膜
Superficial fascia

腹股沟韧带
Inguinal ligament

腹股沟管深环（透过腹壁观）
Deep inguinal ring
(seen through abdominal wall)

腹股沟管
Inguinal canal

腹股沟管浅环
Superficial inguinal ring

腹横筋膜及壁腹膜（已打开）
Transversalis fascia and parietal peritoneum (opened)

精索
Spermatic cord

脐外侧襞内的腹壁下血管
Inferior epigastric vessels
in lateral umbilical fold

脐内侧韧带
Medial umbilical ligament

小肠
Small intestine

图 5-14　腹膜和腹膜腔　Peritoneum and Peritoneal Cavity

A. 大网膜
Greater omentum

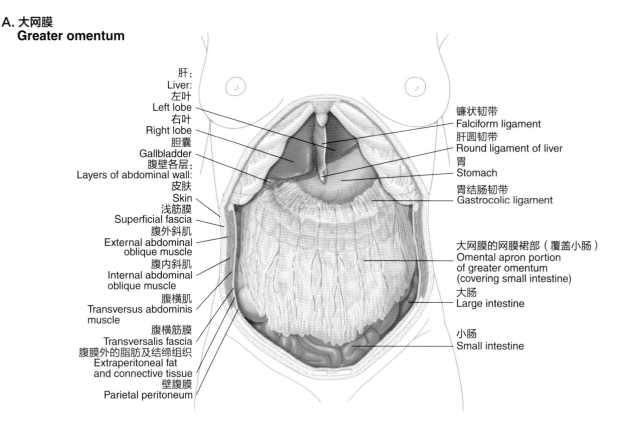

肝：
Liver:
左叶
Left lobe
右叶
Right lobe
胆囊
Gallbladder
腹壁各层：
Layers of abdominal wall:
皮肤
Skin
浅筋膜
Superficial fascia
腹外斜肌
External abdominal oblique muscle
腹内斜肌
Internal abdominal oblique muscle
腹横肌
Transversus abdominis muscle
腹横筋膜
Transversalis fascia
腹膜外的脂肪及结缔组织
Extraperitoneal fat and connective tissue
壁腹膜
Parietal peritoneum

镰状韧带
Falciform ligament
肝圆韧带
Round ligament of liver
胃
Stomach
胃结肠韧带
Gastrocolic ligament
大网膜的网膜裙部（覆盖小肠）
Omental apron portion of greater omentum (covering small intestine)
大肠
Large intestine
小肠
Small intestine

B. 大肠和小肠
Large and small intestines

大肠的特征：
Features of large intestine:
结肠带
Tenia coli
肠脂垂
Omental appendages
结肠袋
Haustra (sacculations)
结肠右（肝）曲
Right colic (hepatic) flexure
升结肠
Ascending colon
盲肠
Cecum
阑尾
Appendix
小肠：
Small intestine:
空肠
Jejunum
回肠
Ileum

大网膜的网膜裙部（翻起）
Omental apron portion of greater omentum (turned up)
横结肠（翻起）
Transverse colon (turned up)
横结肠系膜
Transverse mesocolon
结肠左（脾）区
Left colic (splenic) flexure
十二指肠空肠曲
Duodenojejunal junction
降结肠
Descending colon
乙状结肠
Sigmoid colon

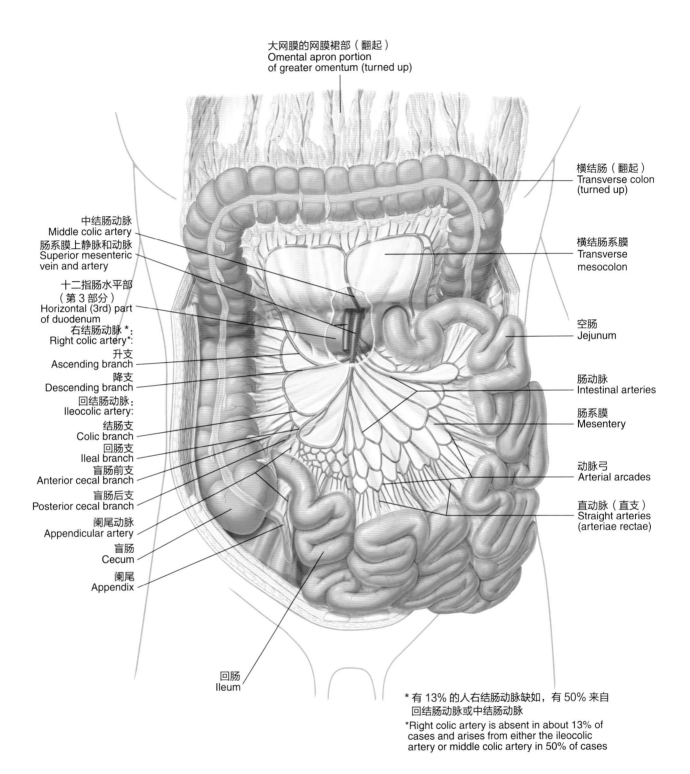

大网膜的网膜裙部（翻起）
Omental apron portion
of greater omentum (turned up)

横结肠（翻起）
Transverse colon
(turned up)

中结肠动脉
Middle colic artery
肠系膜上静脉和动脉
Superior mesenteric
vein and artery

横结肠系膜
Transverse
mesocolon

十二指肠水平部
（第 3 部分）
Horizontal (3rd) part
of duodenum
右结肠动脉 *：
Right colic artery*:
升支
Ascending branch
降支
Descending branch
回结肠动脉：
Ileocolic artery:
结肠支
Colic branch
回肠支
Ileal branch
盲肠前支
Anterior cecal branch
盲肠后支
Posterior cecal branch
阑尾动脉
Appendicular artery
盲肠
Cecum
阑尾
Appendix

空肠
Jejunum

肠动脉
Intestinal arteries

肠系膜
Mesentery

动脉弓
Arterial arcades

直动脉（直支）
Straight arteries
(arteriae rectae)

回肠
Ileum

* 有 13% 的人右结肠动脉缺如，有 50% 来自
回结肠动脉或中结肠动脉
*Right colic artery is absent in about 13% of
cases and arises from either the ileocolic
artery or middle colic artery in 50% of cases

图 5-16 肠系膜下动脉 Inferior Mesenteric Artery

A. 解剖
Dissection

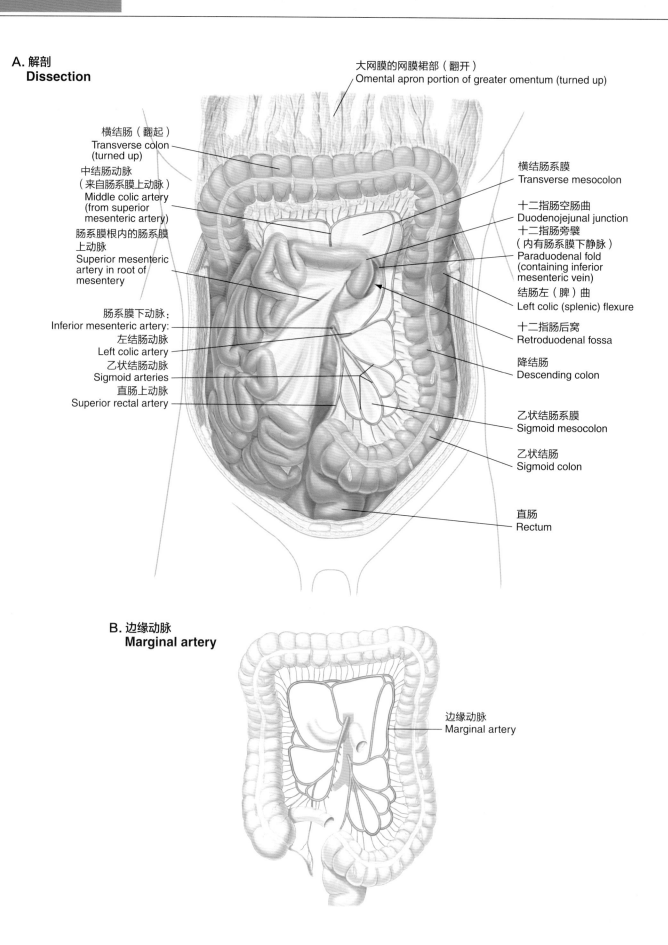

大网膜的网膜裙部（翻开）
Omental apron portion of greater omentum (turned up)

横结肠（翻起）
Transverse colon (turned up)

中结肠动脉
（来自肠系膜上动脉）
Middle colic artery (from superior mesenteric artery)

肠系膜根内的肠系膜上动脉
Superior mesenteric artery in root of mesentery

肠系膜下动脉：
Inferior mesenteric artery:
左结肠动脉
Left colic artery
乙状结肠动脉
Sigmoid arteries
直肠上动脉
Superior rectal artery

横结肠系膜
Transverse mesocolon

十二指肠空肠曲
Duodenojejunal junction

十二指肠旁襞
（内有肠系膜下静脉）
Paraduodenal fold (containing inferior mesenteric vein)

结肠左（脾）曲
Left colic (splenic) flexure

十二指肠后窝
Retroduodenal fossa

降结肠
Descending colon

乙状结肠系膜
Sigmoid mesocolon

乙状结肠
Sigmoid colon

直肠
Rectum

B. 边缘动脉
Marginal artery

边缘动脉
Marginal artery

A. 解剖
Dissection

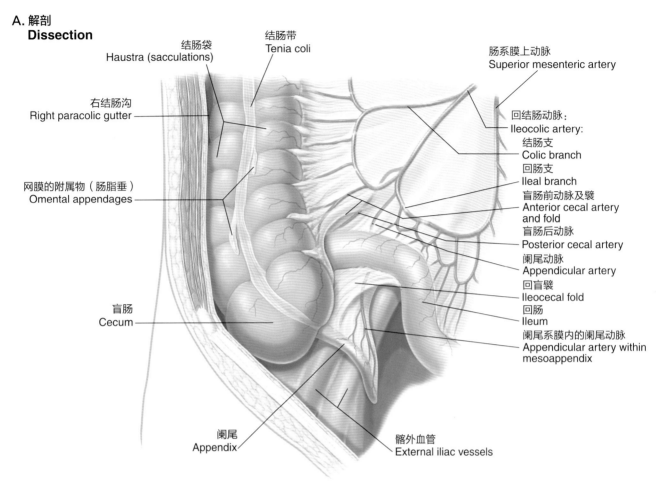

结肠袋
Haustra (sacculations)

结肠带
Tenia coli

肠系膜上动脉
Superior mesenteric artery

右结肠沟
Right paracolic gutter

回结肠动脉：
Ileocolic artery:

结肠支
Colic branch

回肠支
Ileal branch

网膜的附属物（肠脂垂）
Omental appendages

盲肠前动脉及襞
Anterior cecal artery
and fold

盲肠后动脉
Posterior cecal artery

阑尾动脉
Appendicular artery

回盲襞
Ileocecal fold

回肠
Ileum

盲肠
Cecum

阑尾系膜内的阑尾动脉
Appendicular artery within
mesoappendix

阑尾
Appendix

髂外血管
External iliac vessels

B. 回盲瓣
Ileocecal junction

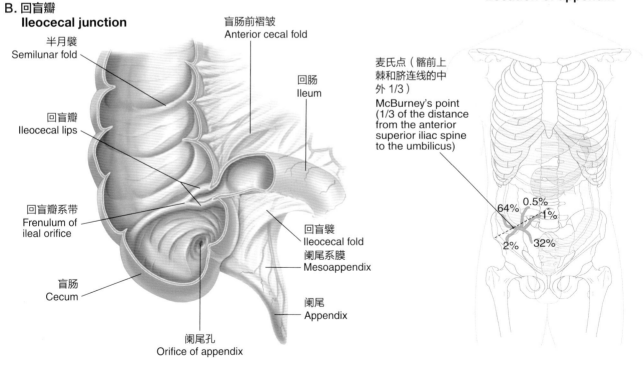

半月襞
Semilunar fold

盲肠前褶皱
Anterior cecal fold

回肠
Ileum

回盲瓣
Ileocecal lips

回盲瓣系带
Frenulum of
ileal orifice

回盲襞
Ileocecal fold

阑尾系膜
Mesoappendix

盲肠
Cecum

阑尾
Appendix

阑尾孔
Orifice of appendix

C. 阑尾位置
Location of appendix

麦氏点（髂前上
棘和脐连线的中
外 1/3）
McBurney's point
(1/3 of the distance
from the anterior
superior iliac spine
to the umbilicus)

64%　0.5%

1%

2%　32%

图 5-18　空肠和回肠　Jejunum and Ileum

A. 定位
Orientation

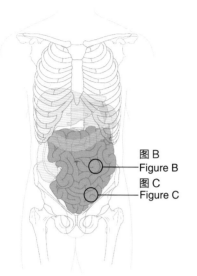

图 B
Figure B

图 C
Figure C

B. 空肠
Jejunum

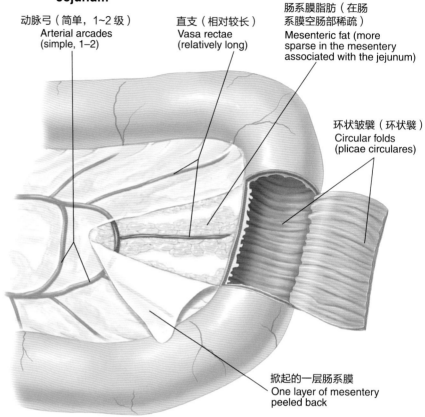

动脉弓（简单，1~2级）
Arterial arcades
(simple, 1–2)

直支（相对较长）
Vasa rectae
(relatively long)

肠系膜脂肪（在肠系膜空肠部稀疏）
Mesenteric fat (more sparse in the mesentery associated with the jejunum)

环状皱襞（环状襞）
Circular folds
(plicae circulares)

掀起的一层肠系膜
One layer of mesentery peeled back

C. 回肠
Ileum

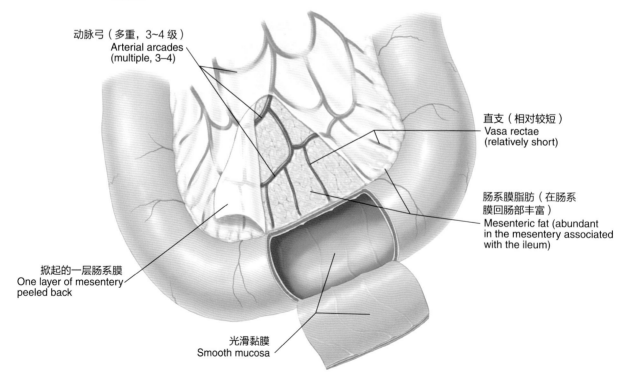

动脉弓（多重，3~4级）
Arterial arcades
(multiple, 3–4)

直支（相对较短）
Vasa rectae
(relatively short)

肠系膜脂肪（在肠系膜回肠部丰富）
Mesenteric fat (abundant in the mesentery associated with the ileum)

掀起的一层肠系膜
One layer of mesentery peeled back

光滑黏膜
Smooth mucosa

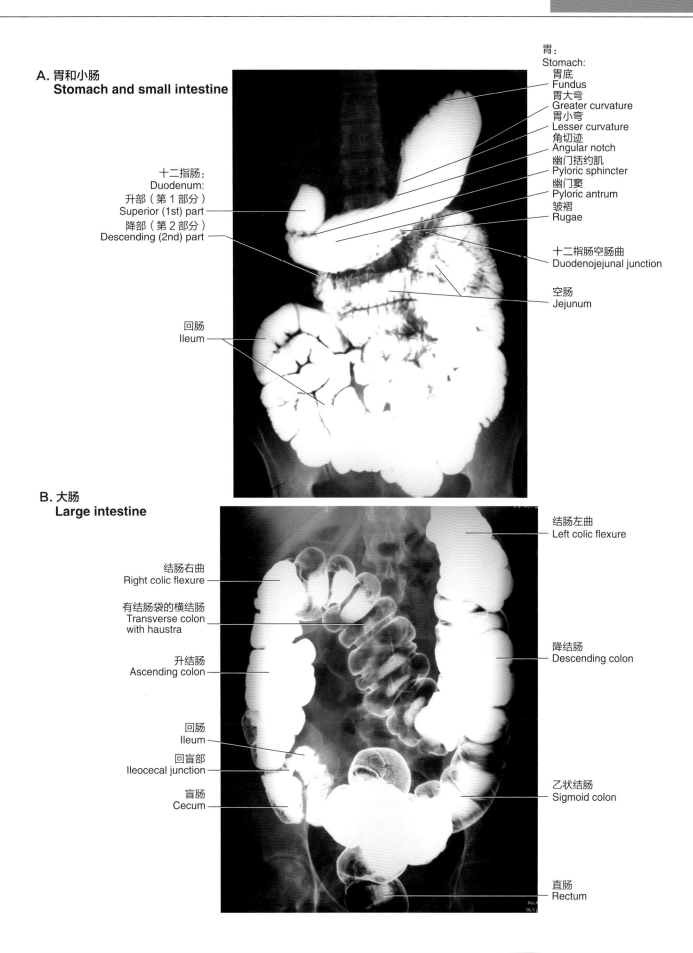

A. 胃和小肠
Stomach and small intestine

胃：
Stomach:

胃底
Fundus

胃大弯
Greater curvature

胃小弯
Lesser curvature

角切迹
Angular notch

幽门括约肌
Pyloric sphincter

幽门窦
Pyloric antrum

皱褶
Rugae

十二指肠：
Duodenum:

升部（第 1 部分）
Superior (1st) part

降部（第 2 部分）
Descending (2nd) part

十二指肠空肠曲
Duodenojejunal junction

空肠
Jejunum

回肠
Ileum

B. 大肠
Large intestine

结肠左曲
Left colic flexure

结肠右曲
Right colic flexure

有结肠袋的横结肠
Transverse colon
with haustra

升结肠
Ascending colon

降结肠
Descending colon

回肠
Ileum

回盲部
Ileocecal junction

盲肠
Cecum

乙状结肠
Sigmoid colon

直肠
Rectum

图 5-20 　胃和小网膜 **Stomach and Lesser Omentum**

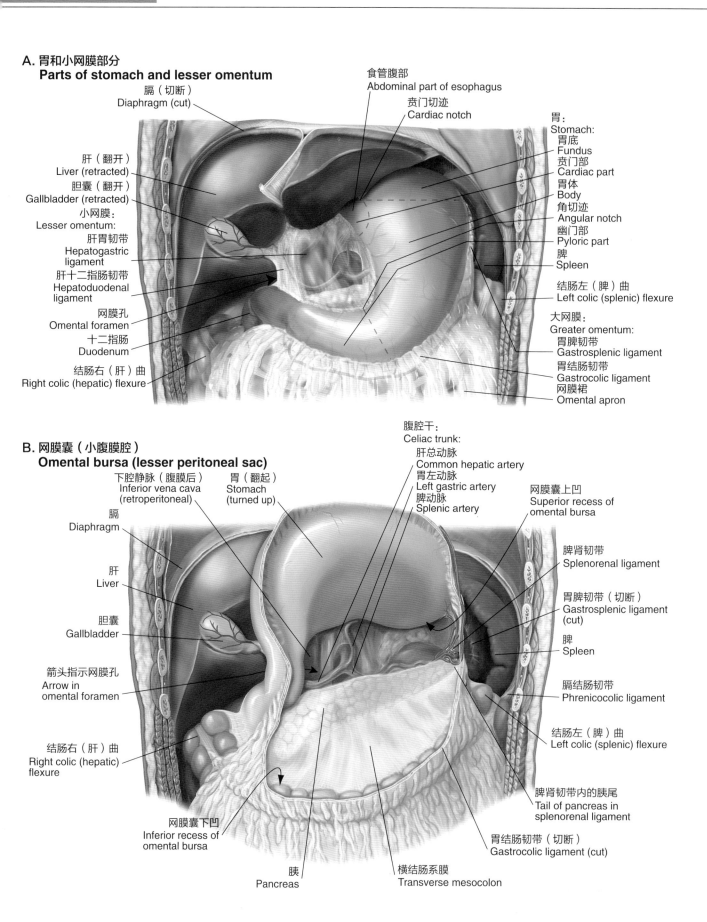

A. 胃和小网膜部分
Parts of stomach and lesser omentum

膈（切断）
Diaphragm (cut)

肝（翻开）
Liver (retracted)

胆囊（翻开）
Gallbladder (retracted)

小网膜：
Lesser omentum:

肝胃韧带
Hepatogastric ligament

肝十二指肠韧带
Hepatoduodenal ligament

网膜孔
Omental foramen

十二指肠
Duodenum

结肠右（肝）曲
Right colic (hepatic) flexure

食管腹部
Abdominal part of esophagus

贲门切迹
Cardiac notch

胃：
Stomach:
胃底
Fundus
贲门部
Cardiac part
胃体
Body
角切迹
Angular notch
幽门部
Pyloric part
脾
Spleen

结肠左（脾）曲
Left colic (splenic) flexure

大网膜：
Greater omentum:
胃脾韧带
Gastrosplenic ligament
胃结肠韧带
Gastrocolic ligament
网膜裙
Omental apron

B. 网膜囊（小腹膜腔）
Omental bursa (lesser peritoneal sac)

下腔静脉（腹膜后）
Inferior vena cava (retroperitoneal)

膈
Diaphragm

肝
Liver

胆囊
Gallbladder

箭头指示网膜孔
Arrow in omental foramen

结肠右（肝）曲
Right colic (hepatic) flexure

网膜囊下凹
Inferior recess of omental bursa

胰
Pancreas

胃（翻起）
Stomach (turned up)

腹腔干：
Celiac trunk:
肝总动脉
Common hepatic artery
胃左动脉
Left gastric artery
脾动脉
Splenic artery

网膜囊上凹
Superior recess of omental bursa

脾肾韧带
Splenorenal ligament

胃脾韧带（切断）
Gastrosplenic ligament (cut)

脾
Spleen

膈结肠韧带
Phrenicocolic ligament

结肠左（脾）曲
Left colic (splenic) flexure

脾肾韧带内的胰尾
Tail of pancreas in splenorenal ligament

胃结肠韧带（切断）
Gastrocolic ligament (cut)

横结肠系膜
Transverse mesocolon

A. 腹腔干
Celiac trunk

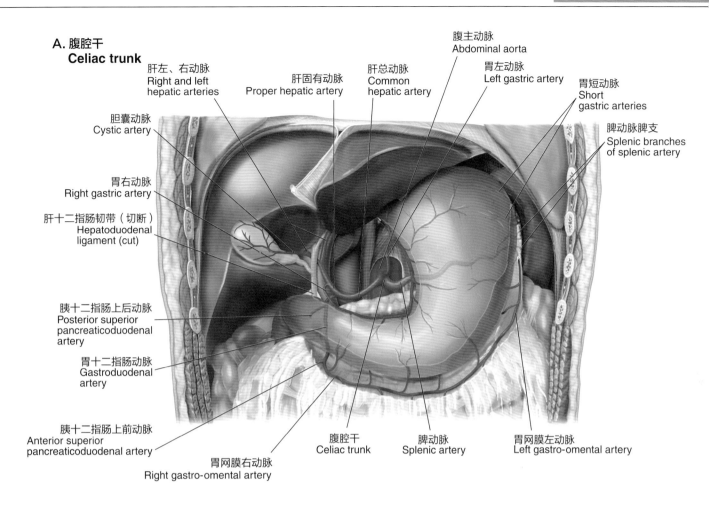

胆囊动脉
Cystic artery

肝左、右动脉
Right and left
hepatic arteries

肝固有动脉
Proper hepatic artery

肝总动脉
Common
hepatic artery

腹主动脉
Abdominal aorta

胃左动脉
Left gastric artery

胃短动脉
Short
gastric arteries

脾动脉脾支
Splenic branches
of splenic artery

胃右动脉
Right gastric artery

肝十二指肠韧带（切断）
Hepatoduodenal
ligament (cut)

胰十二指肠上后动脉
Posterior superior
pancreaticoduodenal
artery

胃十二指肠动脉
Gastroduodenal
artery

胰十二指肠上前动脉
Anterior superior
pancreaticoduodenal artery

胃网膜右动脉
Right gastro-omental artery

腹腔干
Celiac trunk

脾动脉
Splenic artery

胃网膜左动脉
Left gastro-omental artery

B. 胃内面观
Stomach, internal view

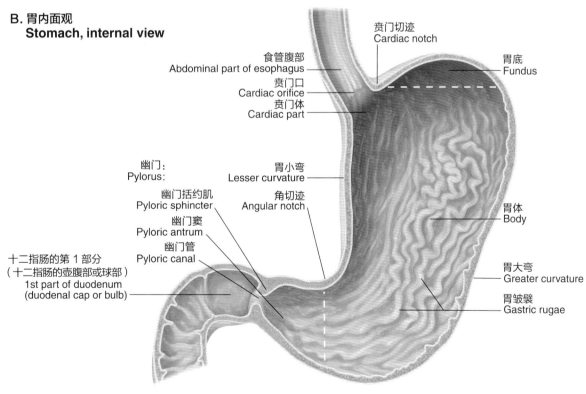

食管腹部
Abdominal part of esophagus

贲门切迹
Cardiac notch

胃底
Fundus

贲门口
Cardiac orifice

贲门体
Cardiac part

幽门:
Pylorus:

胃小弯
Lesser curvature

幽门括约肌
Pyloric sphincter

角切迹
Angular notch

胃体
Body

幽门窦
Pyloric antrum

幽门管
Pyloric canal

十二指肠的第 1 部分
（十二指肠的壶腹部或球部）
1st part of duodenum
(duodenal cap or bulb)

胃大弯
Greater curvature

胃皱襞
Gastric rugae

图 5-22　　脾脏　Spleen

A. 解剖
Dissection

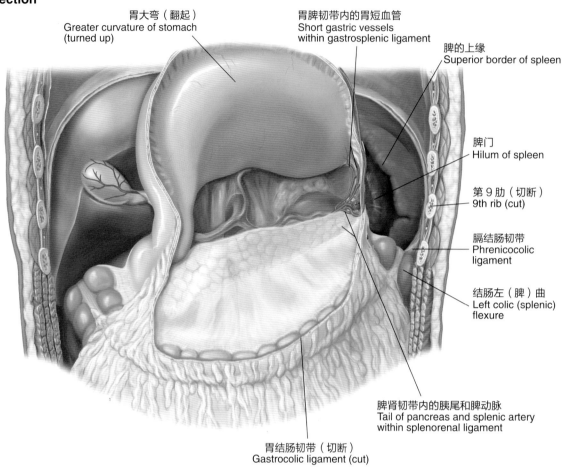

胃大弯（翻起）
Greater curvature of stomach (turned up)

胃脾韧带内的胃短血管
Short gastric vessels within gastrosplenic ligament

脾的上缘
Superior border of spleen

脾门
Hilum of spleen

第 9 肋（切断）
9th rib (cut)

膈结肠韧带
Phrenicocolic ligament

结肠左（脾）曲
Left colic (splenic) flexure

脾肾韧带内的胰尾和脾动脉
Tail of pancreas and splenic artery within splenorenal ligament

胃结肠韧带（切断）
Gastrocolic ligament (cut)

B. 脏面
Visceral surface

C. 膈面
Diaphragmatic surface

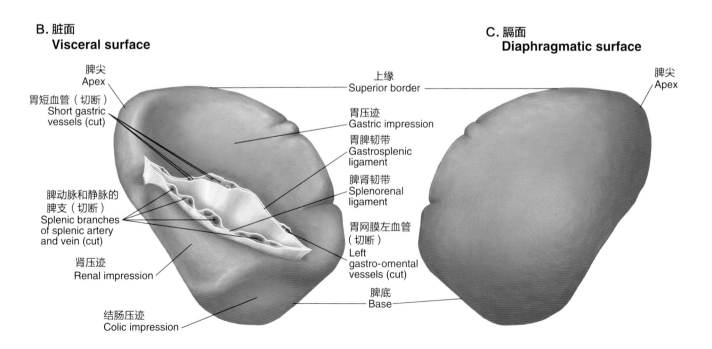

脾尖
Apex

胃短血管（切断）
Short gastric vessels (cut)

脾动脉和静脉的脾支（切断）
Splenic branches of splenic artery and vein (cut)

肾压迹
Renal impression

结肠压迹
Colic impression

上缘
Superior border

胃压迹
Gastric impression

胃脾韧带
Gastrosplenic ligament

脾肾韧带
Splenorenal ligament

胃网膜左血管（切断）
Left gastro-omental vessels (cut)

脾底
Base

脾尖
Apex

A. 定位
Orientation

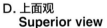

B. 前面观
Anterior view

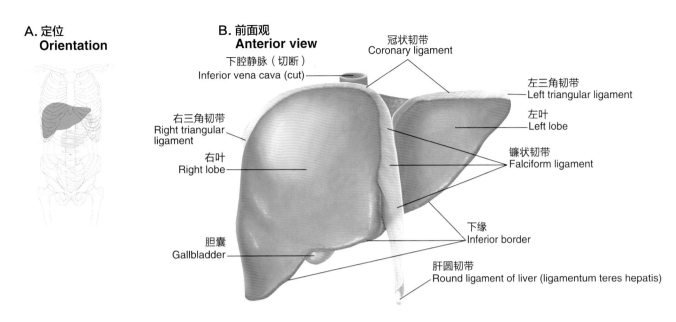

冠状韧带
Coronary ligament

下腔静脉（切断）
Inferior vena cava (cut)

左三角韧带
Left triangular ligament

右三角韧带
Right triangular ligament

左叶
Left lobe

右叶
Right lobe

镰状韧带
Falciform ligament

胆囊
Gallbladder

下缘
Inferior border

肝圆韧带
Round ligament of liver (ligamentum teres hepatis)

C. 下面观
Inferior view

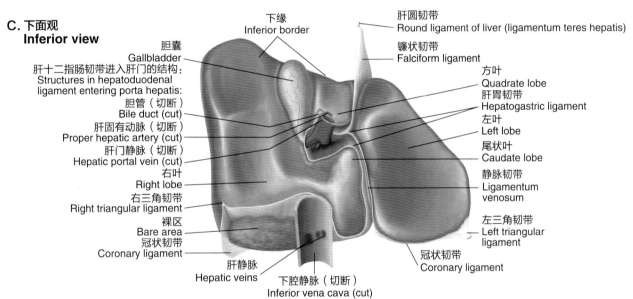

下缘
Inferior border

胆囊
Gallbladder

肝十二指肠韧带进入肝门的结构：
Structures in hepatoduodenal ligament entering porta hepatis:

胆管（切断）
Bile duct (cut)

肝固有动脉（切断）
Proper hepatic artery (cut)

肝门静脉（切断）
Hepatic portal vein (cut)

右叶
Right lobe

右三角韧带
Right triangular ligament

裸区
Bare area

冠状韧带
Coronary ligament

肝静脉
Hepatic veins

下腔静脉（切断）
Inferior vena cava (cut)

肝圆韧带
Round ligament of liver (ligamentum teres hepatis)

镰状韧带
Falciform ligament

方叶
Quadrate lobe

肝胃韧带
Hepatogastric ligament

左叶
Left lobe

尾状叶
Caudate lobe

静脉韧带
Ligamentum venosum

左三角韧带
Left triangular ligament

冠状韧带
Coronary ligament

D. 上面观
Superior view

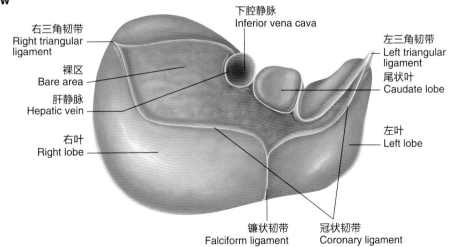

右三角韧带
Right triangular ligament

裸区
Bare area

肝静脉
Hepatic vein

右叶
Right lobe

下腔静脉
Inferior vena cava

左三角韧带
Left triangular ligament

尾状叶
Caudate lobe

左叶
Left lobe

镰状韧带
Falciform ligament

冠状韧带
Coronary ligament

图 5-24　肝，内部结构　Liver, Internal Features

A. 门静脉、肝动脉和胆管系统
Portal vein, hepatic artery, and biliary duct system

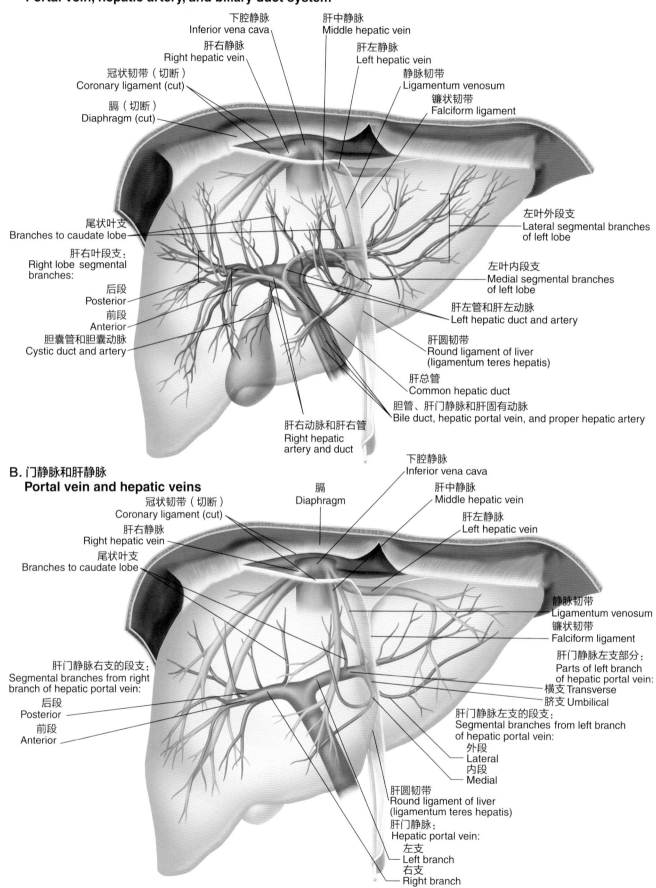

下腔静脉
Inferior vena cava

肝中静脉
Middle hepatic vein

肝右静脉
Right hepatic vein

肝左静脉
Left hepatic vein

冠状韧带（切断）
Coronary ligament (cut)

静脉韧带
Ligamentum venosum

膈（切断）
Diaphragm (cut)

镰状韧带
Falciform ligament

左叶外段支
Lateral segmental branches
of left lobe

尾状叶支
Branches to caudate lobe

肝右叶段支：
Right lobe segmental
branches:

左叶内段支
Medial segmental branches
of left lobe

后段
Posterior

肝左管和肝左动脉
Left hepatic duct and artery

前段
Anterior

肝圆韧带
Round ligament of liver
(ligamentum teres hepatis)

胆囊管和胆囊动脉
Cystic duct and artery

肝总管
Common hepatic duct

胆管、肝门静脉和肝固有动脉
Bile duct, hepatic portal vein, and proper hepatic artery

肝右动脉和肝右管
Right hepatic
artery and duct

B. 门静脉和肝静脉
Portal vein and hepatic veins

下腔静脉
Inferior vena cava

膈
Diaphragm

肝中静脉
Middle hepatic vein

冠状韧带（切断）
Coronary ligament (cut)

肝左静脉
Left hepatic vein

肝右静脉
Right hepatic vein

尾状叶支
Branches to caudate lobe

静脉韧带
Ligamentum venosum

镰状韧带
Falciform ligament

肝门静脉左支部分：
Parts of left branch
of hepatic portal vein:

横支 Transverse

脐支 Umbilical

肝门静脉右支的段支：
Segmental branches from right
branch of hepatic portal vein:

肝门静脉左支的段支：
Segmental branches from left branch
of hepatic portal vein:

后段
Posterior

外段
Lateral

前段
Anterior

内段
Medial

肝圆韧带
Round ligament of liver
(ligamentum teres hepatis)

肝门静脉：
Hepatic portal vein:

左支
Left branch

右支
Right branch

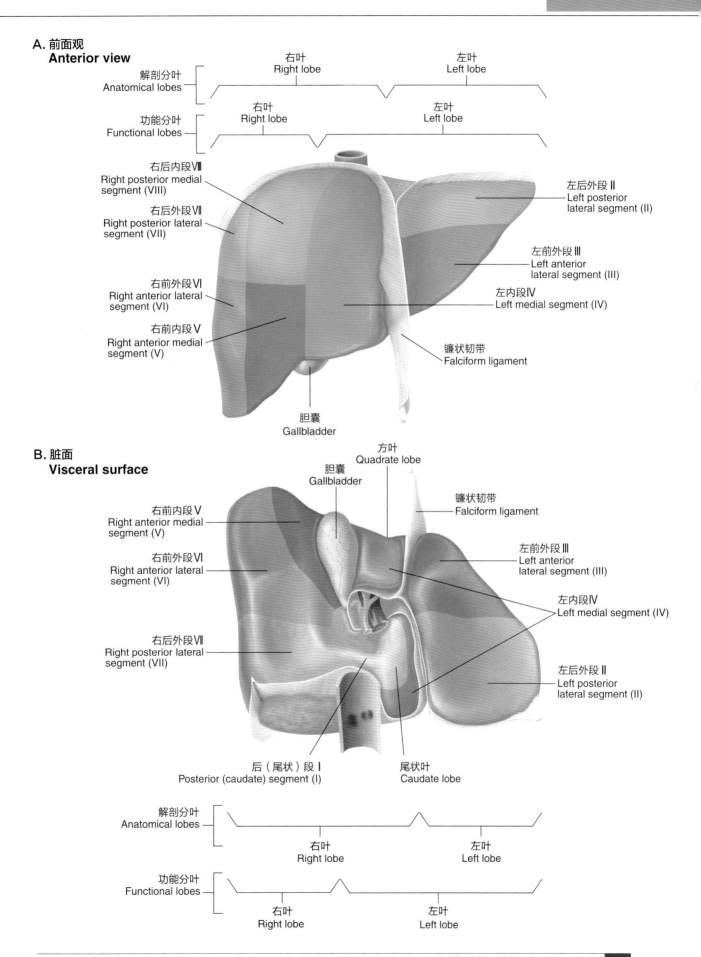

A. 前面观
Anterior view

解剖分叶
Anatomical lobes
右叶 Right lobe　左叶 Left lobe

功能分叶
Functional lobes
右叶 Right lobe　左叶 Left lobe

右后内段 VⅢ
Right posterior medial
segment (VIII)

右后外段 VⅡ
Right posterior lateral
segment (VII)

右前外段 VI
Right anterior lateral
segment (VI)

右前内段 V
Right anterior medial
segment (V)

左后外段 II
Left posterior
lateral segment (II)

左前外段 III
Left anterior
lateral segment (III)

左内段 IV
Left medial segment (IV)

镰状韧带
Falciform ligament

胆囊
Gallbladder

B. 脏面
Visceral surface

胆囊
Gallbladder

方叶
Quadrate lobe

镰状韧带
Falciform ligament

右前内段 V
Right anterior medial
segment (V)

右前外段 VI
Right anterior lateral
segment (VI)

右后外段 VⅡ
Right posterior lateral
segment (VII)

左前外段 III
Left anterior
lateral segment (III)

左内段 IV
Left medial segment (IV)

左后外段 II
Left posterior
lateral segment (II)

后（尾状）段 I
Posterior (caudate) segment (I)

尾状叶
Caudate lobe

解剖分叶
Anatomical lobes
右叶 Right lobe　左叶 Left lobe

功能分叶
Functional lobes
右叶 Right lobe　左叶 Left lobe

图 5-26　胆囊　Gallbladder

A. 定位
Orientation

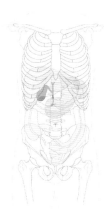

B. 解剖
Dissection

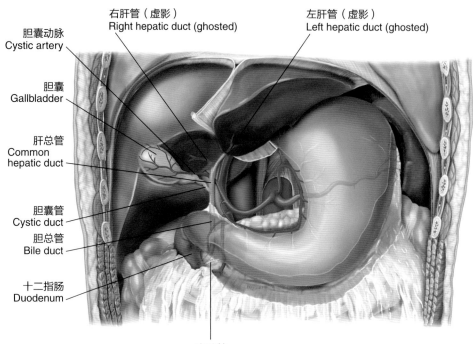

右肝管（虚影）
Right hepatic duct (ghosted)

左肝管（虚影）
Left hepatic duct (ghosted)

胆囊动脉
Cystic artery

胆囊
Gallbladder

肝总管
Common
hepatic duct

胆囊管
Cystic duct

胆总管
Bile duct

十二指肠
Duodenum

主胰管
Main pancreatic duct

C. 内面观
Internal view

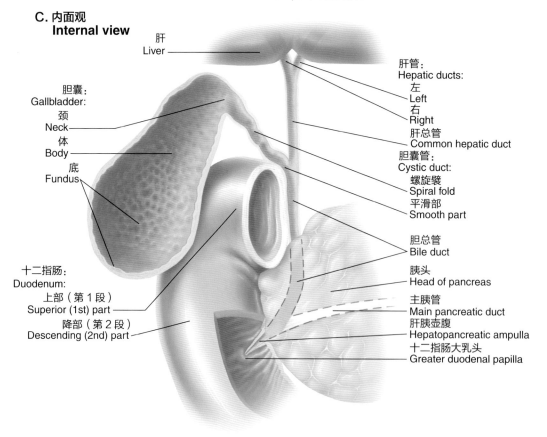

肝
Liver

肝管：
Hepatic ducts:
左
Left
右
Right
肝总管
Common hepatic duct
胆囊管：
Cystic duct:
螺旋襞
Spiral fold
平滑部
Smooth part

胆囊：
Gallbladder:
颈
Neck
体
Body
底
Fundus

胆总管
Bile duct

胰头
Head of pancreas

主胰管
Main pancreatic duct
肝胰壶腹
Hepatopancreatic ampulla
十二指肠大乳头
Greater duodenal papilla

十二指肠：
Duodenum:
上部（第 1 段）
Superior (1st) part
降部（第 2 段）
Descending (2nd) part

A. 肝动脉的变异
Variations in the hepatic arteries

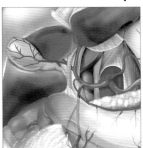 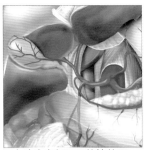 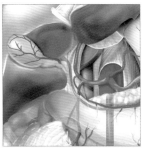 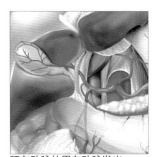

肝左、右动脉从肝固有动脉发出，肝右动脉走行于肝总管后面（64%）
Right and left hepatic arteries arising from proper hepatic artery; right hepatic artery passing posterior to common hepatic duct (64%)

肝右动脉走行于肝总管前面（24%）
Right hepatic artery passing anterior to common hepatic duct (24%)

肝右动脉从肠系膜上动脉发出（12%）
Right hepatic artery arising from superior mesenteric artery (12%)

肝左动脉从胃左动脉发出（11%）
Left hepatic artery arising from left gastric artery (11%)

B. 胆囊动脉的变异
Variations in the cystic artery

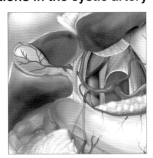 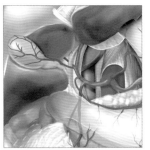 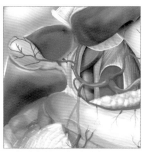

胆囊动脉从肝右动脉发出，并走行于肝总管后面（76%）
Cystic artery arising from right hepatic artery and passing posterior to common hepatic duct (76%)

胆囊动脉从肝右动脉发出，并走行于肝总管前面（13%）
Cystic artery arising from right hepatic artery and passing anterior to common hepatic duct (13%)

胆囊动脉从肝左动脉发出，并走行于肝总管前面（6%）
Cystic artery arising from left hepatic artery and passing anterior to common hepatic duct (6%)

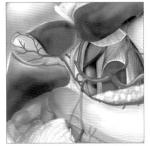 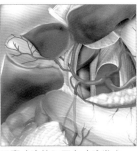

胆囊动脉从胃十二指肠动脉发出，并走行于肝总管前面（3%）
Cystic artery arising from gastroduodenal artery and passing anterior to common hepatic duct (3%)

胆囊动脉从肝固有动脉发出，并走行于肝总管前面（2%）
Cystic artery arising from proper hepatic artery and passing anterior to common hepatic duct (2%)

图 5-28　十二指肠和胰 I　Duodenum and Pancreas I

A. 定位
Orientation

B. 表面特征
Surface features

门脉三联管：
Portal triad:

肝固有动脉
Proper hepatic artery

肝门静脉
Hepatic portal vein

胆管
Bile duct

胆囊
Gallbladder

肝
Liver

右肾（透过腹膜和肾筋膜）
Right kidney (seen through peritoneum and renal fascia)

十二指肠（切断）：
Duodenum (cut):

上部（第 1 段）
Superior (1st) part

降部（第 2 段）
Descending (2nd) part

水平部（第 3 段）
Transverse (3rd) part

结肠右曲（肝曲）
Right colic (hepatic) flexure

网膜囊下凹
Inferior recess of omental bursa

大网膜：
Greater omentum:

胃结肠韧带（切断）
Gastrocolic ligament (cut)

网膜裙（切断）
Omental apron (cut)

下腔静脉和主动脉
Inferior vena cava and aorta

腹腔干
Celiac trunk

脾动脉
Splenic artery

胃（切断）
Stomach (cut)

大网膜：
Greater omentum:

胃结肠韧带（切断）
Gastrosplenic ligament (cut)

脾
Spleen

胰：
Pancreas:

头 Head
颈 Neck
体 Body
尾 Tail

结肠左曲（脾曲）
Left colic (splenic) flexure

横结肠系膜（切断）
Transverse mesocolon (cut)

左肾（透过腹膜和肾筋膜）
Left kidney (seen through peritoneum and renal fascia)

大网膜：
Greater omentum:

胃结肠韧带（切断）
Gastrocolic ligament (cut)

网膜裙（切断）
Omental apron (cut)

十二指肠空肠曲
Duodenojejunal junction

十二指肠升部（第 4 段）
Ascending (4th) part of duodenum

钩突
Uncinate process

横结肠（切断）
Transverse colon (cut)

肠系膜上动脉和静脉（切断）
Superior mesenteric vein and artery (cut)

C. 解剖
Dissection

幽门括约肌
Pyloric sphincter

幽门管
Pyloric canal

十二指肠上部（十二指肠球）（第 1 段）
Superior (1st) part of duodenum (duodenal cap or bulb)

十二指肠降部（第 2 段）
Descending (2nd) part of duodenum

十二指肠小乳头（副胰管开口处）
Lesser duodenal papilla (accessory pancreatic duct)

十二指肠大乳头
Greater duodenal papilla

胆总管和主胰管
Bile duct and main pancreatic duct

环状襞
Circular folds

十二指肠水平部（第 3 段）
Transverse (3rd) part of duodenum

十二指肠悬肌
Suspensory muscle of duodenum

十二指肠空肠曲
Duodenojejunal flexure

横结肠系膜（切断）
Transverse mesocolon (cut)

空肠
Jejunum

十二指肠升部（第 4 段）
Ascending (4th) part of duodenum

肠系膜上动脉和静脉（切断）
Superior mesenteric vein and artery (cut)

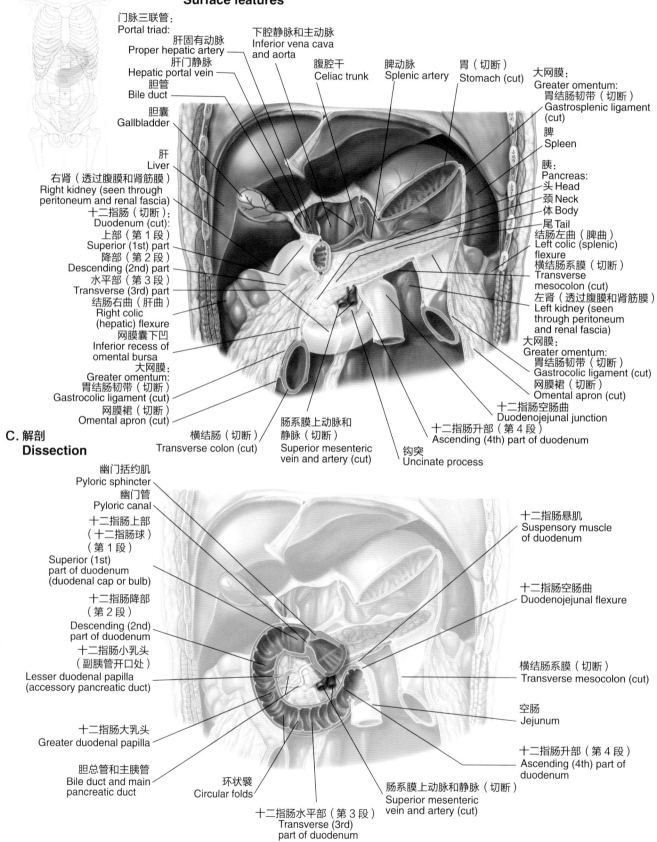

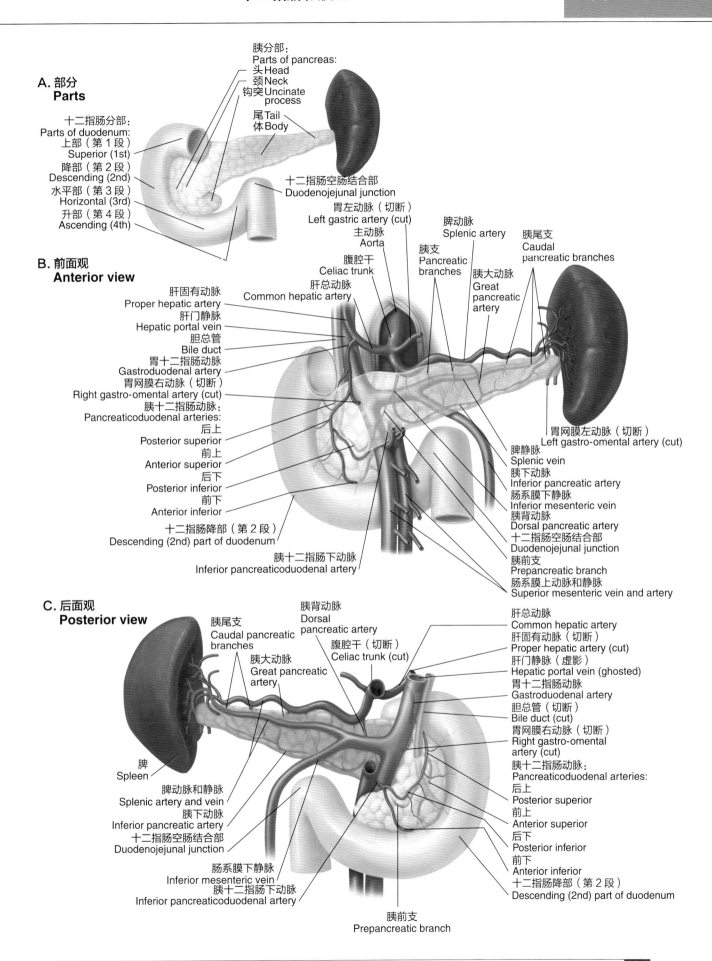

A. 部分
Parts

胰分部：
Parts of pancreas:
头 Head
颈 Neck
钩突 Uncinate process
尾 Tail
体 Body

十二指肠分部：
Parts of duodenum:
上部（第 1 段）
Superior (1st)
降部（第 2 段）
Descending (2nd)
水平部（第 3 段）
Horizontal (3rd)
升部（第 4 段）
Ascending (4th)

十二指肠空肠结合部
Duodenojejunal junction

B. 前面观
Anterior view

胃左动脉（切断）
Left gastric artery (cut)
主动脉
Aorta
腹腔干
Celiac trunk
肝总动脉
Common hepatic artery
胰支
Pancreatic branches
脾动脉
Splenic artery
胰尾支
Caudal pancreatic branches
胰大动脉
Great pancreatic artery

肝固有动脉
Proper hepatic artery
肝门静脉
Hepatic portal vein
胆总管
Bile duct
胃十二指肠动脉
Gastroduodenal artery
胃网膜右动脉（切断）
Right gastro-omental artery (cut)
胰十二指肠动脉：
Pancreaticoduodenal arteries:
后上
Posterior superior
前上
Anterior superior
后下
Posterior inferior
前下
Anterior inferior
十二指肠降部（第 2 段）
Descending (2nd) part of duodenum
胰十二指肠下动脉
Inferior pancreaticoduodenal artery

胃网膜左动脉（切断）
Left gastro-omental artery (cut)
脾静脉
Splenic vein
胰下动脉
Inferior pancreatic artery
肠系膜下静脉
Inferior mesenteric vein
胰背动脉
Dorsal pancreatic artery
十二指肠空肠结合部
Duodenojejunal junction
胰前支
Prepancreatic branch
肠系膜上动脉和静脉
Superior mesenteric vein and artery

C. 后面观
Posterior view

胰背动脉
Dorsal pancreatic artery
腹腔干（切断）
Celiac trunk (cut)
胰尾支
Caudal pancreatic branches
胰大动脉
Great pancreatic artery

肝总动脉
Common hepatic artery
肝固有动脉（切断）
Proper hepatic artery (cut)
肝门静脉（虚影）
Hepatic portal vein (ghosted)
胃十二指肠动脉
Gastroduodenal artery
胆总管（切断）
Bile duct (cut)
胃网膜右动脉（切断）
Right gastro-omental artery (cut)
胰十二指肠动脉：
Pancreaticoduodenal arteries:
后上
Posterior superior
前上
Anterior superior
后下
Posterior inferior
前下
Anterior inferior
十二指肠降部（第 2 段）
Descending (2nd) part of duodenum

脾
Spleen
脾动脉和静脉
Splenic artery and vein
胰下动脉
Inferior pancreatic artery
十二指肠空肠结合部
Duodenojejunal junction
肠系膜下静脉
Inferior mesenteric vein
胰十二指肠下动脉
Inferior pancreaticoduodenal artery

胰前支
Prepancreatic branch

图 5-30　肝门静脉　Hepatic Portal Vein

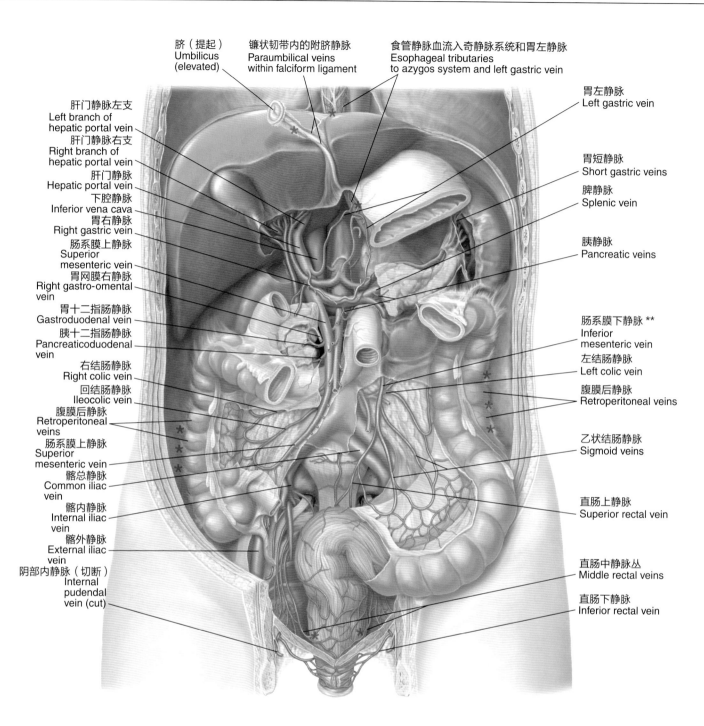

脐（提起）
Umbilicus
(elevated)

镰状韧带内的附脐静脉
Paraumbilical veins
within falciform ligament

食管静脉血流入奇静脉系统和胃左静脉
Esophageal tributaries
to azygos system and left gastric vein

胃左静脉
Left gastric vein

肝门静脉左支
Left branch of
hepatic portal vein

肝门静脉右支
Right branch of
hepatic portal vein

肝门静脉
Hepatic portal vein

下腔静脉
Inferior vena cava

胃右静脉
Right gastric vein

肠系膜上静脉
Superior
mesenteric vein

胃网膜右静脉
Right gastro-omental
vein

胃十二指肠静脉
Gastroduodenal vein

胰十二指肠静脉
Pancreaticoduodenal
vein

右结肠静脉
Right colic vein

回结肠静脉
Ileocolic vein

腹膜后静脉
Retroperitoneal
veins

肠系膜上静脉
Superior
mesenteric vein

髂总静脉
Common iliac
vein

髂内静脉
Internal iliac
vein

髂外静脉
External iliac
vein

阴部内静脉（切断）
Internal
pudendal
vein (cut)

胃短静脉
Short gastric veins

脾静脉
Splenic vein

胰静脉
Pancreatic veins

肠系膜下静脉 **
Inferior
mesenteric vein

左结肠静脉
Left colic vein

腹膜后静脉
Retroperitoneal veins

乙状结肠静脉
Sigmoid veins

直肠上静脉
Superior rectal vein

直肠中静脉丛
Middle rectal veins

直肠下静脉
Inferior rectal vein

✱ 表示门脉高压时门－腔侧支吻合的部位：
Denotes sites of portal-caval anastomosis in cases of portal hypertension:
1. 胃左静脉的食管支与奇静脉食管支之间的交通
Esophageal tributaries of left gastric vein to esophageal tributaries of azygos system of veins
2. 直肠上静脉和直肠中、下静脉之间的交通
Superior rectal vein to middle and inferior rectal veins
3. 肝门静脉左支的脐周静脉和体前壁浅静脉之间的交通
Paraumbilical tributaries of left hepatic portal vein to superficial veins of anterior body wall
4. 腹膜后静脉与体后壁静脉之间的交通
Retroperitoneal veins to veins of posterior body wall

** 肠系膜下静脉可以汇入脾静脉（34%）、肠系膜上静脉（33%）或者脾静脉和肠系膜上静脉交接处（32%）
Inferior mesenteric vein can join the splenic vein (34%), the superior mesenteric vein (33%),
or the junction of the splenic and superior mesenteric veins (32%)

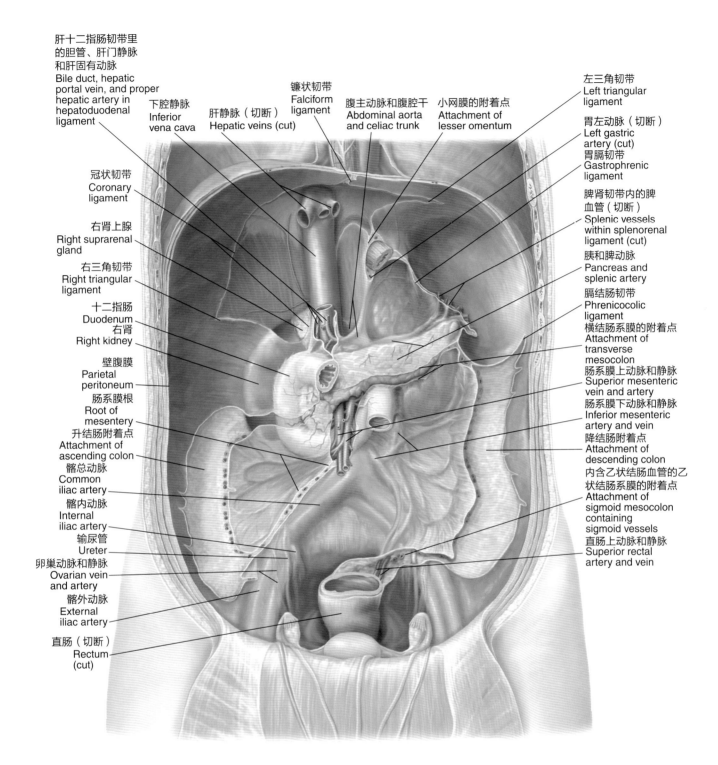

肝十二指肠韧带里的胆管、肝门静脉和肝固有动脉
Bile duct, hepatic portal vein, and proper hepatic artery in hepatoduodenal ligament

下腔静脉
Inferior vena cava

肝静脉（切断）
Hepatic veins (cut)

镰状韧带
Falciform ligament

腹主动脉和腹腔干
Abdominal aorta and celiac trunk

小网膜的附着点
Attachment of lesser omentum

左三角韧带
Left triangular ligament

胃左动脉（切断）
Left gastric artery (cut)

胃膈韧带
Gastrophrenic ligament

脾肾韧带内的脾血管（切断）
Splenic vessels within splenorenal ligament (cut)

胰和脾动脉
Pancreas and splenic artery

膈结肠韧带
Phrenicocolic ligament

横结肠系膜的附着点
Attachment of transverse mesocolon

肠系膜上动脉和静脉
Superior mesenteric vein and artery

肠系膜下动脉和静脉
Inferior mesenteric artery and vein

降结肠附着点
Attachment of descending colon

内含乙状结肠血管的乙状结肠系膜的附着点
Attachment of sigmoid mesocolon containing sigmoid vessels

直肠上动脉和静脉
Superior rectal artery and vein

冠状韧带
Coronary ligament

右肾上腺
Right suprarenal gland

右三角韧带
Right triangular ligament

十二指肠
Duodenum

右肾
Right kidney

壁腹膜
Parietal peritoneum

肠系膜根
Root of mesentery

升结肠附着点
Attachment of ascending colon

髂总动脉
Common iliac artery

髂内动脉
Internal iliac artery

输尿管
Ureter

卵巢动脉和静脉
Ovarian vein and artery

髂外动脉
External iliac artery

直肠（切断）
Rectum (cut)

图 5-32　**肾和腹膜后隙　Kidneys and Retroperitoneum**

A. 定位
Orientation

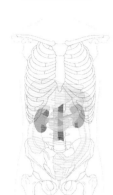

B. 前面观
Anterior view

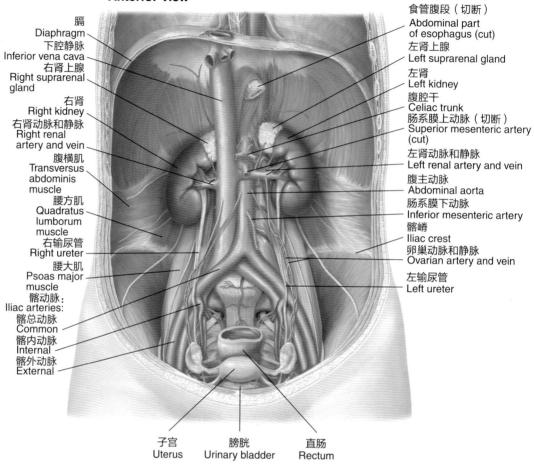

膈
Diaphragm
下腔静脉
Inferior vena cava
右肾上腺
Right suprarenal gland
右肾
Right kidney
右肾动脉和静脉
Right renal artery and vein
腹横肌
Transversus abdominis muscle
腰方肌
Quadratus lumborum muscle
右输尿管
Right ureter
腰大肌
Psoas major muscle
髂动脉：
Iliac arteries:
髂总动脉
Common
髂内动脉
Internal
髂外动脉
External

食管腹段（切断）
Abdominal part of esophagus (cut)
左肾上腺
Left suprarenal gland
左肾
Left kidney
腹腔干
Celiac trunk
肠系膜上动脉（切断）
Superior mesenteric artery (cut)
左肾动脉和静脉
Left renal artery and vein
腹主动脉
Abdominal aorta
肠系膜下动脉
Inferior mesenteric artery
髂嵴
Iliac crest
卵巢动脉和静脉
Ovarian artery and vein
左输尿管
Left ureter

子宫
Uterus
膀胱
Urinary bladder
直肠
Rectum

C. 后面观
Posterior view

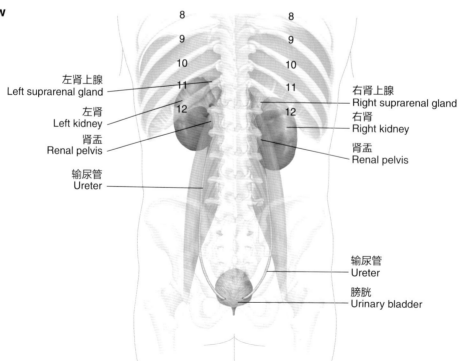

8　8
9　9
10　10
11　11
12　12

左肾上腺
Left suprarenal gland
左肾
Left kidney
肾盂
Renal pelvis
输尿管
Ureter

右肾上腺
Right suprarenal gland
右肾
Right kidney
肾盂
Renal pelvis

输尿管
Ureter
膀胱
Urinary bladder

B. 经 L2 椎体水平的横断面
Cross section through the L2 vertebra

A. 定位
Orientation

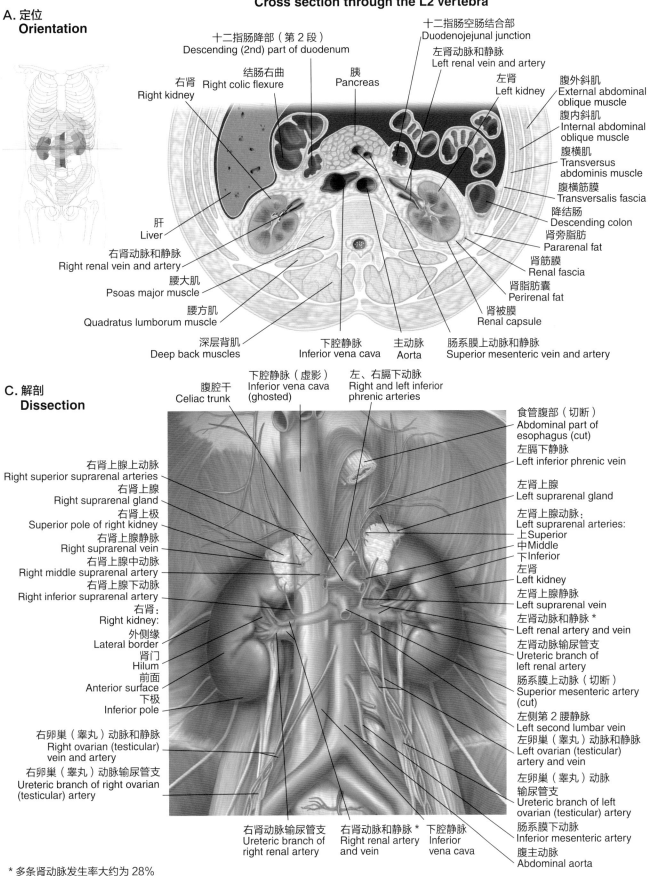

十二指肠降部（第 2 段）
Descending (2nd) part of duodenum

结肠右曲 Right colic flexure

胰 Pancreas

十二指肠空肠结合部
Duodenojejunal junction

左肾动脉和静脉
Left renal vein and artery

左肾 Left kidney

右肾 Right kidney

腹外斜肌 External abdominal oblique muscle

腹内斜肌 Internal abdominal oblique muscle

腹横肌 Transversus abdominis muscle

腹横筋膜 Transversalis fascia

降结肠 Descending colon

肾旁脂肪 Pararenal fat

肾筋膜 Renal fascia

肾脂肪囊 Perirenal fat

肾被膜 Renal capsule

肝 Liver

右肾动脉和静脉 Right renal vein and artery

腰大肌 Psoas major muscle

腰方肌 Quadratus lumborum muscle

深层背肌 Deep back muscles

下腔静脉 Inferior vena cava

主动脉 Aorta

肠系膜上动脉和静脉 Superior mesenteric vein and artery

C. 解剖
Dissection

腹腔干 Celiac trunk

下腔静脉（虚影）Inferior vena cava (ghosted)

左、右膈下动脉 Right and left inferior phrenic arteries

食管腹部（切断）Abdominal part of esophagus (cut)

左膈下静脉 Left inferior phrenic vein

右肾上腺上动脉 Right superior suprarenal arteries

右肾上腺 Right suprarenal gland

右肾上极 Superior pole of right kidney

右肾上腺静脉 Right suprarenal vein

右肾上腺中动脉 Right middle suprarenal artery

右肾上腺下动脉 Right inferior suprarenal artery

右肾：Right kidney:

外侧缘 Lateral border

肾门 Hilum

前面 Anterior surface

下极 Inferior pole

右卵巢（睾丸）动脉和静脉 Right ovarian (testicular) vein and artery

右卵巢（睾丸）动脉输尿管支 Ureteric branch of right ovarian (testicular) artery

左肾上腺 Left suprarenal gland

左肾上腺动脉：Left suprarenal arteries:
上 Superior
中 Middle
下 Inferior

左肾 Left kidney

左肾上腺静脉 Left suprarenal vein

左肾动脉和静脉 * Left renal artery and vein

左肾动脉输尿管支 Ureteric branch of left renal artery

肠系膜上动脉（切断）Superior mesenteric artery (cut)

左侧第 2 腰静脉 Left second lumbar vein

左卵巢（睾丸）动脉和静脉 Left ovarian (testicular) artery and vein

左卵巢（睾丸）动脉输尿管支 Ureteric branch of left ovarian (testicular) artery

肠系膜下动脉 Inferior mesenteric artery

腹主动脉 Abdominal aorta

右肾动脉输尿管支 Ureteric branch of right renal artery

右肾动脉和静脉 * Right renal artery and vein

下腔静脉 Inferior vena cava

* 多条肾动脉发生率大约为 28%
Supernumerary renal arteries occur in approximately 28% of cases

图 5-34　　**肾和肾上腺，内部结构　Kidney and Suprarenal Gland, Internal Features**

A. 动脉
Arteries

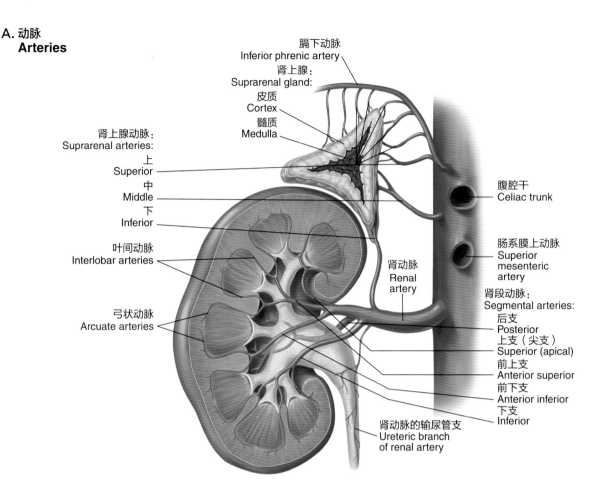

膈下动脉
Inferior phrenic artery

肾上腺：
Suprarenal gland:

皮质
Cortex

髓质
Medulla

肾上腺动脉：
Suprarenal arteries:

上
Superior

中
Middle

下
Inferior

叶间动脉
Interlobar arteries

弓状动脉
Arcuate arteries

腹腔干
Celiac trunk

肠系膜上动脉
Superior mesenteric artery

肾动脉
Renal artery

肾段动脉：
Segmental arteries:

后支
Posterior

上支（尖支）
Superior (apical)

前上支
Anterior superior

前下支
Anterior inferior

下支
Inferior

肾动脉的输尿管支
Ureteric branch of renal artery

B. 肾收集系统
Renal collecting system

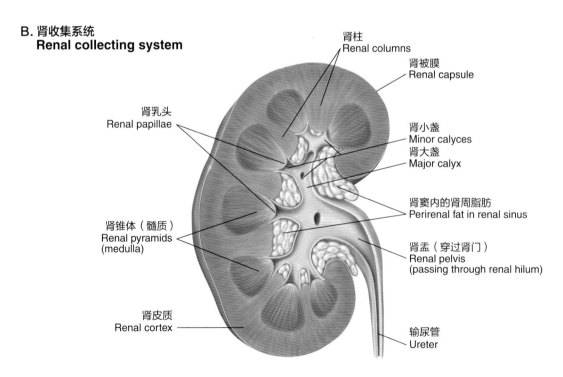

肾柱
Renal columns

肾被膜
Renal capsule

肾乳头
Renal papillae

肾小盏
Minor calyces

肾大盏
Major calyx

肾窦内的肾周脂肪
Perirenal fat in renal sinus

肾锥体（髓质）
Renal pyramids (medulla)

肾盂（穿过肾门）
Renal pelvis (passing through renal hilum)

肾皮质
Renal cortex

输尿管
Ureter

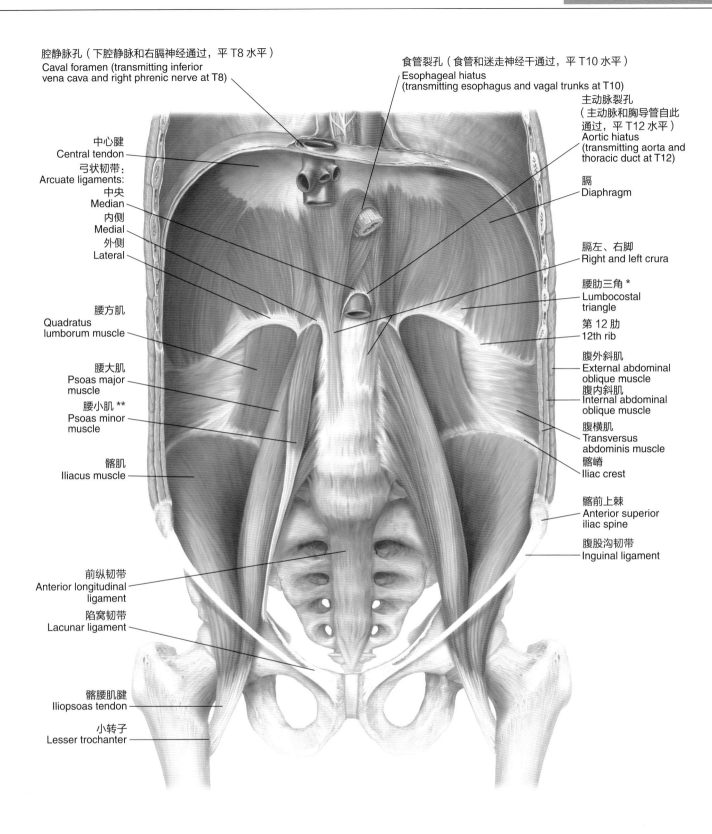

腔静脉孔（下腔静脉和右膈神经通过，平 T8 水平）
Caval foramen (transmitting inferior
vena cava and right phrenic nerve at T8)

食管裂孔（食管和迷走神经干通过，平 T10 水平）
Esophageal hiatus
(transmitting esophagus and vagal trunks at T10)

主动脉裂孔
（主动脉和胸导管自此
通过，平 T12 水平）
Aortic hiatus
(transmitting aorta and
thoracic duct at T12)

膈
Diaphragm

中心腱
Central tendon

弓状韧带：
Arcuate ligaments:
中央
Median
内侧
Medial
外侧
Lateral

膈左、右脚
Right and left crura

腰肋三角 *
Lumbocostal
triangle

第 12 肋
12th rib

腰方肌
Quadratus
lumborum muscle

腹外斜肌
External abdominal
oblique muscle
腹内斜肌
Internal abdominal
oblique muscle

腰大肌
Psoas major
muscle

腰小肌 **
Psoas minor
muscle

腹横肌
Transversus
abdominis muscle
髂嵴
Iliac crest

髂肌
Iliacus muscle

髂前上棘
Anterior superior
iliac spine

腹股沟韧带
Inguinal ligament

前纵韧带
Anterior longitudinal
ligament

陷窝韧带
Lacunar ligament

髂腰肌腱
Iliopsoas tendon

小转子
Lesser trochanter

* 腰肋三角出现的概率约为 80%
Lumbocostal triangle is present in 80% of cases

** 腰小肌出现的概率约为 50%
Psoas minor muscle is present in 50% of cases

图 5-36　腹后壁的血管　Vessels of the Posterior Abdominal Wall

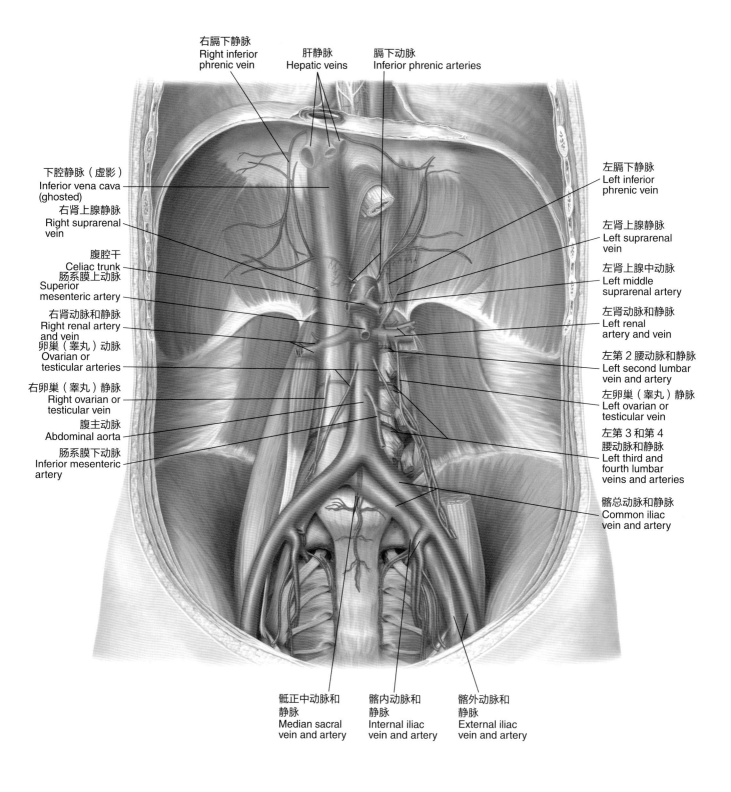

右膈下静脉
Right inferior
phrenic vein

肝静脉
Hepatic veins

膈下动脉
Inferior phrenic arteries

下腔静脉（虚影）
Inferior vena cava
(ghosted)

右肾上腺静脉
Right suprarenal
vein

腹腔干
Celiac trunk
肠系膜上动脉
Superior
mesenteric artery

右肾动脉和静脉
Right renal artery
and vein

卵巢（睾丸）动脉
Ovarian or
testicular arteries

右卵巢（睾丸）静脉
Right ovarian or
testicular vein

腹主动脉
Abdominal aorta

肠系膜下动脉
Inferior mesenteric
artery

左膈下静脉
Left inferior
phrenic vein

左肾上腺静脉
Left suprarenal
vein

左肾上腺中动脉
Left middle
suprarenal artery

左肾动脉和静脉
Left renal
artery and vein

左第 2 腰动脉和静脉
Left second lumbar
vein and artery

左卵巢（睾丸）静脉
Left ovarian or
testicular vein

左第 3 和第 4
腰动脉和静脉
Left third and
fourth lumbar
veins and arteries

髂总动脉和静脉
Common iliac
vein and artery

骶正中动脉和
静脉
Median sacral
vein and artery

髂内动脉和
静脉
Internal iliac
vein and artery

髂外动脉和
静脉
External iliac
vein and artery

A. 浅层解剖
Superficial dissection

肝的膈面淋巴主要汇入膈淋巴结
Diaphragmatic surface of liver drains primarily to phrenic nodes

腹腔淋巴结
Celiac nodes

贲门旁淋巴结
Paracardial nodes

胃左淋巴结
Left gastric nodes

胃（虚影）
Stomach (ghosted)

胰脾淋巴结
Pancreaticosplenic nodes

胆囊淋巴结
Cystic node

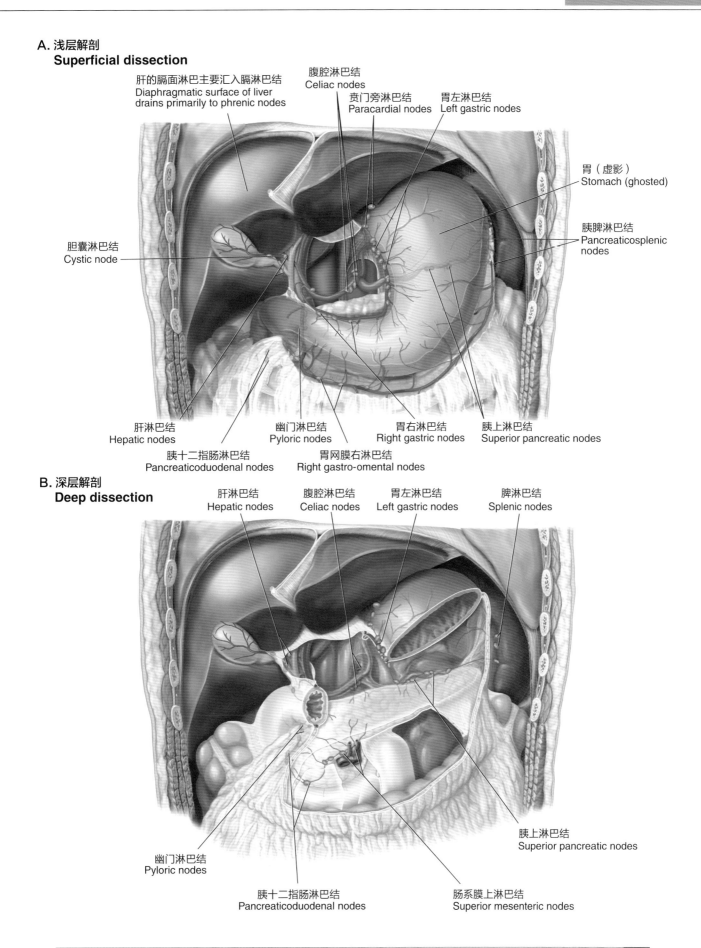

肝淋巴结
Hepatic nodes

幽门淋巴结
Pyloric nodes

胃右淋巴结
Right gastric nodes

胰上淋巴结
Superior pancreatic nodes

胰十二指肠淋巴结
Pancreaticoduodenal nodes

胃网膜右淋巴结
Right gastro-omental nodes

B. 深层解剖
Deep dissection

肝淋巴结
Hepatic nodes

腹腔淋巴结
Celiac nodes

胃左淋巴结
Left gastric nodes

脾淋巴结
Splenic nodes

胰上淋巴结
Superior pancreatic nodes

幽门淋巴结
Pyloric nodes

胰十二指肠淋巴结
Pancreaticoduodenal nodes

肠系膜上淋巴结
Superior mesenteric nodes

A. 小肠、盲肠、升结肠和横结肠
Small intestine, cecum, ascending colon, and transverse colon

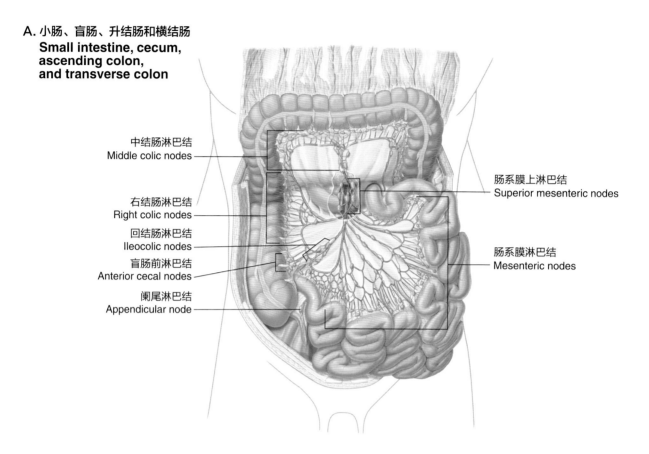

中结肠淋巴结
Middle colic nodes

右结肠淋巴结
Right colic nodes

回结肠淋巴结
Ileocolic nodes

盲肠前淋巴结
Anterior cecal nodes

阑尾淋巴结
Appendicular node

肠系膜上淋巴结
Superior mesenteric nodes

肠系膜淋巴结
Mesenteric nodes

B. 降结肠、乙状结肠和直肠
Descending colon, sigmoid colon, and rectum

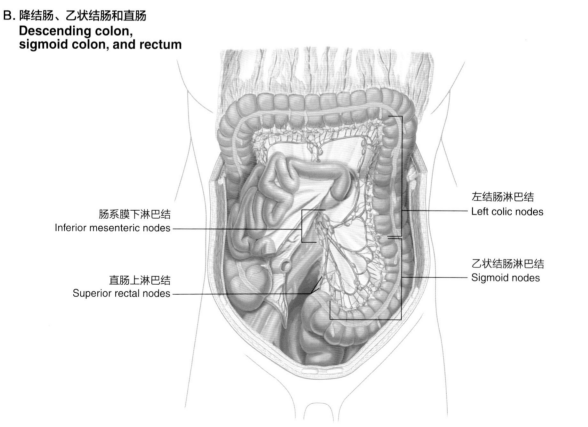

肠系膜下淋巴结
Inferior mesenteric nodes

直肠上淋巴结
Superior rectal nodes

左结肠淋巴结
Left colic nodes

乙状结肠淋巴结
Sigmoid nodes

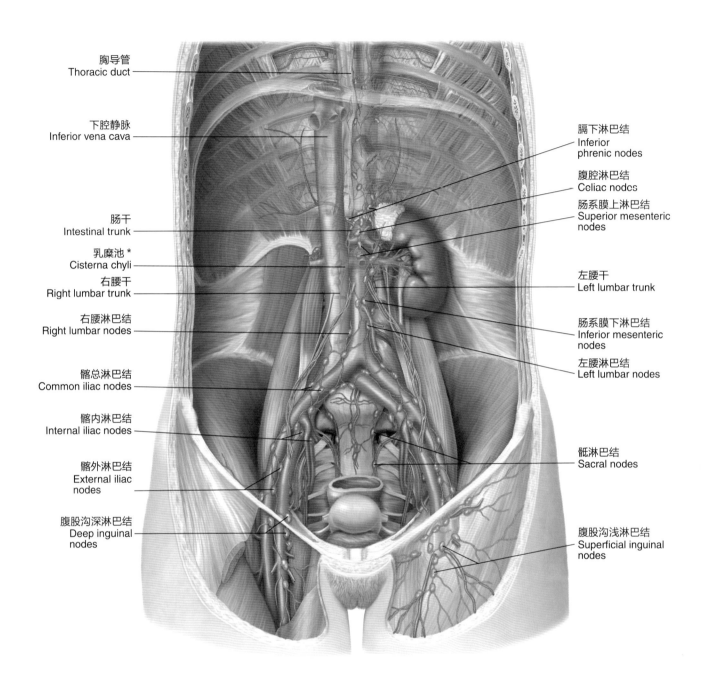

胸导管
Thoracic duct

下腔静脉
Inferior vena cava

肠干
Intestinal trunk

乳糜池 *
Cisterna chyli

右腰干
Right lumbar trunk

右腰淋巴结
Right lumbar nodes

髂总淋巴结
Common iliac nodes

髂内淋巴结
Internal iliac nodes

髂外淋巴结
External iliac nodes

腹股沟深淋巴结
Deep inguinal nodes

膈下淋巴结
Inferior phrenic nodes

腹腔淋巴结
Celiac nodes

肠系膜上淋巴结
Superior mesenteric nodes

左腰干
Left lumbar trunk

肠系膜下淋巴结
Inferior mesenteric nodes

左腰淋巴结
Left lumbar nodes

骶淋巴结
Sacral nodes

腹股沟浅淋巴结
Superficial inguinal nodes

* 乳糜池出现的概率为 25%
Cisterna chyli is present in approximately 25% of cases

图 5-40　　腹后壁的神经　Nerves of the Posterior Abdominal Wall

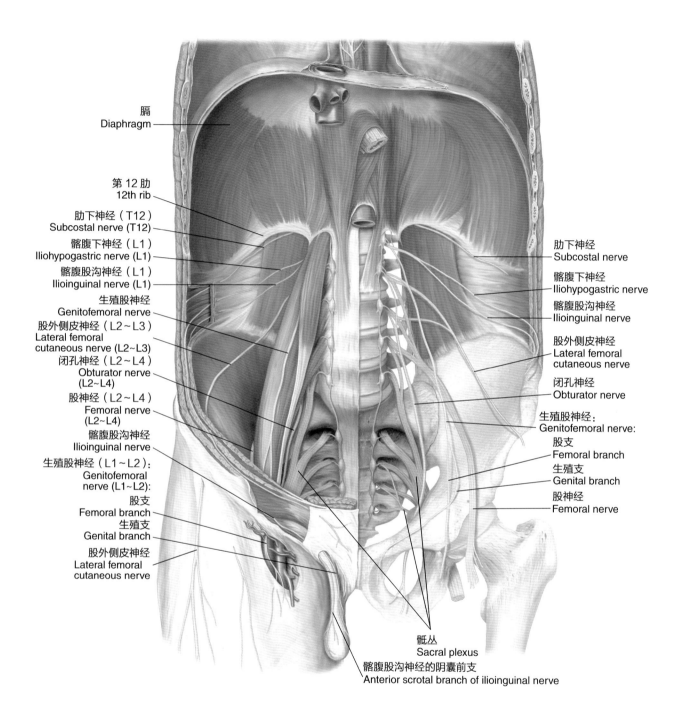

膈
Diaphragm

第 12 肋
12th rib

肋下神经（T12）
Subcostal nerve (T12)

髂腹下神经（L1）
Iliohypogastric nerve (L1)

髂腹股沟神经（L1）
Ilioinguinal nerve (L1)

生殖股神经
Genitofemoral nerve

股外侧皮神经（L2~L3）
Lateral femoral
cutaneous nerve (L2~L3)

闭孔神经（L2~L4）
Obturator nerve
(L2~L4)

股神经（L2~L4）
Femoral nerve
(L2~L4)

髂腹股沟神经
Ilioinguinal nerve

生殖股神经（L1~L2）：
Genitofemoral
nerve (L1~L2):

股支
Femoral branch
生殖支
Genital branch

股外侧皮神经
Lateral femoral
cutaneous nerve

肋下神经
Subcostal nerve

髂腹下神经
Iliohypogastric nerve

髂腹股沟神经
Ilioinguinal nerve

股外侧皮神经
Lateral femoral
cutaneous nerve

闭孔神经
Obturator nerve

生殖股神经：
Genitofemoral nerve:

股支
Femoral branch
生殖支
Genital branch
股神经
Femoral nerve

骶丛
Sacral plexus
髂腹股沟神经的阴囊前支
Anterior scrotal branch of ilioinguinal nerve

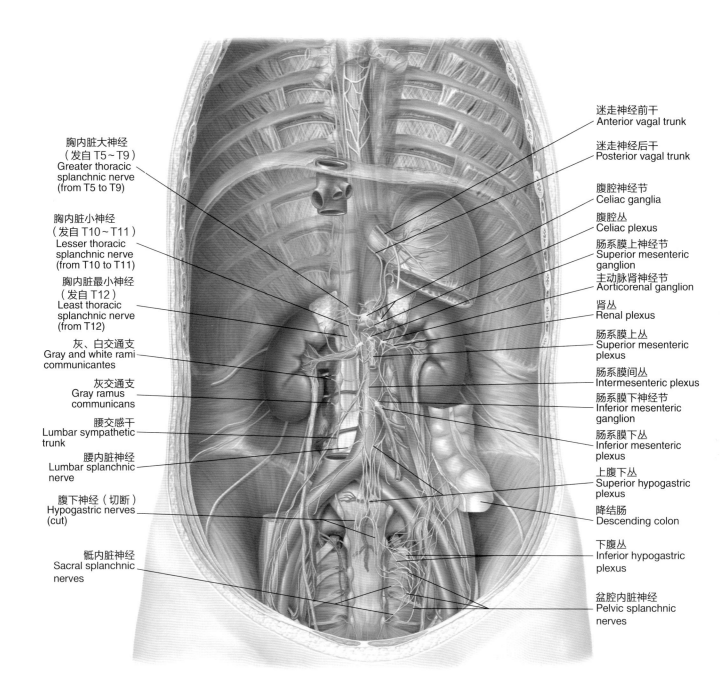

胸内脏大神经
（发自 T5～T9）
Greater thoracic
splanchnic nerve
(from T5 to T9)

胸内脏小神经
（发自 T10～T11）
Lesser thoracic
splanchnic nerve
(from T10 to T11)

胸内脏最小神经
（发自 T12）
Least thoracic
splanchnic nerve
(from T12)

灰、白交通支
Gray and white rami
communicantes

灰交通支
Gray ramus
communicans

腰交感干
Lumbar sympathetic
trunk

腰内脏神经
Lumbar splanchnic
nerve

腹下神经（切断）
Hypogastric nerves
(cut)

骶内脏神经
Sacral splanchnic
nerves

迷走神经前干
Anterior vagal trunk

迷走神经后干
Posterior vagal trunk

腹腔神经节
Celiac ganglia

腹腔丛
Celiac plexus

肠系膜上神经节
Superior mesenteric
ganglion

主动脉肾神经节
Aorticorenal ganglion

肾丛
Renal plexus

肠系膜上丛
Superior mesenteric
plexus

肠系膜间丛
Intermesenteric plexus

肠系膜下神经节
Inferior mesenteric
ganglion

肠系膜下丛
Inferior mesenteric
plexus

上腹下丛
Superior hypogastric
plexus

降结肠
Descending colon

下腹丛
Inferior hypogastric
plexus

盆腔内脏神经
Pelvic splanchnic
nerves

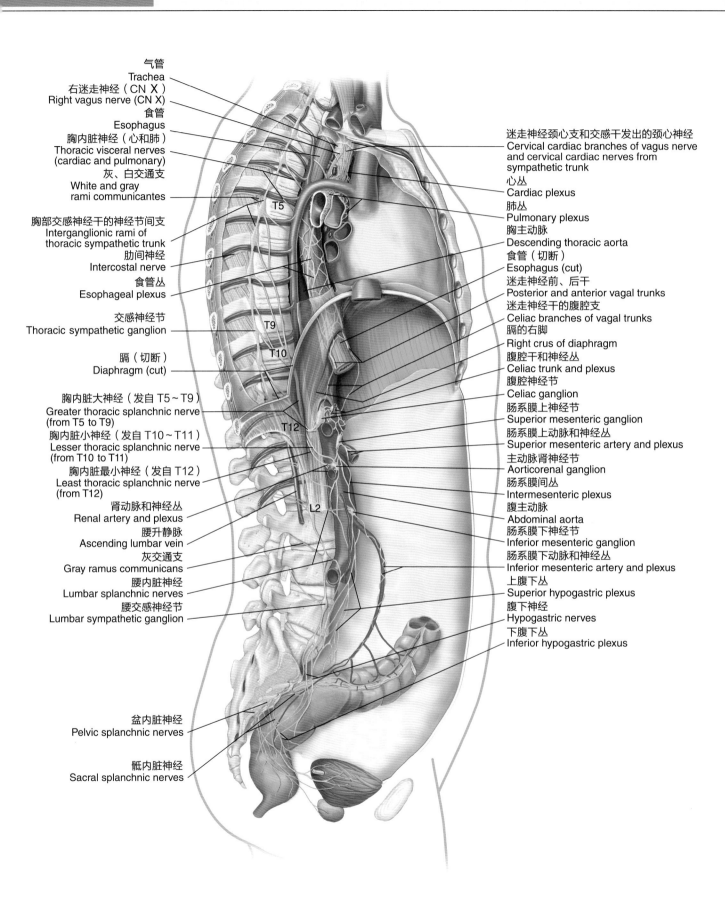

气管
Trachea
右迷走神经（CN X）
Right vagus nerve (CN X)
食管
Esophagus
胸内脏神经（心和肺）
Thoracic visceral nerves
(cardiac and pulmonary)
灰、白交通支
White and gray
rami communicantes

胸部交感神经干的神经节间支
Interganglionic rami of
thoracic sympathetic trunk
肋间神经
Intercostal nerve
食管丛
Esophageal plexus

交感神经节
Thoracic sympathetic ganglion

膈（切断）
Diaphragm (cut)

胸内脏大神经（发自 T5～T9）
Greater thoracic splanchnic nerve
(from T5 to T9)
胸内脏小神经（发自 T10～T11）
Lesser thoracic splanchnic nerve
(from T10 to T11)
胸内脏最小神经（发自 T12）
Least thoracic splanchnic nerve
(from T12)
肾动脉和神经丛
Renal artery and plexus
腰升静脉
Ascending lumbar vein
灰交通支
Gray ramus communicans
腰内脏神经
Lumbar splanchnic nerves
腰交感神经节
Lumbar sympathetic ganglion

盆内脏神经
Pelvic splanchnic nerves

骶内脏神经
Sacral splanchnic nerves

迷走神经颈心支和交感干发出的颈心神经
Cervical cardiac branches of vagus nerve
and cervical cardiac nerves from
sympathetic trunk
心丛
Cardiac plexus
肺丛
Pulmonary plexus
胸主动脉
Descending thoracic aorta
食管（切断）
Esophagus (cut)
迷走神经前、后干
Posterior and anterior vagal trunks
迷走神经干的腹腔支
Celiac branches of vagal trunks
膈的右脚
Right crus of diaphragm
腹腔干和神经丛
Celiac trunk and plexus
腹腔神经节
Celiac ganglion
肠系膜上神经节
Superior mesenteric ganglion
肠系膜上动脉和神经丛
Superior mesenteric artery and plexus
主动脉肾神经节
Aorticorenal ganglion
肠系膜间丛
Intermesenteric plexus
腹主动脉
Abdominal aorta
肠系膜下神经节
Inferior mesenteric ganglion
肠系膜下动脉和神经丛
Inferior mesenteric artery and plexus
上腹下丛
Superior hypogastric plexus
腹下神经
Hypogastric nerves
下腹下丛
Inferior hypogastric plexus

T5
T9
T10
T12
L2

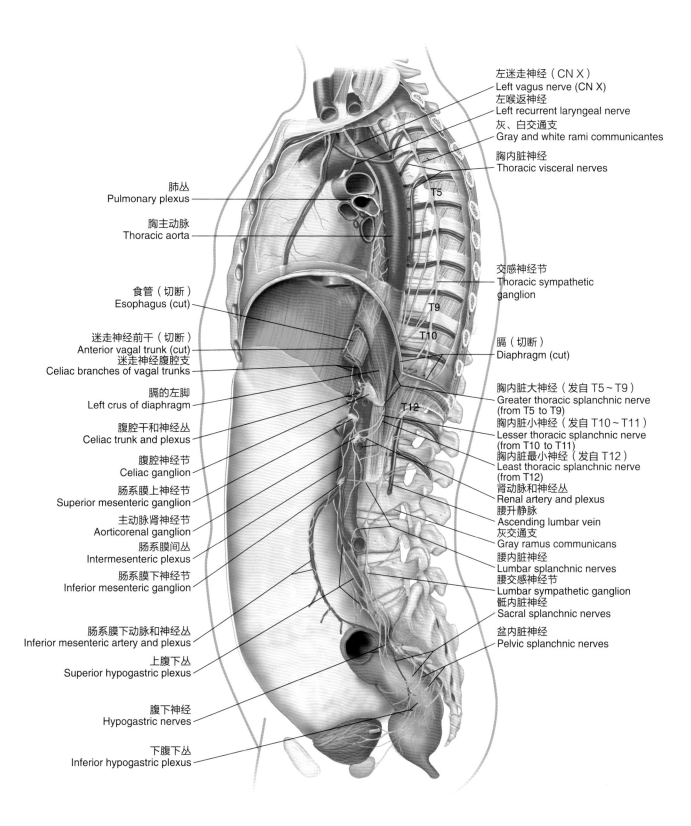

左迷走神经（CN X）
Left vagus nerve (CN X)
左喉返神经
Left recurrent laryngeal nerve
灰、白交通支
Gray and white rami communicantes
胸内脏神经
Thoracic visceral nerves

肺丛
Pulmonary plexus

胸主动脉
Thoracic aorta

T5

交感神经节
Thoracic sympathetic ganglion

食管（切断）
Esophagus (cut)

T9

T10

迷走神经前干（切断）
Anterior vagal trunk (cut)
迷走神经腹腔支
Celiac branches of vagal trunks

膈（切断）
Diaphragm (cut)

膈的左脚
Left crus of diaphragm

胸内脏大神经（发自 T5~T9）
Greater thoracic splanchnic nerve (from T5 to T9)
胸内脏小神经（发自 T10~T11）
Lesser thoracic splanchnic nerve (from T10 to T11)
胸内脏最小神经（发自 T12）
Least thoracic splanchnic nerve (from T12)

腹腔干和神经丛
Celiac trunk and plexus

T12

腹腔神经节
Celiac ganglion

肠系膜上神经节
Superior mesenteric ganglion

肾动脉和神经丛
Renal artery and plexus
腰升静脉
Ascending lumbar vein
灰交通支
Gray ramus communicans
腰内脏神经
Lumbar splanchnic nerves
腰交感神经节
Lumbar sympathetic ganglion
骶内脏神经
Sacral splanchnic nerves

主动脉肾神经节
Aorticorenal ganglion

肠系膜间丛
Intermesenteric plexus

肠系膜下神经节
Inferior mesenteric ganglion

肠系膜下动脉和神经丛
Inferior mesenteric artery and plexus

盆内脏神经
Pelvic splanchnic nerves

上腹下丛
Superior hypogastric plexus

腹下神经
Hypogastric nerves

下腹下丛
Inferior hypogastric plexus

A. T10 椎体水平
T10 vertebral level

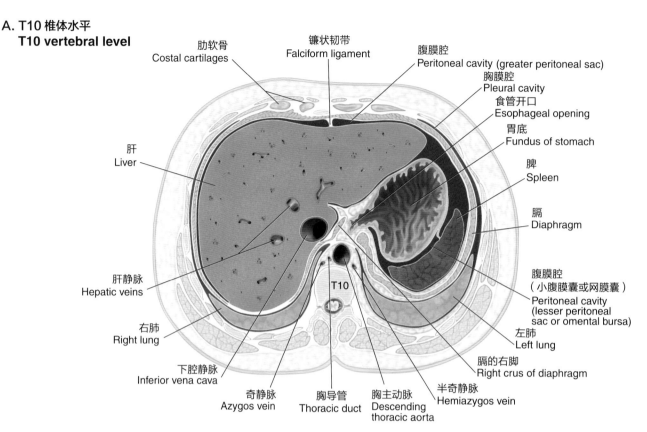

肋软骨
Costal cartilages

镰状韧带
Falciform ligament

腹膜腔
Peritoneal cavity (greater peritoneal sac)

胸膜腔
Pleural cavity

食管开口
Esophageal opening

胃底
Fundus of stomach

脾
Spleen

膈
Diaphragm

腹膜腔
（小腹膜囊或网膜囊）
Peritoneal cavity
(lesser peritoneal
sac or omental bursa)

左肺
Left lung

膈的右脚
Right crus of diaphragm

半奇静脉
Hemiazygos vein

肝
Liver

肝静脉
Hepatic veins

右肺
Right lung

下腔静脉
Inferior vena cava

奇静脉
Azygos vein

胸导管
Thoracic duct

胸主动脉
Descending
thoracic aorta

B. L1 椎体水平
L1 vertebral level

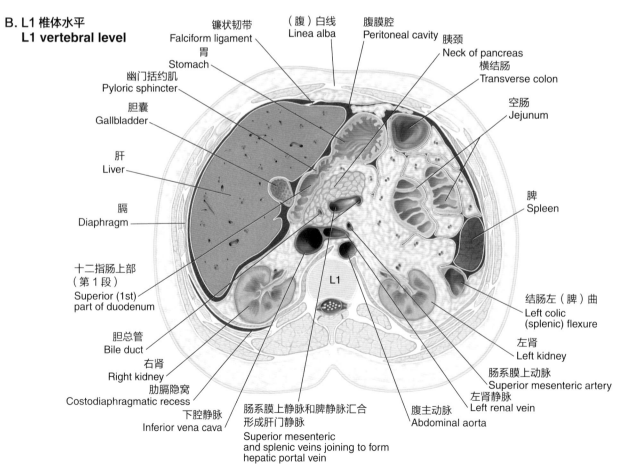

镰状韧带
Falciform ligament

胃
Stomach

幽门括约肌
Pyloric sphincter

胆囊
Gallbladder

肝
Liver

膈
Diaphragm

十二指肠上部
（第 1 段）
Superior (1st)
part of duodenum

胆总管
Bile duct

右肾
Right kidney

肋膈隐窝
Costodiaphragmatic recess

下腔静脉
Inferior vena cava

肠系膜上静脉和脾静脉汇合
形成肝门静脉
Superior mesenteric
and splenic veins joining to form
hepatic portal vein

（腹）白线
Linea alba

腹膜腔
Peritoneal cavity

胰颈
Neck of pancreas

横结肠
Transverse colon

空肠
Jejunum

脾
Spleen

结肠左（脾）曲
Left colic
(splenic) flexure

左肾
Left kidney

肠系膜上动脉
Superior mesenteric artery

左肾静脉
Left renal vein

腹主动脉
Abdominal aorta

A. L3 椎体水平
L3 vertebral level

包含肠内血管的肠系膜
Mesentery containing intestinal vessels

横结肠
Transverse colon

十二指肠水平部
Transverse (3rd) part of duodenum

升结肠
Ascending colon

肠系膜上动脉和静脉
Superior mesenteric vein and artery

右输尿管
Right ureter

下腔静脉
Inferior vena cava

腹主动脉
Abdominal aorta

腹膜腔
Peritoneal cavity

腹白线
Linea alba

大网膜的网膜裙部
Omental apron portion of greater omentum

回肠
Ileum

空肠
Jejunum

降结肠
Descending colon

左输尿管
Left ureter

腰大肌
Psoas major muscle

肠系膜下动脉
Inferior mesenteric artery

B. L5/S1 椎体水平
L5/S1 vertebral level

腹白线
Linea alba

大网膜的网膜裙部
Omental apron portion of greater omentum

肠系膜
Mesentery

空肠
Jejunum

腹膜腔
Peritoneal cavity

降结肠
Descending colon

升结肠
Ascending colon

回肠
Ileum

髂骨
Ilium

右输尿管
Right ureter

腰大肌
Psoas major muscle

左输尿管
Left ureter

髂总动脉
Common iliac arteries

髂总静脉汇合形成下腔静脉
Common iliac veins joining to form inferior vena cava

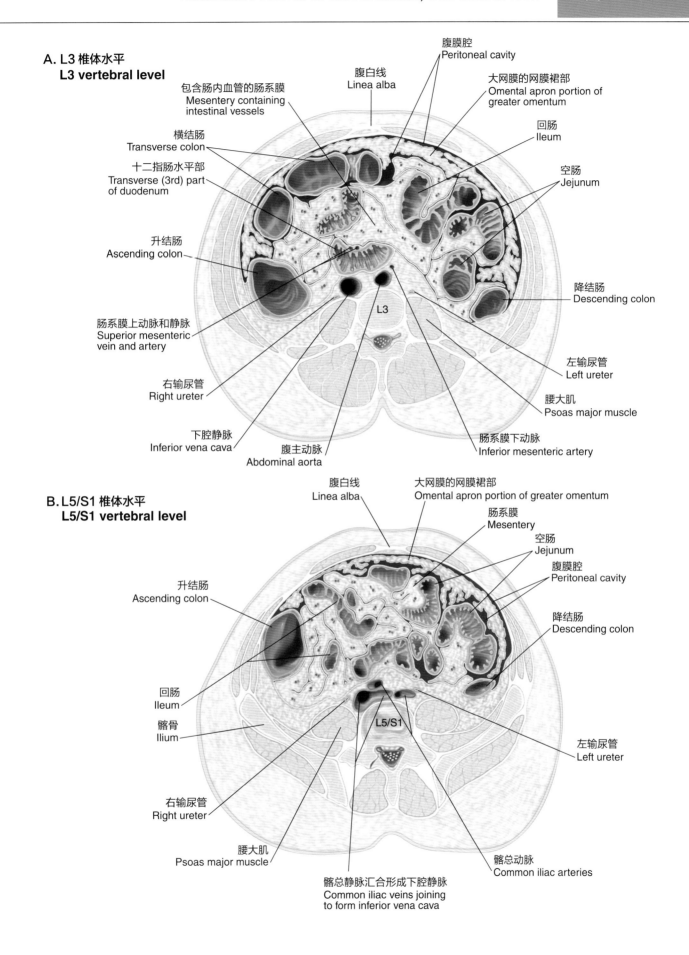

腹部肌群

名称	起点	止点	主要作用	神经支配	动脉	注释
腹外斜肌（图5-04、图5-05和图5-06B及C）	下8肋	白线、耻骨嵴、耻骨结节、髂前上棘和髂嵴的前半	屈曲和侧弯躯干	第7~11肋间神经、肋下神经、髂腹下神经和髂腹股沟神经	肌膈动脉、腹壁上动脉、第7~11肋间动脉、肋下动脉、腰动脉、旋髂浅动脉、旋髂深动脉、腹壁浅动脉、腹壁下动脉、阴部外浅动脉	腹股沟韧带是特化的腹外斜肌腱膜；腹外斜肌参与形成覆盖睾丸和精索的精索外筋膜
腹内斜肌（图5-05和图5-06B及C）	胸腰筋膜、髂嵴的前2/3和腹股沟韧带的外2/3	下3或4肋、白线、耻骨嵴和耻骨梳	屈曲和侧弯躯干	第7~11肋间神经、肋下神经、髂腹下神经和髂腹股沟神经	肌膈动脉、腹壁上动脉、第7~11肋间动脉、肋下动脉、腰动脉、旋髂浅动脉、旋髂深动脉、腹壁浅动脉、腹壁下动脉、阴部外浅动脉	腹内斜肌的前部肌纤维行向内上方，与腹外斜肌的纤维方向垂直；提睾肌和筋膜是腹内斜肌参与覆盖睾丸和精索的结构
腹横肌（图5-05和图5-06B及C）	下6肋、胸腰筋膜、髂嵴的前3/4和腹股沟韧带的外侧1/3	白线、耻骨嵴和耻骨梳	屈曲和侧弯躯干	第7~11肋间神经、肋下神经、髂腹下神经和髂腹股沟神经	肌膈动脉、腹壁上动脉、第7~11肋间动脉、肋下动脉、腰动脉、旋髂浅动脉、旋髂深动脉、腹壁浅动脉、腹壁下动脉、阴部外浅动脉	腹横肌不参与覆盖精索和睾丸；腹横筋膜是覆盖腹横肌内面的深筋膜，形成精索内筋膜
腹直肌（图5-05和图5-06B及C）	耻骨嵴和耻骨联合	胸骨的剑突和第5~7肋软骨	屈曲躯干	第7~11肋间神经和肋下神经	腹壁上动脉、肋间动脉、肋下动脉、腹壁下动脉	腹直肌鞘有腹外斜肌腱膜、腹内斜肌腱膜和腹横肌腱膜构成，内有腹直肌
锥状肌（图5-12）	耻骨嵴，位于腹直肌前方	白线	拉白线向下	肋下神经	肋下动脉，腹壁下动脉	锥状肌存在缺失变异
提睾肌（图5-04、图5-12B和图6-31）	腹股沟韧带	在精索和睾丸周围形成肌筋膜网（或在子宫圆韧带远端）	上提睾丸（女性发育不完全）	生殖股神经的生殖支	腹壁下动脉的分支，提睾肌动脉	腹内斜肌纤维覆盖精索和睾丸形成提睾肌；触摸大腿内侧可引发提睾反射（生殖股神经股支支配皮肤感觉）
肉膜（图5-04和图5-05）	阴囊和阴茎（或大阴唇和阴蒂）的皮下结缔组织	阴囊和阴茎（或大阴唇和阴蒂）的皮肤	上提睾丸（紧张女性阴部皮肤）	交感神经节后纤维通过髂腹股沟神经和阴囊后神经支配	提睾肌动脉、阴囊（阴唇）后动脉	寒冷刺激肉膜上提睾丸（肉膜是特化的竖毛肌纤维，或立毛肌）

腹部肌群						
名称	**起点**	**止点**	**主要作用**	**神经支配**	**动脉**	**注释**
膈 （图 5-35）	剑突、肋缘、覆盖腰方肌和腰大肌的筋膜（内外侧弓状韧带）、L1~L3 椎体	膈的中心腱	向下推腹腔内脏，增加胸腔容积（吸气）	膈神经（C3~C5）	肌膈动脉、膈上动脉、膈下动脉	左膈脚附着于 L1~L2 椎体，右膈脚附着于 L1~L3 椎体
髂肌 （图 5-35）	髂窝和髂嵴；骶骨翼	股骨小转子	屈大腿；在大腿屈曲时，可以屈骨盆靠近大腿	股神经	髂腰动脉	与腰大肌一起形成髂腰肌腱
腰大肌 （图 5-35）	腰椎横突和椎体	股骨小转子（与髂肌一起）借髂腰肌腱	屈大腿；屈曲和侧弯腰椎	L2~L4 脊神经的腹侧主支	肋下动脉，腰动脉	生殖股神经从腰大肌前面穿出
腰小肌 （图 5-35）	T12 和 L1 椎体	髂骨和耻骨上支连接线处的髂耻隆起	屈曲和侧弯腰椎	L1~L2	腰动脉	40% 人群缺如
腰方肌 （图 5-35）	髂嵴后部和髂腰韧带	L1~L4 横突和第 12 肋	侧弯躯干，固定第 12 肋	肋下神经和 L1~L4 脊神经的腹侧主支	肋下动脉，腰动脉	膈的外侧弓状韧带跨过腰方肌前面

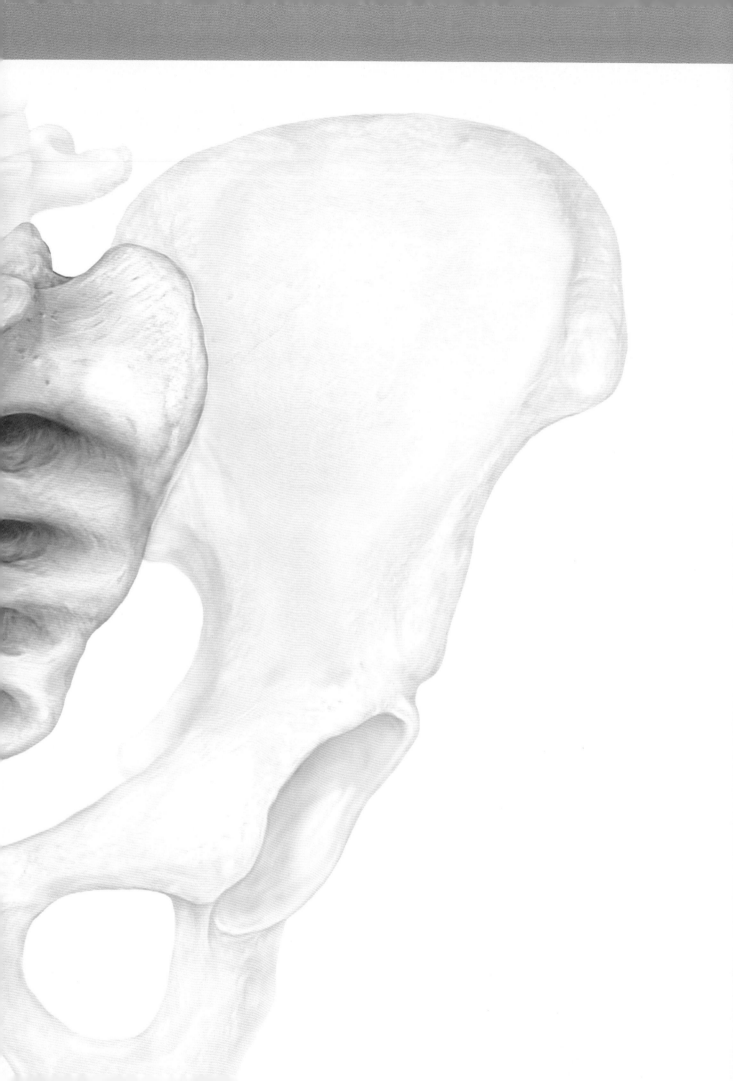

第六章 骨盆和会阴

The Pelvis and Perineum

A. 前面观
Anterior view

可触及的骨性结构
Palpable bony structures

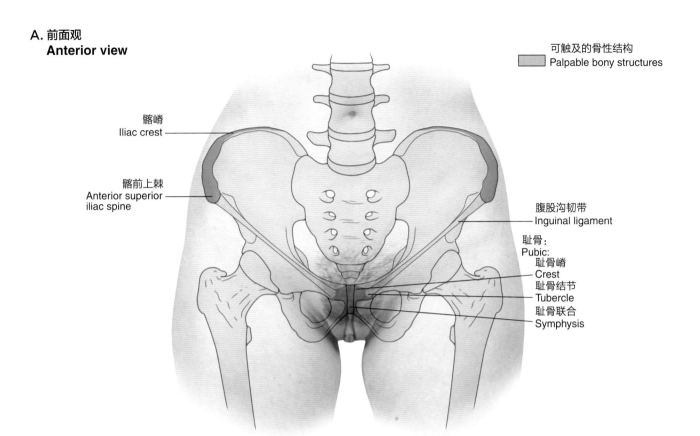

髂嵴
Iliac crest

髂前上棘
Anterior superior
iliac spine

腹股沟韧带
Inguinal ligament

耻骨:
Pubic:
耻骨嵴
Crest
耻骨结节
Tubercle
耻骨联合
Symphysis

B. 后面观
Posterior view

髂嵴
Iliac crest

髂后上棘
Posterior superior
iliac spine

骶骨
Sacrum

尾骨
Coccyx

坐骨结节
Ischial tuberosity

坐骨大切迹
Greater sciatic notch

坐骨棘
Ischial spine

坐骨小切迹
Lesser sciatic notch

A. 前面观
Anterior view

可触及的骨性结构
Palpable bony structures

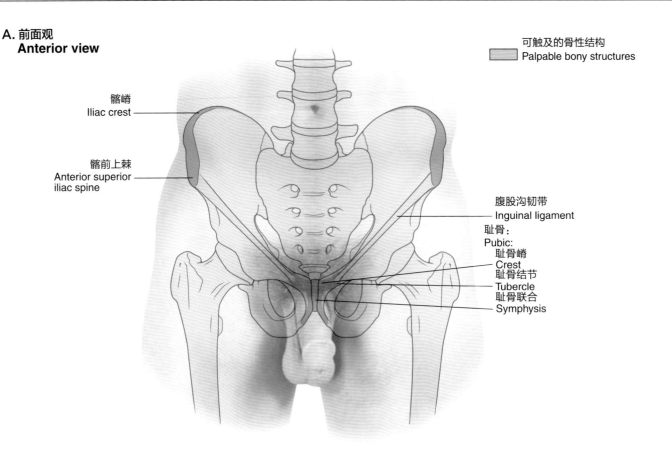

髂嵴
Iliac crest

髂前上棘
Anterior superior
iliac spine

腹股沟韧带
Inguinal ligament

耻骨：
Pubic:
耻骨嵴
Crest
耻骨结节
Tubercle
耻骨联合
Symphysis

B. 后面观
Posterior view

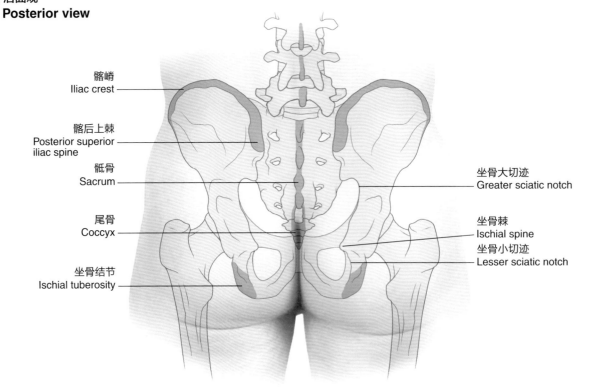

髂嵴
Iliac crest

髂后上棘
Posterior superior
iliac spine

骶骨
Sacrum

尾骨
Coccyx

坐骨结节
Ischial tuberosity

坐骨大切迹
Greater sciatic notch

坐骨棘
Ischial spine

坐骨小切迹
Lesser sciatic notch

A. 内侧面观
Medial view

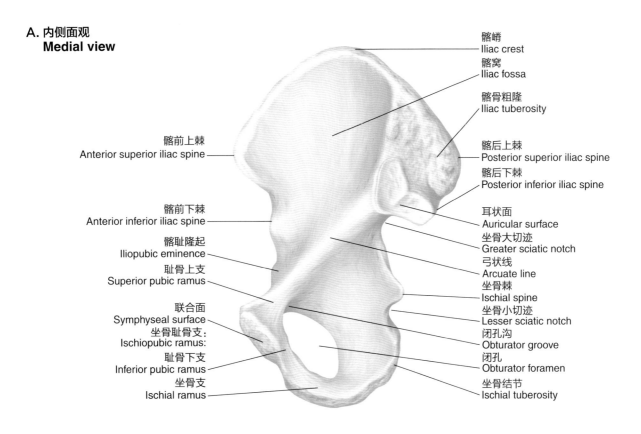

髂嵴
Iliac crest

髂窝
Iliac fossa

髂骨粗隆
Iliac tuberosity

髂前上棘
Anterior superior iliac spine

髂后上棘
Posterior superior iliac spine

髂后下棘
Posterior inferior iliac spine

髂前下棘
Anterior inferior iliac spine

耳状面
Auricular surface

髂耻隆起
Iliopubic eminence

坐骨大切迹
Greater sciatic notch

耻骨上支
Superior pubic ramus

弓状线
Arcuate line

坐骨棘
Ischial spine

联合面
Symphyseal surface

坐骨小切迹
Lesser sciatic notch

坐骨耻骨支：
Ischiopubic ramus:

闭孔沟
Obturator groove

耻骨下支
Inferior pubic ramus

闭孔
Obturator foramen

坐骨支
Ischial ramus

坐骨结节
Ischial tuberosity

B. 外侧面观
Lateral view

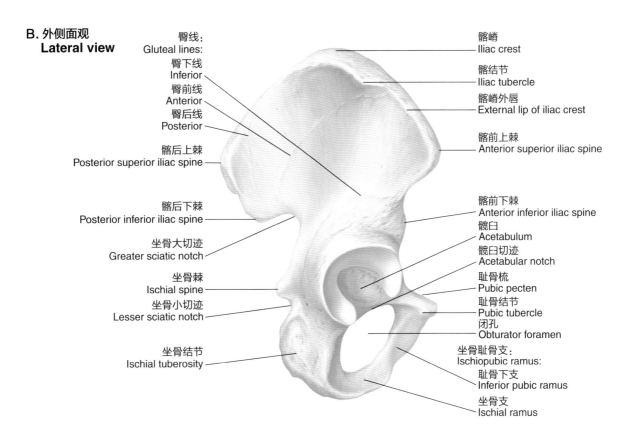

臀线：
Gluteal lines:

髂嵴
Iliac crest

臀下线
Inferior

髂结节
Iliac tubercle

臀前线
Anterior

髂嵴外唇
External lip of iliac crest

臀后线
Posterior

髂后上棘
Posterior superior iliac spine

髂前上棘
Anterior superior iliac spine

髂后下棘
Posterior inferior iliac spine

髂前下棘
Anterior inferior iliac spine

髋臼
Acetabulum

坐骨大切迹
Greater sciatic notch

髋臼切迹
Acetabular notch

坐骨棘
Ischial spine

耻骨梳
Pubic pecten

坐骨小切迹
Lesser sciatic notch

耻骨结节
Pubic tubercle

闭孔
Obturator foramen

坐骨结节
Ischial tuberosity

坐骨耻骨支：
Ischiopubic ramus:

耻骨下支
Inferior pubic ramus

坐骨支
Ischial ramus

图 6-04　男性骨盆连接　Articulated Pelvis, Male

A. 前面观
Anterior view

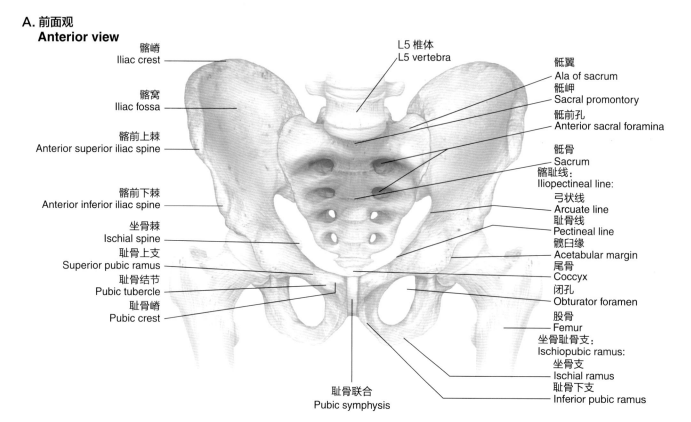

髂嵴
Iliac crest

髂窝
Iliac fossa

髂前上棘
Anterior superior iliac spine

髂前下棘
Anterior inferior iliac spine

坐骨棘
Ischial spine

耻骨上支
Superior pubic ramus

耻骨结节
Pubic tubercle

耻骨嵴
Pubic crest

L5 椎体
L5 vertebra

骶翼
Ala of sacrum

骶岬
Sacral promontory

骶前孔
Anterior sacral foramina

骶骨
Sacrum

髂耻线：
Iliopectineal line:

弓状线
Arcuate line

耻骨线
Pectineal line

髋臼缘
Acetabular margin

尾骨
Coccyx

闭孔
Obturator foramen

股骨
Femur

坐骨耻骨支：
Ischiopubic ramus:

坐骨支
Ischial ramus

耻骨下支
Inferior pubic ramus

耻骨联合
Pubic symphysis

B. 后面观
Posterior view

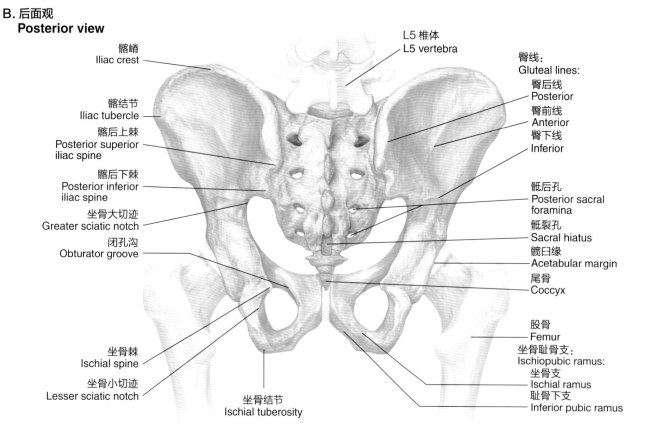

髂嵴
Iliac crest

髂结节
Iliac tubercle

髂后上棘
Posterior superior iliac spine

髂后下棘
Posterior inferior iliac spine

坐骨大切迹
Greater sciatic notch

闭孔沟
Obturator groove

坐骨棘
Ischial spine

坐骨小切迹
Lesser sciatic notch

坐骨结节
Ischial tuberosity

L5 椎体
L5 vertebra

臀线：
Gluteal lines:

臀后线
Posterior

臀前线
Anterior

臀下线
Inferior

骶后孔
Posterior sacral foramina

骶裂孔
Sacral hiatus

髋臼缘
Acetabular margin

尾骨
Coccyx

股骨
Femur

坐骨耻骨支：
Ischiopubic ramus:

坐骨支
Ischial ramus

耻骨下支
Inferior pubic ramus

A. 女性，前面观
Female, anterior view

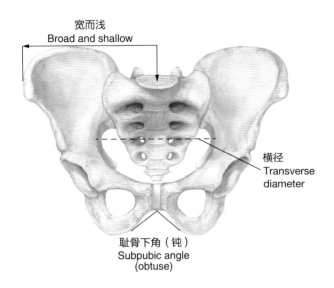

宽而浅
Broad and shallow

横径
Transverse diameter

耻骨下角（钝）
Subpubic angle (obtuse)

B. 男性，前面观
Male, anterior view

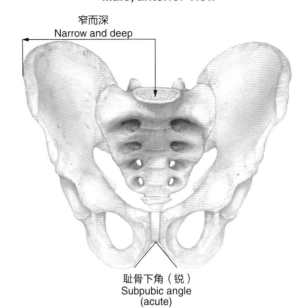

窄而深
Narrow and deep

耻骨下角（锐）
Subpubic angle (acute)

C. 女性，上面观
Female, superior view

D. 男性，上面观
Male, superior view

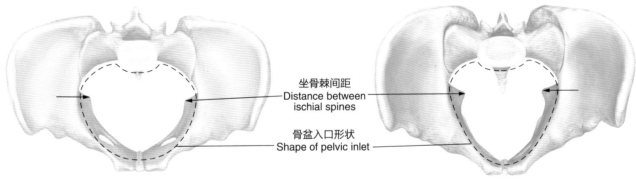

坐骨棘间距
Distance between ischial spines

骨盆入口形状
Shape of pelvic inlet

E. 女性，内侧面观
Female, medial view

F. 男性，内侧面观
Male, medial view

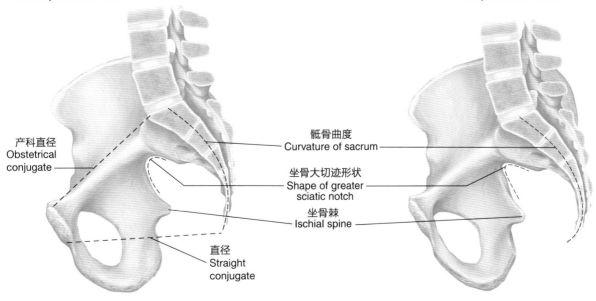

产科直径
Obstetrical conjugate

骶骨曲度
Curvature of sacrum

坐骨大切迹形状
Shape of greater sciatic notch

坐骨棘
Ischial spine

直径
Straight conjugate

图 6-06　　骨盆韧带　Ligaments of the Pelvis

A. 前面观
Anterior view

L5 横突
Transverse process of L5 vertebra

前纵韧带
Anterior longitudinal ligament

髂嵴
Iliac crest

髂窝
Iliac fossa

髂前上棘
Anterior superior
iliac spine

骨盆界限（终线）
Pelvic brim
(linea terminalis)

髂前下棘
Anterior inferior iliac spine

坐骨大孔
Greater sciatic foramen

闭膜管
Obturator canal

股骨
Femur

髂腰韧带
Iliolumbar ligament

骶髂前韧带
Anterior sacroiliac
ligament

骶翼
Ala of sacrum

骶前孔
Anterior sacral foramina

骶结节韧带
Sacrotuberous ligament

骶棘韧带
Sacrospinous ligament

骶尾前韧带
Anterior
sacrococcygeal ligament

闭孔膜
Obturator membrane

耻骨联合
Pubic symphysis

B. 后面观
Posterior view

髂腰韧带
Iliolumbar ligament

棘上韧带
Supraspinous
ligament

骶髂后韧带
Posterior sacroiliac
ligament

骶结节韧带
Sacrotuberous ligament

骶棘韧带
Sacrospinous
ligament

闭膜管
Obturator canal

髂后上棘
Posterior superior
iliac spine

骶后孔
Posterior sacral
foramina

坐骨大孔
Greater sciatic foramen

骶管裂孔
Sacral hiatus

骶棘韧带
Sacrospinous
ligament

坐骨棘
Ischial spine

坐骨小孔
Lesser sciatic
foramen

坐骨结节
Ischial tuberosity

股骨
Femur

骶尾后韧带
Posterior
sacrococcygeal
ligaments

闭孔膜
Obturator
membrane

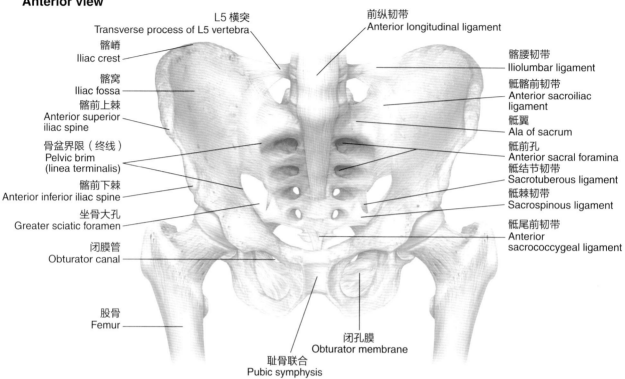

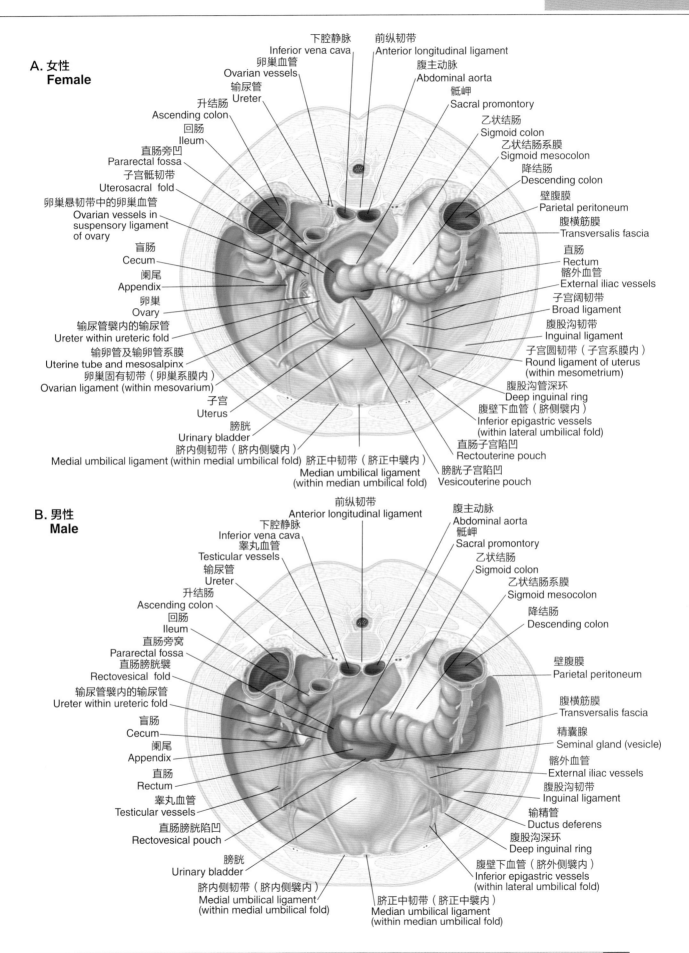

A. 女性
Female

下腔静脉
Inferior vena cava

前纵韧带
Anterior longitudinal ligament

卵巢血管
Ovarian vessels

腹主动脉
Abdominal aorta

输尿管
Ureter

骶岬
Sacral promontory

升结肠
Ascending colon

乙状结肠
Sigmoid colon

回肠
Ileum

乙状结肠系膜
Sigmoid mesocolon

直肠旁凹
Pararectal fossa

降结肠
Descending colon

子宫骶韧带
Uterosacral fold

壁腹膜
Parietal peritoneum

卵巢悬韧带中的卵巢血管
Ovarian vessels in suspensory ligament of ovary

腹横筋膜
Transversalis fascia

盲肠
Cecum

直肠
Rectum

阑尾
Appendix

髂外血管
External iliac vessels

卵巢
Ovary

子宫阔韧带
Broad ligament

输尿管襞内的输尿管
Ureter within ureteric fold

腹股沟韧带
Inguinal ligament

输卵管及输卵管系膜
Uterine tube and mesosalpinx

子宫圆韧带（子宫系膜内）
Round ligament of uterus (within mesometrium)

卵巢固有韧带（卵巢系膜内）
Ovarian ligament (within mesovarium)

腹股沟管深环
Deep inguinal ring

子宫
Uterus

腹壁下血管（脐侧襞内）
Inferior epigastric vessels (within lateral umbilical fold)

膀胱
Urinary bladder

直肠子宫陷凹
Rectouterine pouch

脐内侧韧带（脐内侧襞内）
Medial umbilical ligament (within medial umbilical fold)

脐正中韧带（脐正中襞内）
Median umbilical ligament (within median umbilical fold)

膀胱子宫陷凹
Vesicouterine pouch

B. 男性
Male

前纵韧带
Anterior longitudinal ligament

腹主动脉
Abdominal aorta

下腔静脉
Inferior vena cava

骶岬
Sacral promontory

睾丸血管
Testicular vessels

乙状结肠
Sigmoid colon

输尿管
Ureter

乙状结肠系膜
Sigmoid mesocolon

升结肠
Ascending colon

降结肠
Descending colon

回肠
Ileum

直肠旁窝
Pararectal fossa

直肠膀胱襞
Rectovesical fold

壁腹膜
Parietal peritoneum

输尿管襞内的输尿管
Ureter within ureteric fold

腹横筋膜
Transversalis fascia

盲肠
Cecum

精囊腺
Seminal gland (vesicle)

阑尾
Appendix

髂外血管
External iliac vessels

直肠
Rectum

腹股沟韧带
Inguinal ligament

睾丸血管
Testicular vessels

输精管
Ductus deferens

直肠膀胱陷凹
Rectovesical pouch

腹股沟深环
Deep inguinal ring

膀胱
Urinary bladder

腹壁下血管（脐外侧襞内）
Inferior epigastric vessels (within lateral umbilical fold)

脐内侧韧带（脐内侧襞内）
Medial umbilical ligament (within medial umbilical fold)

脐正中韧带（脐正中襞内）
Median umbilical ligament (within median umbilical fold)

图 6-08 　盆腹膜，矢状面观　Pelvic Peritoneum, Sagittal View

A. 女性 Female

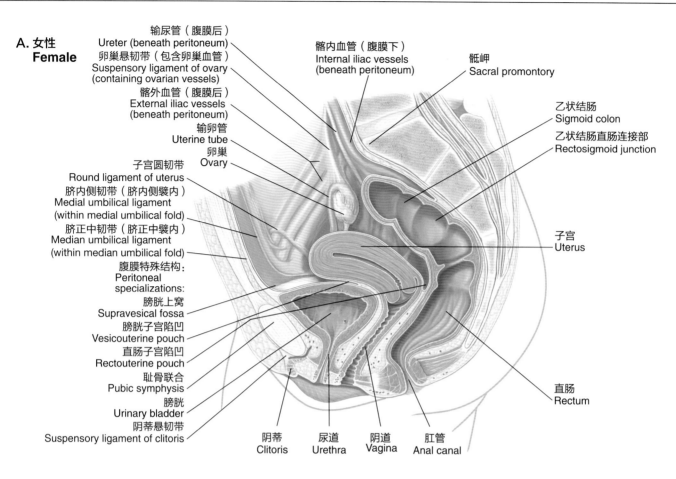

输尿管（腹膜后）
Ureter (beneath peritoneum)

卵巢悬韧带（包含卵巢血管）
Suspensory ligament of ovary
(containing ovarian vessels)

髂外血管（腹膜后）
External iliac vessels
(beneath peritoneum)

输卵管
Uterine tube

卵巢
Ovary

子宫圆韧带
Round ligament of uterus

脐内侧韧带（脐内侧襞内）
Medial umbilical ligament
(within medial umbilical fold)

脐正中韧带（脐正中襞内）
Median umbilical ligament
(within median umbilical fold)

腹膜特殊结构：
Peritoneal
specializations:

膀胱上窝
Supravesical fossa

膀胱子宫陷凹
Vesicouterine pouch

直肠子宫陷凹
Rectouterine pouch

耻骨联合
Pubic symphysis

膀胱
Urinary bladder

阴蒂悬韧带
Suspensory ligament of clitoris

髂内血管（腹膜下）
Internal iliac vessels
(beneath peritoneum)

骶岬
Sacral promontory

乙状结肠
Sigmoid colon

乙状结肠直肠连接部
Rectosigmoid junction

子宫
Uterus

直肠
Rectum

阴蒂
Clitoris

尿道
Urethra

阴道
Vagina

肛管
Anal canal

B. 男性 Male

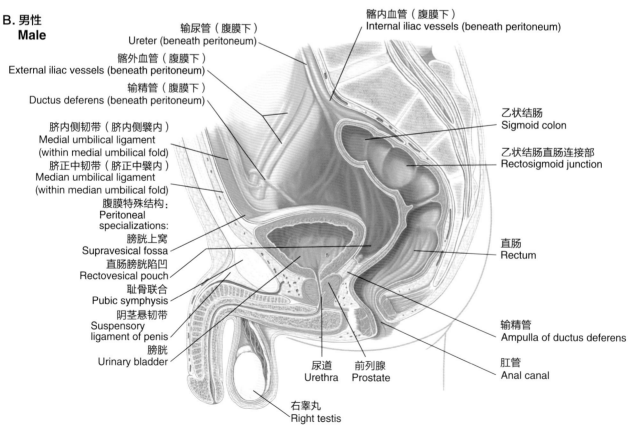

输尿管（腹膜下）
Ureter (beneath peritoneum)

髂外血管（腹膜下）
External iliac vessels (beneath peritoneum)

输精管（腹膜下）
Ductus deferens (beneath peritoneum)

脐内侧韧带（脐内侧襞内）
Medial umbilical ligament
(within medial umbilical fold)

脐正中韧带（脐正中襞内）
Median umbilical ligament
(within median umbilical fold)

腹膜特殊结构：
Peritoneal
specializations:

膀胱上窝
Supravesical fossa

直肠膀胱陷凹
Rectovesical pouch

耻骨联合
Pubic symphysis

阴茎悬韧带
Suspensory
ligament of penis

膀胱
Urinary bladder

髂内血管（腹膜下）
Internal iliac vessels (beneath peritoneum)

乙状结肠
Sigmoid colon

乙状结肠直肠连接部
Rectosigmoid junction

直肠
Rectum

输精管
Ampulla of ductus deferens

肛管
Anal canal

尿道
Urethra

前列腺
Prostate

右睾丸
Right testis

A. 女性
Female

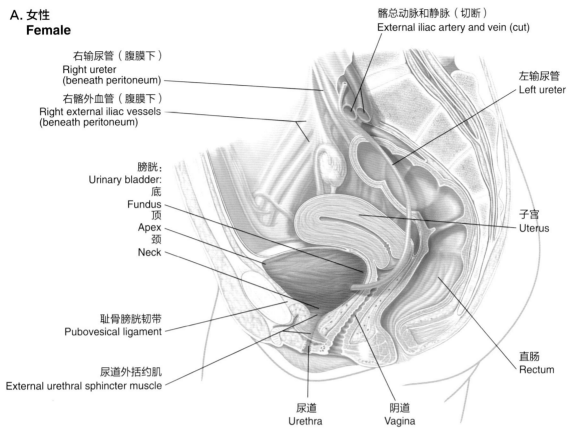

右输尿管（腹膜下）
Right ureter
(beneath peritoneum)

右髂外血管（腹膜下）
Right external iliac vessels
(beneath peritoneum)

髂总动脉和静脉（切断）
External iliac artery and vein (cut)

左输尿管
Left ureter

膀胱：
Urinary bladder:
底
Fundus
顶
Apex
颈
Neck

子宫
Uterus

耻骨膀胱韧带
Pubovesical ligament

直肠
Rectum

尿道外括约肌
External urethral sphincter muscle

尿道
Urethra

阴道
Vagina

B. 男性
Male

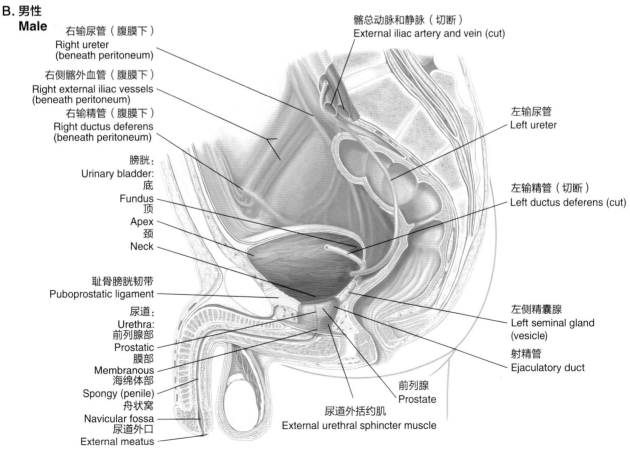

右输尿管（腹膜下）
Right ureter
(beneath peritoneum)

右侧髂外血管（腹膜下）
Right external iliac vessels
(beneath peritoneum)

右输精管（腹膜下）
Right ductus deferens
(beneath peritoneum)

髂总动脉和静脉（切断）
External iliac artery and vein (cut)

左输尿管
Left ureter

膀胱：
Urinary bladder:
底
Fundus
顶
Apex
颈
Neck

左输精管（切断）
Left ductus deferens (cut)

耻骨膀胱韧带
Puboprostatic ligament

尿道：
Urethra:
前列腺部
Prostatic
膜部
Membranous
海绵体部
Spongy (penile)
舟状窝
Navicular fossa
尿道外口
External meatus

左侧精囊腺
Left seminal gland
(vesicle)

射精管
Ejaculatory duct

前列腺
Prostate

尿道外括约肌
External urethral sphincter muscle

图 6-10　　膀胱，前面观　Urinary Bladder, Anterior View

A. 女性
Female

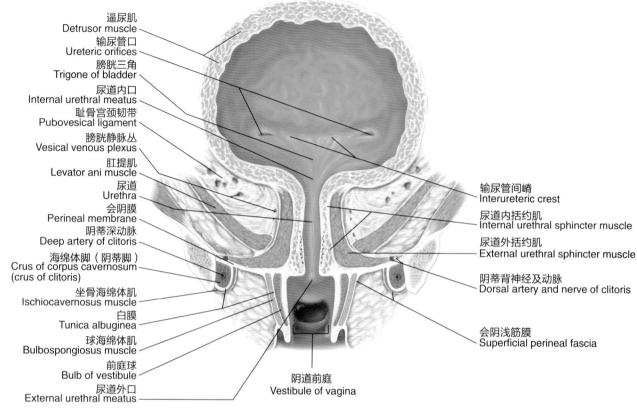

逼尿肌
Detrusor muscle

输尿管口
Ureteric orifices

膀胱三角
Trigone of bladder

尿道内口
Internal urethral meatus

耻骨宫颈韧带
Pubovesical ligament

膀胱静脉丛
Vesical venous plexus

肛提肌
Levator ani muscle

尿道
Urethra

会阴膜
Perineal membrane

阴蒂深动脉
Deep artery of clitoris

海绵体脚（阴蒂脚）
Crus of corpus cavernosum
(crus of clitoris)

坐骨海绵体肌
Ischiocavernosus muscle

白膜
Tunica albuginea

球海绵体肌
Bulbospongiosus muscle

前庭球
Bulb of vestibule

尿道外口
External urethral meatus

输尿管间嵴
Interureteric crest

尿道内括约肌
Internal urethral sphincter muscle

尿道外括约肌
External urethral sphincter muscle

阴蒂背神经及动脉
Dorsal artery and nerve of clitoris

会阴浅筋膜
Superficial perineal fascia

阴道前庭
Vestibule of vagina

B. 男性
Male

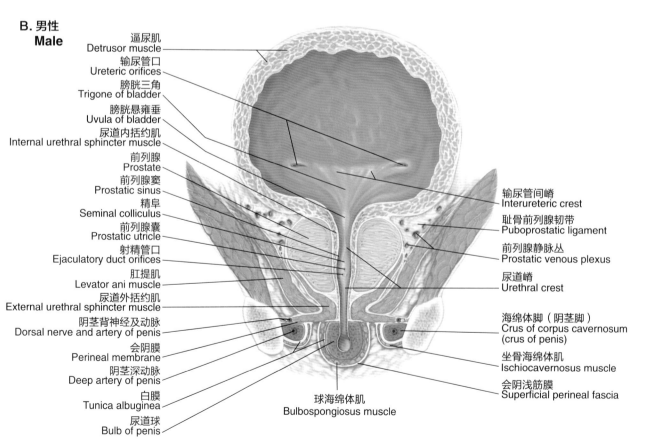

逼尿肌
Detrusor muscle

输尿管口
Ureteric orifices

膀胱三角
Trigone of bladder

膀胱悬雍垂
Uvula of bladder

尿道内括约肌
Internal urethral sphincter muscle

前列腺
Prostate

前列腺窦
Prostatic sinus

精阜
Seminal colliculus

前列腺囊
Prostatic utricle

射精管口
Ejaculatory duct orifices

肛提肌
Levator ani muscle

尿道外括约肌
External urethral sphincter muscle

阴茎背神经及动脉
Dorsal nerve and artery of penis

会阴膜
Perineal membrane

阴茎深动脉
Deep artery of penis

白膜
Tunica albuginea

尿道球
Bulb of penis

输尿管间嵴
Interureteric crest

耻骨前列腺韧带
Puboprostatic ligament

前列腺静脉丛
Prostatic venous plexus

尿道嵴
Urethral crest

海绵体脚（阴茎脚）
Crus of corpus cavernosum
(crus of penis)

坐骨海绵体肌
Ischiocavernosus muscle

会阴浅筋膜
Superficial perineal fascia

球海绵体肌
Bulbospongiosus muscle

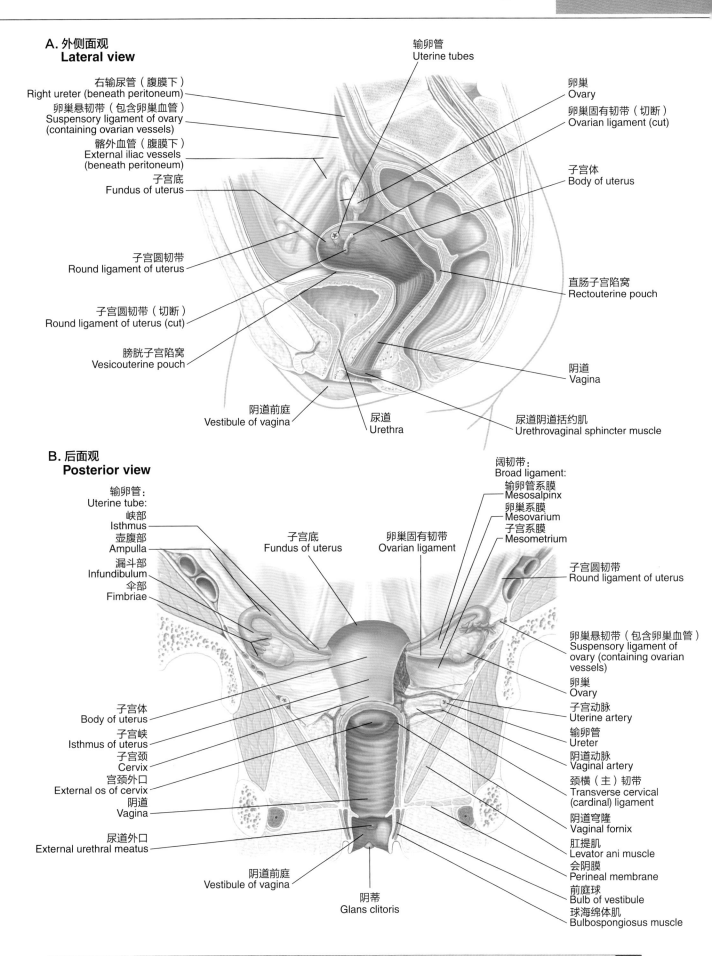

A. 外侧面观
Lateral view

输卵管
Uterine tubes

右输尿管（腹膜下）
Right ureter (beneath peritoneum)

卵巢悬韧带（包含卵巢血管）
Suspensory ligament of ovary
(containing ovarian vessels)

髂外血管（腹膜下）
External iliac vessels
(beneath peritoneum)

子宫底
Fundus of uterus

子宫圆韧带
Round ligament of uterus

子宫圆韧带（切断）
Round ligament of uterus (cut)

膀胱子宫陷窝
Vesicouterine pouch

阴道前庭
Vestibule of vagina

尿道
Urethra

卵巢
Ovary

卵巢固有韧带（切断）
Ovarian ligament (cut)

子宫体
Body of uterus

直肠子宫陷窝
Rectouterine pouch

阴道
Vagina

尿道阴道括约肌
Urethrovaginal sphincter muscle

B. 后面观
Posterior view

阔韧带：
Broad ligament:
输卵管系膜
Mesosalpinx
卵巢系膜
Mesovarium
子宫系膜
Mesometrium

输卵管：
Uterine tube:
峡部
Isthmus
壶腹部
Ampulla
漏斗部
Infundibulum
伞部
Fimbriae

子宫底
Fundus of uterus

卵巢固有韧带
Ovarian ligament

子宫圆韧带
Round ligament of uterus

卵巢悬韧带（包含卵巢血管）
Suspensory ligament of
ovary (containing ovarian
vessels)

卵巢
Ovary

子宫动脉
Uterine artery

输卵管
Ureter

阴道动脉
Vaginal artery

颈横（主）韧带
Transverse cervical
(cardinal) ligament

阴道穹隆
Vaginal fornix

肛提肌
Levator ani muscle

会阴膜
Perineal membrane

前庭球
Bulb of vestibule

球海绵体肌
Bulbospongiosus muscle

子宫体
Body of uterus

子宫峡
Isthmus of uterus

子宫颈
Cervix

宫颈外口
External os of cervix

阴道
Vagina

尿道外口
External urethral meatus

阴道前庭
Vestibule of vagina

阴蒂
Glans clitoris

图 6-12　子宫与阴道 II　Uterus and Vagina II

A. 后面观 Posterior view

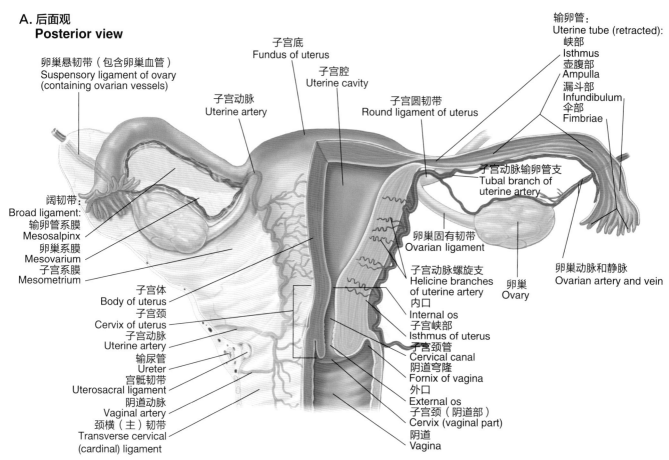

卵巢悬韧带（包含卵巢血管）
Suspensory ligament of ovary (containing ovarian vessels)

子宫底
Fundus of uterus

子宫腔
Uterine cavity

子宫动脉
Uterine artery

子宫圆韧带
Round ligament of uterus

输卵管：
Uterine tube (retracted):
峡部
Isthmus
壶腹部
Ampulla
漏斗部
Infundibulum
伞部
Fimbriae

阔韧带：
Broad ligament:
输卵管系膜
Mesosalpinx
卵巢系膜
Mesovarium
子宫系膜
Mesometrium

子宫动脉输卵管支
Tubal branch of uterine artery

卵巢固有韧带
Ovarian ligament

子宫动脉螺旋支
Helicine branches of uterine artery

卵巢
Ovary

卵巢动脉和静脉
Ovarian artery and vein

子宫体
Body of uterus

子宫颈
Cervix of uterus

子宫动脉
Uterine artery

输尿管
Ureter

宫骶韧带
Uterosacral ligament

阴道动脉
Vaginal artery

颈横（主）韧带
Transverse cervical (cardinal) ligament

内口
Internal os

子宫峡部
Isthmus of uterus

子宫颈管
Cervical canal

阴道穹隆
Fornix of vagina

外口
External os

子宫颈（阴道部）
Cervix (vaginal part)

阴道
Vagina

B. 子宫输卵管造影 Hysterosalpingogram

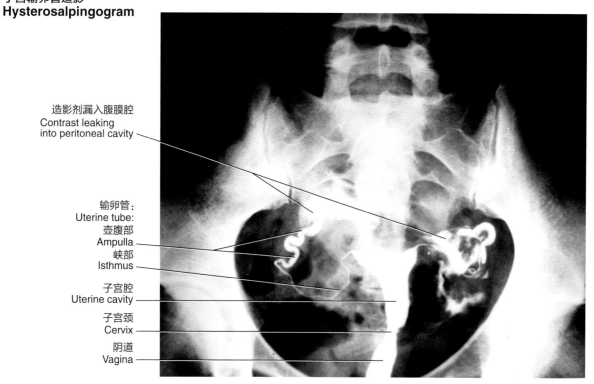

造影剂漏入腹膜腔
Contrast leaking into peritoneal cavity

输卵管：
Uterine tube:
壶腹部
Ampulla
峡部
Isthmus

子宫腔
Uterine cavity

子宫颈
Cervix

阴道
Vagina

A. 正常位置
Normal positions

前屈 **Anteflexed**

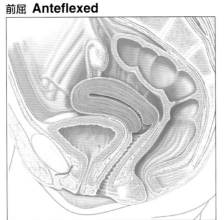

前倾 **Anteverted**

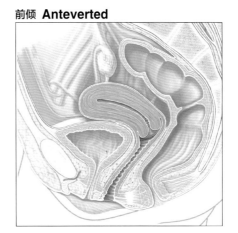

B. 异常位置
Abnormal positions

后屈 **Retroflexed**

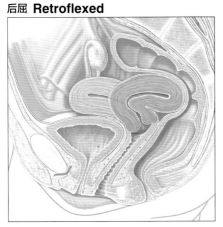

后倾 **Retroverted**

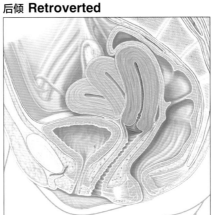

脱垂 **Prolapsed**

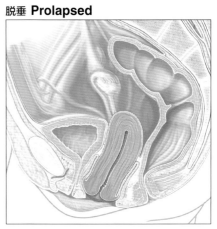

C. 子宫的固定结构，上面观
Supporting structures of the uterus, superior view

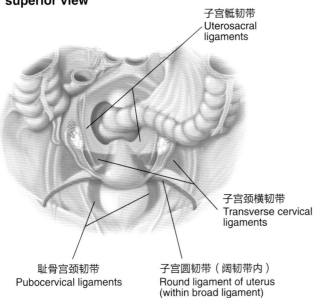

子宫骶韧带
Uterosacral ligaments

子宫颈横韧带
Transverse cervical ligaments

耻骨宫颈韧带
Pubocervical ligaments

子宫圆韧带（阔韧带内）
Round ligament of uterus (within broad ligament)

D. 子宫的固定结构，外侧面观
Supporting structures of the uterus, lateral view

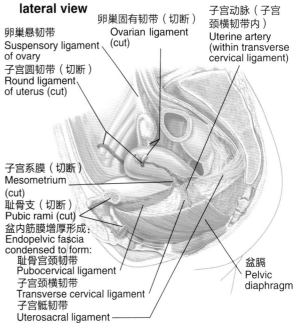

卵巢悬韧带
Suspensory ligament of ovary

子宫圆韧带（切断）
Round ligament of uterus (cut)

卵巢固有韧带（切断）
Ovarian ligament (cut)

子宫动脉（子宫颈横韧带内）
Uterine artery (within transverse cervical ligament)

子宫系膜（切断）
Mesometrium (cut)

耻骨支（切断）
Pubic rami (cut)

盆内筋膜增厚形成：
Endopelvic fascia condensed to form:
　耻骨宫颈韧带
　Pubocervical ligament
　子宫颈横韧带
　Transverse cervical ligament
　子宫骶韧带
　Uterosacral ligament

盆膈
Pelvic diaphragm

图 6-14　男性内生殖器 **Male Internal Genitalia**

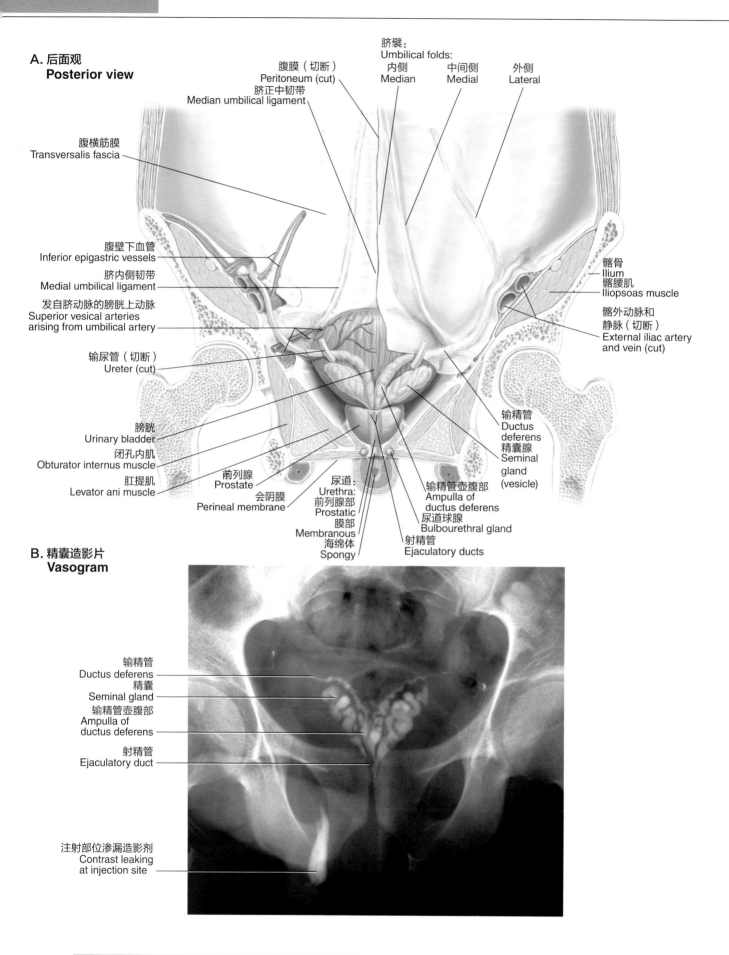

A. 后面观
Posterior view

脐襞：
Umbilical folds:
内侧　　　中间侧　　　外侧
Median　　Medial　　　Lateral

腹膜（切断）
Peritoneum (cut)
脐正中韧带
Median umbilical ligament

腹横筋膜
Transversalis fascia

腹壁下血管
Inferior epigastric vessels

脐内侧韧带
Medial umbilical ligament

发自脐动脉的膀胱上动脉
Superior vesical arteries
arising from umbilical artery

输尿管（切断）
Ureter (cut)

膀胱
Urinary bladder

闭孔内肌
Obturator internus muscle

肛提肌
Levator ani muscle

前列腺
Prostate

会阴膜
Perineal membrane

尿道：
Urethra:
前列腺部
Prostatic
膜部
Membranous
海绵体
Spongy

髂骨
Ilium
髂腰肌
Iliopsoas muscle

髂外动脉和
静脉（切断）
External iliac artery
and vein (cut)

输精管
Ductus
deferens
精囊腺
Seminal
gland
(vesicle)

输精管壶腹部
Ampulla of
ductus deferens
尿道球腺
Bulbourethral gland
射精管
Ejaculatory ducts

B. 精囊造影片
Vasogram

输精管
Ductus deferens
精囊
Seminal gland
输精管壶腹部
Ampulla of
ductus deferens
射精管
Ejaculatory duct

注射部位渗漏造影剂
Contrast leaking
at injection site

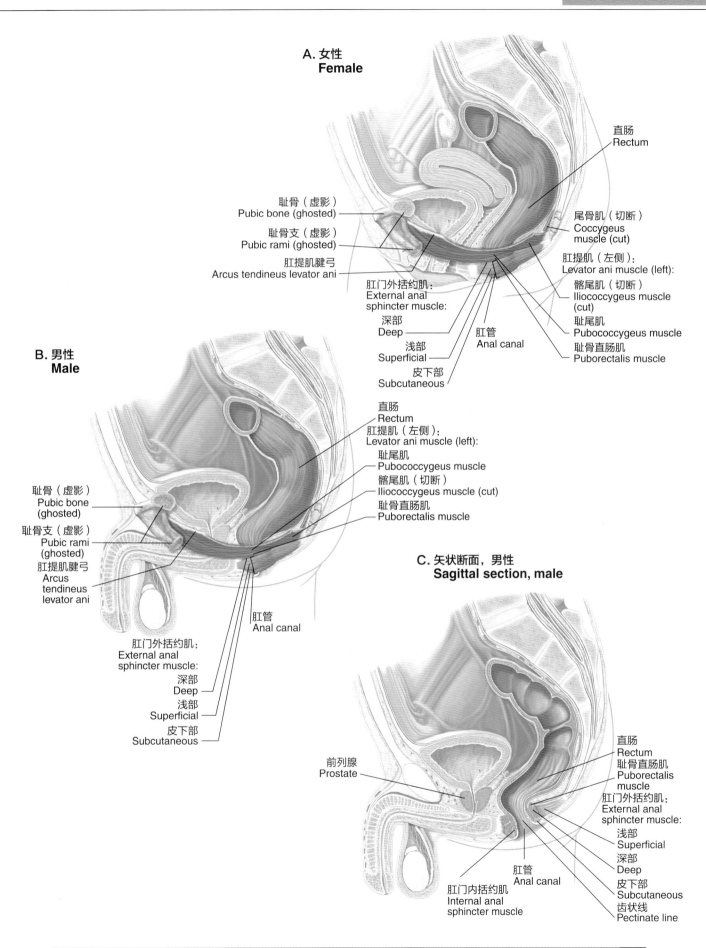

A. 女性
Female

直肠
Rectum

耻骨（虚影）
Pubic bone (ghosted)

耻骨支（虚影）
Pubic rami (ghosted)

肛提肌腱弓
Arcus tendineus levator ani

尾骨肌（切断）
Coccygeus
muscle (cut)

肛提肌（左侧）：
Levator ani muscle (left):

髂尾肌（切断）
Iliococcygeus muscle
(cut)

耻尾肌
Pubococcygeus muscle

耻骨直肠肌
Puborectalis muscle

肛门外括约肌：
External anal
sphincter muscle:

深部
Deep

浅部
Superficial

皮下部
Subcutaneous

肛管
Anal canal

B. 男性
Male

直肠
Rectum

肛提肌（左侧）：
Levator ani muscle (left):

耻尾肌
Pubococcygeus muscle

髂尾肌（切断）
Iliococcygeus muscle (cut)

耻骨直肠肌
Puborectalis muscle

耻骨（虚影）
Pubic bone
(ghosted)

耻骨支（虚影）
Pubic rami
(ghosted)

肛提肌腱弓
Arcus
tendineus
levator ani

肛管
Anal canal

肛门外括约肌：
External anal
sphincter muscle:

深部
Deep

浅部
Superficial

皮下部
Subcutaneous

C. 矢状断面，男性
Sagittal section, male

前列腺
Prostate

直肠
Rectum

耻骨直肠肌
Puborectalis
muscle

肛门外括约肌：
External anal
sphincter muscle:

浅部
Superficial

深部
Deep

皮下部
Subcutaneous

齿状线
Pectinate line

肛管
Anal canal

肛门内括约肌
Internal anal
sphincter muscle

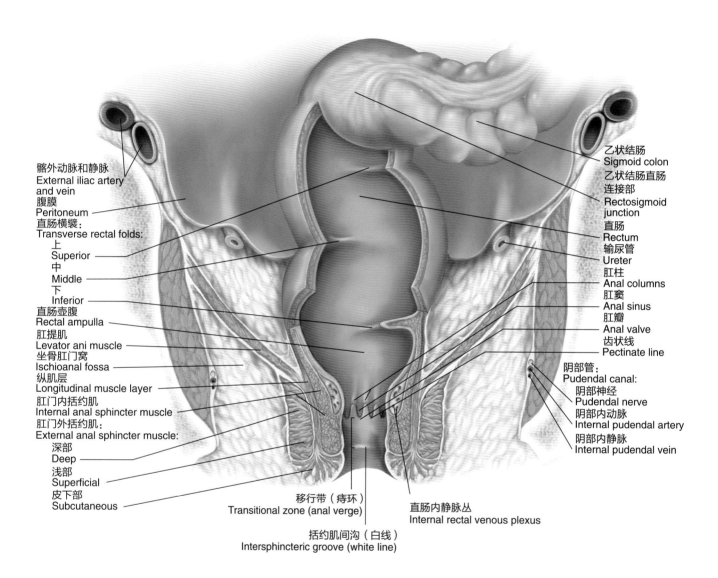

髂外动脉和静脉
External iliac artery and vein
腹膜
Peritoneum
直肠横襞：
Transverse rectal folds:
上
Superior
中
Middle
下
Inferior
直肠壶腹
Rectal ampulla
肛提肌
Levator ani muscle
坐骨肛门窝
Ischioanal fossa
纵肌层
Longitudinal muscle layer
肛门内括约肌
Internal anal sphincter muscle
肛门外括约肌：
External anal sphincter muscle:
深部
Deep
浅部
Superficial
皮下部
Subcutaneous

乙状结肠
Sigmoid colon
乙状结肠直肠连接部
Rectosigmoid junction
直肠
Rectum
输尿管
Ureter
肛柱
Anal columns
肛窦
Anal sinus
肛瓣
Anal valve
齿状线
Pectinate line
阴部管：
Pudendal canal:
阴部神经
Pudendal nerve
阴部内动脉
Internal pudendal artery
阴部内静脉
Internal pudendal vein

移行带（痔环）
Transitional zone (anal verge)
直肠内静脉丛
Internal rectal venous plexus
括约肌间沟（白线）
Intersphincteric groove (white line)

A. 女性 Female

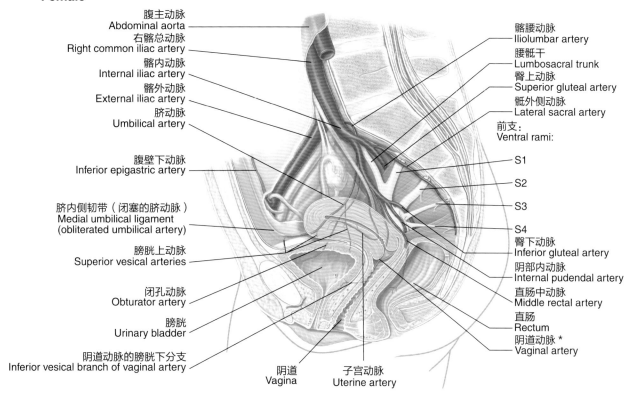

腹主动脉
Abdominal aorta

右髂总动脉
Right common iliac artery

髂内动脉
Internal iliac artery

髂外动脉
External iliac artery

脐动脉
Umbilical artery

腹壁下动脉
Inferior epigastric artery

脐内侧韧带（闭塞的脐动脉）
Medial umbilical ligament
(obliterated umbilical artery)

膀胱上动脉
Superior vesical arteries

闭孔动脉
Obturator artery

膀胱
Urinary bladder

阴道动脉的膀胱下分支
Inferior vesical branch of vaginal artery

髂腰动脉
Iliolumbar artery

腰骶干
Lumbosacral trunk

臀上动脉
Superior gluteal artery

骶外侧动脉
Lateral sacral artery

前支：
Ventral rami:

S1

S2

S3

S4

臀下动脉
Inferior gluteal artery

阴部内动脉
Internal pudendal artery

直肠中动脉
Middle rectal artery

直肠
Rectum

阴道动脉 *
Vaginal artery

阴道
Vagina

子宫动脉
Uterine artery

*11% 的阴道动脉来源于子宫动脉
Vaginal artery arises from uterine artery in 11% of cases

B. 男性 Male

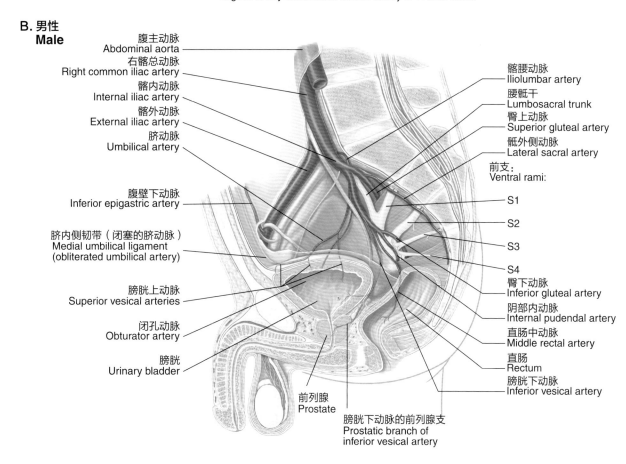

腹主动脉
Abdominal aorta

右髂总动脉
Right common iliac artery

髂内动脉
Internal iliac artery

髂外动脉
External iliac artery

脐动脉
Umbilical artery

腹壁下动脉
Inferior epigastric artery

脐内侧韧带（闭塞的脐动脉）
Medial umbilical ligament
(obliterated umbilical artery)

膀胱上动脉
Superior vesical arteries

闭孔动脉
Obturator artery

膀胱
Urinary bladder

髂腰动脉
Iliolumbar artery

腰骶干
Lumbosacral trunk

臀上动脉
Superior gluteal artery

骶外侧动脉
Lateral sacral artery

前支：
Ventral rami:

S1

S2

S3

S4

臀下动脉
Inferior gluteal artery

阴部内动脉
Internal pudendal artery

直肠中动脉
Middle rectal artery

直肠
Rectum

膀胱下动脉
Inferior vesical artery

前列腺
Prostate

膀胱下动脉的前列腺支
Prostatic branch of
inferior vesical artery

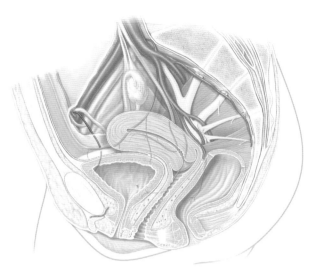

A. 闭孔动脉变异
Aberrant obturator artery

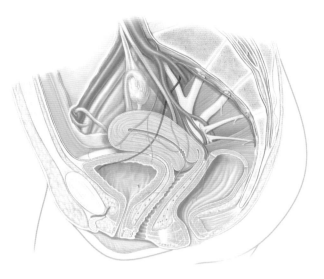

B. 闭孔动脉发自后干
Obturator artery from posterior division

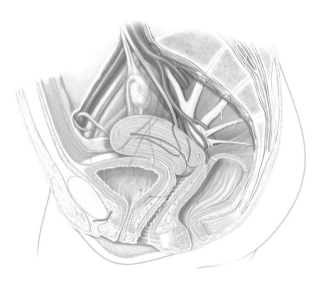

C. 子宫阴道干
Uterovaginal trunk

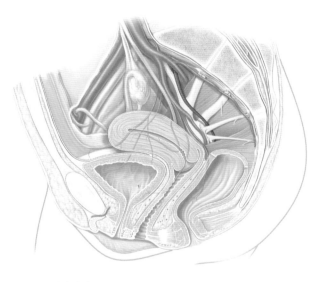

D. 臀下动脉发自后干
Inferior gluteal artery from posterior division

A. 女性 Female

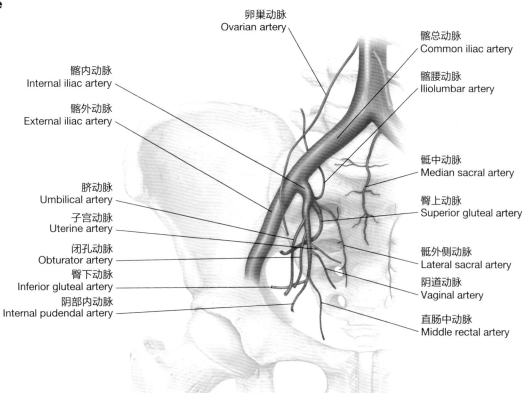

卵巢动脉
Ovarian artery

髂总动脉
Common iliac artery

髂内动脉
Internal iliac artery

髂腰动脉
Iliolumbar artery

髂外动脉
External iliac artery

骶中动脉
Median sacral artery

脐动脉
Umbilical artery

臀上动脉
Superior gluteal artery

子宫动脉
Uterine artery

闭孔动脉
Obturator artery

骶外侧动脉
Lateral sacral artery

臀下动脉
Inferior gluteal artery

阴道动脉
Vaginal artery

阴部内动脉
Internal pudendal artery

直肠中动脉
Middle rectal artery

B. 男性 Male

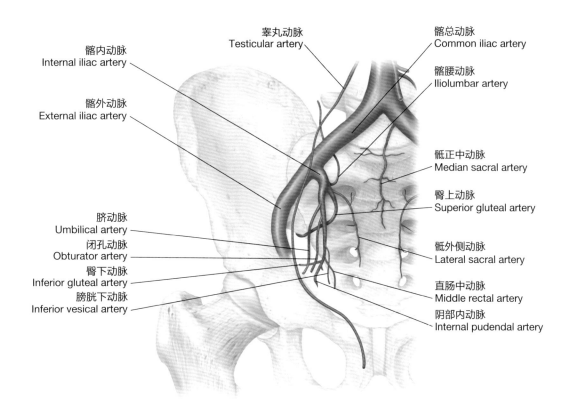

睾丸动脉
Testicular artery

髂总动脉
Common iliac artery

髂内动脉
Internal iliac artery

髂腰动脉
Iliolumbar artery

髂外动脉
External iliac artery

骶正中动脉
Median sacral artery

臀上动脉
Superior gluteal artery

脐动脉
Umbilical artery

闭孔动脉
Obturator artery

骶外侧动脉
Lateral sacral artery

臀下动脉
Inferior gluteal artery

直肠中动脉
Middle rectal artery

膀胱下动脉
Inferior vesical artery

阴部内动脉
Internal pudendal artery

图 6-20 盆腔的静脉回流 **Venous Drainage of the Pelvis**

A. 矢状位观（女性）
Sagittal view (female)

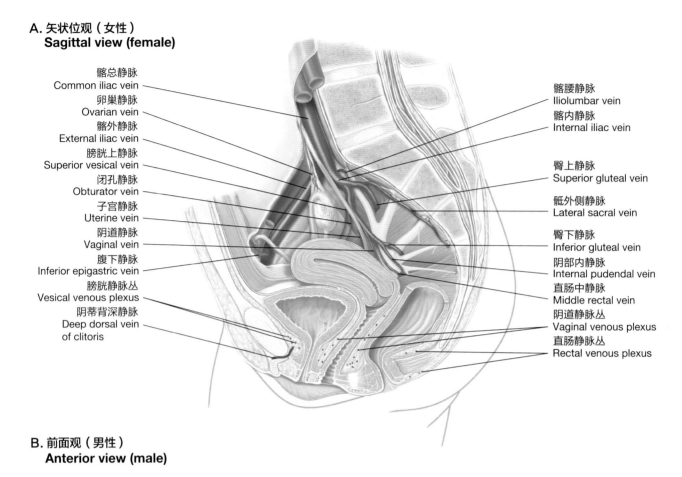

髂总静脉
Common iliac vein

卵巢静脉
Ovarian vein

髂外静脉
External iliac vein

膀胱上静脉
Superior vesical vein

闭孔静脉
Obturator vein

子宫静脉
Uterine vein

阴道静脉
Vaginal vein

腹下静脉
Inferior epigastric vein

膀胱静脉丛
Vesical venous plexus

阴蒂背深静脉
Deep dorsal vein
of clitoris

髂腰静脉
Iliolumbar vein

髂内静脉
Internal iliac vein

臀上静脉
Superior gluteal vein

骶外侧静脉
Lateral sacral vein

臀下静脉
Inferior gluteal vein

阴部内静脉
Internal pudendal vein

直肠中静脉
Middle rectal vein

阴道静脉丛
Vaginal venous plexus

直肠静脉丛
Rectal venous plexus

B. 前面观（男性）
Anterior view (male)

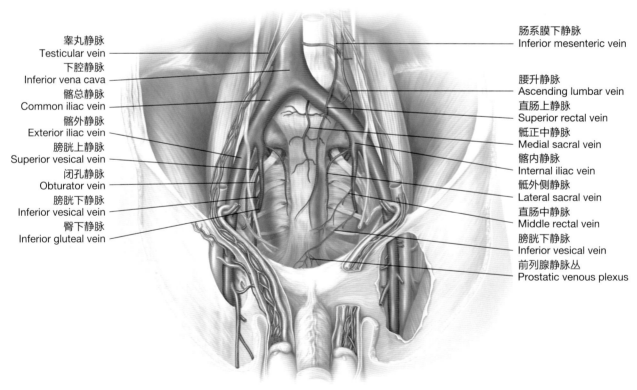

睾丸静脉
Testicular vein

下腔静脉
Inferior vena cava

髂总静脉
Common iliac vein

髂外静脉
Exterior iliac vein

膀胱上静脉
Superior vesical vein

闭孔静脉
Obturator vein

膀胱下静脉
Inferior vesical vein

臀下静脉
Inferior gluteal vein

肠系膜下静脉
Inferior mesenteric vein

腰升静脉
Ascending lumbar vein

直肠上静脉
Superior rectal vein

骶正中静脉
Medial sacral vein

髂内静脉
Internal iliac vein

骶外侧静脉
Lateral sacral vein

直肠中静脉
Middle rectal vein

膀胱下静脉
Inferior vesical vein

前列腺静脉丛
Prostatic venous plexus

A. 内侧面观
Medial view

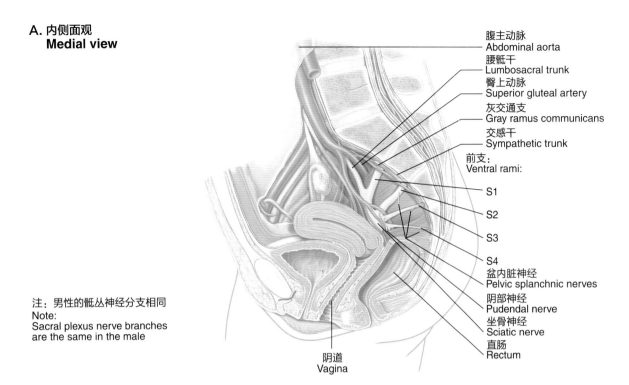

腹主动脉
Abdominal aorta

腰骶干
Lumbosacral trunk

臀上动脉
Superior gluteal artery

灰交通支
Gray ramus communicans

交感干
Sympathetic trunk

前支：
Ventral rami:

S1

S2

S3

S4

盆内脏神经
Pelvic splanchnic nerves

阴部神经
Pudendal nerve

坐骨神经
Sciatic nerve

直肠
Rectum

注：男性的骶丛神经分支相同
Note:
Sacral plexus nerve branches
are the same in the male

阴道
Vagina

B. 前面观
Anterior view

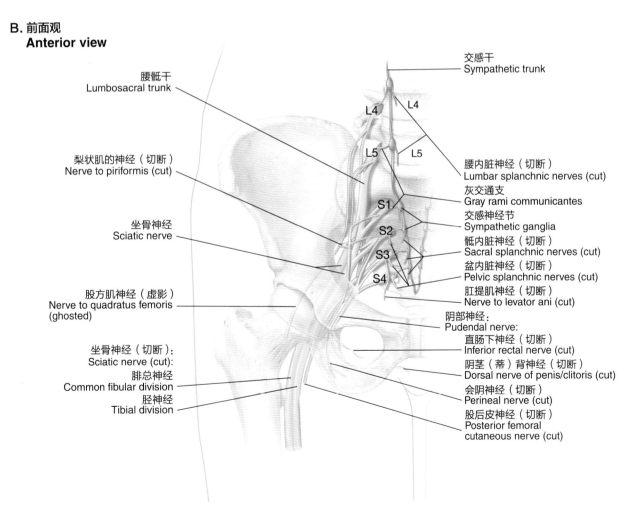

腰骶干
Lumbosacral trunk

交感干
Sympathetic trunk

L4

L4

梨状肌的神经（切断）
Nerve to piriformis (cut)

L5

L5

坐骨神经
Sciatic nerve

S1

S2

S3

S4

腰内脏神经（切断）
Lumbar splanchnic nerves (cut)

灰交通支
Gray rami communicantes

交感神经节
Sympathetic ganglia

骶内脏神经（切断）
Sacral splanchnic nerves (cut)

盆内脏神经（切断）
Pelvic splanchnic nerves (cut)

肛提肌神经（切断）
Nerve to levator ani (cut)

股方肌神经（虚影）
Nerve to quadratus femoris
(ghosted)

阴部神经：
Pudendal nerve:

直肠下神经（切断）
Inferior rectal nerve (cut)

坐骨神经（切断）：
Sciatic nerve (cut):

腓总神经
Common fibular division

胫神经
Tibial division

阴茎（蒂）背神经（切断）
Dorsal nerve of penis/clitoris (cut)

会阴神经（切断）
Perineal nerve (cut)

股后皮神经（切断）
Posterior femoral
cutaneous nerve (cut)

图 6-22 　盆腔自主神经 **Autonomic Nerves of the Pelvis**

A. 女性
Female

交感干
Sympathetic trunk

腰内脏神经
Lumbar splanchnic nerve

上腹下丛
Superior hypogastric plexus

起于下腹下丛分布于乙状结
肠和降结肠的神经（副交感）
Nerve from inferior hypogastric
plexus to sigmoid colon and
descending colon (parasympathetic)

S1 腹侧支（切断）
S1 ventral ramus (cut)

腹下神经
Hypogastric nerves

灰交通支
Gray ramus communicans

盆内脏神经
Pelvic splanchnic nerves

骶内脏神经
Sacral splanchnic nerves

下腹下丛
Inferior hypogastric plexus

子宫阴道丛
Uterovaginal plexus

阴部神经（S2～S4，躯体
神经，非自主神经）
Pudendal nerve
(S2~S4, somatic nerve,
not autonomic)

直肠下神经
Inferior rectal nerve

膀胱丛
Vesical plexus

阴蒂背神经
Dorsal nerve of clitoris

海绵体神经（切断）
Cavernous nerves (cut)

阴唇后神经（切断）
Posterior labial nerve (cut)

B. 男性
Male

上腹下丛
Superior hypogastric plexus

腹下神经
Hypogastric nerves

起于下腹下丛分布于乙状结
肠和降结肠的神经（副交感）
Nerve from inferior hypogastric plexus
to sigmoid colon and descending colon
(parasympathetic)

输精管（切断）和输精管丛
Ductus deferens (cut)
and plexus

膀胱丛
Vesical plexus

前列腺丛
Prostatic plexus

阴茎海绵体神经
Cavernous nerves of penis

腰内脏神经
Lumbar splanchnic nerve

L5 腹侧支（切断）
L5 ventral ramus (cut)

灰交通支
Gray rami communicantes

S1 腹侧支（切断）
S1 ventral ramus (cut)

交感干和神经节
Sympathetic trunk and ganglia

盆内脏神经
Pelvic splanchnic nerves

骶内脏神经
Sacral splanchnic nerves

下腹下（盆）丛
Inferior hypogastric (pelvic) plexus

直肠丛
Rectal plexus

阴部神经（S2～S4，躯体神经，
非自主神经）
Pudendal nerve
(S2~S4, somatic nerve, not autonomic)

直肠下神经
Inferior rectal nerve

会阴神经
Perineal nerve

肛提肌（切断）
Levator ani muscle (cut)

阴茎背神经
Dorsal nerve of penis

阴囊后神经
Posterior scrotal nerve

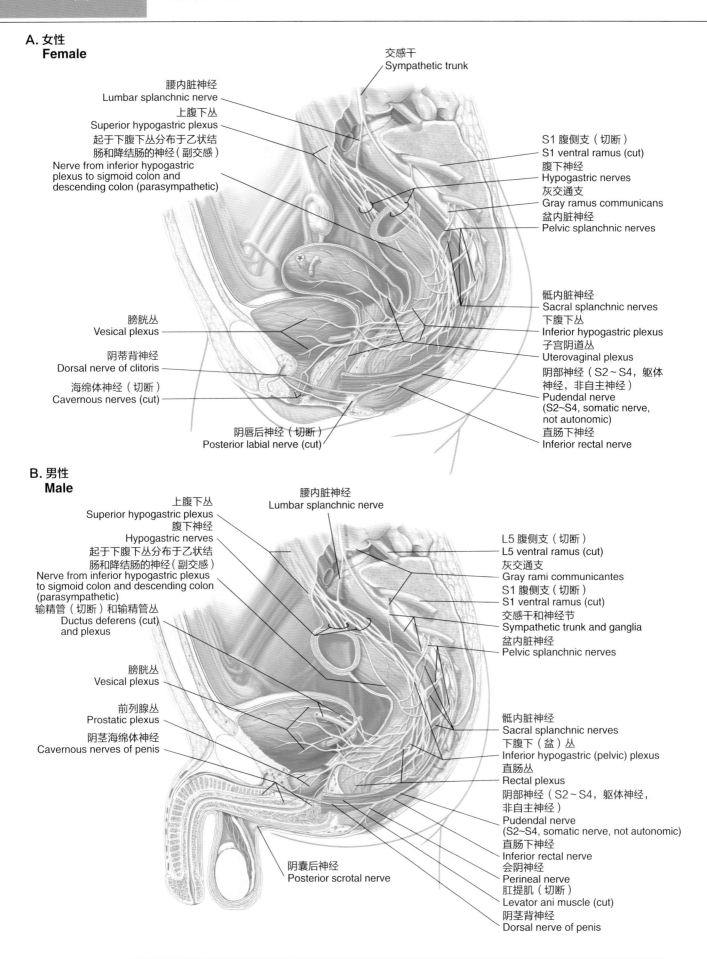

A. 女性
Female

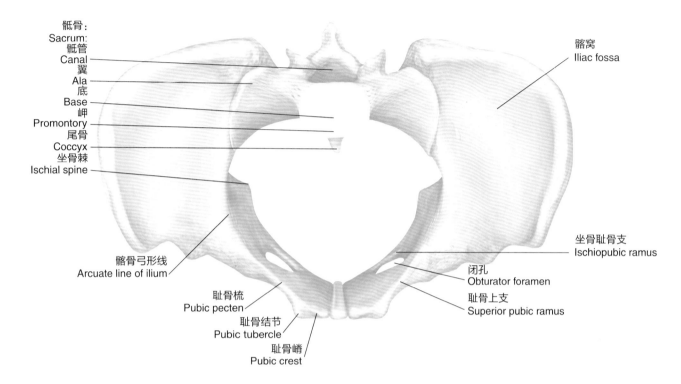

骶骨：
Sacrum:
骶管
Canal
翼
Ala
底
Base
岬
Promontory
尾骨
Coccyx
坐骨棘
Ischial spine

髂窝
Iliac fossa

坐骨耻骨支
Ischiopubic ramus

闭孔
Obturator foramen

耻骨上支
Superior pubic ramus

髂骨弓形线
Arcuate line of ilium

耻骨梳
Pubic pecten

耻骨结节
Pubic tubercle

耻骨嵴
Pubic crest

B. 男性
Male

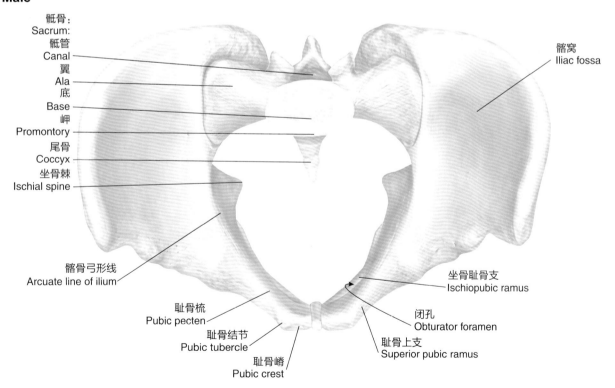

骶骨：
Sacrum:
骶管
Canal
翼
Ala
底
Base
岬
Promontory
尾骨
Coccyx
坐骨棘
Ischial spine

髂窝
Iliac fossa

坐骨耻骨支
Ischiopubic ramus

闭孔
Obturator foramen

耻骨上支
Superior pubic ramus

髂骨弓形线
Arcuate line of ilium

耻骨梳
Pubic pecten

耻骨结节
Pubic tubercle

耻骨嵴
Pubic crest

图 6-24 盆膈，上面观 Pelvic Diaphragm, Superior View

A. 女性
Female

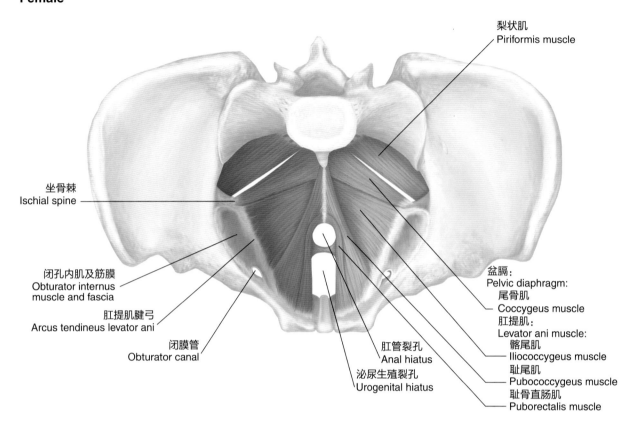

梨状肌
Piriformis muscle

坐骨棘
Ischial spine

闭孔内肌及筋膜
Obturator internus
muscle and fascia

肛提肌腱弓
Arcus tendineus levator ani

闭膜管
Obturator canal

肛管裂孔
Anal hiatus

泌尿生殖裂孔
Urogenital hiatus

盆膈：
Pelvic diaphragm:
尾骨肌
Coccygeus muscle
肛提肌：
Levator ani muscle:
髂尾肌
Iliococcygeus muscle
耻尾肌
Pubococcygeus muscle
耻骨直肠肌
Puborectalis muscle

B. 男性
Male

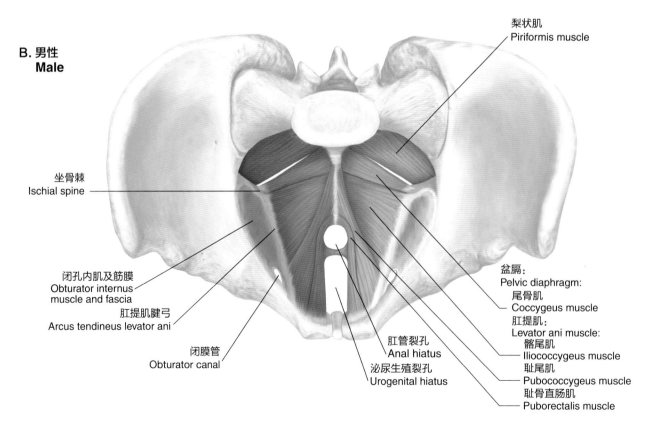

梨状肌
Piriformis muscle

坐骨棘
Ischial spine

闭孔内肌及筋膜
Obturator internus
muscle and fascia

肛提肌腱弓
Arcus tendineus levator ani

闭膜管
Obturator canal

肛管裂孔
Anal hiatus

泌尿生殖裂孔
Urogenital hiatus

盆膈：
Pelvic diaphragm:
尾骨肌
Coccygeus muscle
肛提肌：
Levator ani muscle:
髂尾肌
Iliococcygeus muscle
耻尾肌
Pubococcygeus muscle
耻骨直肠肌
Puborectalis muscle

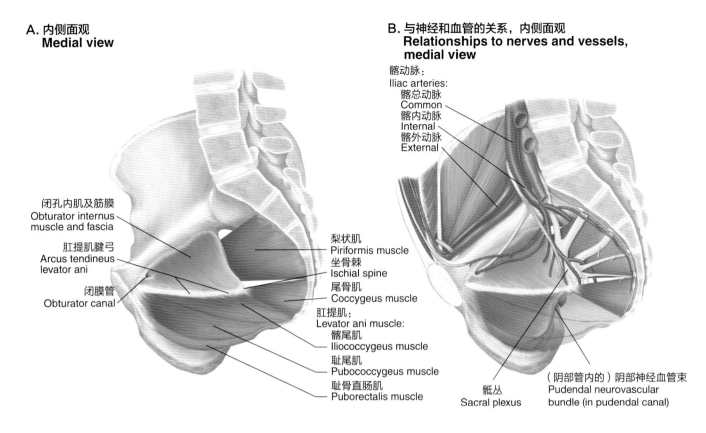

A. 内侧面观
Medial view

闭孔内肌及筋膜
Obturator internus
muscle and fascia

肛提肌腱弓
Arcus tendineus
levator ani

闭膜管
Obturator canal

梨状肌
Piriformis muscle

坐骨棘
Ischial spine

尾骨肌
Coccygeus muscle

肛提肌：
Levator ani muscle:

髂尾肌
Iliococcygeus muscle

耻尾肌
Pubococcygeus muscle

耻骨直肠肌
Puborectalis muscle

B. 与神经和血管的关系，内侧面观
**Relationships to nerves and vessels,
medial view**

髂动脉：
Iliac arteries:
　髂总动脉
　Common
　髂内动脉
　Internal
　髂外动脉
　External

骶丛
Sacral plexus

（阴部管内的）阴部神经血管束
Pudendal neurovascular
bundle (in pudendal canal)

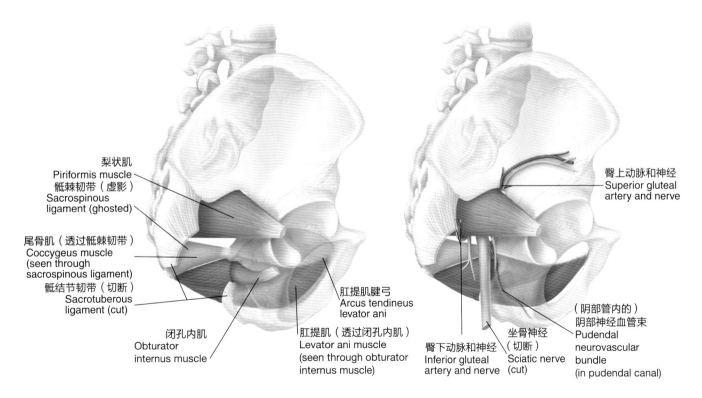

C. 外侧面观
Lateral view

梨状肌
Piriformis muscle

骶棘韧带（虚影）
Sacrospinous
ligament (ghosted)

尾骨肌（透过骶棘韧带）
Coccygeus muscle
(seen through
sacrospinous ligament)

骶结节韧带（切断）
Sacrotuberous
ligament (cut)

闭孔内肌
Obturator
internus muscle

肛提肌腱弓
Arcus tendineus
levator ani

肛提肌（透过闭孔内肌）
Levator ani muscle
(seen through obturator
internus muscle)

D. 与神经和血管的关系，外侧面观
**Relationships to nerves and vessels,
lateral view**

臀上动脉和神经
Superior gluteal
artery and nerve

臀下动脉和神经
Inferior gluteal
artery and nerve

坐骨神经
（切断）
Sciatic nerve
(cut)

（阴部管内的）
阴部神经血管束
Pudendal
neurovascular
bundle
(in pudendal canal)

图 6-26　盆膈，下面观　Pelvic Diaphragm, Inferior View

A. 女性
Female

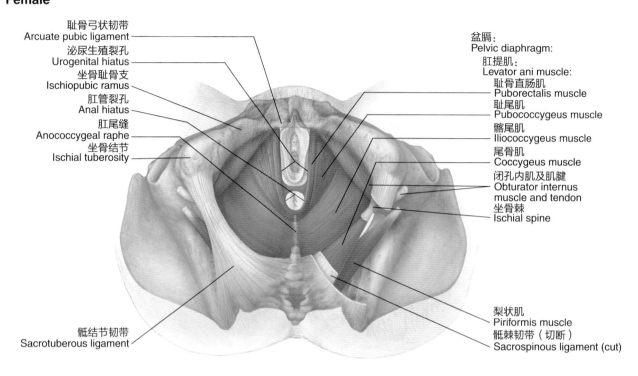

耻骨弓状韧带
Arcuate pubic ligament

泌尿生殖裂孔
Urogenital hiatus

坐骨耻骨支
Ischiopubic ramus

肛管裂孔
Anal hiatus

肛尾缝
Anococcygeal raphe

坐骨结节
Ischial tuberosity

骶结节韧带
Sacrotuberous ligament

盆膈：
Pelvic diaphragm:
肛提肌：
Levator ani muscle:
耻骨直肠肌
Puborectalis muscle
耻尾肌
Pubococcygeus muscle
髂尾肌
Iliococcygeus muscle
尾骨肌
Coccygeus muscle
闭孔内肌及肌腱
Obturator internus muscle and tendon
坐骨棘
Ischial spine

梨状肌
Piriformis muscle
骶棘韧带（切断）
Sacrospinous ligament (cut)

B. 男性
Male

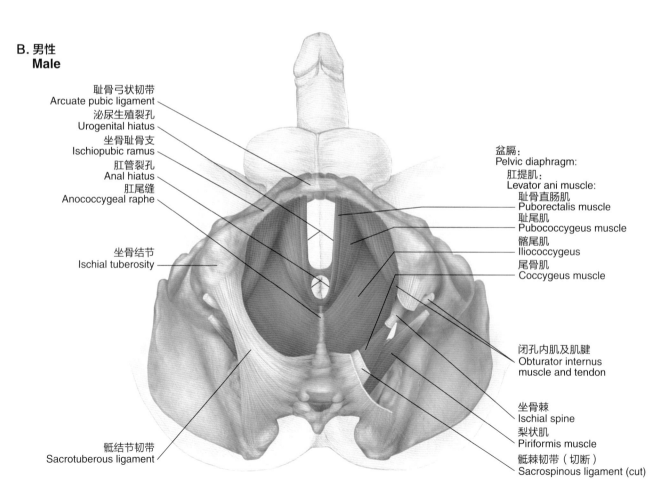

耻骨弓状韧带
Arcuate pubic ligament

泌尿生殖裂孔
Urogenital hiatus

坐骨耻骨支
Ischiopubic ramus

肛管裂孔
Anal hiatus

肛尾缝
Anococcygeal raphe

坐骨结节
Ischial tuberosity

骶结节韧带
Sacrotuberous ligament

盆膈：
Pelvic diaphragm:
肛提肌：
Levator ani muscle:
耻骨直肠肌
Puborectalis muscle
耻尾肌
Pubococcygeus muscle
髂尾肌
Iliococcygeus
尾骨肌
Coccygeus muscle

闭孔内肌及肌腱
Obturator internus muscle and tendon

坐骨棘
Ischial spine
梨状肌
Piriformis muscle
骶棘韧带（切断）
Sacrospinous ligament (cut)

A. 女性 Female

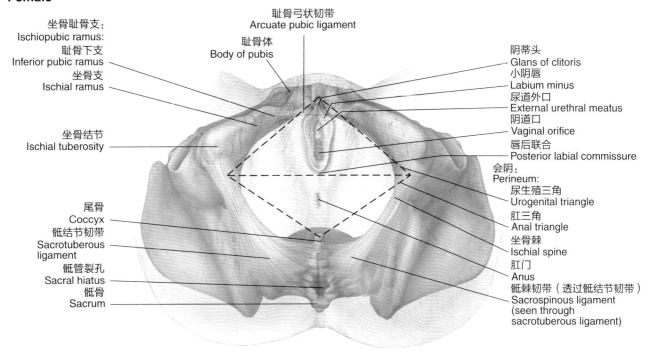

坐骨耻骨支：
Ischiopubic ramus:
耻骨下支
Inferior pubic ramus
坐骨支
Ischial ramus

耻骨弓状韧带
Arcuate pubic ligament

耻骨体
Body of pubis

阴蒂头
Glans of clitoris

小阴唇
Labium minus

尿道外口
External urethral meatus

阴道口
Vaginal orifice

唇后联合
Posterior labial commissure

坐骨结节
Ischial tuberosity

会阴：
Perineum:

尿生殖三角
Urogenital triangle

肛三角
Anal triangle

坐骨棘
Ischial spine

肛门
Anus

骶棘韧带（透过骶结节韧带）
Sacrospinous ligament
(seen through
sacrotuberous ligament)

尾骨
Coccyx

骶结节韧带
Sacrotuberous
ligament

骶管裂孔
Sacral hiatus

骶骨
Sacrum

B. 男性 Male

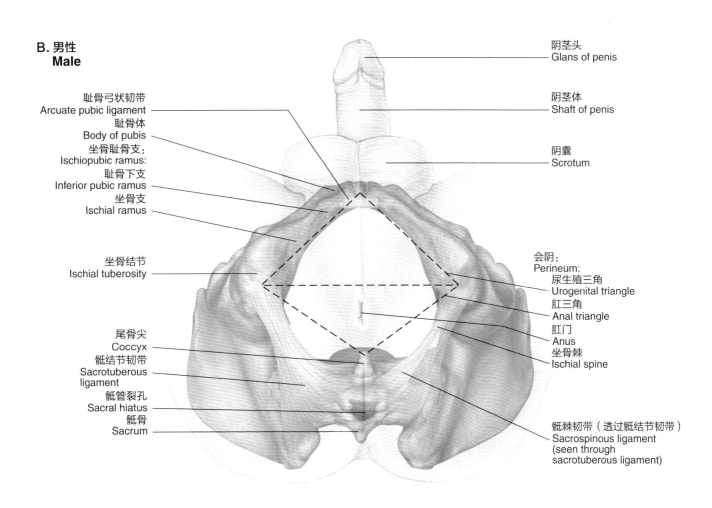

耻骨弓状韧带
Arcuate pubic ligament

耻骨体
Body of pubis

坐骨耻骨支：
Ischiopubic ramus:

耻骨下支
Inferior pubic ramus

坐骨支
Ischial ramus

阴茎头
Glans of penis

阴茎体
Shaft of penis

阴囊
Scrotum

坐骨结节
Ischial tuberosity

会阴：
Perineum:

尿生殖三角
Urogenital triangle

肛三角
Anal triangle

肛门
Anus

坐骨棘
Ischial spine

尾骨尖
Coccyx

骶结节韧带
Sacrotuberous
ligament

骶管裂孔
Sacral hiatus

骶骨
Sacrum

骶棘韧带（透过骶结节韧带）
Sacrospinous ligament
(seen through
sacrotuberous ligament)

图 6-28　会阴，表面解剖　Perineum, Surface Anatomy

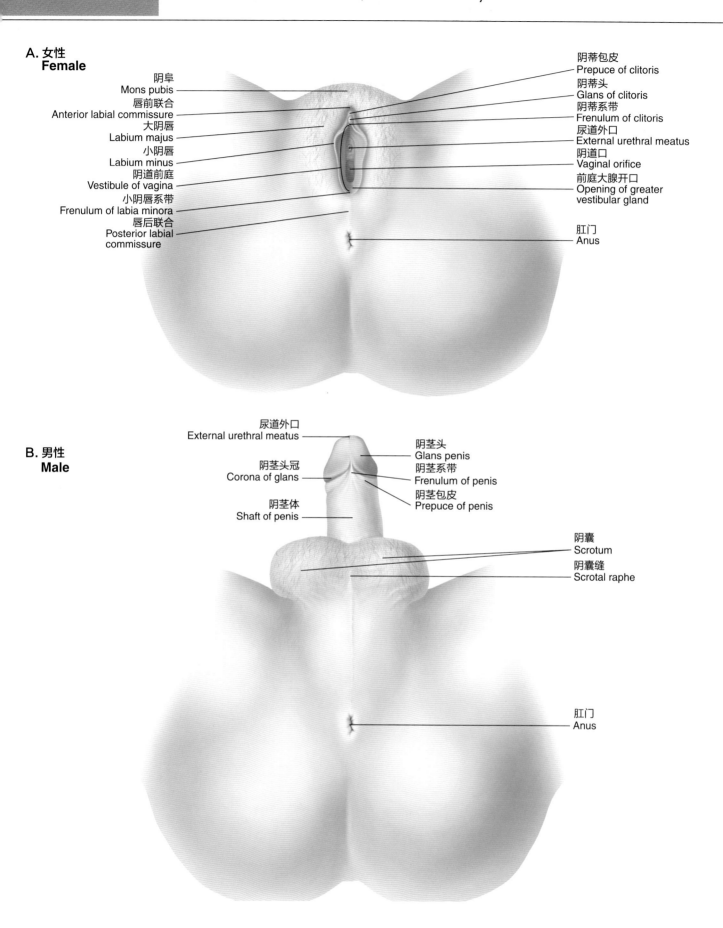

A. 女性
Female

阴阜
Mons pubis

唇前联合
Anterior labial commissure

大阴唇
Labium majus

小阴唇
Labium minus

阴道前庭
Vestibule of vagina

小阴唇系带
Frenulum of labia minora

唇后联合
Posterior labial commissure

阴蒂包皮
Prepuce of clitoris

阴蒂头
Glans of clitoris

阴蒂系带
Frenulum of clitoris

尿道外口
External urethral meatus

阴道口
Vaginal orifice

前庭大腺开口
Opening of greater vestibular gland

肛门
Anus

B. 男性
Male

尿道外口
External urethral meatus

阴茎头冠
Corona of glans

阴茎体
Shaft of penis

阴茎头
Glans penis

阴茎系带
Frenulum of penis

阴茎包皮
Prepuce of penis

阴囊
Scrotum

阴囊缝
Scrotal raphe

肛门
Anus

A. 女性
Female

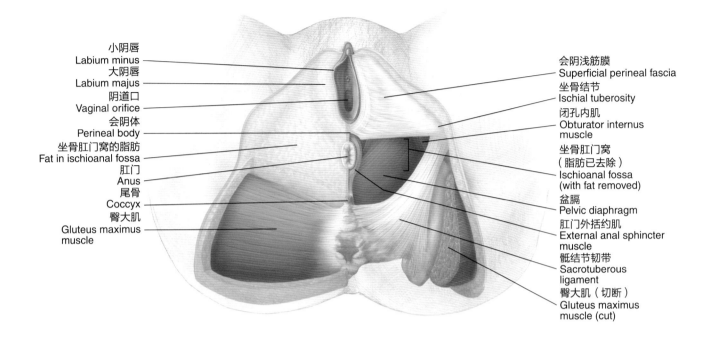

小阴唇
Labium minus

大阴唇
Labium majus

阴道口
Vaginal orifice

会阴体
Perineal body

坐骨肛门窝的脂肪
Fat in ischioanal fossa

肛门
Anus

尾骨
Coccyx

臀大肌
Gluteus maximus
muscle

会阴浅筋膜
Superficial perineal fascia

坐骨结节
Ischial tuberosity

闭孔内肌
Obturator internus
muscle

坐骨肛门窝
（脂肪已去除）
Ischioanal fossa
(with fat removed)

盆膈
Pelvic diaphragm

肛门外括约肌
External anal sphincter
muscle

骶结节韧带
Sacrotuberous
ligament

臀大肌（切断）
Gluteus maximus
muscle (cut)

B. 男性
Male

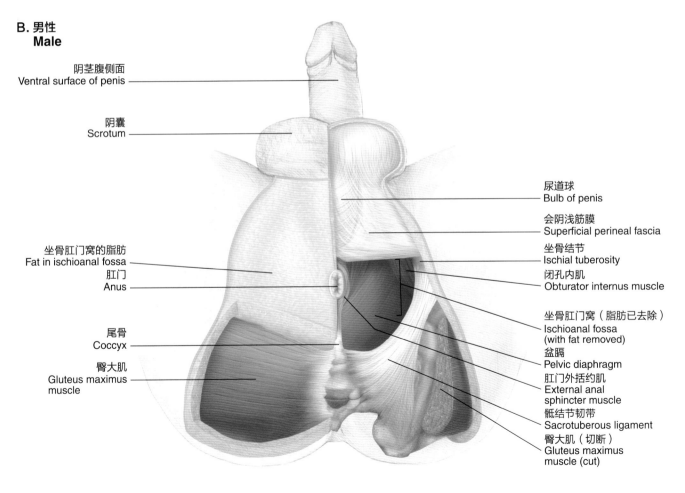

阴茎腹侧面
Ventral surface of penis

阴囊
Scrotum

坐骨肛门窝的脂肪
Fat in ischioanal fossa

肛门
Anus

尾骨
Coccyx

臀大肌
Gluteus maximus
muscle

尿道球
Bulb of penis

会阴浅筋膜
Superficial perineal fascia

坐骨结节
Ischial tuberosity

闭孔内肌
Obturator internus muscle

坐骨肛门窝（脂肪已去除）
Ischioanal fossa
(with fat removed)

盆膈
Pelvic diaphragm

肛门外括约肌
External anal
sphincter muscle

骶结节韧带
Sacrotuberous ligament

臀大肌（切断）
Gluteus maximus
muscle (cut)

图 6-30　会阴，中层解剖　Perineum, Intermediate Dissection

A. 女性
Female

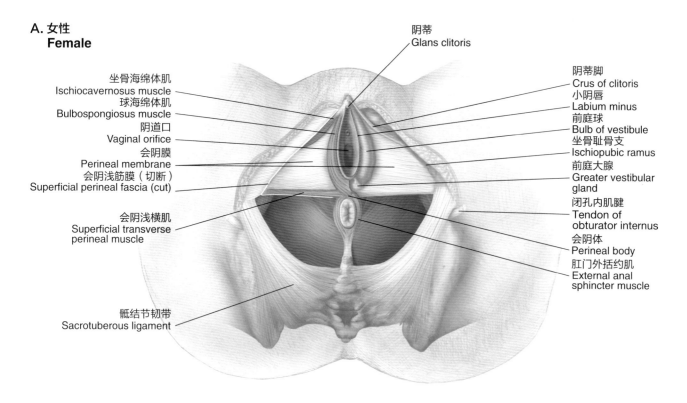

阴蒂
Glans clitoris

坐骨海绵体肌
Ischiocavernosus muscle

球海绵体肌
Bulbospongiosus muscle

阴道口
Vaginal orifice

会阴膜
Perineal membrane

会阴浅筋膜（切断）
Superficial perineal fascia (cut)

会阴浅横肌
Superficial transverse perineal muscle

骶结节韧带
Sacrotuberous ligament

阴蒂脚
Crus of clitoris

小阴唇
Labium minus

前庭球
Bulb of vestibule

坐骨耻骨支
Ischiopubic ramus

前庭大腺
Greater vestibular gland

闭孔内肌腱
Tendon of obturator internus

会阴体
Perineal body

肛门外括约肌
External anal sphincter muscle

B. 男性
Male

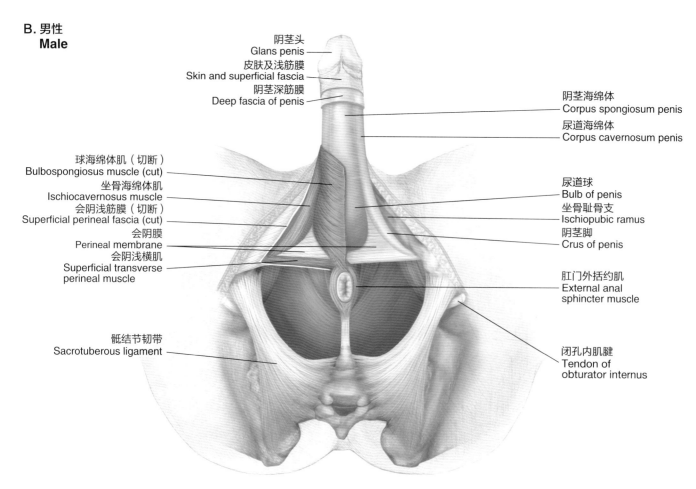

阴茎头
Glans penis

皮肤及浅筋膜
Skin and superficial fascia

阴茎深筋膜
Deep fascia of penis

球海绵体肌（切断）
Bulbospongiosus muscle (cut)

坐骨海绵体肌
Ischiocavernosus muscle

会阴浅筋膜（切断）
Superficial perineal fascia (cut)

会阴膜
Perineal membrane

会阴浅横肌
Superficial transverse perineal muscle

骶结节韧带
Sacrotuberous ligament

阴茎海绵体
Corpus spongiosum penis

尿道海绵体
Corpus cavernosum penis

尿道球
Bulb of penis

坐骨耻骨支
Ischiopubic ramus

阴茎脚
Crus of penis

肛门外括约肌
External anal sphincter muscle

闭孔内肌腱
Tendon of obturator internus

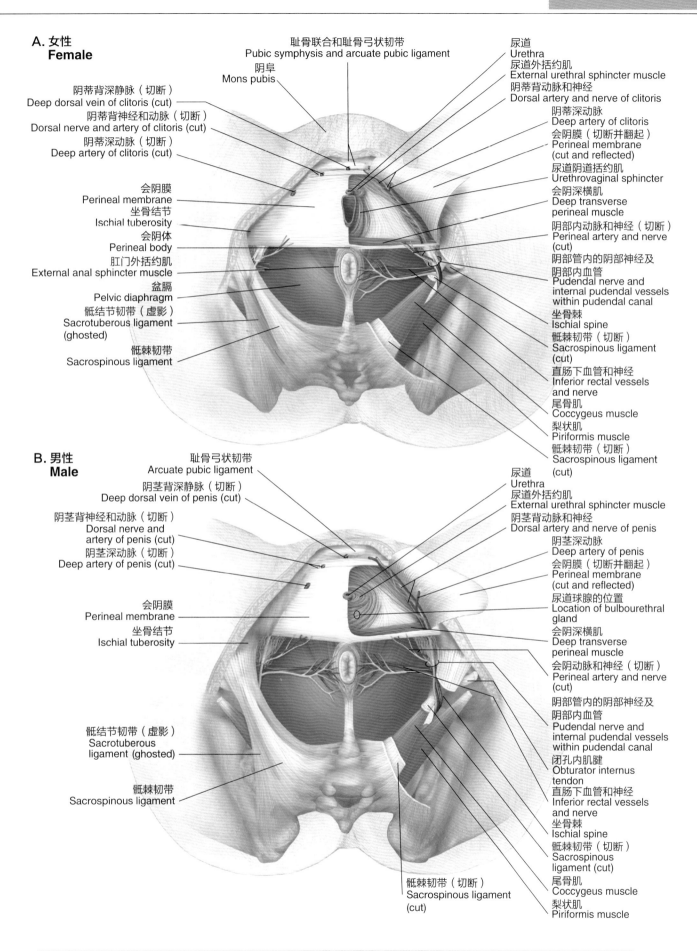

A. 女性
Female

耻骨联合和耻骨弓状韧带
Pubic symphysis and arcuate pubic ligament

阴阜
Mons pubis

阴蒂背深静脉（切断）
Deep dorsal vein of clitoris (cut)

阴蒂背神经和动脉（切断）
Dorsal nerve and artery of clitoris (cut)

阴蒂深动脉（切断）
Deep artery of clitoris (cut)

会阴膜
Perineal membrane

坐骨结节
Ischial tuberosity

会阴体
Perineal body

肛门外括约肌
External anal sphincter muscle

盆膈
Pelvic diaphragm

骶结节韧带（虚影）
Sacrotuberous ligament
(ghosted)

骶棘韧带
Sacrospinous ligament

尿道
Urethra

尿道外括约肌
External urethral sphincter muscle

阴蒂背动脉和神经
Dorsal artery and nerve of clitoris

阴蒂深动脉
Deep artery of clitoris

会阴膜（切断并翻起）
Perineal membrane
(cut and reflected)

尿道阴道括约肌
Urethrovaginal sphincter

会阴深横肌
Deep transverse
perineal muscle

阴部内动脉和神经（切断）
Perineal artery and nerve
(cut)

阴部管内的阴部神经及
阴部内血管
Pudendal nerve and
internal pudendal vessels
within pudendal canal

坐骨棘
Ischial spine

骶棘韧带（切断）
Sacrospinous ligament
(cut)

直肠下血管和神经
Inferior rectal vessels
and nerve

尾骨肌
Coccygeus muscle

梨状肌
Piriformis muscle

骶棘韧带（切断）
Sacrospinous ligament
(cut)

B. 男性
Male

耻骨弓状韧带
Arcuate pubic ligament

阴茎背深静脉（切断）
Deep dorsal vein of penis (cut)

阴茎背神经和动脉（切断）
Dorsal nerve and
artery of penis (cut)

阴茎深动脉（切断）
Deep artery of penis (cut)

会阴膜
Perineal membrane

坐骨结节
Ischial tuberosity

骶结节韧带（虚影）
Sacrotuberous
ligament (ghosted)

骶棘韧带
Sacrospinous ligament

尿道
Urethra

尿道外括约肌
External urethral sphincter muscle

阴茎背动脉和神经
Dorsal artery and nerve of penis

阴茎深动脉
Deep artery of penis

会阴膜（切断并翻起）
Perineal membrane
(cut and reflected)

尿道球腺的位置
Location of bulbourethral
gland

会阴深横肌
Deep transverse
perineal muscle

会阴动脉和神经（切断）
Perineal artery and nerve
(cut)

阴部管内的阴部神经及
阴部内血管
Pudendal nerve and
internal pudendal vessels
within pudendal canal

闭孔内肌腱
Obturator internus
tendon

直肠下血管和神经
Inferior rectal vessels
and nerve

坐骨棘
Ischial spine

骶棘韧带（切断）
Sacrospinous
ligament (cut)

尾骨肌
Coccygeus muscle

梨状肌
Piriformis muscle

图 6-32 **会阴的动脉 Arteries of the Perineum**

A. 女性
Female

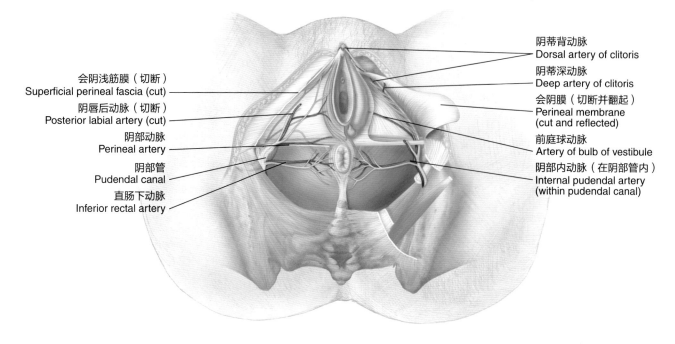

阴蒂背动脉
Dorsal artery of clitoris

会阴浅筋膜（切断）
Superficial perineal fascia (cut)

阴蒂深动脉
Deep artery of clitoris

阴唇后动脉（切断）
Posterior labial artery (cut)

会阴膜（切断并翻起）
Perineal membrane
(cut and reflected)

阴部动脉
Perineal artery

前庭球动脉
Artery of bulb of vestibule

阴部管
Pudendal canal

阴部内动脉（在阴部管内）
Internal pudendal artery
(within pudendal canal)

直肠下动脉
Inferior rectal artery

B. 男性
Male

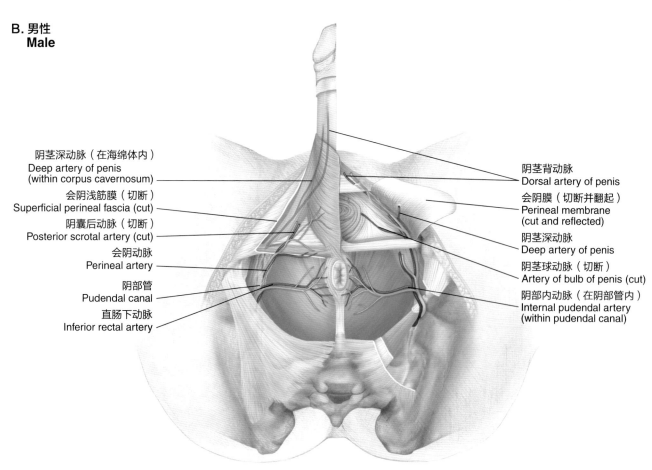

阴茎深动脉（在海绵体内）
Deep artery of penis
(within corpus cavernosum)

阴茎背动脉
Dorsal artery of penis

会阴浅筋膜（切断）
Superficial perineal fascia (cut)

会阴膜（切断并翻起）
Perineal membrane
(cut and reflected)

阴囊后动脉（切断）
Posterior scrotal artery (cut)

阴茎深动脉
Deep artery of penis

会阴动脉
Perineal artery

阴茎球动脉（切断）
Artery of bulb of penis (cut)

阴部管
Pudendal canal

阴部内动脉（在阴部管内）
Internal pudendal artery
(within pudendal canal)

直肠下动脉
Inferior rectal artery

A. 女性
Female

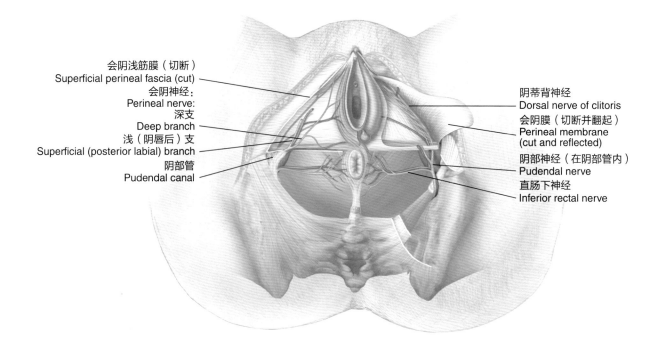

会阴浅筋膜（切断）
Superficial perineal fascia (cut)
会阴神经：
Perineal nerve:
深支
Deep branch
浅（阴唇后）支
Superficial (posterior labial) branch
阴部管
Pudendal canal

阴蒂背神经
Dorsal nerve of clitoris
会阴膜（切断并翻起）
Perineal membrane
(cut and reflected)
阴部神经（在阴部管内）
Pudendal nerve
直肠下神经
Inferior rectal nerve

B. 男性
Male

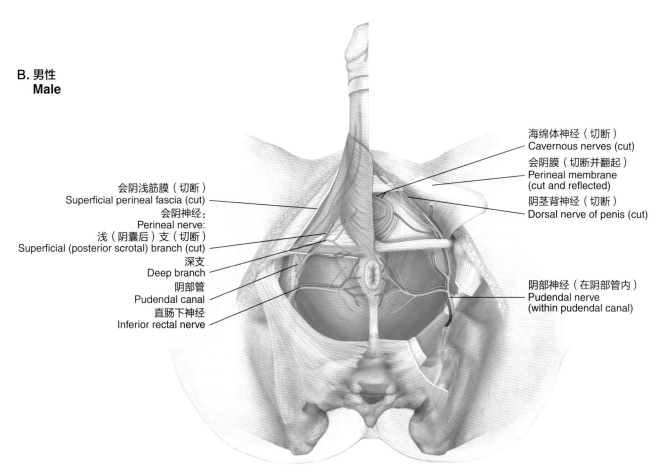

会阴浅筋膜（切断）
Superficial perineal fascia (cut)
会阴神经：
Perineal nerve:
浅（阴囊后）支（切断）
Superficial (posterior scrotal) branch (cut)
深支
Deep branch
阴部管
Pudendal canal
直肠下神经
Inferior rectal nerve

海绵体神经（切断）
Cavernous nerves (cut)
会阴膜（切断并翻起）
Perineal membrane
(cut and reflected)
阴茎背神经（切断）
Dorsal nerve of penis (cut)
阴部神经（在阴部管内）
Pudendal nerve
(within pudendal canal)

图 6-34　阴茎与睾丸　Penis and Testis

A. 前面观
Anterior view

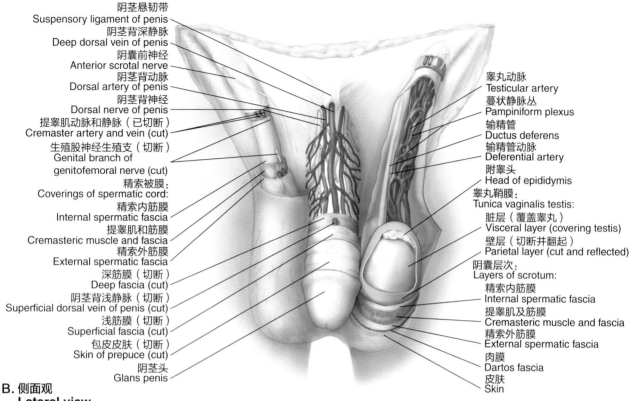

阴茎悬韧带
Suspensory ligament of penis

阴茎背深静脉
Deep dorsal vein of penis

阴囊前神经
Anterior scrotal nerve

阴茎背动脉
Dorsal artery of penis

阴茎背神经
Dorsal nerve of penis

提睾肌动脉和静脉（已切断）
Cremaster artery and vein (cut)

生殖股神经生殖支（切断）
Genital branch of
genitofemoral nerve (cut)

精索被膜：
Coverings of spermatic cord:

精索内筋膜
Internal spermatic fascia

提睾肌和筋膜
Cremasteric muscle and fascia

精索外筋膜
External spermatic fascia

深筋膜（切断）
Deep fascia (cut)

阴茎背浅静脉（切断）
Superficial dorsal vein of penis (cut)

浅筋膜（切断）
Superficial fascia (cut)

包皮皮肤（切断）
Skin of prepuce (cut)

阴茎头
Glans penis

睾丸动脉
Testicular artery

蔓状静脉丛
Pampiniform plexus

输精管
Ductus deferens

输精管动脉
Deferential artery

附睾头
Head of epididymis

睾丸鞘膜：
Tunica vaginalis testis:

脏层（覆盖睾丸）
Visceral layer (covering testis)

壁层（切断并翻起）
Parietal layer (cut and reflected)

阴囊层次：
Layers of scrotum:

精索内筋膜
Internal spermatic fascia

提睾肌及筋膜
Cremasteric muscle and fascia

精索外筋膜
External spermatic fascia

肉膜
Dartos fascia

皮肤
Skin

B. 侧面观
Lateral view

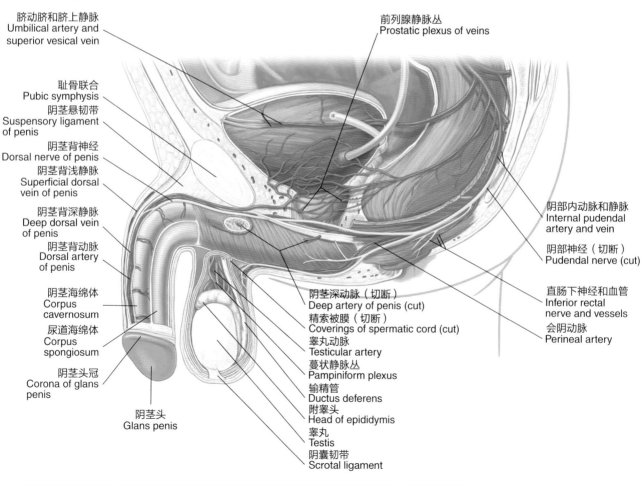

脐动脐和脐上静脉
Umbilical artery and
superior vesical vein

耻骨联合
Pubic symphysis

阴茎悬韧带
Suspensory ligament
of penis

阴茎背神经
Dorsal nerve of penis

阴茎背浅静脉
Superficial dorsal
vein of penis

阴茎背深静脉
Deep dorsal vein
of penis

阴茎背动脉
Dorsal artery
of penis

阴茎海绵体
Corpus
cavernosum

尿道海绵体
Corpus
spongiosum

阴茎头冠
Corona of glans
penis

阴茎头
Glans penis

前列腺静脉丛
Prostatic plexus of veins

阴部内动脉和静脉
Internal pudendal
artery and vein

阴部神经（切断）
Pudendal nerve (cut)

直肠下神经和血管
Inferior rectal
nerve and vessels

会阴动脉
Perineal artery

阴茎深动脉（切断）
Deep artery of penis (cut)

精索被膜（切断）
Coverings of spermatic cord (cut)

睾丸动脉
Testicular artery

蔓状静脉丛
Pampiniform plexus

输精管
Ductus deferens

附睾头
Head of epididymis

睾丸
Testis

阴囊韧带
Scrotal ligament

A. 定位
Orientation

图 B 所在平面
Plane of section B

B. 阴茎断面
Section through penis

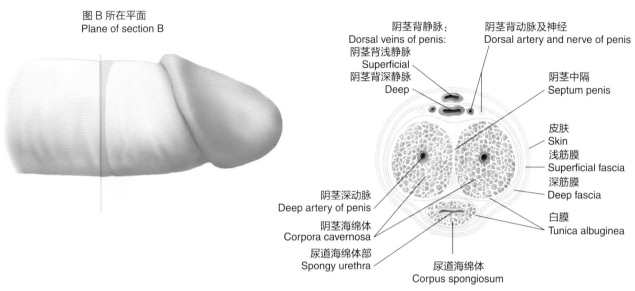

阴茎背静脉：
Dorsal veins of penis:
阴茎背浅静脉
Superficial
阴茎背深静脉
Deep

阴茎背动脉及神经
Dorsal artery and nerve of penis

阴茎中隔
Septum penis

皮肤
Skin
浅筋膜
Superficial fascia
深筋膜
Deep fascia

白膜
Tunica albuginea

阴茎深动脉
Deep artery of penis

阴茎海绵体
Corpora cavernosa

尿道海绵体部
Spongy urethra

尿道海绵体
Corpus spongiosum

C. 睾丸断面
Section through testis

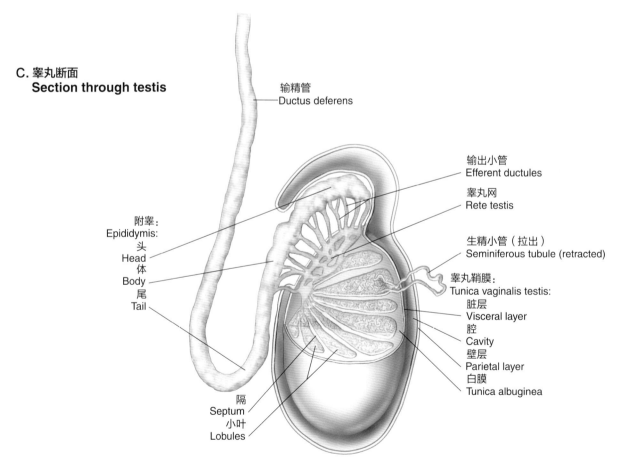

输精管
Ductus deferens

输出小管
Efferent ductules

睾丸网
Rete testis

生精小管（拉出）
Seminiferous tubule (retracted)

睾丸鞘膜：
Tunica vaginalis testis:
脏层
Visceral layer
腔
Cavity
壁层
Parietal layer
白膜
Tunica albuginea

附睾：
Epididymis:
头
Head
体
Body
尾
Tail

隔
Septum
小叶
Lobules

图 6-36　**女性盆腔与会阴部的淋巴　Lymphatics of the Pelvis and Perineum, Female**

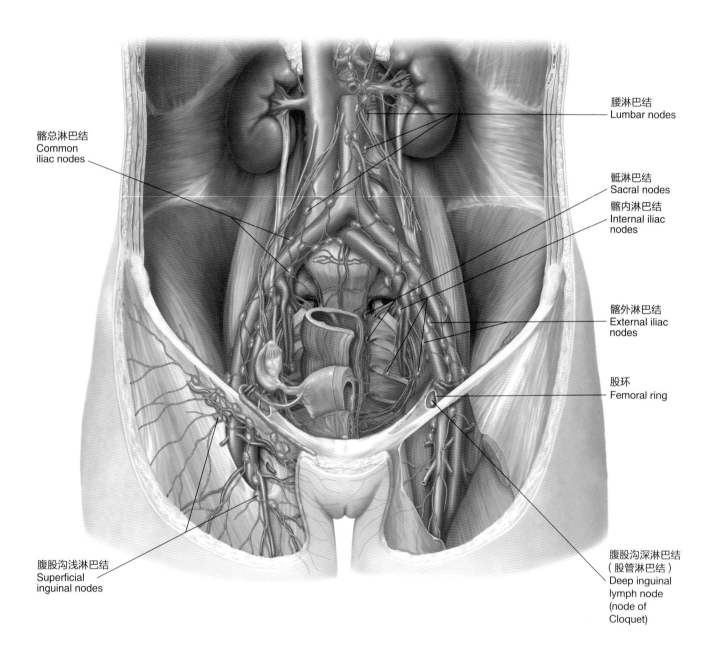

髂总淋巴结
Common
iliac nodes

腰淋巴结
Lumbar nodes

骶淋巴结
Sacral nodes

髂内淋巴结
Internal iliac
nodes

髂外淋巴结
External iliac
nodes

股环
Femoral ring

腹股沟深淋巴结
（股管淋巴结）
Deep inguinal
lymph node
(node of
Cloquet)

腹股沟浅淋巴结
Superficial
inguinal nodes

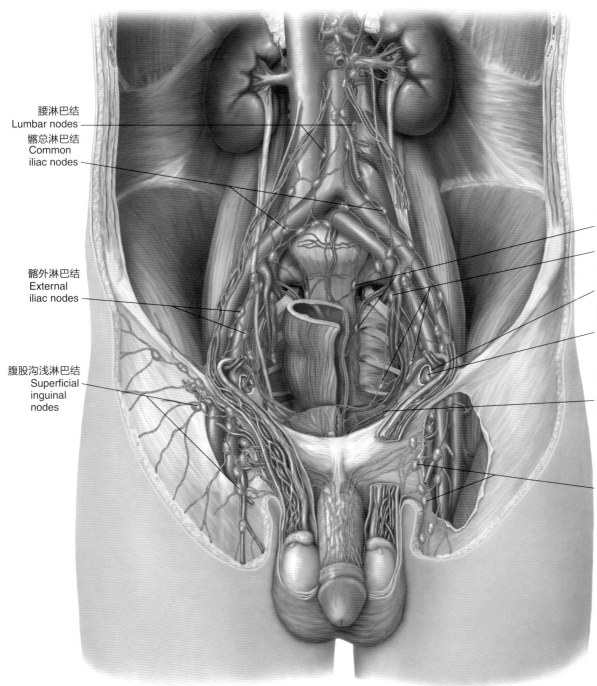

腰淋巴结
Lumbar nodes

髂总淋巴结
Common
iliac nodes

髂外淋巴结
External
iliac nodes

腹股沟浅淋巴结
Superficial
inguinal
nodes

骶淋巴结
Sacral nodes

髂内淋巴结
Internal iliac
nodes

股环
Femoral ring

腹股沟深淋巴结
（股管淋巴结）
Deep inguinal
lymph node
(node of Cloquet)

前列腺淋巴沿膀胱
下血管引流
Lymphatic
drainage
from prostate
follows inferior
vesical vessels

腹股沟浅淋巴结
Superficial
inguinal
nodes

图 6-38　　**女性骨盆的横断面　Cross Section of the Female Pelvis**

A. 定位
Orientation

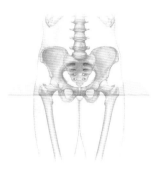

B. 横断面
Cross section

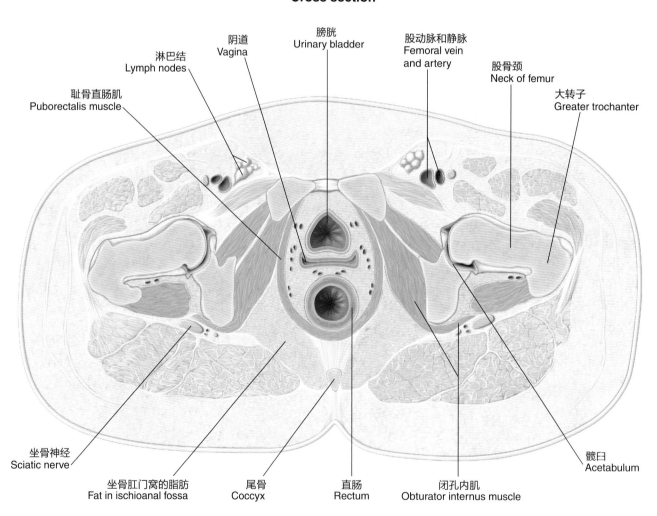

淋巴结
Lymph nodes

阴道
Vagina

膀胱
Urinary bladder

股动脉和静脉
Femoral vein
and artery

股骨颈
Neck of femur

耻骨直肠肌
Puborectalis muscle

大转子
Greater trochanter

坐骨神经
Sciatic nerve

坐骨肛门窝的脂肪
Fat in ischioanal fossa

尾骨
Coccyx

直肠
Rectum

闭孔内肌
Obturator internus muscle

髋臼
Acetabulum

A. 定位
Orientation

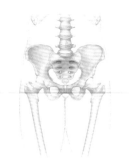

B. 横断面
Cross section

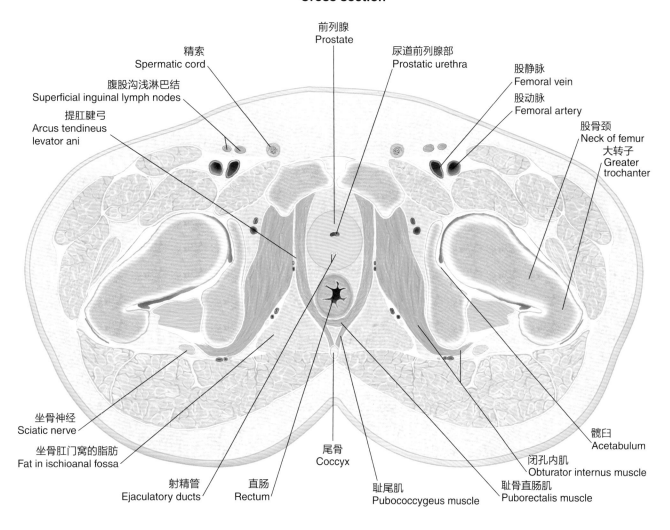

前列腺
Prostate

精索
Spermatic cord

尿道前列腺部
Prostatic urethra

股静脉
Femoral vein

腹股沟浅淋巴结
Superficial inguinal lymph nodes

股动脉
Femoral artery

提肛腱弓
Arcus tendineus
levator ani

股骨颈
Neck of femur

大转子
Greater
trochanter

坐骨神经
Sciatic nerve

髋臼
Acetabulum

坐骨肛门窝的脂肪
Fat in ischioanal fossa

闭孔内肌
Obturator internus muscle

射精管
Ejaculatory ducts

直肠
Rectum

尾骨
Coccyx

耻尾肌
Pubococcygeus muscle

耻骨直肠肌
Puborectalis muscle

盆部肌群

名称	起点	止点	主要作用	神经支配	动脉	注释
肛提肌 （图 6-15， 图 6-21 和 图 6-23）	耻骨体后面、闭孔内肌筋膜（肛提肌腱弓）、坐骨棘	肛尾缝和尾骨	上提盆底	S3~S4 脊神经的腹侧主支	臀下动脉	耻骨直肠肌、耻尾肌和髂尾肌组成肛提肌；尾骨肌和肛提肌共同组成盆膈
耻骨直肠肌 （图 6-15， 图 6-24， 图 6-25， 图 6-26， 图 6-38 和 图 6-39）	耻骨体后面	在直肠后方与对侧的耻骨直肠肌汇合	向前上方拉直肠远端；辅助控制排便	S3~S4 脊神经的腹侧主支	臀下动脉	耻骨直肠肌、耻尾肌和髂尾肌组成肛提肌
耻骨阴道肌	耻骨体后面	阴道筋膜和会阴体	向前上方拉阴道	S3~S4 脊神经的腹侧主支	臀下动脉	耻骨阴道肌是肛提肌的一部分
耻尾肌 （图 6-15， 图 6-24， 图 6-25， 图 6-26， 图 6-38 和 图 6-39）	耻骨上支后面	尾骨	上提盆底	S3~S4 脊神经的腹侧主支	臀下动脉	耻骨直肠肌、耻尾肌和髂尾肌组成肛提肌
髂尾肌 （图 6-15， 图 6-24 和 图 6-26）	肛提肌腱弓和坐骨棘	肛尾缝和尾骨	上提盆底	S3~S4 脊神经的腹侧主支	臀下动脉	耻骨直肠肌、耻尾肌和髂尾肌组成肛提肌
尾骨肌 （图 6-15， 图 6-24 和 图 6-26）	坐骨棘	尾骨侧面和骶骨下面	上提盆底	S3~S4 脊神经的腹侧主支	臀下动脉	尾骨肌和肛提肌构成盆膈
闭孔内肌 （图 3-13， 图 5-07， 图 6-14， 图 6-24 和 图 3-28）	闭孔膜内面和闭孔边缘	转子窝上方的大转子内面	外旋和外展大腿	闭孔内肌神经	闭孔动脉	闭孔内肌穿坐骨小孔离开骨盆；上孖肌和下孖肌附着于闭孔内肌腱上
梨状肌 （图 3-12， 图 6-24 和 图 6-26）	骶骨前面	股骨大转子上缘	外旋和外展大腿	S1~S2 脊神经腹侧支		梨状肌穿坐骨大孔离开骨盆
女性尿道括约肌 （图 6-08， 图 6-10 和 图 6-31）	环绕尿道	环绕尿道和阴道；沿尿道向上伸展直到膀胱下面	压迫尿道和阴道	阴部神经发出的会阴神经深支	阴部内动脉	属骨骼肌（名字"sphincter"来源于希腊语，意为紧密连接）
男性尿道括约肌 （图 6-08， 图 6-10 和 图 6-31）	环绕尿道	环绕尿道，连接前列腺侧面和膀胱下方	压迫尿道	阴部神经发出的会阴神经深支	阴部内动脉	属骨骼肌（名字"sphincter"来源于希腊语，意为紧密连接）

盆部肌群						
名称	起点	止点	主要作用	神经支配	动脉	注释
肛门外括约肌（图6-15和图6-30）	会阴体或会阴中心腱	环绕肛管；浅层肌纤维附着于尾骨	收缩肛管	直肠下神经（发自阴部神经）	直肠下动脉	属骨骼（随意）肌，相反，肛门内括约肌属于平滑（不随意）肌；肛门外括约肌属于盆膈的一部分
肛门内括约肌（图6-15）	环绕肛管	环绕肛管	收缩肛管	S4 的副交感神经	直肠中动脉	属平滑（不随意）肌，相反肛门外括约肌属于骨骼（随意）肌
女性的球海绵体肌（图6-30）	会阴体和前庭球的筋膜	会阴膜和阴蒂海绵体	压迫前庭球并收缩阴道口	阴部神经发出的会阴神经深支	会阴动脉	属骨骼肌
男性的球海绵体肌（图6-30）	会阴中心腱和尿道球中缝	会阴膜、阴茎海绵体背面、阴茎深筋膜	压迫尿道球，压迫尿道海绵体	阴部神经发出的会阴神经深支	会阴动脉	排空尿道最后几滴尿液；射精时排出精液
坐骨海绵体肌（图6-30）	坐骨结节内面和坐骨耻骨支	阴茎海绵体和阴茎 / 阴蒂脚	压迫阴茎海绵体	阴部神经发出的会阴神经深支	会阴动脉	坐骨海绵体肌紧贴阴茎 / 阴蒂脚表面

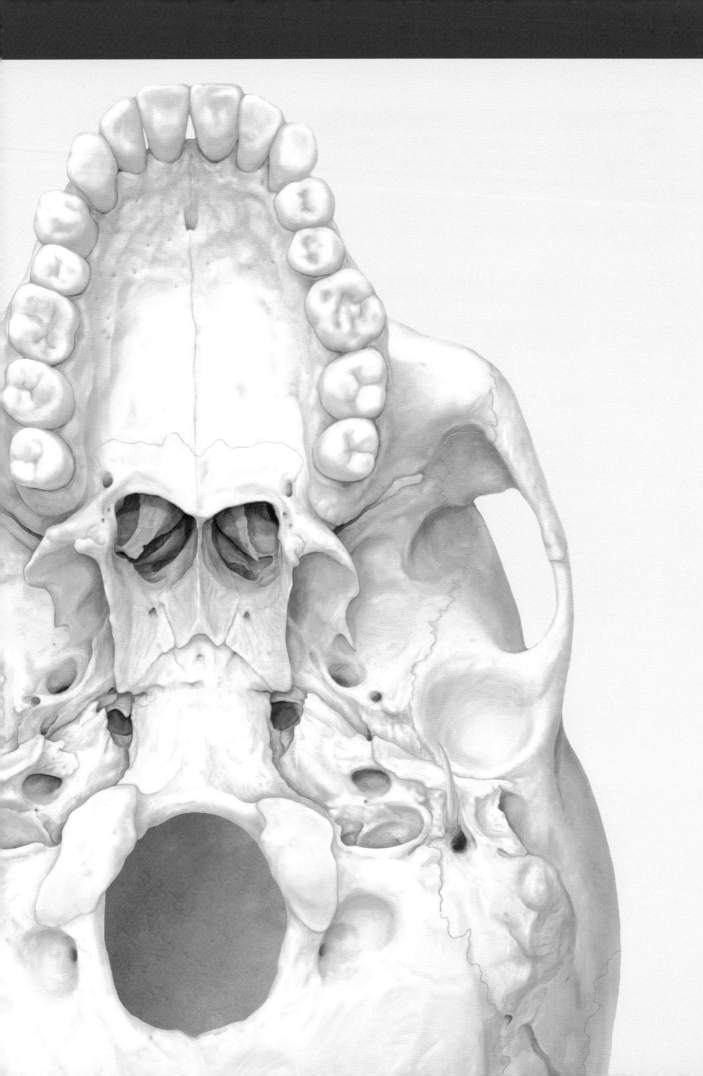

A. 解剖位置
Anatomic position

可触及的骨性结构
Palpable bony structures

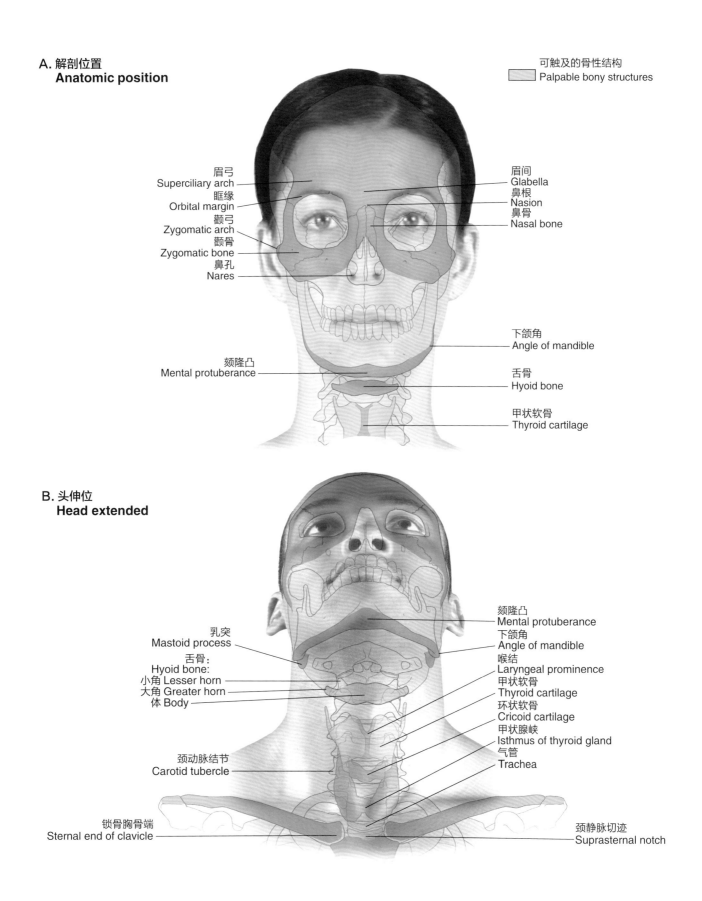

眉弓
Superciliary arch

眉间
Glabella

眶缘
Orbital margin

鼻根
Nasion

鼻骨
Nasal bone

颧弓
Zygomatic arch

颧骨
Zygomatic bone

鼻孔
Nares

下颌角
Angle of mandible

颏隆凸
Mental protuberance

舌骨
Hyoid bone

甲状软骨
Thyroid cartilage

B. 头伸位
Head extended

乳突
Mastoid process

颏隆凸
Mental protuberance

下颌角
Angle of mandible

喉结
Laryngeal prominence

舌骨：
Hyoid bone:

小角 Lesser horn

大角 Greater horn

体 Body

甲状软骨
Thyroid cartilage

环状软骨
Cricoid cartilage

甲状腺峡
Isthmus of thyroid gland

气管
Trachea

颈动脉结节
Carotid tubercle

锁骨胸骨端
Sternal end of clavicle

颈静脉切迹
Suprasternal notch

图 7-02　头部分区及颈部三角　Regions of the Head and Triangles of the Neck

A. 前面观
Anterior view

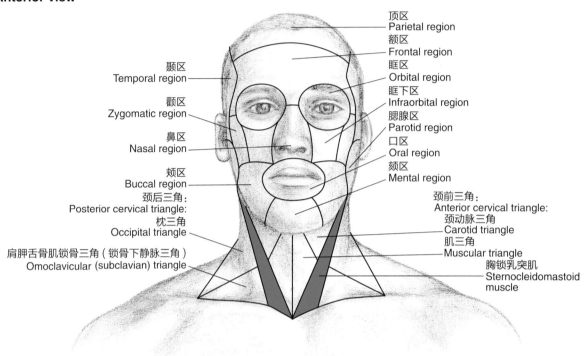

顶区
Parietal region

额区
Frontal region

眶区
Orbital region

眶下区
Infraorbital region

腮腺区
Parotid region

口区
Oral region

颏区
Mental region

颞区
Temporal region

颧区
Zygomatic region

鼻区
Nasal region

颊区
Buccal region

颈后三角：
Posterior cervical triangle:

枕三角
Occipital triangle

肩胛舌骨肌锁骨三角（锁骨下静脉三角）
Omoclavicular (subclavian) triangle

颈前三角：
Anterior cervical triangle:

颈动脉三角
Carotid triangle

肌三角
Muscular triangle

胸锁乳突肌
Sternocleidomastoid muscle

B. 侧面观
Lateral view

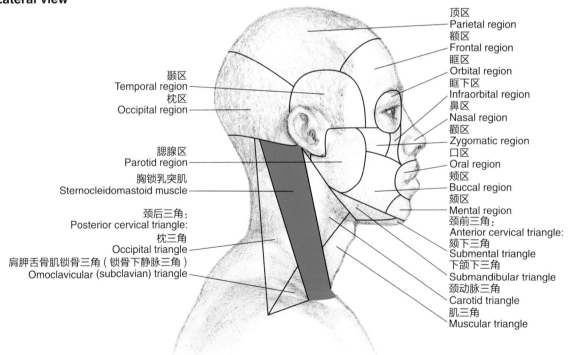

顶区
Parietal region

额区
Frontal region

眶区
Orbital region

眶下区
Infraorbital region

鼻区
Nasal region

颧区
Zygomatic region

口区
Oral region

颊区
Buccal region

颏区
Mental region

颈前三角：
Anterior cervical triangle:

颏下三角
Submental triangle

下颌下三角
Submandibular triangle

颈动脉三角
Carotid triangle

肌三角
Muscular triangle

颞区
Temporal region

枕区
Occipital region

腮腺区
Parotid region

胸锁乳突肌
Sternocleidomastoid muscle

颈后三角：
Posterior cervical triangle:

枕三角
Occipital triangle

肩胛舌骨肌锁骨三角（锁骨下静脉三角）
Omoclavicular (subclavian) triangle

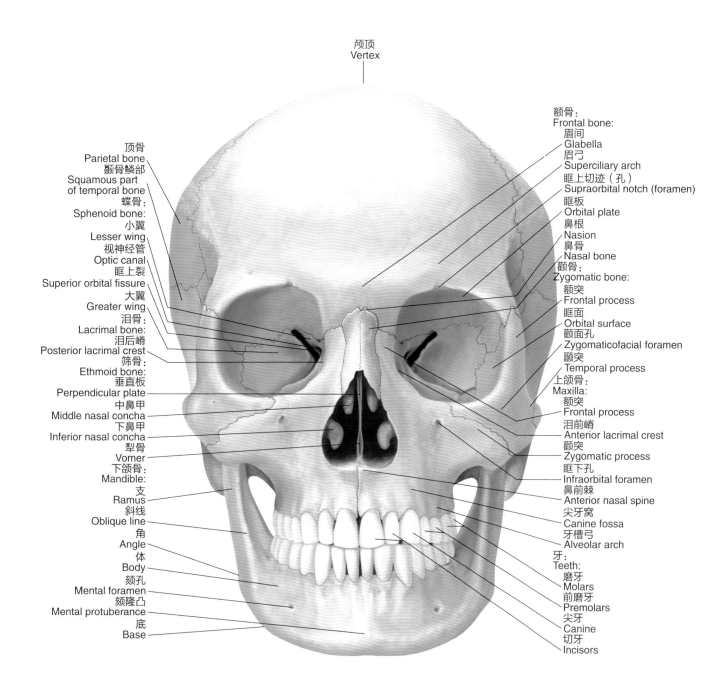

颅顶
Vertex

顶骨
Parietal bone
颞骨鳞部
Squamous part
of temporal bone
蝶骨：
Sphenoid bone:
小翼
Lesser wing
视神经管
Optic canal
眶上裂
Superior orbital fissure
大翼
Greater wing
泪骨：
Lacrimal bone:
泪后嵴
Posterior lacrimal crest
筛骨：
Ethmoid bone:
垂直板
Perpendicular plate
中鼻甲
Middle nasal concha
下鼻甲
Inferior nasal concha
犁骨
Vomer
下颌骨：
Mandible:
支
Ramus
斜线
Oblique line
角
Angle
体
Body
颏孔
Mental foramen
颏隆凸
Mental protuberance
底
Base

额骨：
Frontal bone:
眉间
Glabella
眉弓
Superciliary arch
眶上切迹（孔）
Supraorbital notch (foramen)
眶板
Orbital plate
鼻根
Nasion
鼻骨
Nasal bone
颧骨：
Zygomatic bone:
额突
Frontal process
眶面
Orbital surface
颧面孔
Zygomaticofacial foramen
颞突
Temporal process
上颌骨：
Maxilla:
额突
Frontal process
泪前嵴
Anterior lacrimal crest
颧突
Zygomatic process
眶下孔
Infraorbital foramen
鼻前棘
Anterior nasal spine
尖牙窝
Canine fossa
牙槽弓
Alveolar arch
牙：
Teeth:
磨牙
Molars
前磨牙
Premolars
尖牙
Canine
切牙
Incisors

图 7-04　颅骨，肌肉起止点　Skull, Origins and Insertions

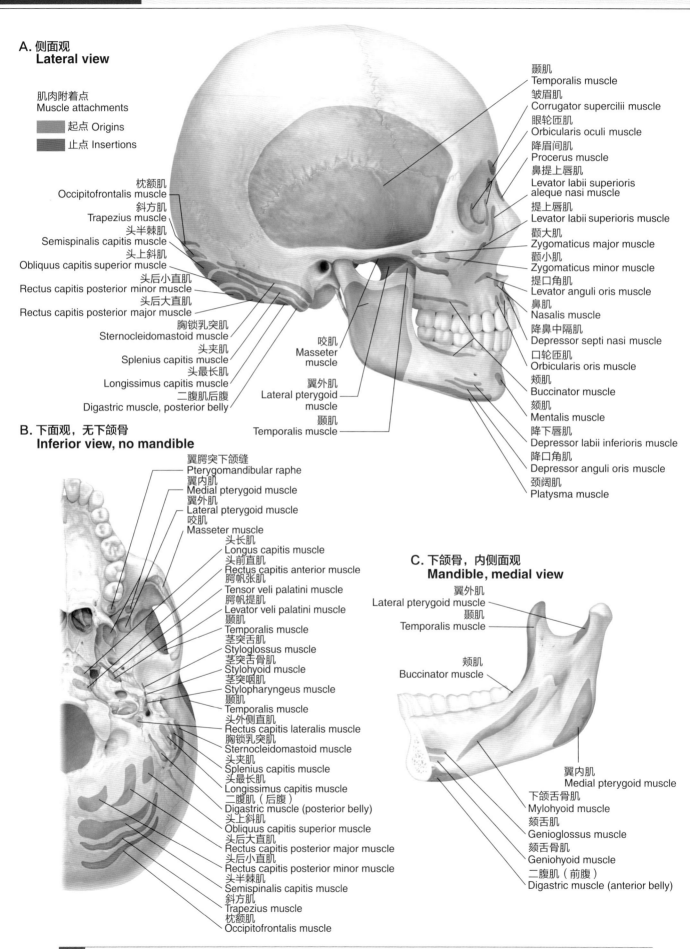

A. 侧面观
Lateral view

肌肉附着点
Muscle attachments
　起点 Origins
　止点 Insertions

枕额肌
Occipitofrontalis muscle
斜方肌
Trapezius muscle
头半棘肌
Semispinalis capitis muscle
头上斜肌
Obliquus capitis superior muscle
头后小直肌
Rectus capitis posterior minor muscle
头后大直肌
Rectus capitis posterior major muscle
胸锁乳突肌
Sternocleidomastoid muscle
头夹肌
Splenius capitis muscle
头最长肌
Longissimus capitis muscle
二腹肌后腹
Digastric muscle, posterior belly

颞肌
Temporalis muscle
皱眉肌
Corrugator supercilii muscle
眼轮匝肌
Orbicularis oculi muscle
降眉间肌
Procerus muscle
鼻提上唇肌
Levator labii superioris aleque nasi muscle
提上唇肌
Levator labii superioris muscle
颧大肌
Zygomaticus major muscle
颧小肌
Zygomaticus minor muscle
提口角肌
Levator anguli oris muscle
鼻肌
Nasalis muscle
降鼻中隔肌
Depressor septi nasi muscle
口轮匝肌
Orbicularis oris muscle
颊肌
Buccinator muscle
颏肌
Mentalis muscle
降下唇肌
Depressor labii inferioris muscle
降口角肌
Depressor anguli oris muscle
颈阔肌
Platysma muscle

咬肌
Masseter muscle
翼外肌
Lateral pterygoid muscle
颞肌
Temporalis muscle

B. 下面观，无下颌骨
Inferior view, no mandible

翼腭突下颌缝
Pterygomandibular raphe
翼内肌
Medial pterygoid muscle
翼外肌
Lateral pterygoid muscle
咬肌
Masseter muscle
头长肌
Longus capitis muscle
头前直肌
Rectus capitis anterior muscle
腭帆张肌
Tensor veli palatini muscle
腭帆提肌
Levator veli palatini muscle
颞肌
Temporalis muscle
茎突舌肌
Styloglossus muscle
茎突舌骨肌
Stylohyoid muscle
茎突咽肌
Stylopharyngeus muscle
颞肌
Temporalis muscle
头外侧直肌
Rectus capitis lateralis muscle
胸锁乳突肌
Sternocleidomastoid muscle
头夹肌
Splenius capitis muscle
头最长肌
Longissimus capitis muscle
二腹肌（后腹）
Digastric muscle (posterior belly)
头上斜肌
Obliquus capitis superior muscle
头后大直肌
Rectus capitis posterior major muscle
头后小直肌
Rectus capitis posterior minor muscle
头半棘肌
Semispinalis capitis muscle
斜方肌
Trapezius muscle
枕额肌
Occipitofrontalis muscle

C. 下颌骨，内侧面观
Mandible, medial view

翼外肌
Lateral pterygoid muscle
颞肌
Temporalis muscle
颊肌
Buccinator muscle
翼内肌
Medial pterygoid muscle
下颌舌骨肌
Mylohyoid muscle
颏舌肌
Genioglossus muscle
颏舌骨肌
Geniohyoid muscle
二腹肌（前腹）
Digastric muscle (anterior belly)

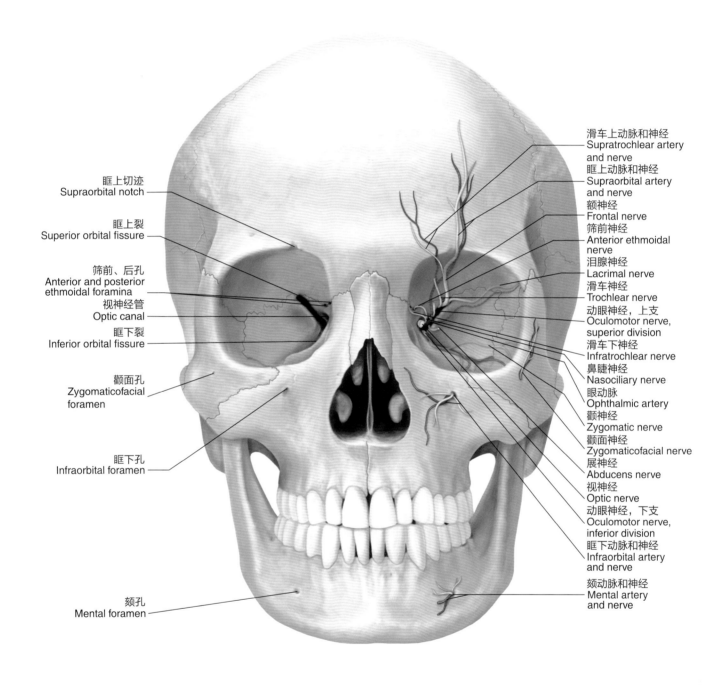

眶上切迹
Supraorbital notch

眶上裂
Superior orbital fissure

筛前、后孔
Anterior and posterior
ethmoidal foramina

视神经管
Optic canal

眶下裂
Inferior orbital fissure

颧面孔
Zygomaticofacial
foramen

眶下孔
Infraorbital foramen

颏孔
Mental foramen

滑车上动脉和神经
Supratrochlear artery
and nerve

眶上动脉和神经
Supraorbital artery
and nerve

额神经
Frontal nerve

筛前神经
Anterior ethmoidal
nerve

泪腺神经
Lacrimal nerve

滑车神经
Trochlear nerve

动眼神经，上支
Oculomotor nerve,
superior division

滑车下神经
Infratrochlear nerve

鼻睫神经
Nasociliary nerve

眼动脉
Ophthalmic artery

颧神经
Zygomatic nerve

颧面神经
Zygomaticofacial nerve

展神经
Abducens nerve

视神经
Optic nerve

动眼神经，下支
Oculomotor nerve,
inferior division

眶下动脉和神经
Infraorbital artery
and nerve

颏动脉和神经
Mental artery
and nerve

图 7-06 颅骨的骨 **Bones of the Skull**

A. 前面观
Anterior view

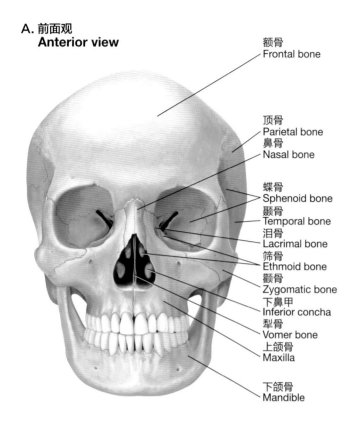

额骨
Frontal bone

顶骨
Parietal bone

鼻骨
Nasal bone

蝶骨
Sphenoid bone

颞骨
Temporal bone

泪骨
Lacrimal bone

筛骨
Ethmoid bone

颧骨
Zygomatic bone

下鼻甲
Inferior concha

犁骨
Vomer bone

上颌骨
Maxilla

下颌骨
Mandible

C. 下面观
Inferior view

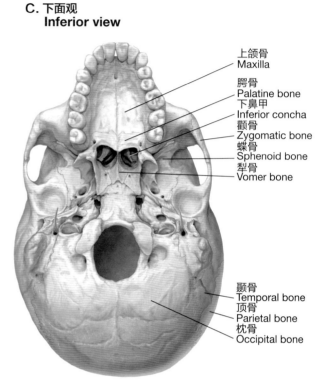

上颌骨
Maxilla

腭骨
Palatine bone

下鼻甲
Inferior concha

颧骨
Zygomatic bone

蝶骨
Sphenoid bone

犁骨
Vomer bone

颞骨
Temporal bone

顶骨
Parietal bone

枕骨
Occipital bone

B. 侧面观
Lateral view

顶骨
Parietal bone

额骨
Frontal bone

颞骨
Temporal bone

蝶骨
Sphenoid bone

筛骨
Ethmoid bone

鼻骨
Nasal bone

泪骨
Lacrimal bone

颧骨
Zygomatic bone

上颌骨
Maxilla

枕骨
Occipital bone

下颌骨
Mandible

D. 内面观
Interior view

筛骨
Ethmoid bone

额骨
Frontal bone

蝶骨
Sphenoid bone

颞骨
Temporal bone

顶骨
Parietal bone

枕骨
Occipital bone

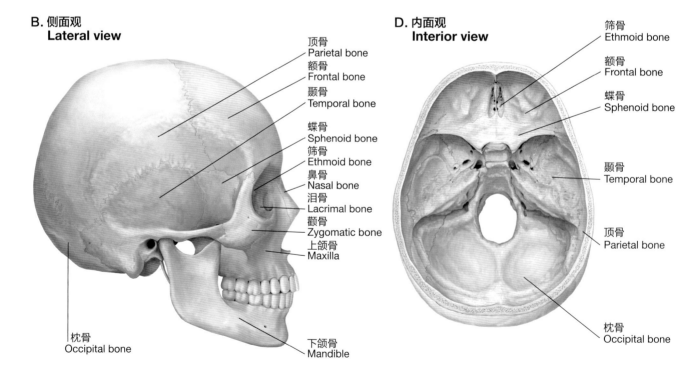

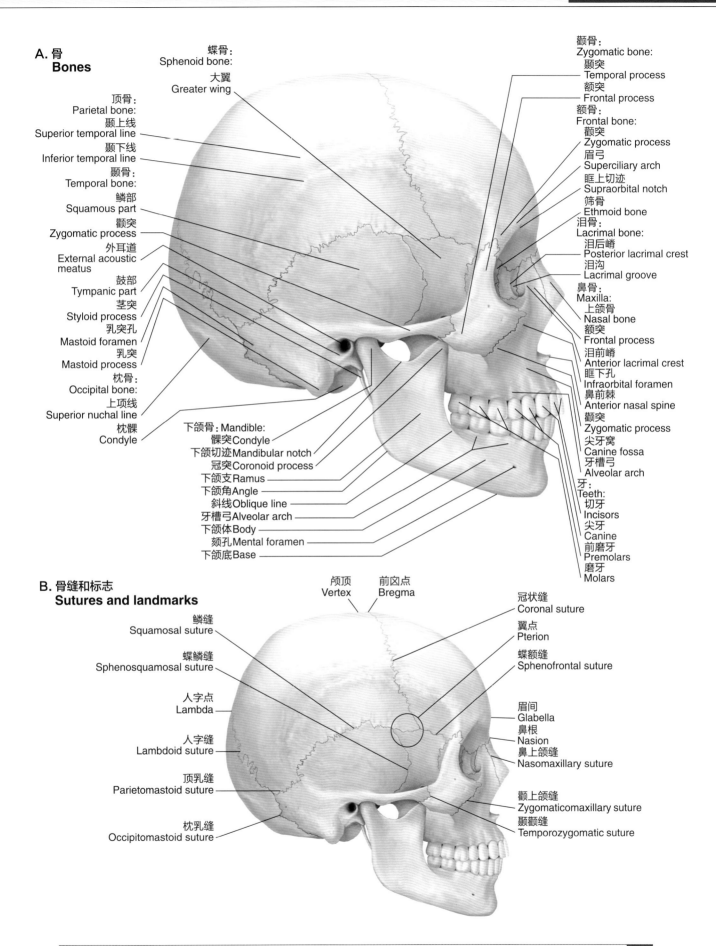

A. 骨
Bones

蝶骨：
Sphenoid bone:
大翼
Greater wing

顶骨：
Parietal bone:
颞上线
Superior temporal line
颞下线
Inferior temporal line
颞骨：
Temporal bone:
鳞部
Squamous part
颧突
Zygomatic process
外耳道
External acoustic meatus
鼓部
Tympanic part
茎突
Styloid process
乳突孔
Mastoid foramen
乳突
Mastoid process
枕骨：
Occipital bone:
上项线
Superior nuchal line
枕髁
Condyle

颧骨：
Zygomatic bone:
颞突
Temporal process
额突
Frontal process
额骨：
Frontal bone:
颧突
Zygomatic process
眉弓
Superciliary arch
眶上切迹
Supraorbital notch
筛骨
Ethmoid bone
泪骨：
Lacrimal bone:
泪后嵴
Posterior lacrimal crest
泪沟
Lacrimal groove
鼻骨：
Maxilla:
上颌骨
Nasal bone
额突
Frontal process
泪前嵴
Anterior lacrimal crest
眶下孔
Infraorbital foramen
鼻前棘
Anterior nasal spine
颧突
Zygomatic process
尖牙窝
Canine fossa
牙槽弓
Alveolar arch
牙：
Teeth:
切牙
Incisors
尖牙
Canine
前磨牙
Premolars
磨牙
Molars

下颌骨：Mandible:
髁突 Condyle
下颌切迹 Mandibular notch
冠突 Coronoid process
下颌支 Ramus
下颌角 Angle
斜线 Oblique line
牙槽弓 Alveolar arch
下颌体 Body
颏孔 Mental foramen
下颌底 Base

B. 骨缝和标志
Sutures and landmarks

颅顶
Vertex
前囟点
Bregma

鳞缝
Squamosal suture
蝶鳞缝
Sphenosquamosal suture
人字点
Lambda
人字缝
Lambdoid suture
顶乳缝
Parietomastoid suture
枕乳缝
Occipitomastoid suture

冠状缝
Coronal suture
翼点
Pterion
蝶额缝
Sphenofrontal suture
眉间
Glabella
鼻根
Nasion
鼻上颌缝
Nasomaxillary suture
颧上颌缝
Zygomaticomaxillary suture
颞颧缝
Temporozygomatic suture

图 7-08　　颅骨和颅顶　Skull and Calvaria

A. 后面观
Posterior view

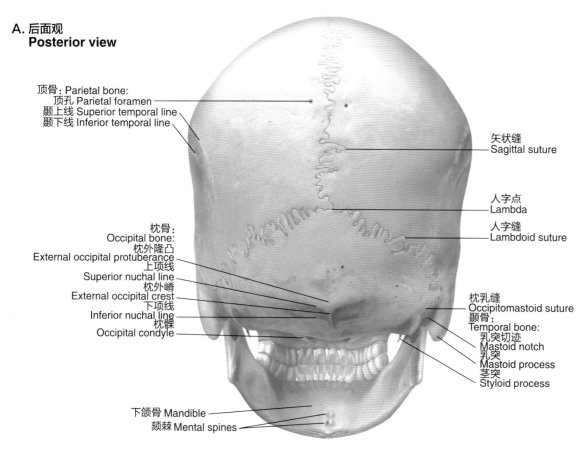

顶骨：Parietal bone:
　顶孔 Parietal foramen
　颞上线 Superior temporal line
　颞下线 Inferior temporal line

矢状缝
Sagittal suture

人字点
Lambda

人字缝
Lambdoid suture

枕骨：
Occipital bone:
枕外隆凸
External occipital protuberance
上项线
Superior nuchal line
枕外嵴
External occipital crest
下项线
Inferior nuchal line
枕髁
Occipital condyle

枕乳缝
Occipitomastoid suture
颞骨：
Temporal bone:
乳突切迹
Mastoid notch
乳突
Mastoid process
茎突
Styloid process

下颌骨 Mandible
颏棘 Mental spines

B. 颅顶上面观
Calvaria, superior view

C. 颅顶内面观
Calvaria, internal surface

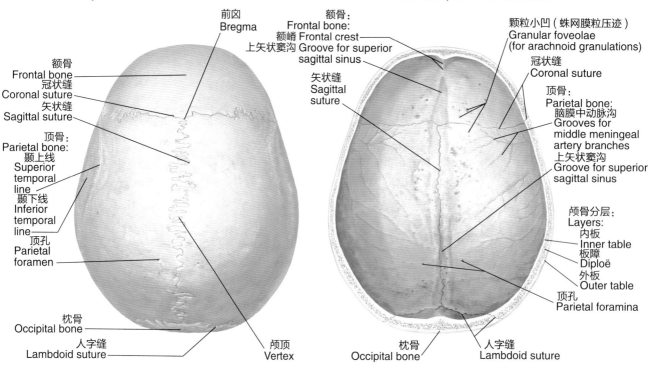

前囟
Bregma

额骨
Frontal bone
冠状缝
Coronal suture
矢状缝
Sagittal suture
顶骨：
Parietal bone:
颞上线
Superior
temporal
line
颞下线
Inferior
temporal
line
顶孔
Parietal
foramen

枕骨
Occipital bone
人字缝
Lambdoid suture

颅顶
Vertex

额骨：
Frontal bone:
额嵴 Frontal crest
上矢状窦沟 Groove for superior
sagittal sinus

矢状缝
Sagittal
suture

颗粒小凹（蛛网膜粒压迹）
Granular foveolae
(for arachnoid granulations)

冠状缝
Coronal suture

顶骨：
Parietal bone:
脑膜中动脉沟
Grooves for
middle meningeal
artery branches
上矢状窦沟
Groove for superior
sagittal sinus

颅骨分层：
Layers:
内板
Inner table
板障
Diploë
外板
Outer table

顶孔
Parietal foramina

枕骨
Occipital bone
人字缝
Lambdoid suture

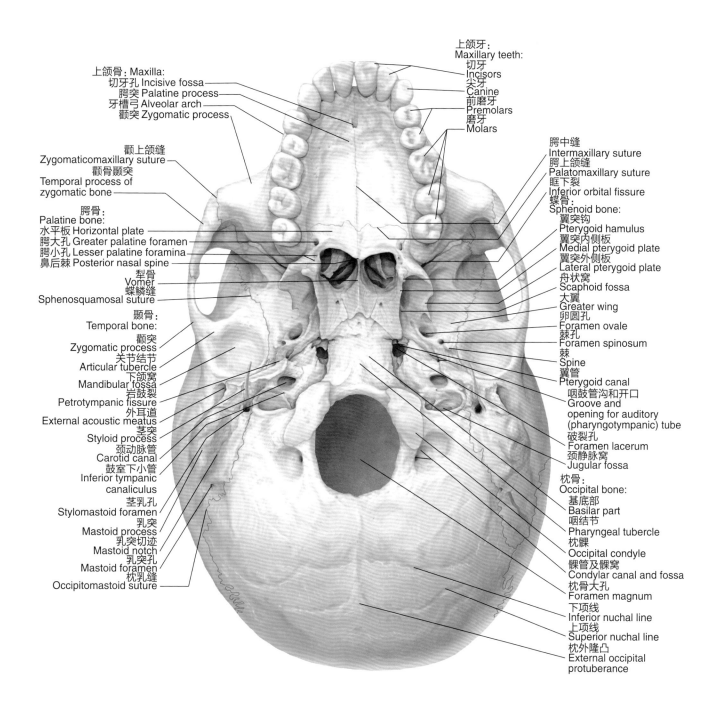

上颌骨：Maxilla:
切牙孔 Incisive fossa
腭突 Palatine process
牙槽弓 Alveolar arch
颧突 Zygomatic process

颧上颌缝
Zygomaticomaxillary suture
颧骨颞突
Temporal process of
zygomatic bone

腭骨：
Palatine bone:
水平板 Horizontal plate
腭大孔 Greater palatine foramen
腭小孔 Lesser palatine foramina
鼻后棘 Posterior nasal spine
犁骨
Vomer
蝶鳞缝
Sphenosquamosal suture

颞骨：
Temporal bone:
颧突
Zygomatic process
关节结节
Articular tubercle
下颌窝
Mandibular fossa
岩鼓裂
Petrotympanic fissure
外耳道
External acoustic meatus
茎突
Styloid process
颈动脉管
Carotid canal
鼓室下小管
Inferior tympanic
canaliculus
茎乳孔
Stylomastoid foramen
乳突
Mastoid process
乳突切迹
Mastoid notch
乳突孔
Mastoid foramen
枕乳缝
Occipitomastoid suture

上颌牙：
Maxillary teeth:
切牙
Incisors
尖牙
Canine
前磨牙
Premolars
磨牙
Molars

腭中缝
Intermaxillary suture
腭上颌缝
Palatomaxillary suture
眶下裂
Inferior orbital fissure
蝶骨：
Sphenoid bone:
翼突钩
Pterygoid hamulus
翼突内侧板
Medial pterygoid plate
翼突外侧板
Lateral pterygoid plate
舟状窝
Scaphoid fossa
大翼
Greater wing
卵圆孔
Foramen ovale
棘孔
Foramen spinosum
棘
Spine
翼管
Pterygoid canal
咽鼓管沟和开口
Groove and
opening for auditory
(pharyngotympanic) tube
破裂孔
Foramen lacerum
颈静脉窝
Jugular fossa

枕骨：
Occipital bone:
基底部
Basilar part
咽结节
Pharyngeal tubercle
枕髁
Occipital condyle
髁管及髁窝
Condylar canal and fossa
枕骨大孔
Foramen magnum
下项线
Inferior nuchal line
上项线
Superior nuchal line
枕外隆凸
External occipital
protuberance

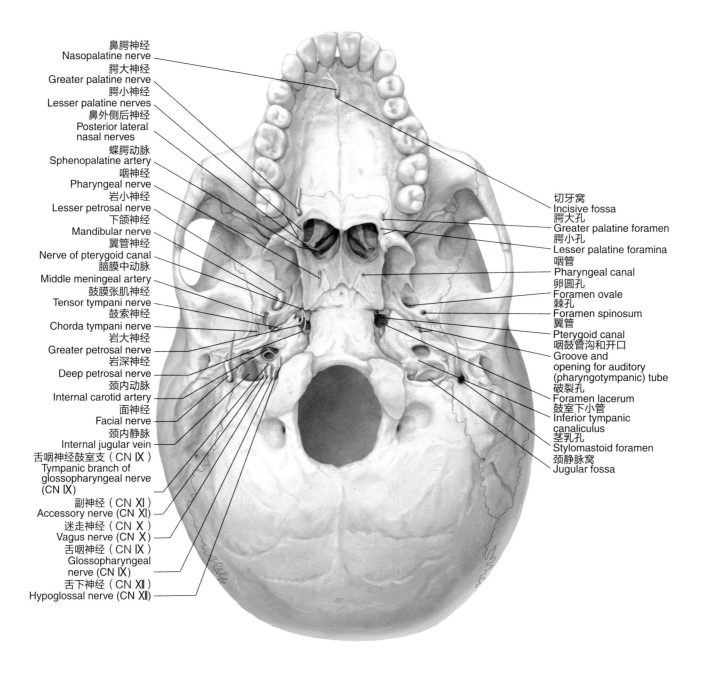

鼻腭神经
Nasopalatine nerve
腭大神经
Greater palatine nerve
腭小神经
Lesser palatine nerves
鼻外侧后神经
Posterior lateral
nasal nerves
蝶腭动脉
Sphenopalatine artery
咽神经
Pharyngeal nerve
岩小神经
Lesser petrosal nerve
下颌神经
Mandibular nerve
翼管神经
Nerve of pterygoid canal
脑膜中动脉
Middle meningeal artery
鼓膜张肌神经
Tensor tympani nerve
鼓索神经
Chorda tympani nerve
岩大神经
Greater petrosal nerve
岩深神经
Deep petrosal nerve
颈内动脉
Internal carotid artery
面神经
Facial nerve
颈内静脉
Internal jugular vein
舌咽神经鼓室支（CN IX）
Tympanic branch of
glossopharyngeal nerve
(CN IX)
副神经（CN XI）
Accessory nerve (CN XI)
迷走神经（CN X）
Vagus nerve (CN X)
舌咽神经（CN IX）
Glossopharyngeal
nerve (CN IX)
舌下神经（CN XII）
Hypoglossal nerve (CN XII)

切牙窝
Incisive fossa
腭大孔
Greater palatine foramen
腭小孔
Lesser palatine foramina
咽管
Pharyngeal canal
卵圆孔
Foramen ovale
棘孔
Foramen spinosum
翼管
Pterygoid canal
咽鼓管沟和开口
Groove and
opening for auditory
(pharyngotympanic) tube
破裂孔
Foramen lacerum
鼓室下小管
Inferior tympanic
canaliculus
茎乳孔
Stylomastoid foramen
颈静脉窝
Jugular fossa

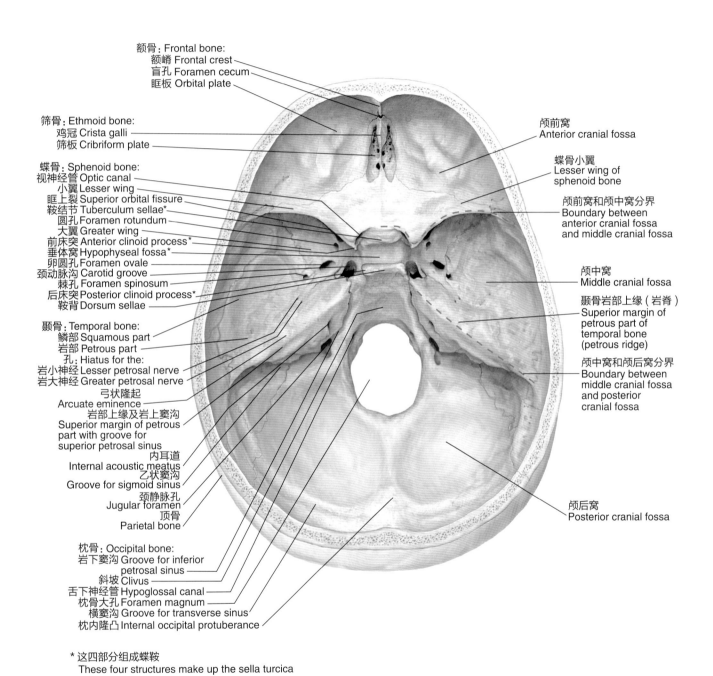

额骨：Frontal bone:
额嵴 Frontal crest
盲孔 Foramen cecum
眶板 Orbital plate

筛骨：Ethmoid bone:
鸡冠 Crista galli
筛板 Cribriform plate

蝶骨：Sphenoid bone:
视神经管 Optic canal
小翼 Lesser wing
眶上裂 Superior orbital fissure
鞍结节 Tuberculum sellae*
圆孔 Foramen rotundum
大翼 Greater wing
前床突 Anterior clinoid process*
垂体窝 Hypophyseal fossa*
卵圆孔 Foramen ovale
颈动脉沟 Carotid groove
棘孔 Foramen spinosum
后床突 Posterior clinoid process*
鞍背 Dorsum sellae

颞骨：Temporal bone:
鳞部 Squamous part
岩部 Petrous part
孔：Hiatus for the:
岩小神经 Lesser petrosal nerve
岩大神经 Greater petrosal nerve
弓状隆起 Arcuate eminence
岩部上缘及岩上窦沟 Superior margin of petrous part with groove for superior petrosal sinus
内耳道 Internal acoustic meatus
乙状窦沟 Groove for sigmoid sinus
颈静脉孔 Jugular foramen
顶骨 Parietal bone

枕骨：Occipital bone:
岩下窦沟 Groove for inferior petrosal sinus
斜坡 Clivus
舌下神经管 Hypoglossal canal
枕骨大孔 Foramen magnum
横窦沟 Groove for transverse sinus
枕内隆凸 Internal occipital protuberance

颅前窝 Anterior cranial fossa

蝶骨小翼 Lesser wing of sphenoid bone

颅前窝和颅中窝分界 Boundary between anterior cranial fossa and middle cranial fossa

颅中窝 Middle cranial fossa

颞骨岩部上缘（岩脊）Superior margin of petrous part of temporal bone (petrous ridge)

颅中窝和颅后窝分界 Boundary between middle cranial fossa and posterior cranial fossa

颅后窝 Posterior cranial fossa

* 这四部分组成蝶鞍
These four structures make up the sella turcica

图 7-12　颅骨矢状断面　Skull, Sagittal Section

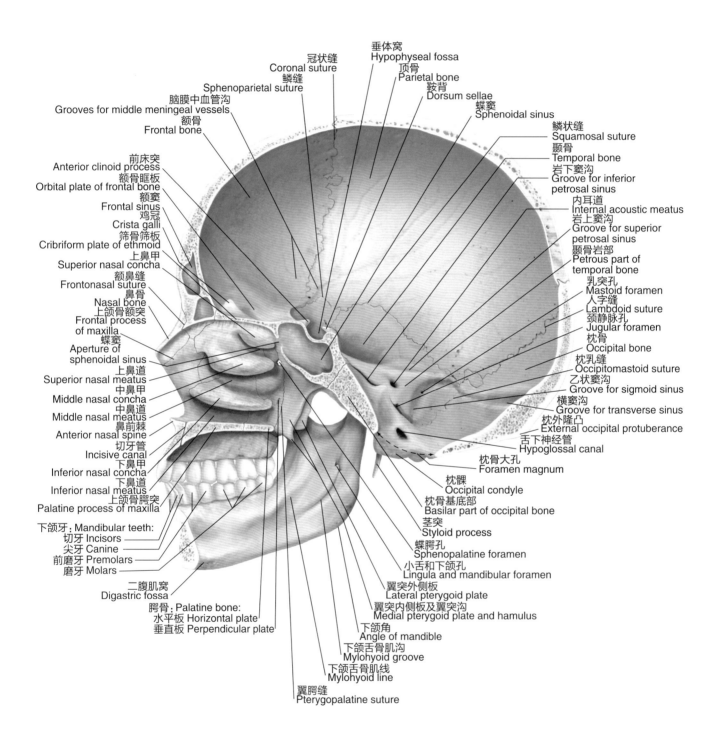

冠状缝
Coronal suture

垂体窝
Hypophyseal fossa

顶骨
Parietal bone

鞍背
Dorsum sellae

蝶窦
Sphenoidal sinus

鳞缝
Sphenoparietal suture

脑膜中血管沟
Grooves for middle meningeal vessels

额骨
Frontal bone

鳞状缝
Squamosal suture

颞骨
Temporal bone

岩下窦沟
Groove for inferior petrosal sinus

内耳道
Internal acoustic meatus

岩上窦沟
Groove for superior petrosal sinus

颞骨岩部
Petrous part of temporal bone

乳突孔
Mastoid foramen

人字缝
Lambdoid suture

颈静脉孔
Jugular foramen

枕骨
Occipital bone

枕乳缝
Occipitomastoid suture

乙状窦沟
Groove for sigmoid sinus

横窦沟
Groove for transverse sinus

枕外隆凸
External occipital protuberance

舌下神经管
Hypoglossal canal

枕骨大孔
Foramen magnum

枕髁
Occipital condyle

枕骨基底部
Basilar part of occipital bone

茎突
Styloid process

蝶腭孔
Sphenopalatine foramen

小舌和下颌孔
Lingula and mandibular foramen

翼突外侧板
Lateral pterygoid plate

翼突内侧板及翼突沟
Medial pterygoid plate and hamulus

下颌角
Angle of mandible

下颌舌骨肌沟
Mylohyoid groove

下颌舌骨肌线
Mylohyoid line

翼腭缝
Pterygopalatine suture

前床突
Anterior clinoid process

额骨眶板
Orbital plate of frontal bone

额窦
Frontal sinus

鸡冠
Crista galli

筛骨筛板
Cribriform plate of ethmoid

上鼻甲
Superior nasal concha

额鼻缝
Frontonasal suture

鼻骨
Nasal bone

上颌骨额突
Frontal process of maxilla

蝶窦
Aperture of sphenoidal sinus

上鼻道
Superior nasal meatus

中鼻甲
Middle nasal concha

中鼻道
Middle nasal meatus

鼻前棘
Anterior nasal spine

切牙管
Incisive canal

下鼻甲
Inferior nasal concha

下鼻道
Inferior nasal meatus

上颌骨腭突
Palatine process of maxilla

下颌牙：Mandibular teeth:
切牙 Incisors
尖牙 Canine
前磨牙 Premolars
磨牙 Molars

二腹肌窝
Digastric fossa

腭骨：Palatine bone:
水平板 Horizontal plate
垂直板 Perpendicular plate

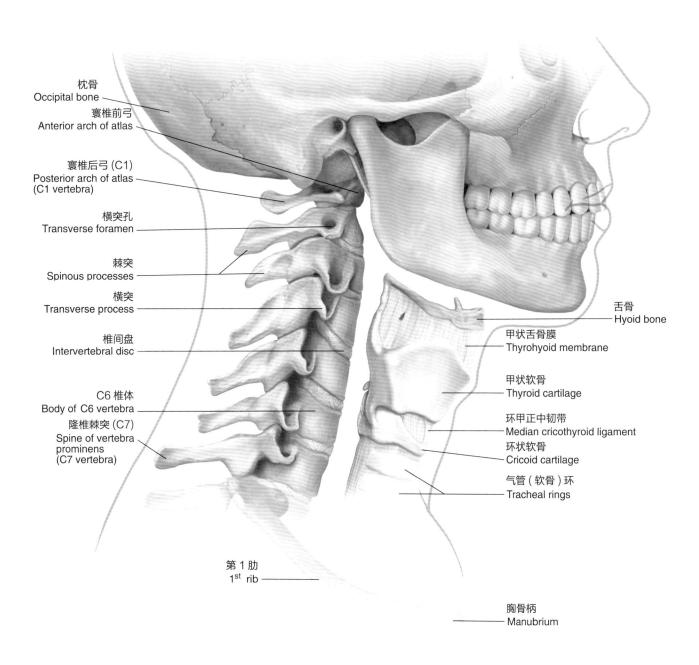

枕骨
Occipital bone

寰椎前弓
Anterior arch of atlas

寰椎后弓 (C1)
Posterior arch of atlas
(C1 vertebra)

横突孔
Transverse foramen

棘突
Spinous processes

横突
Transverse process

椎间盘
Intervertebral disc

C6 椎体
Body of C6 vertebra

隆椎棘突 (C7)
Spine of vertebra
prominens
(C7 vertebra)

第 1 肋
1st rib

舌骨
Hyoid bone

甲状舌骨膜
Thyrohyoid membrane

甲状软骨
Thyroid cartilage

环甲正中韧带
Median cricothyroid ligament

环状软骨
Cricoid cartilage

气管（软骨）环
Tracheal rings

胸骨柄
Manubrium

图 7-14　颈筋膜　Cervical Fascia

A. 矢状断面
Sagittal section

枕骨
Occipital bone

咽
Pharynx

颈深筋膜浅层
Superficial layer of
deep cervical fascia

椎前筋膜
Prevertebral fascia

颊咽筋膜
Buccopharyngeal fascia

气管
Trachea

食管
Esophagus

图 B 所在平面
Plane of cross section B

下颌骨
Mandible

舌骨
Hyoid bone

喉
Larynx
浅筋膜
Superficial fascia
甲状腺峡
Thyroid isthmus
气管前筋膜
Pretracheal fascia
舌骨下筋膜
Infrahyoid fascia
颈深筋膜浅层
Superficial layer of
deep cervical fascia
胸骨上间隙
Suprasternal space
胸骨柄
Manubrium of sternum

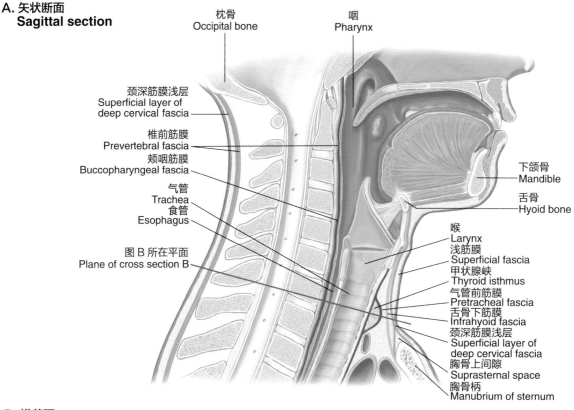

B. 横截面
Cross section

颈部器官：Cervical viscera:
甲状腺 Thyroid gland
气管 Trachea
食管 Esophagus

皮肤
Skin

浅筋膜：
Superficial fascia:
颈阔肌
Platysma muscle

颈深筋膜：
Deep cervical fascia:
浅层
Superficial layer
舌骨下筋膜
Infrahyoid fascia

内脏筋膜：
Visceral fascia:
气管前筋膜
Pretracheal
颊咽筋膜
Buccopharyngeal
颈动脉鞘
Carotid sheath
翼状筋膜
Alar fascia
椎前筋膜
Prevertebral fascia

舌骨下肌：Infrahyoid muscles:
胸骨舌骨肌 Sternohyoid
胸骨甲状肌 Sternothyroid
肩胛舌骨肌 Omohyoid

胸锁乳突肌
Sternocleidomastoid muscle
颈总动脉
Common carotid artery
颈内静脉
Internal jugular vein
迷走神经（CN X）
Vagus nerve (CN X)
交感干
Sympathetic trunk
颈长肌
Longus colli muscle
前斜角肌
Anterior scalene muscle

中斜角肌
Middle scalene muscle

斜方肌
Trapezius muscle

第 7 颈椎椎弓
Vertebral arch of C7

项韧带
Nuchal ligament

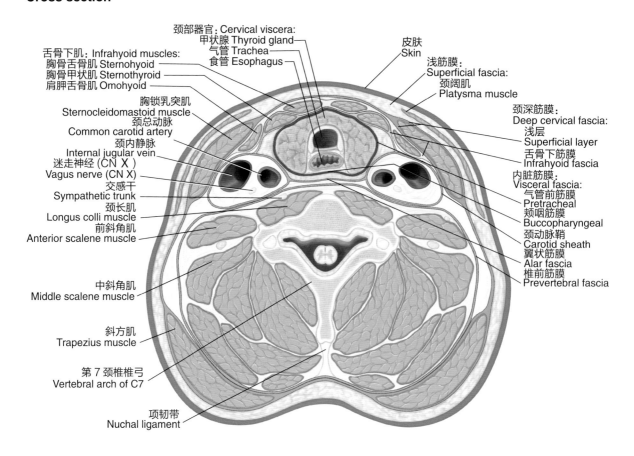

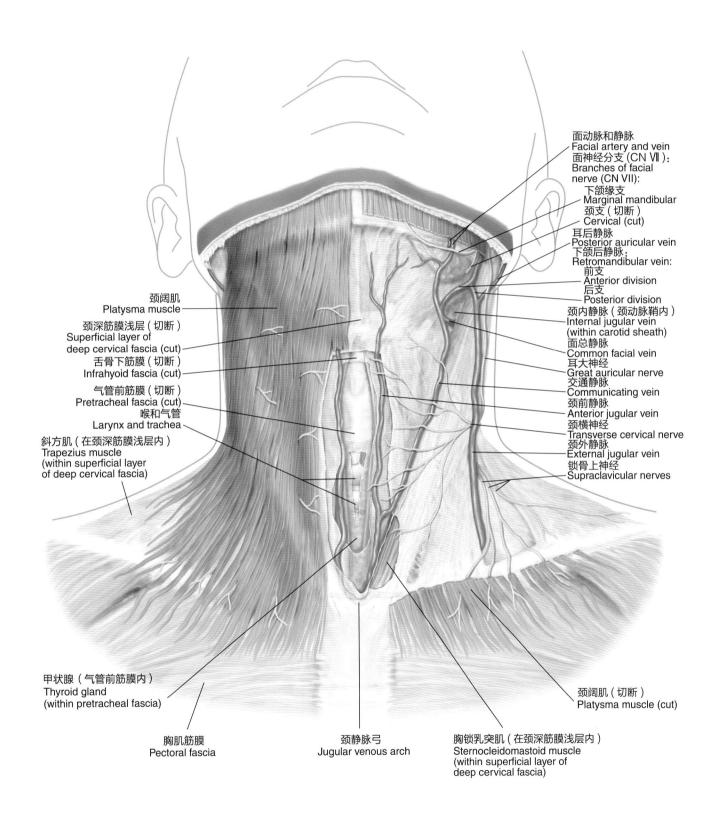

颈阔肌
Platysma muscle

颈深筋膜浅层（切断）
Superficial layer of
deep cervical fascia (cut)

舌骨下筋膜（切断）
Infrahyoid fascia (cut)

气管前筋膜（切断）
Pretracheal fascia (cut)

喉和气管
Larynx and trachea

斜方肌（在颈深筋膜浅层内）
Trapezius muscle
(within superficial layer
of deep cervical fascia)

面动脉和静脉
Facial artery and vein
面神经分支 (CN Ⅶ)：
Branches of facial
nerve (CN VII)：
下颌缘支
Marginal mandibular
颈支（切断）
Cervical (cut)
耳后静脉
Posterior auricular vein
下颌后静脉：
Retromandibular vein：
前支
Anterior division
后支
Posterior division
颈内静脉（颈动脉鞘内）
Internal jugular vein
(within carotid sheath)
面总静脉
Common facial vein
耳大神经
Great auricular nerve
交通静脉
Communicating vein
颈前静脉
Anterior jugular vein
颈横神经
Transverse cervical nerve
颈外静脉
External jugular vein
锁骨上神经
Supraclavicular nerves

甲状腺（气管前筋膜内）
Thyroid gland
(within pretracheal fascia)

胸肌筋膜
Pectoral fascia

颈静脉弓
Jugular venous arch

胸锁乳突肌（在颈深筋膜浅层内）
Sternocleidomastoid muscle
(within superficial layer of
deep cervical fascia)

颈阔肌（切断）
Platysma muscle (cut)

图 7-16　颈部，中层结构　Neck, Intermediate Dissection

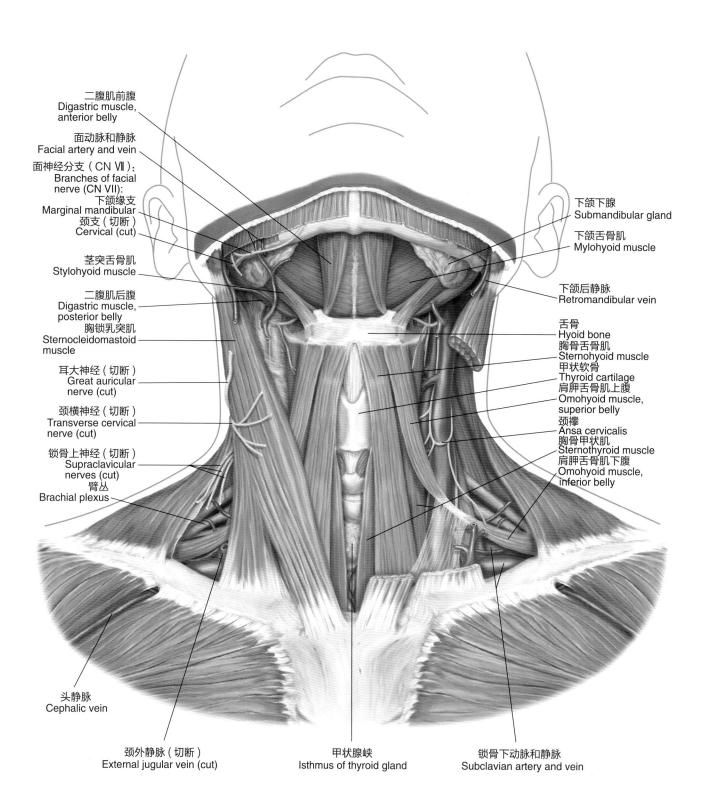

二腹肌前腹
Digastric muscle,
anterior belly

面动脉和静脉
Facial artery and vein

面神经分支（CN Ⅶ）：
Branches of facial
nerve (CN VII):
下颌缘支
Marginal mandibular
颈支（切断）
Cervical (cut)

茎突舌骨肌
Stylohyoid muscle

二腹肌后腹
Digastric muscle,
posterior belly

胸锁乳突肌
Sternocleidomastoid
muscle

耳大神经（切断）
Great auricular
nerve (cut)

颈横神经（切断）
Transverse cervical
nerve (cut)

锁骨上神经（切断）
Supraclavicular
nerves (cut)

臂丛
Brachial plexus

头静脉
Cephalic vein

下颌下腺
Submandibular gland

下颌舌骨肌
Mylohyoid muscle

下颌后静脉
Retromandibular vein

舌骨
Hyoid bone
胸骨舌骨肌
Sternohyoid muscle
甲状软骨
Thyroid cartilage
肩胛舌骨肌上腹
Omohyoid muscle,
superior belly
颈襻
Ansa cervicalis
胸骨甲状肌
Sternothyroid muscle
肩胛舌骨肌下腹
Omohyoid muscle,
inferior belly

颈外静脉（切断）
External jugular vein (cut)

甲状腺峡
Isthmus of thyroid gland

锁骨下动脉和静脉
Subclavian artery and vein

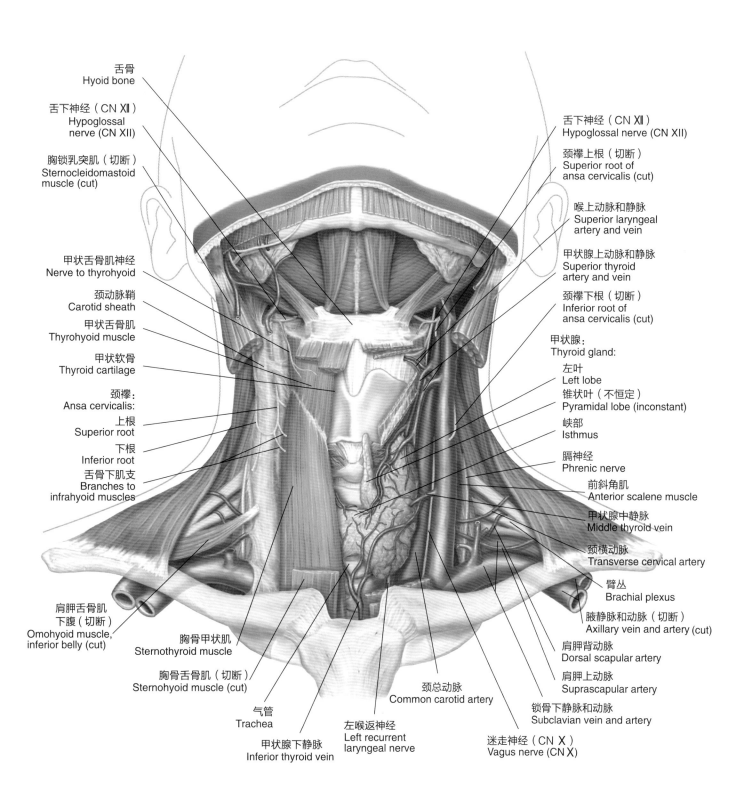

舌骨
Hyoid bone

舌下神经（CN XII）
Hypoglossal
nerve (CN XII)

胸锁乳突肌（切断）
Sternocleidomastoid
muscle (cut)

甲状舌骨肌神经
Nerve to thyrohyoid

颈动脉鞘
Carotid sheath

甲状舌骨肌
Thyrohyoid muscle

甲状软骨
Thyroid cartilage

颈襻：
Ansa cervicalis:

上根
Superior root

下根
Inferior root

舌骨下肌支
Branches to
infrahyoid muscles

肩胛舌骨肌
下腹（切断）
Omohyoid muscle,
inferior belly (cut)

胸骨甲状肌
Sternothyroid muscle

胸骨舌骨肌（切断）
Sternohyoid muscle (cut)

气管
Trachea

甲状腺下静脉
Inferior thyroid vein

左喉返神经
Left recurrent
laryngeal nerve

颈总动脉
Common carotid artery

迷走神经（CN X）
Vagus nerve (CN X)

舌下神经（CN XII）
Hypoglossal nerve (CN XII)

颈襻上根（切断）
Superior root of
ansa cervicalis (cut)

喉上动脉和静脉
Superior laryngeal
artery and vein

甲状腺上动脉和静脉
Superior thyroid
artery and vein

颈襻下根（切断）
Inferior root of
ansa cervicalis (cut)

甲状腺：
Thyroid gland:

左叶
Left lobe

锥状叶（不恒定）
Pyramidal lobe (inconstant)

峡部
Isthmus

膈神经
Phrenic nerve

前斜角肌
Anterior scalene muscle

甲状腺中静脉
Middle thyroid vein

颈横动脉
Transverse cervical artery

臂丛
Brachial plexus

腋静脉和动脉（切断）
Axillary vein and artery (cut)

肩胛背动脉
Dorsal scapular artery

肩胛上动脉
Suprascapular artery

锁骨下静脉和动脉
Subclavian vein and artery

图 7-18　**颈根　Root of Neck**

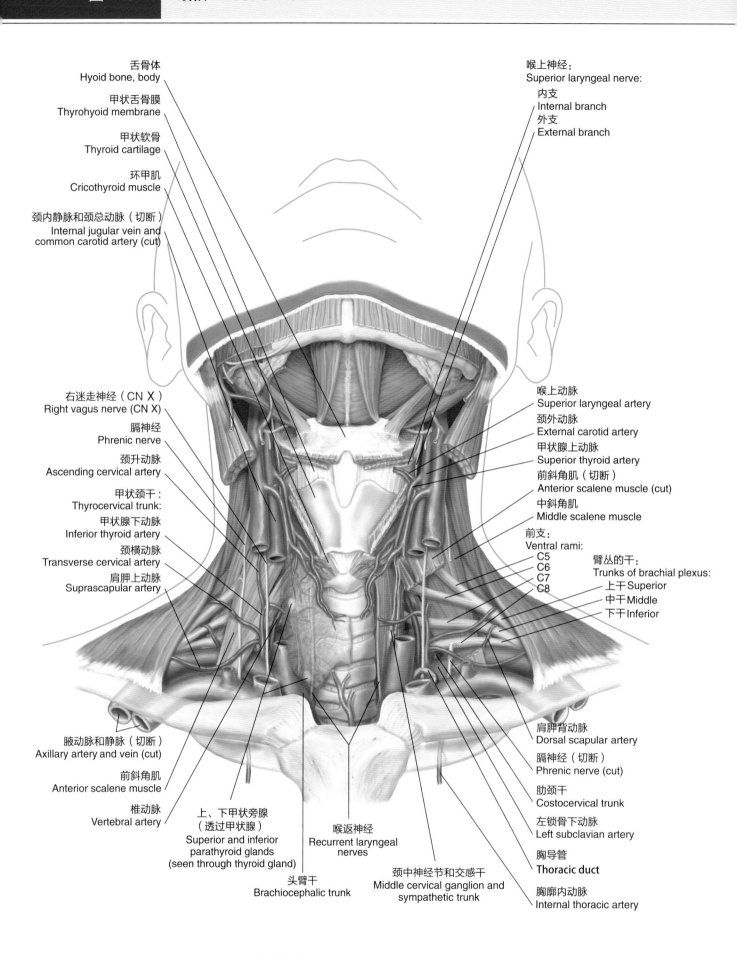

舌骨体
Hyoid bone, body

甲状舌骨膜
Thyrohyoid membrane

甲状软骨
Thyroid cartilage

环甲肌
Cricothyroid muscle

颈内静脉和颈总动脉（切断）
Internal jugular vein and
common carotid artery (cut)

喉上神经：
Superior laryngeal nerve:

内支
Internal branch

外支
External branch

右迷走神经（CN X）
Right vagus nerve (CN X)

膈神经
Phrenic nerve

颈升动脉
Ascending cervical artery

甲状颈干：
Thyrocervical trunk:

甲状腺下动脉
Inferior thyroid artery

颈横动脉
Transverse cervical artery

肩胛上动脉
Suprascapular artery

喉上动脉
Superior laryngeal artery

颈外动脉
External carotid artery

甲状腺上动脉
Superior thyroid artery

前斜角肌（切断）
Anterior scalene muscle (cut)

中斜角肌
Middle scalene muscle

前支：
Ventral rami:
C5
C6
C7
C8

臂丛的干：
Trunks of brachial plexus:
上干 Superior
中干 Middle
下干 Inferior

腋动脉和静脉（切断）
Axillary artery and vein (cut)

前斜角肌
Anterior scalene muscle

椎动脉
Vertebral artery

上、下甲状旁腺
（透过甲状腺）
Superior and inferior
parathyroid glands
(seen through thyroid gland)

喉返神经
Recurrent laryngeal
nerves

头臂干
Brachiocephalic trunk

颈中神经节和交感干
Middle cervical ganglion and
sympathetic trunk

肩胛背动脉
Dorsal scapular artery

膈神经（切断）
Phrenic nerve (cut)

肋颈干
Costocervical trunk

左锁骨下动脉
Left subclavian artery

胸导管
Thoracic duct

胸廓内动脉
Internal thoracic artery

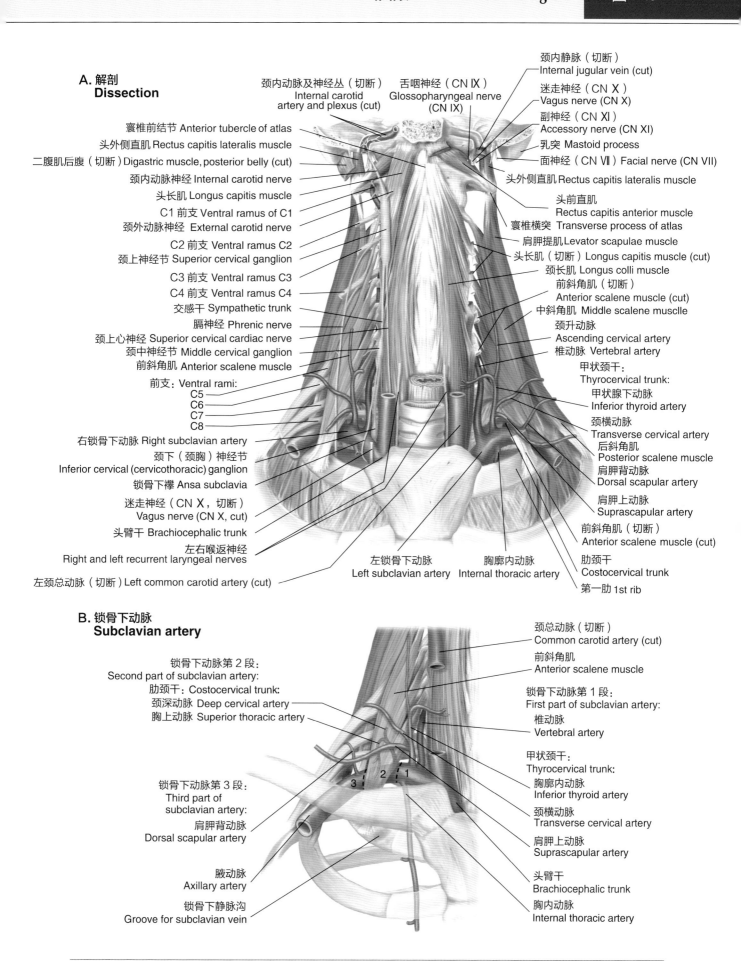

A. 解剖
Dissection

颈内动脉及神经丛（切断）Internal carotid artery and plexus (cut)
舌咽神经（CN IX）Glossopharyngeal nerve (CN IX)
颈内静脉（切断）Internal jugular vein (cut)
迷走神经（CN X）Vagus nerve (CN X)
副神经（CN XI）Accessory nerve (CN XI)
乳突 Mastoid process
面神经（CN VII）Facial nerve (CN VII)

寰椎前结节 Anterior tubercle of atlas
头外侧直肌 Rectus capitis lateralis muscle
二腹肌后腹（切断）Digastric muscle, posterior belly (cut)
颈内动脉神经 Internal carotid nerve
头长肌 Longus capitis muscle
C1 前支 Ventral ramus of C1
颈外动脉神经 External carotid nerve
C2 前支 Ventral ramus C2
颈上神经节 Superior cervical ganglion
C3 前支 Ventral ramus C3
C4 前支 Ventral ramus C4
交感干 Sympathetic trunk
膈神经 Phrenic nerve
颈上心神经 Superior cervical cardiac nerve
颈中神经节 Middle cervical ganglion
前斜角肌 Anterior scalene muscle
前支：Ventral rami:
C5
C6
C7
C8
右锁骨下动脉 Right subclavian artery
颈下（颈胸）神经节 Inferior cervical (cervicothoracic) ganglion
锁骨下襻 Ansa subclavia
迷走神经（CN X，切断）Vagus nerve (CN X, cut)
头臂干 Brachiocephalic trunk
左右喉返神经 Right and left recurrent laryngeal nerves
左颈总动脉（切断）Left common carotid artery (cut)

头外侧直肌 Rectus capitis lateralis muscle
头前直肌 Rectus capitis anterior muscle
寰椎横突 Transverse process of atlas
肩胛提肌 Levator scapulae muscle
头长肌（切断）Longus capitis muscle (cut)
颈长肌 Longus colli muscle
前斜角肌（切断）Anterior scalene muscle (cut)
中斜角肌 Middle scalene musclle
颈升动脉 Ascending cervical artery
椎动脉 Vertebral artery
甲状颈干：Thyrocervical trunk:
甲状腺下动脉 Inferior thyroid artery
颈横动脉 Transverse cervical artery
后斜角肌 Posterior scalene muscle
肩胛背动脉 Dorsal scapular artery
肩胛上动脉 Suprascapular artery
前斜角肌（切断）Anterior scalene muscle (cut)
肋颈干 Costocervical trunk
第一肋 1st rib

左锁骨下动脉 Left subclavian artery
胸廓内动脉 Internal thoracic artery

B. 锁骨下动脉
Subclavian artery

锁骨下动脉第 2 段：Second part of subclavian artery:
肋颈干：Costocervical trunk:
颈深动脉 Deep cervical artery
胸上动脉 Superior thoracic artery

锁骨下动脉第 3 段：Third part of subclavian artery:
肩胛背动脉 Dorsal scapular artery

腋动脉 Axillary artery
锁骨下静脉沟 Groove for subclavian vein

颈总动脉（切断）Common carotid artery (cut)
前斜角肌 Anterior scalene muscle
锁骨下动脉第 1 段：First part of subclavian artery:
椎动脉 Vertebral artery
甲状颈干：Thyrocervical trunk:
胸廓内动脉 Internal thoracic artery
甲状腺下动脉 Inferior thyroid artery
颈横动脉 Transverse cervical artery
肩胛上动脉 Suprascapular artery
头臂干 Brachiocephalic trunk
胸内动脉 Internal thoracic artery

3 2 1

图 7-20　颈部侧面观　Neck, Lateral View

A. 浅层解剖
Superficial dissection

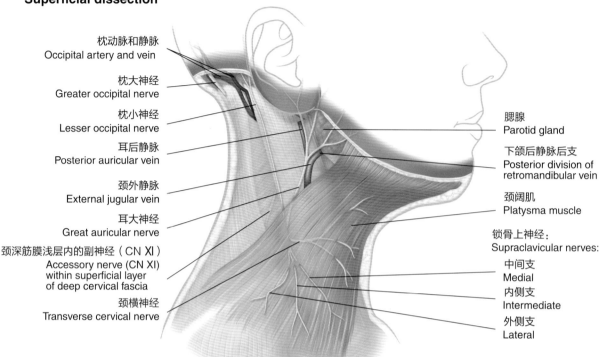

枕动脉和静脉
Occipital artery and vein

枕大神经
Greater occipital nerve

枕小神经
Lesser occipital nerve

耳后静脉
Posterior auricular vein

颈外静脉
External jugular vein

耳大神经
Great auricular nerve

颈深筋膜浅层内的副神经（CN XI）
Accessory nerve (CN XI)
within superficial layer
of deep cervical fascia

颈横神经
Transverse cervical nerve

腮腺
Parotid gland

下颌后静脉后支
Posterior division of
retromandibular vein

颈阔肌
Platysma muscle

锁骨上神经：
Supraclavicular nerves:

中间支
Medial

内侧支
Intermediate

外侧支
Lateral

B. 中层解剖
Intermediate dissection

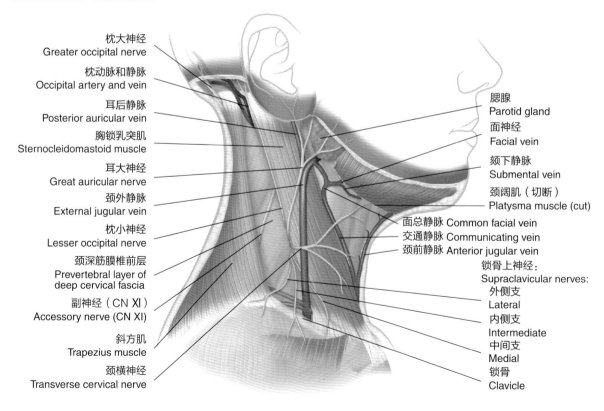

枕大神经
Greater occipital nerve

枕动脉和静脉
Occipital artery and vein

耳后静脉
Posterior auricular vein

胸锁乳突肌
Sternocleidomastoid muscle

耳大神经
Great auricular nerve

颈外静脉
External jugular vein

枕小神经
Lesser occipital nerve

颈深筋膜椎前层
Prevertebral layer of
deep cervical fascia

副神经（CN XI）
Accessory nerve (CN XI)

斜方肌
Trapezius muscle

颈横神经
Transverse cervical nerve

腮腺
Parotid gland

面神经
Facial vein

颏下静脉
Submental vein

颈阔肌（切断）
Platysma muscle (cut)

面总静脉 Common facial vein
交通静脉 Communicating vein
颈前静脉 Anterior jugular vein

锁骨上神经：
Supraclavicular nerves:

外侧支
Lateral

内侧支
Intermediate

中间支
Medial

锁骨
Clavicle

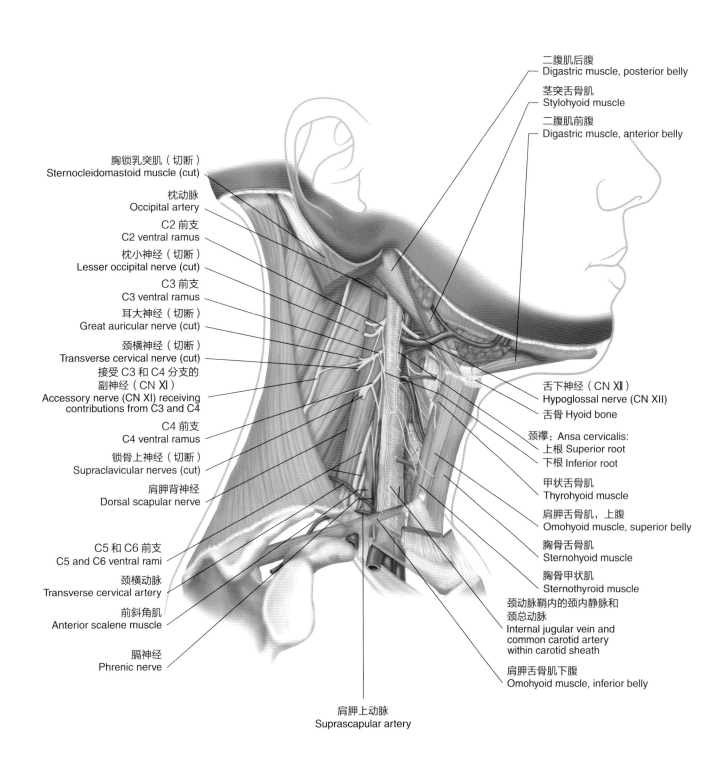

胸锁乳突肌（切断）
Sternocleidomastoid muscle (cut)

枕动脉
Occipital artery

C2 前支
C2 ventral ramus

枕小神经（切断）
Lesser occipital nerve (cut)

C3 前支
C3 ventral ramus

耳大神经（切断）
Great auricular nerve (cut)

颈横神经（切断）
Transverse cervical nerve (cut)

接受 C3 和 C4 分支的
副神经（CN XI）
Accessory nerve (CN XI) receiving
contributions from C3 and C4

C4 前支
C4 ventral ramus

锁骨上神经（切断）
Supraclavicular nerves (cut)

肩胛背神经
Dorsal scapular nerve

C5 和 C6 前支
C5 and C6 ventral rami

颈横动脉
Transverse cervical artery

前斜角肌
Anterior scalene muscle

膈神经
Phrenic nerve

二腹肌后腹
Digastric muscle, posterior belly

茎突舌骨肌
Stylohyoid muscle

二腹肌前腹
Digastric muscle, anterior belly

舌下神经（CN XII）
Hypoglossal nerve (CN XII)

舌骨 Hyoid bone

颈襻：Ansa cervicalis:
上根 Superior root
下根 Inferior root

甲状舌骨肌
Thyrohyoid muscle

肩胛舌骨肌，上腹
Omohyoid muscle, superior belly

胸骨舌骨肌
Sternohyoid muscle

胸骨甲状肌
Sternothyroid muscle

颈动脉鞘内的颈内静脉和
颈总动脉
Internal jugular vein and
common carotid artery
within carotid sheath

肩胛舌骨肌下腹
Omohyoid muscle, inferior belly

肩胛上动脉
Suprascapular artery

图 7-22　　**颈部侧面观，最深层解剖**　**Neck, Lateral View, Deepest Dissection**

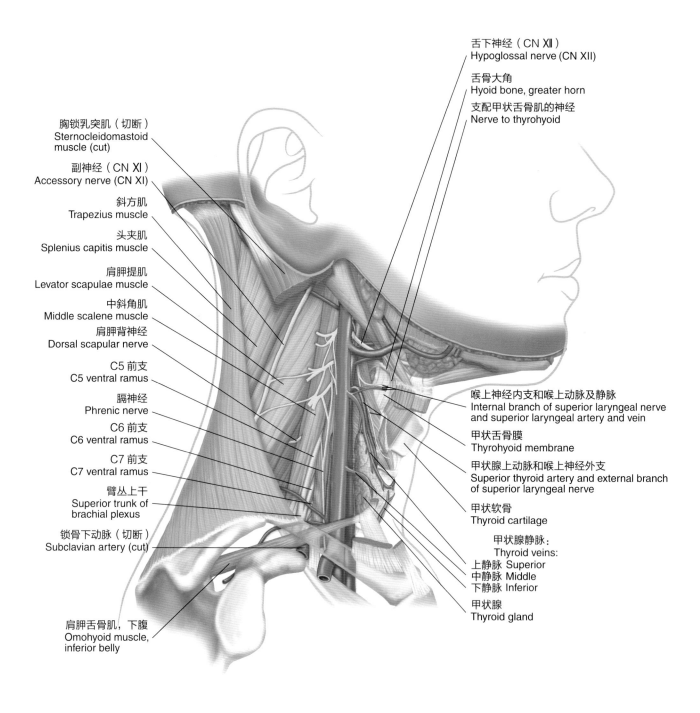

舌下神经（CN XII）
Hypoglossal nerve (CN XII)

舌骨大角
Hyoid bone, greater horn

支配甲状舌骨肌的神经
Nerve to thyrohyoid

胸锁乳突肌（切断）
Sternocleidomastoid
muscle (cut)

副神经（CN XI）
Accessory nerve (CN XI)

斜方肌
Trapezius muscle

头夹肌
Splenius capitis muscle

肩胛提肌
Levator scapulae muscle

中斜角肌
Middle scalene muscle

肩胛背神经
Dorsal scapular nerve

C5 前支
C5 ventral ramus

膈神经
Phrenic nerve

C6 前支
C6 ventral ramus

C7 前支
C7 ventral ramus

臂丛上干
Superior trunk of
brachial plexus

锁骨下动脉（切断）
Subclavian artery (cut)

肩胛舌骨肌，下腹
Omohyoid muscle,
inferior belly

喉上神经内支和喉上动脉及静脉
Internal branch of superior laryngeal nerve
and superior laryngeal artery and vein

甲状舌骨膜
Thyrohyoid membrane

甲状腺上动脉和喉上神经外支
Superior thyroid artery and external branch
of superior laryngeal nerve

甲状软骨
Thyroid cartilage

甲状腺静脉：
Thyroid veins:
上静脉 Superior
中静脉 Middle
下静脉 Inferior

甲状腺
Thyroid gland

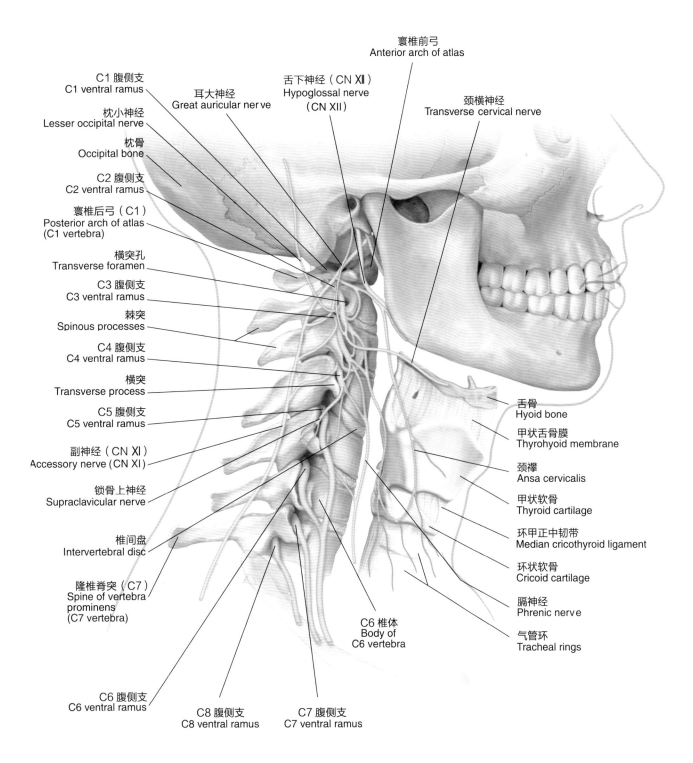

寰椎前弓
Anterior arch of atlas

舌下神经（CN XII）
Hypoglossal nerve
(CN XII)

颈横神经
Transverse cervical nerve

C1 腹侧支
C1 ventral ramus

耳大神经
Great auricular nerve

枕小神经
Lesser occipital nerve

枕骨
Occipital bone

C2 腹侧支
C2 ventral ramus

寰椎后弓（C1）
Posterior arch of atlas
(C1 vertebra)

横突孔
Transverse foramen

C3 腹侧支
C3 ventral ramus

棘突
Spinous processes

C4 腹侧支
C4 ventral ramus

横突
Transverse process

C5 腹侧支
C5 ventral ramus

副神经（CN XI）
Accessory nerve (CN XI)

锁骨上神经
Supraclavicular nerve

椎间盘
Intervertebral disc

隆椎脊突（C7）
Spine of vertebra
prominens
(C7 vertebra)

C6 腹侧支
C6 ventral ramus

C8 腹侧支
C8 ventral ramus

C7 腹侧支
C7 ventral ramus

C6 椎体
Body of
C6 vertebra

舌骨
Hyoid bone

甲状舌骨膜
Thyrohyoid membrane

颈襻
Ansa cervicalis

甲状软骨
Thyroid cartilage

环甲正中韧带
Median cricothyroid ligament

环状软骨
Cricoid cartilage

膈神经
Phrenic nerve

气管环
Tracheal rings

图 7-24　颈部侧面观，喉和咽　Neck, Lateral View, Larynx and Pharynx

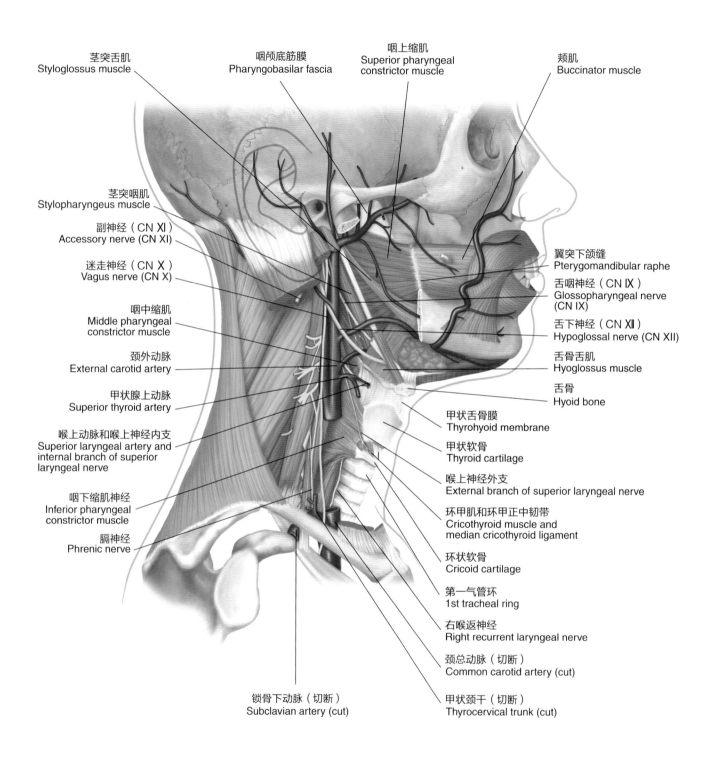

茎突舌肌
Styloglossus muscle

咽颅底筋膜
Pharyngobasilar fascia

咽上缩肌
Superior pharyngeal
constrictor muscle

颊肌
Buccinator muscle

茎突咽肌
Stylopharyngeus muscle

副神经（CN XI）
Accessory nerve (CN XI)

迷走神经（CN X）
Vagus nerve (CN X)

咽中缩肌
Middle pharyngeal
constrictor muscle

颈外动脉
External carotid artery

甲状腺上动脉
Superior thyroid artery

喉上动脉和喉上神经内支
Superior laryngeal artery and
internal branch of superior
laryngeal nerve

咽下缩肌神经
Inferior pharyngeal
constrictor muscle

膈神经
Phrenic nerve

翼突下颌缝
Pterygomandibular raphe

舌咽神经（CN IX）
Glossopharyngeal nerve
(CN IX)

舌下神经（CN XII）
Hypoglossal nerve (CN XII)

舌骨舌肌
Hyoglossus muscle

舌骨
Hyoid bone

甲状舌骨膜
Thyrohyoid membrane

甲状软骨
Thyroid cartilage

喉上神经外支
External branch of superior laryngeal nerve

环甲肌和环甲正中韧带
Cricothyroid muscle and
median cricothyroid ligament

环状软骨
Cricoid cartilage

第一气管环
1st tracheal ring

右喉返神经
Right recurrent laryngeal nerve

颈总动脉（切断）
Common carotid artery (cut)

甲状颈干（切断）
Thyrocervical trunk (cut)

锁骨下动脉（切断）
Subclavian artery (cut)

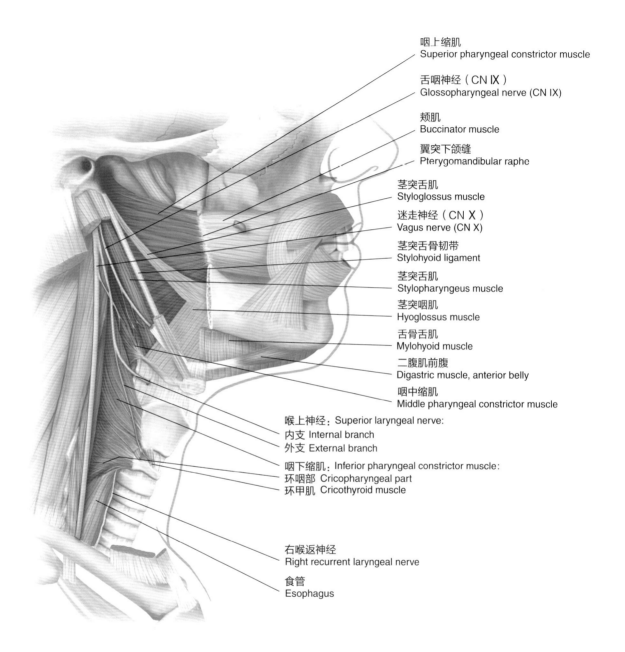

咽上缩肌
Superior pharyngeal constrictor muscle

舌咽神经（CN IX）
Glossopharyngeal nerve (CN IX)

颊肌
Buccinator muscle

翼突下颌缝
Pterygomandibular raphe

茎突舌肌
Styloglossus muscle

迷走神经（CN X）
Vagus nerve (CN X)

茎突舌骨韧带
Stylohyoid ligament

茎突舌肌
Stylopharyngeus muscle

茎突咽肌
Hyoglossus muscle

舌骨舌肌
Mylohyoid muscle

二腹肌前腹
Digastric muscle, anterior belly

咽中缩肌
Middle pharyngeal constrictor muscle

喉上神经：Superior laryngeal nerve:

内支 Internal branch

外支 External branch

咽下缩肌：Inferior pharyngeal constrictor muscle:

环咽部 Cricopharyngeal part

环甲肌 Cricothyroid muscle

右喉返神经
Right recurrent laryngeal nerve

食管
Esophagus

图 7-26　咽，后面观　Pharynx, Posterior View

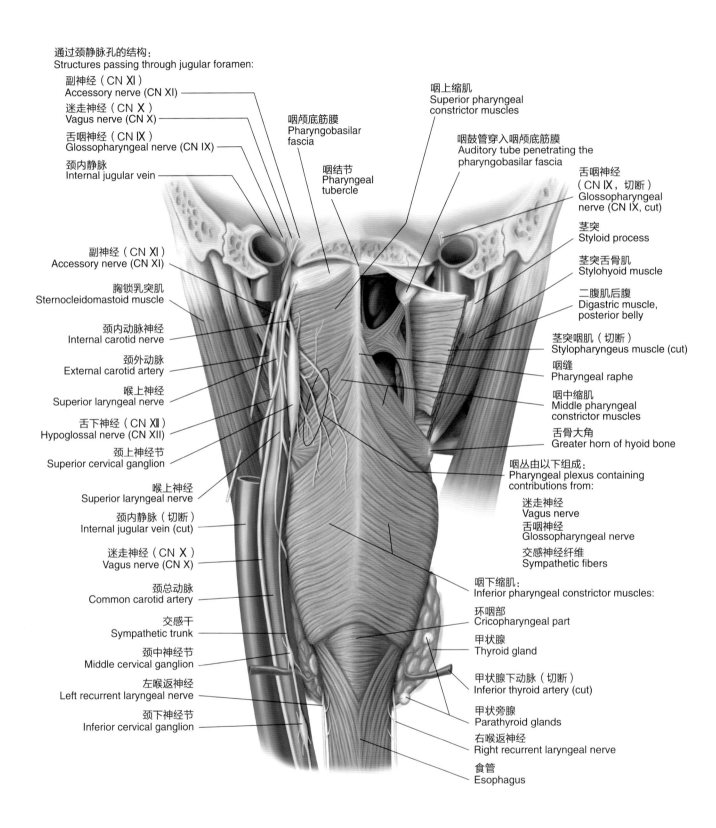

通过颈静脉孔的结构：
Structures passing through jugular foramen:

副神经（CN XI）
Accessory nerve (CN XI)

迷走神经（CN X）
Vagus nerve (CN X)

舌咽神经（CN IX）
Glossopharyngeal nerve (CN IX)

颈内静脉
Internal jugular vein

副神经（CN XI）
Accessory nerve (CN XI)

胸锁乳突肌
Sternocleidomastoid muscle

颈内动脉神经
Internal carotid nerve

颈外动脉
External carotid artery

喉上神经
Superior laryngeal nerve

舌下神经（CN XII）
Hypoglossal nerve (CN XII)

颈上神经节
Superior cervical ganglion

喉上神经
Superior laryngeal nerve

颈内静脉（切断）
Internal jugular vein (cut)

迷走神经（CN X）
Vagus nerve (CN X)

颈总动脉
Common carotid artery

交感干
Sympathetic trunk

颈中神经节
Middle cervical ganglion

左喉返神经
Left recurrent laryngeal nerve

颈下神经节
Inferior cervical ganglion

咽颅底筋膜
Pharyngobasilar fascia

咽结节
Pharyngeal tubercle

咽上缩肌
Superior pharyngeal constrictor muscles

咽鼓管穿入咽颅底筋膜
Auditory tube penetrating the pharyngobasilar fascia

舌咽神经
（CN IX，切断）
Glossopharyngeal nerve (CN IX, cut)

茎突
Styloid process

茎突舌骨肌
Stylohyoid muscle

二腹肌后腹
Digastric muscle, posterior belly

茎突咽肌（切断）
Stylopharyngeus muscle (cut)

咽缝
Pharyngeal raphe

咽中缩肌
Middle pharyngeal constrictor muscles

舌骨大角
Greater horn of hyoid bone

咽丛由以下组成：
Pharyngeal plexus containing contributions from:

迷走神经
Vagus nerve

舌咽神经
Glossopharyngeal nerve

交感神经纤维
Sympathetic fibers

咽下缩肌：
Inferior pharyngeal constrictor muscles:

环咽部
Cricopharyngeal part

甲状腺
Thyroid gland

甲状腺下动脉（切断）
Inferior thyroid artery (cut)

甲状旁腺
Parathyroid glands

右喉返神经
Right recurrent laryngeal nerve

食管
Esophagus

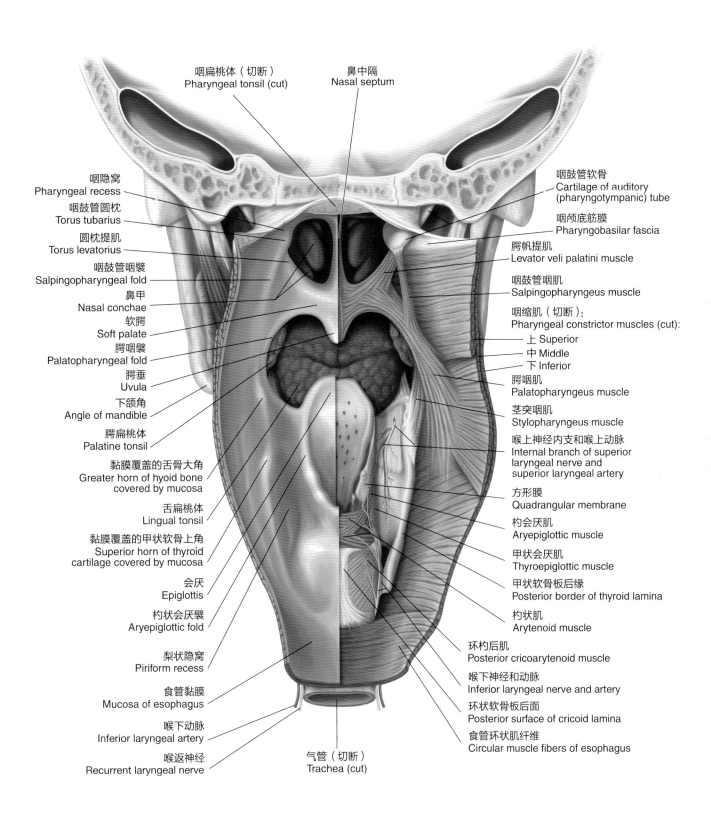

咽扁桃体（切断）
Pharyngeal tonsil (cut)

鼻中隔
Nasal septum

咽隐窝
Pharyngeal recess

咽鼓管圆枕
Torus tubarius

圆枕提肌
Torus levatorius

咽鼓管咽襞
Salpingopharyngeal fold

鼻甲
Nasal conchae

软腭
Soft palate

腭咽襞
Palatopharyngeal fold

腭垂
Uvula

下颌角
Angle of mandible

腭扁桃体
Palatine tonsil

黏膜覆盖的舌骨大角
Greater horn of hyoid bone
covered by mucosa

舌扁桃体
Lingual tonsil

黏膜覆盖的甲状软骨上角
Superior horn of thyroid
cartilage covered by mucosa

会厌
Epiglottis

杓状会厌襞
Aryepiglottic fold

梨状隐窝
Piriform recess

食管黏膜
Mucosa of esophagus

喉下动脉
Inferior laryngeal artery

喉返神经
Recurrent laryngeal nerve

气管（切断）
Trachea (cut)

咽鼓管软骨
Cartilage of auditory
(pharyngotympanic) tube

咽颅底筋膜
Pharyngobasilar fascia

腭帆提肌
Levator veli palatini muscle

咽鼓管咽肌
Salpingopharyngeus muscle

咽缩肌（切断）：
Pharyngeal constrictor muscles (cut):

上 Superior

中 Middle

下 Inferior

腭咽肌
Palatopharyngeus muscle

茎突咽肌
Stylopharyngeus muscle

喉上神经内支和喉上动脉
Internal branch of superior
laryngeal nerve and
superior laryngeal artery

方形膜
Quadrangular membrane

杓会厌肌
Aryepiglottic muscle

甲状会厌肌
Thyroepiglottic muscle

甲状软骨板后缘
Posterior border of thyroid lamina

杓状肌
Arytenoid muscle

环杓后肌
Posterior cricoarytenoid muscle

喉下神经和动脉
Inferior laryngeal nerve and artery

环状软骨板后面
Posterior surface of cricoid lamina

食管环状肌纤维
Circular muscle fibers of esophagus

图 7-28 　咽内部，内侧面观　Interior of the Pharynx, Medial View

A. 分区
Regions

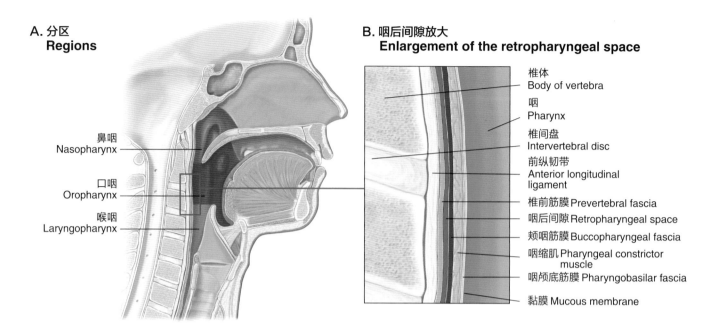

鼻咽
Nasopharynx

口咽
Oropharynx

喉咽
Laryngopharynx

B. 咽后间隙放大
Enlargement of the retropharyngeal space

椎体
Body of vertebra

咽
Pharynx

椎间盘
Intervertebral disc

前纵韧带
Anterior longitudinal ligament

椎前筋膜 Prevertebral fascia

咽后间隙 Retropharyngeal space

颊咽筋膜 Buccopharyngeal fascia

咽缩肌 Pharyngeal constrictor muscle

咽颅底筋膜 Pharyngobasilar fascia

黏膜 Mucous membrane

C. 黏膜结构
Mucosal features

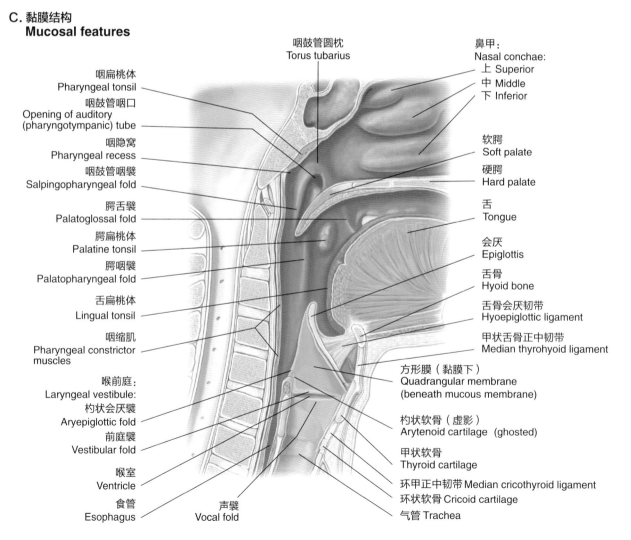

咽扁桃体
Pharyngeal tonsil

咽鼓管咽口
Opening of auditory (pharyngotympanic) tube

咽隐窝
Pharyngeal recess

咽鼓管咽襞
Salpingopharyngeal fold

腭舌襞
Palatoglossal fold

腭扁桃体
Palatine tonsil

腭咽襞
Palatopharyngeal fold

舌扁桃体
Lingual tonsil

咽缩肌
Pharyngeal constrictor muscles

喉前庭：
Laryngeal vestibule:
杓状会厌襞
Aryepiglottic fold
前庭襞
Vestibular fold

喉室
Ventricle

食管
Esophagus

咽鼓管圆枕
Torus tubarius

声襞
Vocal fold

鼻甲：
Nasal conchae:
上 Superior
中 Middle
下 Inferior

软腭
Soft palate

硬腭
Hard palate

舌
Tongue

会厌
Epiglottis

舌骨
Hyoid bone

舌骨会厌韧带
Hyoepiglottic ligament

甲状舌骨正中韧带
Median thyrohyoid ligament

方形膜（黏膜下）
Quadrangular membrane (beneath mucous membrane)

杓状软骨（虚影）
Arytenoid cartilage (ghosted)

甲状软骨
Thyroid cartilage

环甲正中韧带 Median cricothyroid ligament

环状软骨 Cricoid cartilage

气管 Trachea

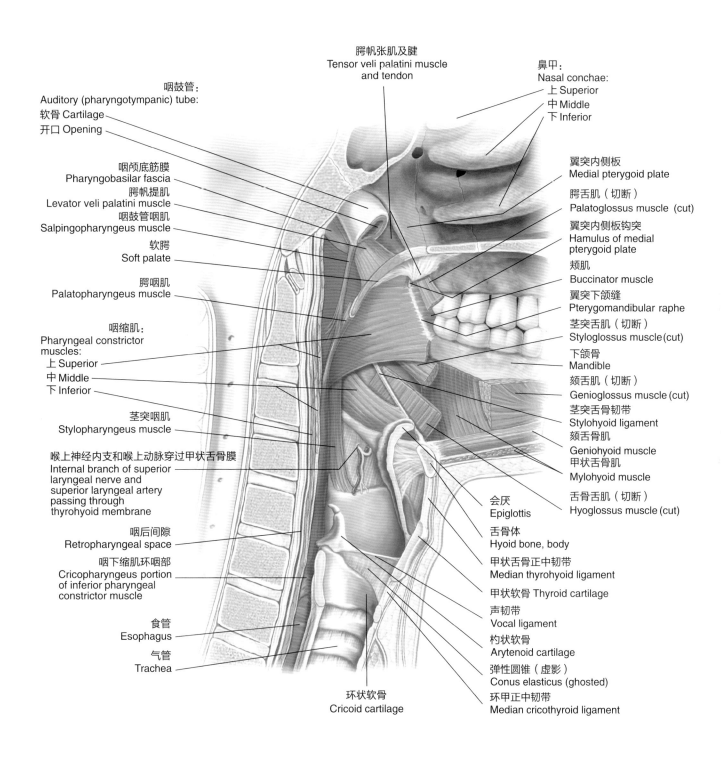

腭帆张肌及腱
Tensor veli palatini muscle
and tendon

鼻甲：
Nasal conchae:
上 Superior
中 Middle
下 Inferior

咽鼓管：
Auditory (pharyngotympanic) tube:
软骨 Cartilage
开口 Opening

翼突内侧板
Medial pterygoid plate

咽颅底筋膜
Pharyngobasilar fascia

腭帆提肌
Levator veli palatini muscle

咽鼓管咽肌
Salpingopharyngeus muscle

软腭
Soft palate

腭咽肌
Palatopharyngeus muscle

腭舌肌（切断）
Palatoglossus muscle (cut)

翼突内侧板钩突
Hamulus of medial
pterygoid plate

颊肌
Buccinator muscle

翼突下颌缝
Pterygomandibular raphe

茎突舌肌（切断）
Styloglossus muscle (cut)

下颌骨
Mandible

颏舌肌（切断）
Genioglossus muscle (cut)

茎突舌骨韧带
Stylohyoid ligament

颏舌骨肌
Geniohyoid muscle

甲状舌骨肌
Mylohyoid muscle

舌骨舌肌（切断）
Hyoglossus muscle (cut)

咽缩肌：
Pharyngeal constrictor
muscles:
上 Superior
中 Middle
下 Inferior

茎突咽肌
Stylopharyngeus muscle

喉上神经内支和喉上动脉穿过甲状舌骨膜
Internal branch of superior
laryngeal nerve and
superior laryngeal artery
passing through
thyrohyoid membrane

咽后间隙
Retropharyngeal space

咽下缩肌环咽部
Cricopharyngeus portion
of inferior pharyngeal
constrictor muscle

食管
Esophagus

气管
Trachea

环状软骨
Cricoid cartilage

会厌
Epiglottis

舌骨体
Hyoid bone, body

甲状舌骨正中韧带
Median thyrohyoid ligament

甲状软骨 Thyroid cartilage

声韧带
Vocal ligament

杓状软骨
Arytenoid cartilage

弹性圆锥（虚影）
Conus elasticus (ghosted)

环甲正中韧带
Median cricothyroid ligament

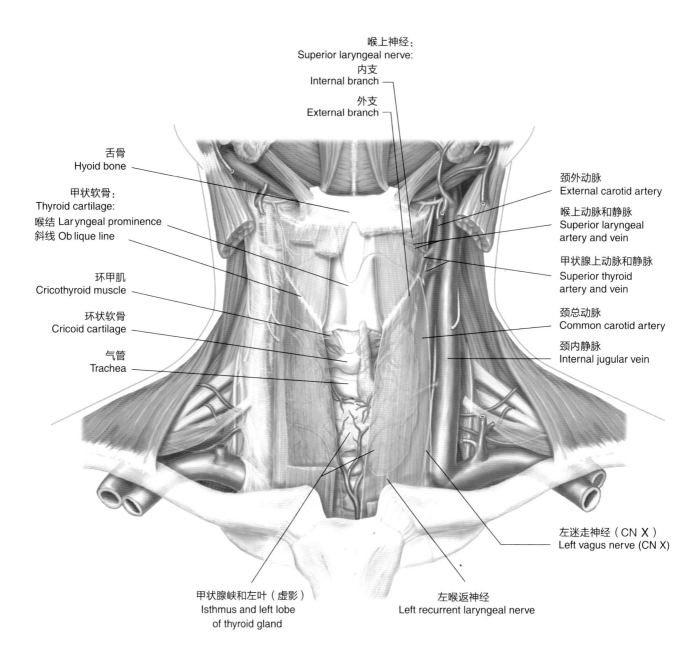

图 7-30　原位喉，前面观　Larynx In Situ, Anterior View

喉上神经：
Superior laryngeal nerve:

内支
Internal branch

外支
External branch

舌骨
Hyoid bone

甲状软骨：
Thyroid cartilage:

喉结 Laryngeal prominence
斜线 Oblique line

环甲肌
Cricothyroid muscle

环状软骨
Cricoid cartilage

气管
Trachea

颈外动脉
External carotid artery

喉上动脉和静脉
Superior laryngeal
artery and vein

甲状腺上动脉和静脉
Superior thyroid
artery and vein

颈总动脉
Common carotid artery

颈内静脉
Internal jugular vein

左迷走神经（CN X）
Left vagus nerve (CN X)

甲状腺峡和左叶（虚影）
Isthmus and left lobe
of thyroid gland

左喉返神经
Left recurrent laryngeal nerve

A. 前面观
Anterior view

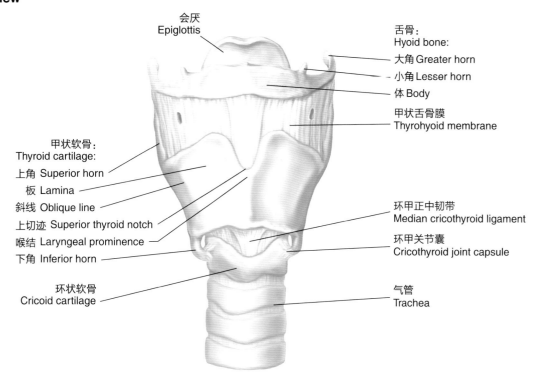

会厌
Epiglottis

舌骨：
Hyoid bone:

大角 Greater horn

小角 Lesser horn

体 Body

甲状舌骨膜
Thyrohyoid membrane

甲状软骨：
Thyroid cartilage:

上角 Superior horn

板 Lamina

斜线 Oblique line

上切迹 Superior thyroid notch

喉结 Laryngeal prominence

下角 Inferior horn

环甲正中韧带
Median cricothyroid ligament

环甲关节囊
Cricothyroid joint capsule

环状软骨
Cricoid cartilage

气管
Trachea

B. 侧面观
Lateral view

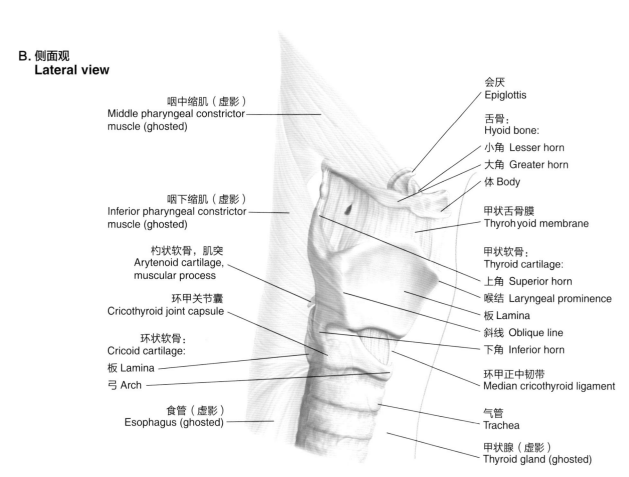

咽中缩肌（虚影）
Middle pharyngeal constrictor
muscle (ghosted)

咽下缩肌（虚影）
Inferior pharyngeal constrictor
muscle (ghosted)

枸状软骨，肌突
Arytenoid cartilage,
muscular process

环甲关节囊
Cricothyroid joint capsule

环状软骨：
Cricoid cartilage:

板 Lamina

弓 Arch

食管（虚影）
Esophagus (ghosted)

会厌
Epiglottis

舌骨：
Hyoid bone:

小角 Lesser horn

大角 Greater horn

体 Body

甲状舌骨膜
Thyrohyoid membrane

甲状软骨：
Thyroid cartilage:

上角 Superior horn

喉结 Laryngeal prominence

板 Lamina

斜线 Oblique line

下角 Inferior horn

环甲正中韧带
Median cricothyroid ligament

气管
Trachea

甲状腺（虚影）
Thyroid gland (ghosted)

图 7-32　喉肌　**Laryngeal Muscles**

A. 前面观
Lateral view

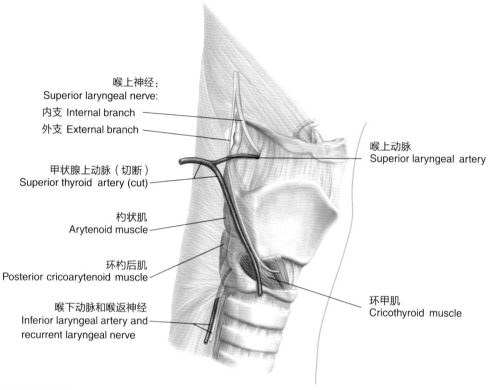

喉上神经：
Superior laryngeal nerve:

内支 Internal branch

外支 External branch

甲状腺上动脉（切断）
Superior thyroid artery (cut)

杓状肌
Arytenoid muscle

环杓后肌
Posterior cricoarytenoid muscle

喉下动脉和喉返神经
Inferior laryngeal artery and
recurrent laryngeal nerve

喉上动脉
Superior laryngeal artery

环甲肌
Cricothyroid muscle

B. 外侧面观，甲状软骨板切除
Lateral view,
thyroid lamina removed

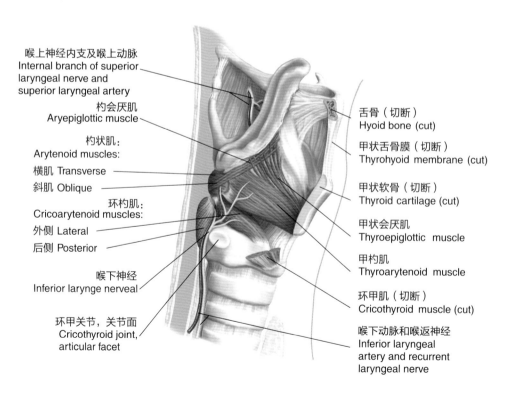

喉上神经内支及喉上动脉
Internal branch of superior
laryngeal nerve and
superior laryngeal artery

杓会厌肌
Aryepiglottic muscle

杓状肌：
Arytenoid muscles:

横肌 Transverse

斜肌 Oblique

环杓肌：
Cricoarytenoid muscles:

外侧 Lateral

后侧 Posterior

喉下神经
Inferior larynge nerveal

环甲关节，关节面
Cricothyroid joint,
articular facet

舌骨（切断）
Hyoid bone (cut)

甲状舌骨膜（切断）
Thyrohyoid membrane (cut)

甲状软骨（切断）
Thyroid cartilage (cut)

甲状会厌肌
Thyroepiglottic muscle

甲杓肌
Thyroarytenoid muscle

环甲肌（切断）
Cricothyroid muscle (cut)

喉下动脉和喉返神经
Inferior laryngeal
artery and recurrent
laryngeal nerve

A. 软骨
Cartilages

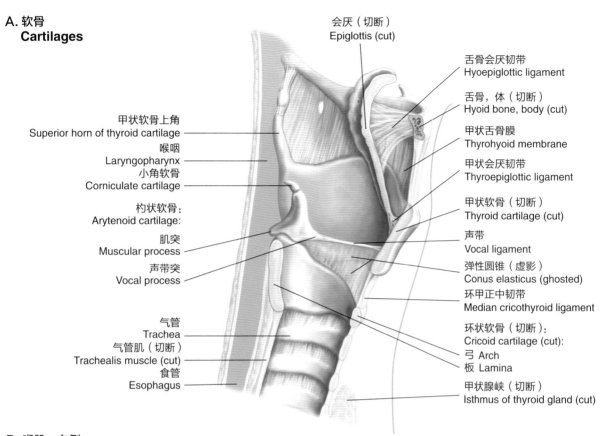

会厌（切断）
Epiglottis (cut)

舌骨会厌韧带
Hyoepiglottic ligament

舌骨，体（切断）
Hyoid bone, body (cut)

甲状舌骨膜
Thyrohyoid membrane

甲状会厌韧带
Thyroepiglottic ligament

甲状软骨（切断）
Thyroid cartilage (cut)

声带
Vocal ligament

弹性圆锥（虚影）
Conus elasticus (ghosted)

环甲正中韧带
Median cricothyroid ligament

环状软骨（切断）:
Cricoid cartilage (cut):

弓 Arch
板 Lamina

甲状腺峡（切断）
Isthmus of thyroid gland (cut)

甲状软骨上角
Superior horn of thyroid cartilage

喉咽
Laryngopharynx

小角软骨
Corniculate cartilage

杓状软骨:
Arytenoid cartilage:

肌突
Muscular process

声带突
Vocal process

气管
Trachea

气管肌（切断）
Trachealis muscle (cut)

食管
Esophagus

B. 喉肌，左侧
Muscles, left side of larynx

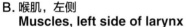

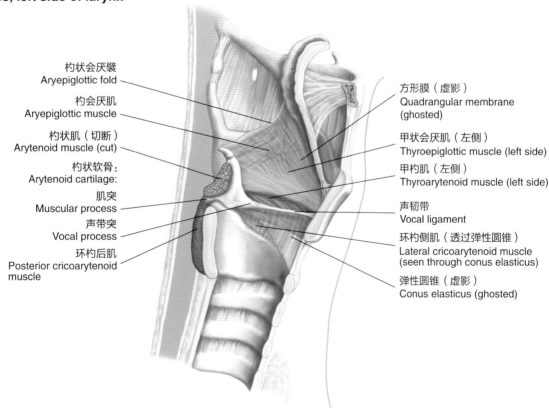

杓状会厌襞
Aryepiglottic fold

杓会厌肌
Aryepiglottic muscle

杓状肌（切断）
Arytenoid muscle (cut)

杓状软骨:
Arytenoid cartilage:

肌突
Muscular process

声带突
Vocal process

环杓后肌
Posterior cricoarytenoid
muscle

方形膜（虚影）
Quadrangular membrane
(ghosted)

甲状会厌肌（左侧）
Thyroepiglottic muscle (left side)

甲杓肌（左侧）
Thyroarytenoid muscle (left side)

声韧带
Vocal ligament

环杓侧肌（透过弹性圆锥）
Lateral cricoarytenoid muscle
(seen through conus elasticus)

弹性圆锥（虚影）
Conus elasticus (ghosted)

图 7-34　　喉，后面观　Larynx, Posterior View

A. 软骨
Cartilages

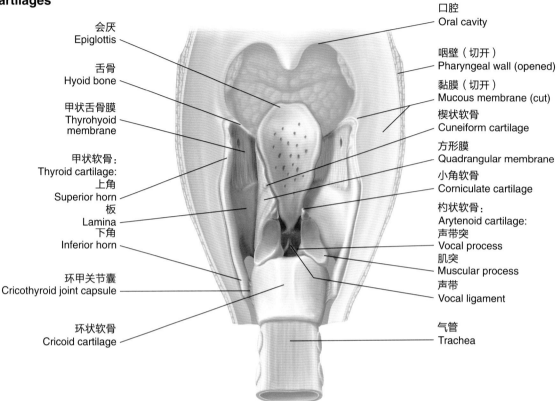

会厌
Epiglottis

舌骨
Hyoid bone

甲状舌骨膜
Thyrohyoid
membrane

甲状软骨：
Thyroid cartilage:
上角
Superior horn
板
Lamina
下角
Inferior horn

环甲关节囊
Cricothyroid joint capsule

环状软骨
Cricoid cartilage

口腔
Oral cavity

咽壁（切开）
Pharyngeal wall (opened)

黏膜（切开）
Mucous membrane (cut)

楔状软骨
Cuneiform cartilage

方形膜
Quadrangular membrane

小角软骨
Corniculate cartilage

杓状软骨：
Arytenoid cartilage:
声带突
Vocal process
肌突
Muscular process
声带
Vocal ligament

气管
Trachea

B. 肌肉
Muscles

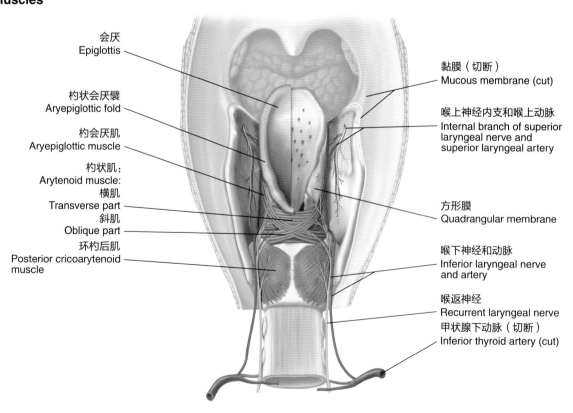

会厌
Epiglottis

杓状会厌襞
Aryepiglottic fold

杓会厌肌
Aryepiglottic muscle

杓状肌：
Arytenoid muscle:
横肌
Transverse part
斜肌
Oblique part

环杓后肌
Posterior cricoarytenoid
muscle

黏膜（切断）
Mucous membrane (cut)

喉上神经内支和喉上动脉
Internal branch of superior
laryngeal nerve and
superior laryngeal artery

方形膜
Quadrangular membrane

喉下神经和动脉
Inferior laryngeal nerve
and artery

喉返神经
Recurrent laryngeal nerve
甲状腺下动脉（切断）
Inferior thyroid artery (cut)

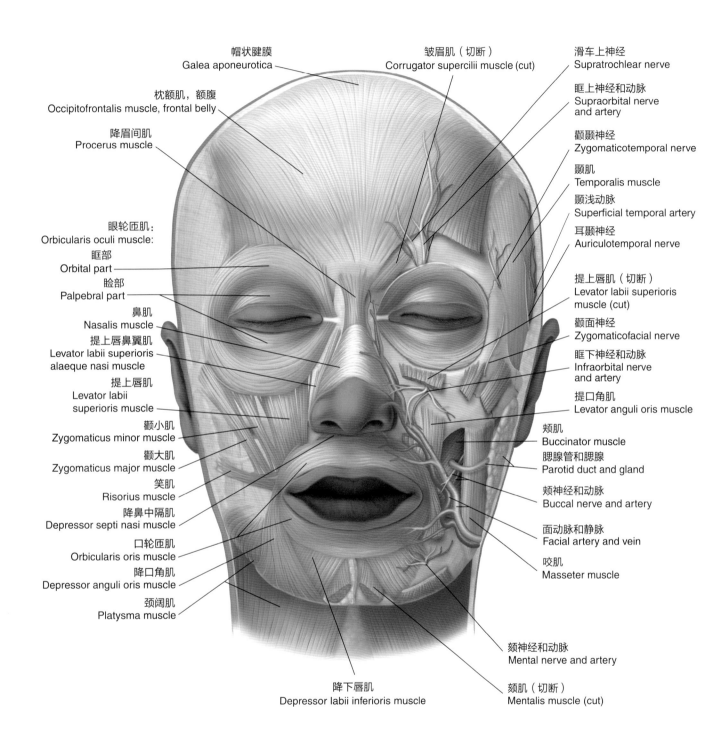

帽状腱膜
Galea aponeurotica

枕额肌，额腹
Occipitofrontalis muscle, frontal belly

降眉间肌
Procerus muscle

眼轮匝肌：
Orbicularis oculi muscle:

眶部
Orbital part

睑部
Palpebral part

鼻肌
Nasalis muscle

提上唇鼻翼肌
Levator labii superioris
alaeque nasi muscle

提上唇肌
Levator labii
superioris muscle

颧小肌
Zygomaticus minor muscle

颧大肌
Zygomaticus major muscle

笑肌
Risorius muscle

降鼻中隔肌
Depressor septi nasi muscle

口轮匝肌
Orbicularis oris muscle

降口角肌
Depressor anguli oris muscle

颈阔肌
Platysma muscle

皱眉肌（切断）
Corrugator supercilii muscle (cut)

降下唇肌
Depressor labii inferioris muscle

滑车上神经
Supratrochlear nerve

眶上神经和动脉
Supraorbital nerve
and artery

颧颞神经
Zygomaticotemporal nerve

颞肌
Temporalis muscle

颞浅动脉
Superficial temporal artery

耳颞神经
Auriculotemporal nerve

提上唇肌（切断）
Levator labii superioris
muscle (cut)

颧面神经
Zygomaticofacial nerve

眶下神经和动脉
Infraorbital nerve
and artery

提口角肌
Levator anguli oris muscle

颊肌
Buccinator muscle

腮腺管和腮腺
Parotid duct and gland

颊神经和动脉
Buccal nerve and artery

面动脉和静脉
Facial artery and vein

咬肌
Masseter muscle

颏神经和动脉
Mental nerve and artery

颏肌（切断）
Mentalis muscle (cut)

图 7-36　面部，外侧面观 I　Face, Lateral View I

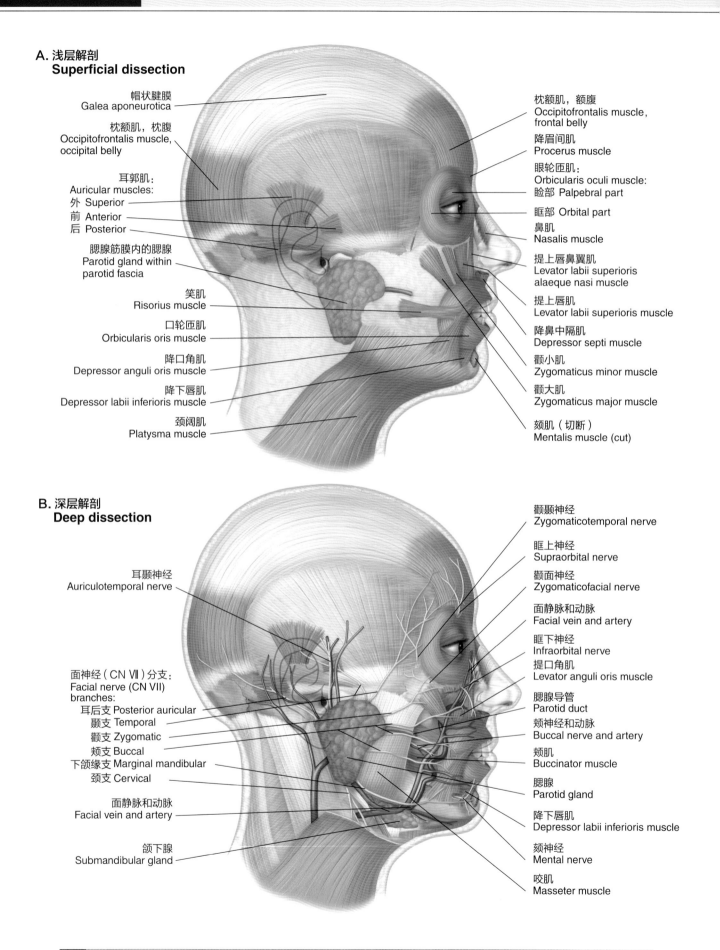

A. 浅层解剖
Superficial dissection

帽状腱膜
Galea aponeurotica

枕额肌，枕腹
Occipitofrontalis muscle,
occipital belly

耳郭肌：
Auricular muscles:
外 Superior
前 Anterior
后 Posterior

腮腺筋膜内的腮腺
Parotid gland within
parotid fascia

笑肌
Risorius muscle

口轮匝肌
Orbicularis oris muscle

降口角肌
Depressor anguli oris muscle

降下唇肌
Depressor labii inferioris muscle

颈阔肌
Platysma muscle

枕额肌，额腹
Occipitofrontalis muscle,
frontal belly

降眉间肌
Procerus muscle

眼轮匝肌：
Orbicularis oculi muscle:
睑部 Palpebral part
眶部 Orbital part

鼻肌
Nasalis muscle

提上唇鼻翼肌
Levator labii superioris
alaeque nasi muscle

提上唇肌
Levator labii superioris muscle

降鼻中隔肌
Depressor septi muscle

颧小肌
Zygomaticus minor muscle

颧大肌
Zygomaticus major muscle

颏肌（切断）
Mentalis muscle (cut)

B. 深层解剖
Deep dissection

耳颞神经
Auriculotemporal nerve

面神经（CN Ⅶ）分支：
Facial nerve (CN VII)
branches:
耳后支 Posterior auricular
颞支 Temporal
颧支 Zygomatic
颊支 Buccal
下颌缘支 Marginal mandibular
颈支 Cervical

面静脉和动脉
Facial vein and artery

颌下腺
Submandibular gland

颧颞神经
Zygomaticotemporal nerve

眶上神经
Supraorbital nerve

颧面神经
Zygomaticofacial nerve

面静脉和动脉
Facial vein and artery

眶下神经
Infraorbital nerve

提口角肌
Levator anguli oris muscle

腮腺导管
Parotid duct

颊神经和动脉
Buccal nerve and artery

颊肌
Buccinator muscle

腮腺
Parotid gland

降下唇肌
Depressor labii inferioris muscle

颏神经
Mental nerve

咬肌
Masseter muscle

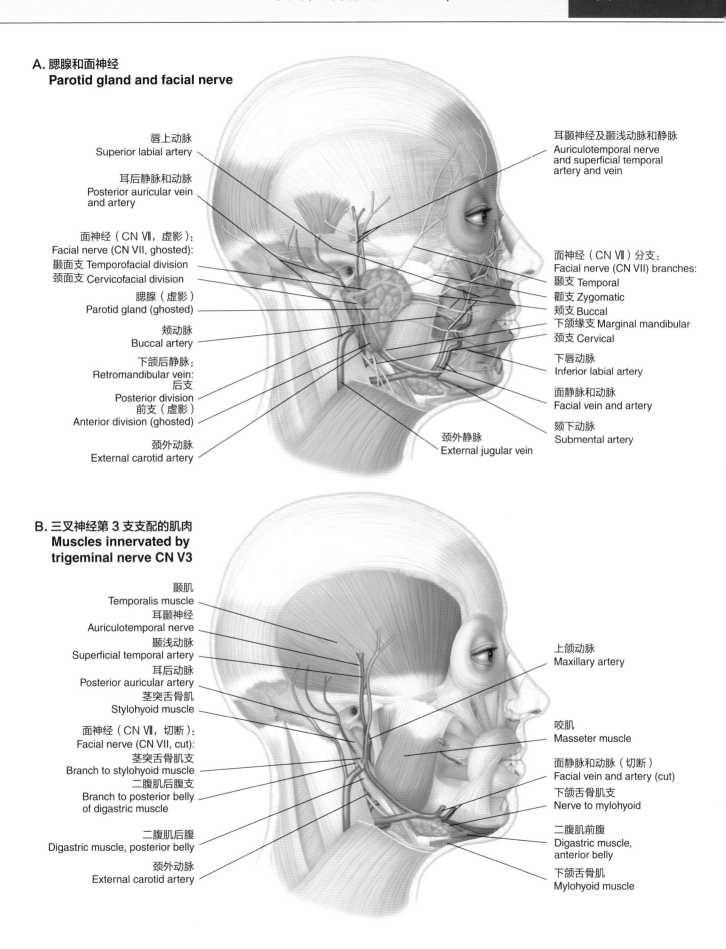

A. 腮腺和面神经
Parotid gland and facial nerve

唇上动脉
Superior labial artery

耳后静脉和动脉
Posterior auricular vein
and artery

面神经（CN VII，虚影）：
Facial nerve (CN VII, ghosted):
颞面支 Temporofacial division
颈面支 Cervicofacial division

腮腺（虚影）
Parotid gland (ghosted)

颊动脉
Buccal artery

下颌后静脉：
Retromandibular vein:
后支
Posterior division
前支（虚影）
Anterior division (ghosted)

颈外动脉
External carotid artery

耳颞神经及颞浅动脉和静脉
Auriculotemporal nerve
and superficial temporal
artery and vein

面神经（CN VII）分支：
Facial nerve (CN VII) branches:
颞支 Temporal
颧支 Zygomatic
颊支 Buccal
下颌缘支 Marginal mandibular
颈支 Cervical

下唇动脉
Inferior labial artery

面静脉和动脉
Facial vein and artery

颏下动脉
Submental artery

颈外静脉
External jugular vein

B. 三叉神经第 3 支支配的肌肉
Muscles innervated by
trigeminal nerve CN V3

颞肌
Temporalis muscle

耳颞神经
Auriculotemporal nerve

颞浅动脉
Superficial temporal artery

耳后动脉
Posterior auricular artery

茎突舌骨肌
Stylohyoid muscle

面神经（CN VII，切断）：
Facial nerve (CN VII, cut):

茎突舌骨肌支
Branch to stylohyoid muscle

二腹肌后腹支
Branch to posterior belly
of digastric muscle

二腹肌后腹
Digastric muscle, posterior belly

颈外动脉
External carotid artery

上颌动脉
Maxillary artery

咬肌
Masseter muscle

面静脉和动脉（切断）
Facial vein and artery (cut)

下颌舌骨肌支
Nerve to mylohyoid

二腹肌前腹
Digastric muscle,
anterior belly

下颌舌骨肌
Mylohyoid muscle

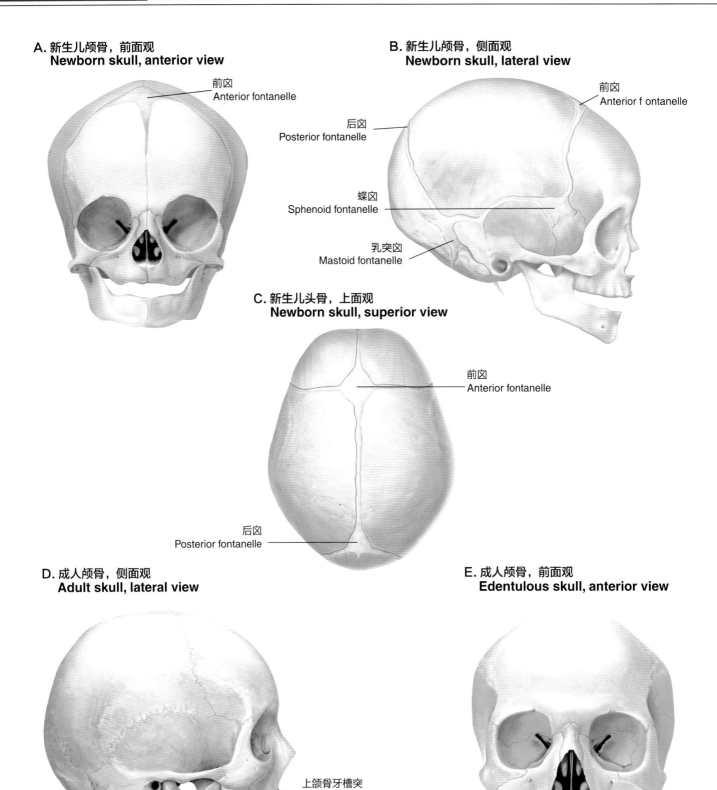

A. 新生儿颅骨，前面观
Newborn skull, anterior view

前囟
Anterior fontanelle

B. 新生儿颅骨，侧面观
Newborn skull, lateral view

前囟
Anterior f ontanelle

后囟
Posterior fontanelle

蝶囟
Sphenoid fontanelle

乳突囟
Mastoid fontanelle

C. 新生儿头骨，上面观
Newborn skull, superior view

前囟
Anterior fontanelle

后囟
Posterior fontanelle

D. 成人颅骨，侧面观
Adult skull, lateral view

上颌骨牙槽突
Alveolar process
of maxilla

下颌骨牙槽突
Alveolar process
of mandible

E. 成人颅骨，前面观
Edentulous skull, anterior view

牙槽骨（骨丢
失后再吸收）
Alveolar bone
(resorbed following
bone loss)

A. 颞区和颞下窝
Temporal and infratemporal fossae

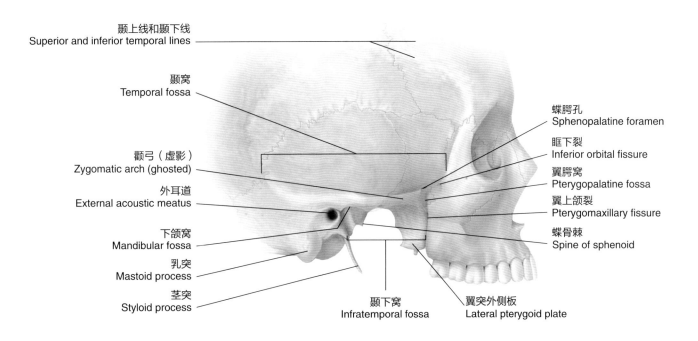

颞上线和颞下线
Superior and inferior temporal lines

颞窝
Temporal fossa

颧弓（虚影）
Zygomatic arch (ghosted)

外耳道
External acoustic meatus

下颌窝
Mandibular fossa

乳突
Mastoid process

茎突
Styloid process

蝶腭孔
Sphenopalatine foramen

眶下裂
Inferior orbital fissure

翼腭窝
Pterygopalatine fossa

翼上颌裂
Pterygomaxillary fissure

蝶骨棘
Spine of sphenoid

颞下窝
Infratemporal fossa

翼突外侧板
Lateral pterygoid plate

C. 下颌骨，内侧面观
Mandible, medial view

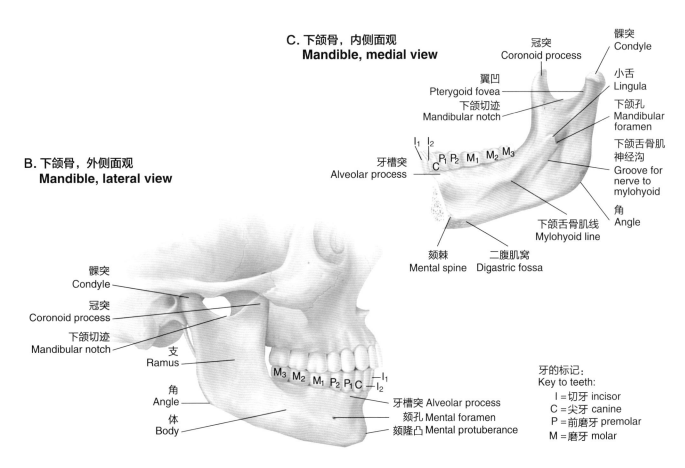

冠突
Coronoid process

髁突
Condyle

翼凹
Pterygoid fovea

下颌切迹
Mandibular notch

小舌
Lingula

下颌孔
Mandibular foramen

下颌舌骨肌神经沟
Groove for nerve to mylohyoid

角
Angle

牙槽突
Alveolar process

下颌舌骨肌线
Mylohyoid line

颏棘
Mental spine

二腹肌窝
Digastric fossa

B. 下颌骨，外侧面观
Mandible, lateral view

髁突
Condyle

冠突
Coronoid process

下颌切迹
Mandibular notch

支
Ramus

角
Angle

体
Body

牙槽突 Alveolar process

颏孔 Mental foramen

颏隆凸 Mental protuberance

牙的标记：
Key to teeth:
I = 切牙 incisor
C = 尖牙 canine
P = 前磨牙 premolar
M = 磨牙 molar

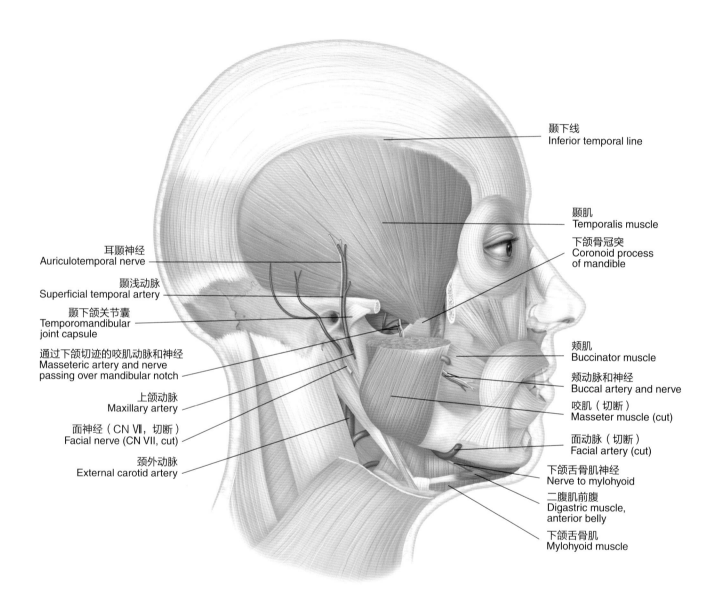

颞下线
Inferior temporal line

颞肌
Temporalis muscle

下颌骨冠突
Coronoid process
of mandible

耳颞神经
Auriculotemporal nerve

颞浅动脉
Superficial temporal artery

颞下颌关节囊
Temporomandibular
joint capsule

通过下颌切迹的咬肌动脉和神经
Masseteric artery and nerve
passing over mandibular notch

上颌动脉
Maxillary artery

面神经（CN VII，切断）
Facial nerve (CN VII, cut)

颈外动脉
External carotid artery

颊肌
Buccinator muscle

颊动脉和神经
Buccal artery and nerve

咬肌（切断）
Masseter muscle (cut)

面动脉（切断）
Facial artery (cut)

下颌舌骨肌神经
Nerve to mylohyoid

二腹肌前腹
Digastric muscle,
anterior belly

下颌舌骨肌
Mylohyoid muscle

A. 颞区和颞下区，深层解剖
Temporal and infratemporal regions, deep dissection

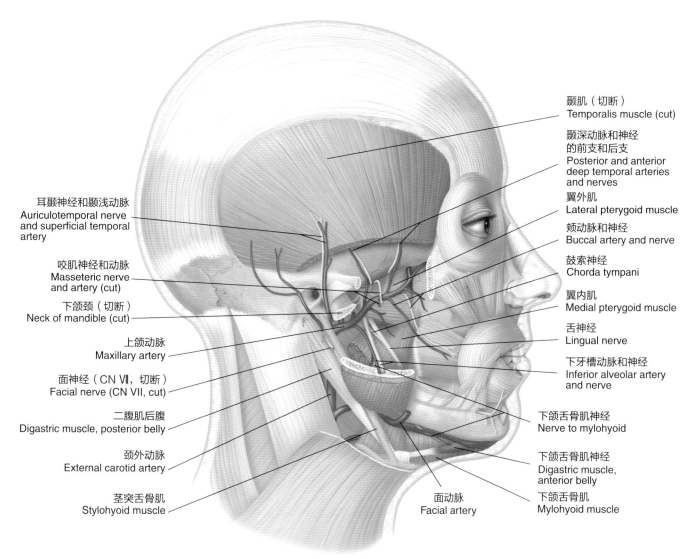

颞肌（切断）
Temporalis muscle (cut)

颞深动脉和神经
的前支和后支
Posterior and anterior
deep temporal arteries
and nerves

翼外肌
Lateral pterygoid muscle

颊动脉和神经
Buccal artery and nerve

鼓索神经
Chorda tympani

翼内肌
Medial pterygoid muscle

舌神经
Lingual nerve

下牙槽动脉和神经
Inferior alveolar artery
and nerve

下颌舌骨肌神经
Nerve to mylohyoid

下颌舌骨肌神经
Digastric muscle,
anterior belly

下颌舌骨肌
Mylohyoid muscle

面动脉
Facial artery

耳颞神经和颞浅动脉
Auriculotemporal nerve
and superficial temporal
artery

咬肌神经和动脉
Masseteric nerve
and artery (cut)

下颌颈（切断）
Neck of mandible (cut)

上颌动脉
Maxillary artery

面神经（CN Ⅶ，切断）
Facial nerve (CN VII, cut)

二腹肌后腹
Digastric muscle, posterior belly

颈外动脉
External carotid artery

茎突舌骨肌
Stylohyoid muscle

B. 颞下颌关节
Temporomandibular joint

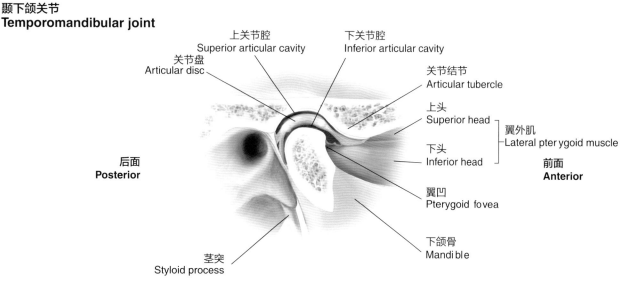

上关节腔
Superior articular cavity

下关节腔
Inferior articular cavity

关节盘
Articular disc

关节结节
Articular tubercle

上头
Superior head

翼外肌
Lateral pterygoid muscle

下头
Inferior head

后面
Posterior

前面
Anterior

翼凹
Pterygoid fovea

下颌骨
Mandible

茎突
Styloid process

图 7-42　颞下区的动脉　Arteries of the Infratemporal Region

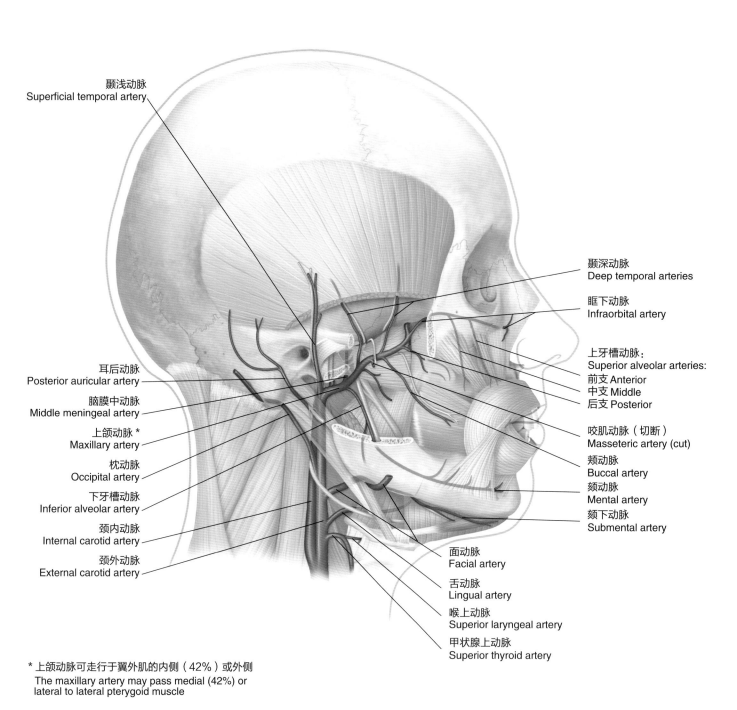

颞浅动脉
Superficial temporal artery

耳后动脉
Posterior auricular artery

脑膜中动脉
Middle meningeal artery

上颌动脉 *
Maxillary artery

枕动脉
Occipital artery

下牙槽动脉
Inferior alveolar artery

颈内动脉
Internal carotid artery

颈外动脉
External carotid artery

颞深动脉
Deep temporal arteries

眶下动脉
Infraorbital artery

上牙槽动脉：
Superior alveolar arteries:
前支 Anterior
中支 Middle
后支 Posterior

咬肌动脉（切断）
Masseteric artery (cut)

颊动脉
Buccal artery

颏动脉
Mental artery

颏下动脉
Submental artery

面动脉
Facial artery

舌动脉
Lingual artery

喉上动脉
Superior laryngeal artery

甲状腺上动脉
Superior thyroid artery

* 上颌动脉可走行于翼外肌的内侧（42%）或外侧
The maxillary artery may pass medial (42%) or
lateral to lateral pterygoid muscle

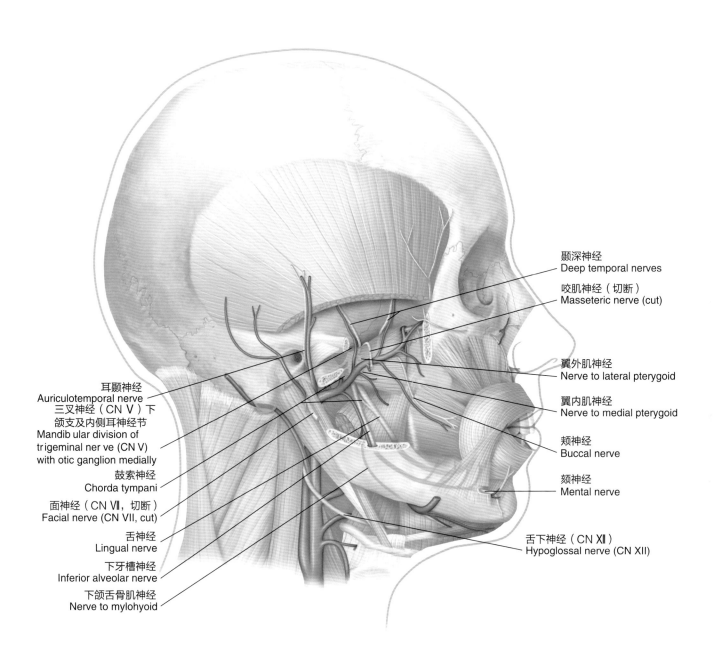

耳颞神经
Auriculotemporal nerve
三叉神经（CN V）下
颌支及内侧耳神经节
Mandib ular division of
tri geminal ner ve (CN V)
with otic ganglion medially

鼓索神经
Chorda tympani

面神经（CN Ⅶ，切断）
Facial nerve (CN VII, cut)

舌神经
Lingual nerve

下牙槽神经
Inferior alveolar nerve

下颌舌骨肌神经
Nerve to mylohyoid

颞深神经
Deep temporal nerves

咬肌神经（切断）
Masseteric nerve (cut)

翼外肌神经
Nerve to lateral pterygoid

翼内肌神经
Nerve to medial pterygoid

颊神经
Buccal nerve

颏神经
Mental nerve

舌下神经（CN Ⅻ）
Hypoglossal nerve (CN XII)

图 7-44　下颌下区和舌下区　Submandibular and Sublingual Regions

A. 外侧观
Lateral view

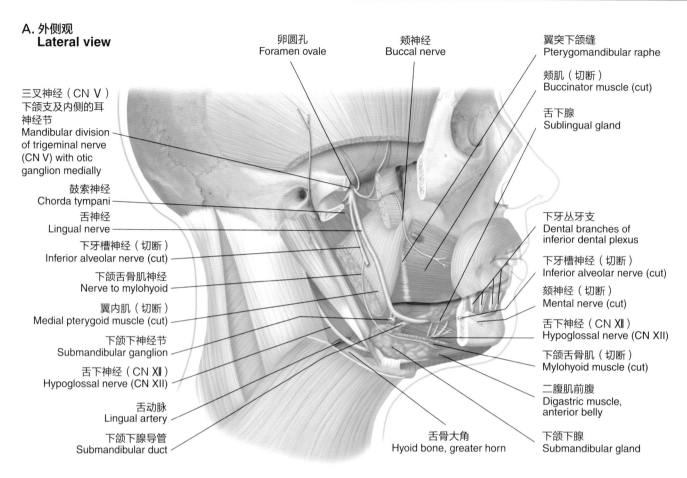

卵圆孔
Foramen ovale

颊神经
Buccal nerve

翼突下颌缝
Pterygomandibular raphe

颊肌（切断）
Buccinator muscle (cut)

舌下腺
Sublingual gland

三叉神经（CN V）
下颌支及内侧的耳
神经节
Mandibular division
of trigeminal nerve
(CN V) with otic
ganglion medially

鼓索神经
Chorda tympani

舌神经
Lingual nerve

下牙槽神经（切断）
Inferior alveolar nerve (cut)

下颌舌骨肌神经
Nerve to mylohyoid

翼内肌（切断）
Medial pterygoid muscle (cut)

下颌下神经节
Submandibular ganglion

舌下神经（CN Ⅻ）
Hypoglossal nerve (CN XII)

舌动脉
Lingual artery

下颌下腺导管
Submandibular duct

下牙丛牙支
Dental branches of
inferior dental plexus

下牙槽神经（切断）
Inferior alveolar nerve (cut)

颏神经（切断）
Mental nerve (cut)

舌下神经（CN Ⅻ）
Hypoglossal nerve (CN XII)

下颌舌骨肌（切断）
Mylohyoid muscle (cut)

二腹肌前腹
Digastric muscle,
anterior belly

下颌下腺
Submandibular gland

舌骨大角
Hyoid bone, greater horn

B. 内侧观
Medial view

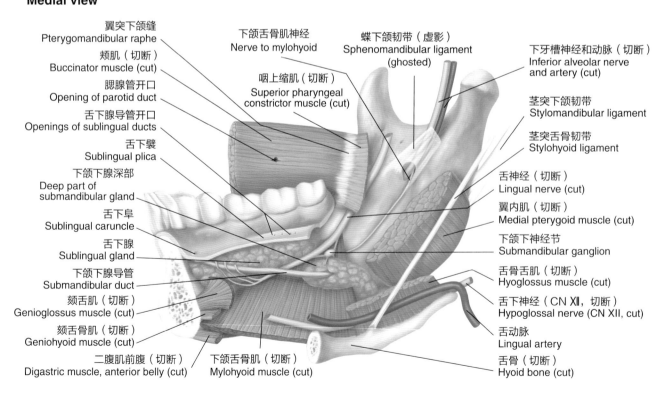

翼突下颌缝
Pterygomandibular raphe

颊肌（切断）
Buccinator muscle (cut)

腮腺管开口
Opening of parotid duct

舌下腺导管开口
Openings of sublingual ducts

舌下襞
Sublingual plica

下颌下腺深部
Deep part of
submandibular gland

舌下阜
Sublingual caruncle

舌下腺
Sublingual gland

下颌下腺导管
Submandibular duct

颏舌肌（切断）
Genioglossus muscle (cut)

颏舌骨肌（切断）
Geniohyoid muscle (cut)

二腹肌前腹（切断）
Digastric muscle, anterior belly (cut)

下颌舌骨肌神经
Nerve to mylohyoid

咽上缩肌（切断）
Superior pharyngeal
constrictor muscle (cut)

下颌舌骨肌（切断）
Mylohyoid muscle (cut)

蝶下颌韧带（虚影）
Sphenomandibular ligament
(ghosted)

下牙槽神经和动脉（切断）
Inferior alveolar nerve
and artery (cut)

茎突下颌韧带
Stylomandibular ligament

茎突舌骨韧带
Stylohyoid ligament

舌神经（切断）
Lingual nerve (cut)

翼内肌（切断）
Medial pterygoid muscle (cut)

下颌下神经节
Submandibular ganglion

舌骨舌肌（切断）
Hyoglossus muscle (cut)

舌下神经（CN Ⅻ，切断）
Hypoglossal nerve (CN XII, cut)

舌动脉
Lingual artery

舌骨（切断）
Hyoid bone (cut)

A. 黏膜特征
Mucosal features

上唇系带
Frenulum of upper lip

牙龈
Gingiva

腮腺乳头
Parotid papilla

伞襞
Fimbriated fold

舌系带
Lingual frenulum

舌下襞
Sublingual plica

舌下阜
Sublingual caruncle

牙龈
Gingiva

下唇系带
Frenulum of lower lip

B. 腭和咽
Palate and fauces

软腭
Soft palate

悬雍垂
Uvula

口咽
Oropharynx

舌背
Dorsum of tongue

咽门：
Fauces:

腭咽襞
Palatopharyngeal fold

腭扁桃体
Palatine tonsil

腭舌襞
Palatoglossal fold

C. 冠状断面
Coronal section

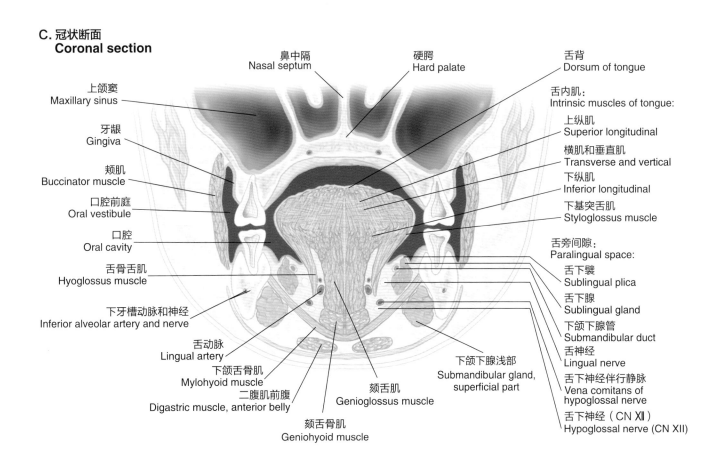

鼻中隔
Nasal septum

硬腭
Hard palate

舌背
Dorsum of tongue

上颌窦
Maxillary sinus

牙龈
Gingiva

颊肌
Buccinator muscle

口腔前庭
Oral vestibule

口腔
Oral cavity

舌骨舌肌
Hyoglossus muscle

下牙槽动脉和神经
Inferior alveolar artery and nerve

舌动脉
Lingual artery

下颌舌骨肌
Mylohyoid muscle

二腹肌前腹
Digastric muscle, anterior belly

颏舌骨肌
Geniohyoid muscle

颏舌肌
Genioglossus muscle

下颌下腺浅部
Submandibular gland, superficial part

舌内肌：
Intrinsic muscles of tongue:

上纵肌
Superior longitudinal

横肌和垂直肌
Transverse and vertical

下纵肌
Inferior longitudinal

下基突舌肌
Styloglossus muscle

舌旁间隙：
Paralingual space:

舌下襞
Sublingual plica

舌下腺
Sublingual gland

下颌下腺管
Submandibular duct

舌神经
Lingual nerve

舌下神经伴行静脉
Vena comitans of hypoglossal nerve

舌下神经（CN XII）
Hypoglossal nerve (CN XII)

图 7-46　舌背　Dorsum of Tongue

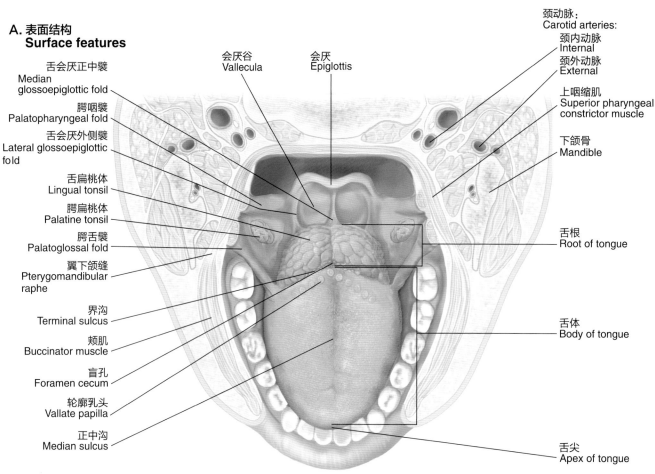

A. 表面结构
Surface features

舌会厌正中襞
Median glossoepiglottic fold

腭咽襞
Palatopharyngeal fold

舌会厌外侧襞
Lateral glossoepiglottic fold

舌扁桃体
Lingual tonsil

腭扁桃体
Palatine tonsil

腭舌襞
Palatoglossal fold

翼下颌缝
Pterygomandibular raphe

界沟
Terminal sulcus

颊肌
Buccinator muscle

盲孔
Foramen cecum

轮廓乳头
Vallate papilla

正中沟
Median sulcus

会厌谷
Vallecula

会厌
Epiglottis

颈动脉：
Carotid arteries:

颈内动脉
Internal

颈外动脉
External

上咽缩肌
Superior pharyngeal constrictor muscle

下颌骨
Mandible

舌根
Root of tongue

舌体
Body of tongue

舌尖
Apex of tongue

B. 神经支配
Innervation

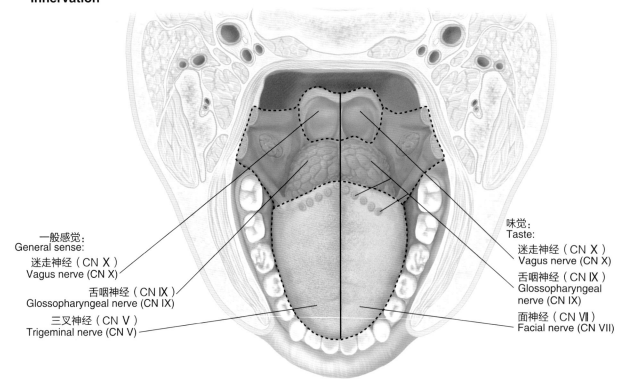

一般感觉：
General sense:

迷走神经（CN Ⅹ）
Vagus nerve (CN X)

舌咽神经（CN Ⅸ）
Glossopharyngeal nerve (CN IX)

三叉神经（CN Ⅴ）
Trigeminal nerve (CN V)

味觉：
Taste:

迷走神经（CN Ⅹ）
Vagus nerve (CN X)

舌咽神经（CN Ⅸ）
Glossopharyngeal nerve (CN IX)

面神经（CN Ⅶ）
Facial nerve (CN VII)

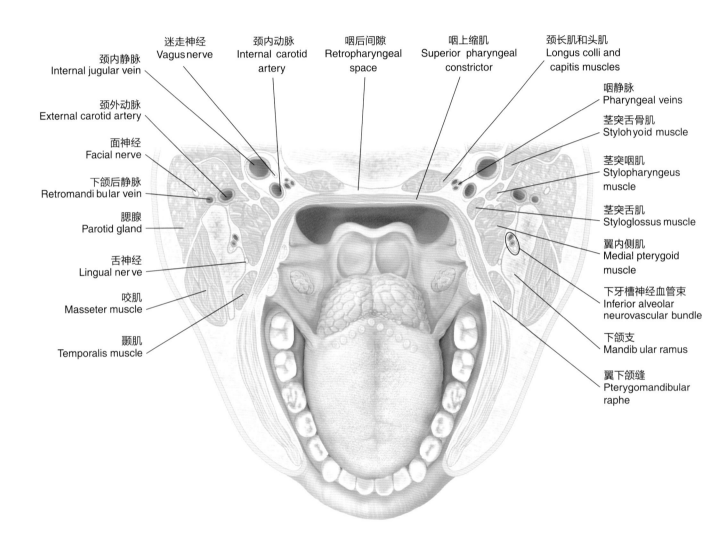

颈内静脉
Internal jugular vein

迷走神经
Vagus nerve

颈内动脉
Internal carotid
artery

咽后间隙
Retropharyngeal
space

咽上缩肌
Superior pharyngeal
constrictor

颈长肌和头肌
Longus colli and
capitis muscles

颈外动脉
External carotid artery

面神经
Facial nerve

下颌后静脉
Retromandibular vein

腮腺
Parotid gland

舌神经
Lingual nerve

咬肌
Masseter muscle

颞肌
Temporalis muscle

咽静脉
Pharyngeal veins

茎突舌骨肌
Stylohyoid muscle

茎突咽肌
Stylopharyngeus
muscle

茎突舌肌
Styloglossus muscle

翼内侧肌
Medial pterygoid
muscle

下牙槽神经血管束
Inferior alveolar
neurovascular bundle

下颌支
Mandibular ramus

翼下颌缝
Pterygomandibular
raphe

图 7-48　　舌，舌外肌　Tongue, Extrinsic Muscles

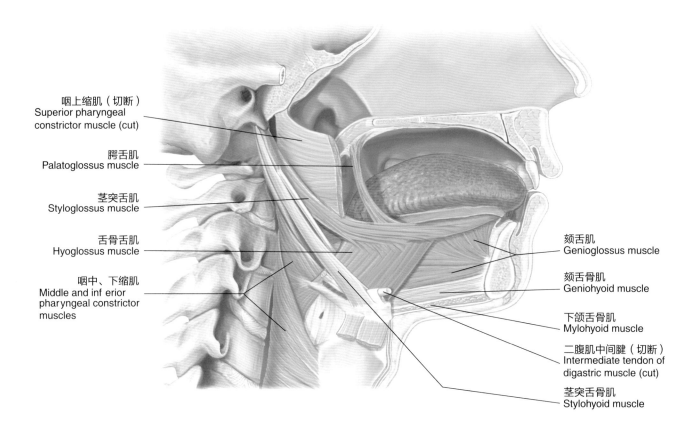

咽上缩肌（切断）
Superior pharyngeal
constrictor muscle (cut)

腭舌肌
Palatoglossus muscle

茎突舌肌
Styloglossus muscle

舌骨舌肌
Hyoglossus muscle

咽中、下缩肌
Middle and inf erior
pharyngeal constrictor
muscles

颏舌肌
Genioglossus muscle

颏舌骨肌
Geniohyoid muscle

下颌舌骨肌
Mylohyoid muscle

二腹肌中间腱（切断）
Intermediate tendon of
digastric muscle (cut)

茎突舌骨肌
Stylohyoid muscle

A. 血供
Blood supply

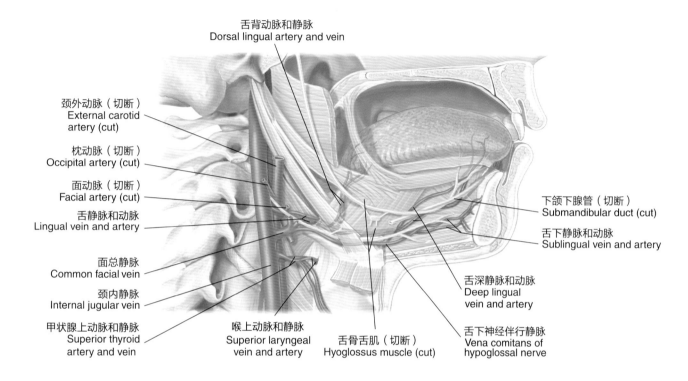

舌背动脉和静脉
Dorsal lingual artery and vein

颈外动脉（切断）
External carotid
artery (cut)

枕动脉（切断）
Occipital artery (cut)

面动脉（切断）
Facial artery (cut)

舌静脉和动脉
Lingual vein and artery

面总静脉
Common facial vein

颈内静脉
Internal jugular vein

甲状腺上动脉和静脉
Superior thyroid
artery and vein

喉上动脉和静脉
Superior laryngeal
vein and artery

舌骨舌肌（切断）
Hyoglossus muscle (cut)

下颌下腺管（切断）
Submandibular duct (cut)

舌下静脉和动脉
Sublingual vein and artery

舌深静脉和动脉
Deep lingual
vein and artery

舌下神经伴行静脉
Vena comitans of
hypoglossal nerve

B. 神经支配
Nerve supply

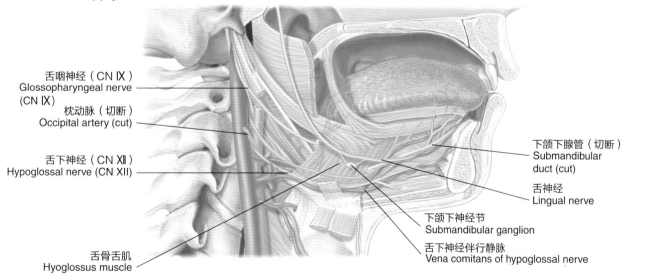

舌咽神经（CN IX）
Glossopharyngeal nerve
(CN IX)

枕动脉（切断）
Occipital artery (cut)

舌下神经（CN XII）
Hypoglossal nerve (CN XII)

舌骨舌肌
Hyoglossus muscle

下颌下腺管（切断）
Submandibular
duct (cut)

舌神经
Lingual nerve

下颌下神经节
Submandibular ganglion

舌下神经伴行静脉
Vena comitans of hypoglossal nerve

图 7-50　鼻中隔和腭　Nasal Septum and Palate

A. 骨和软骨
Bones and cartilages

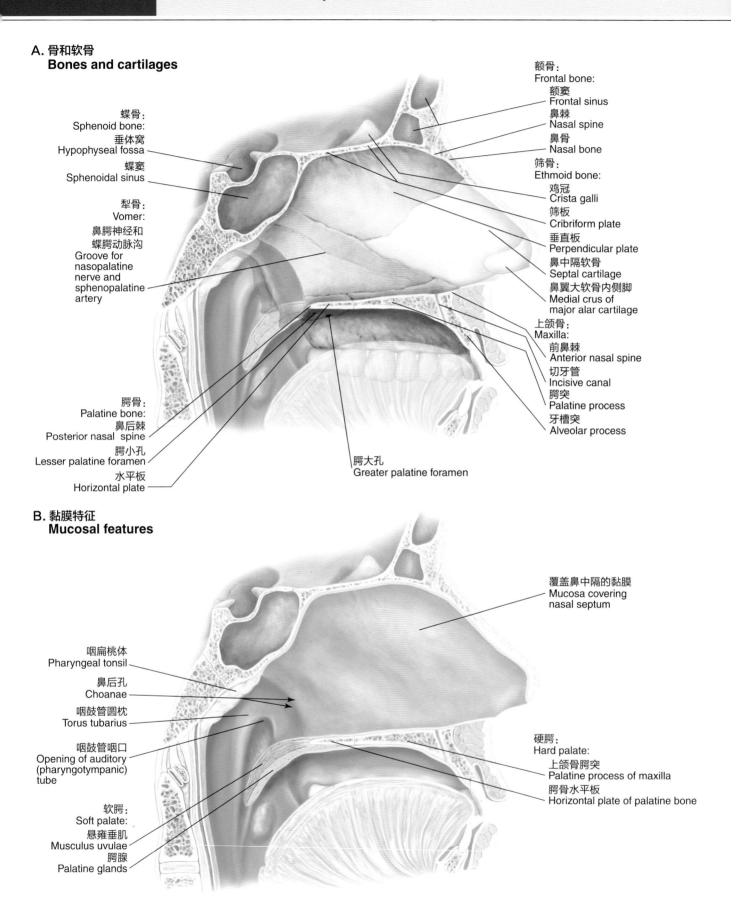

蝶骨:
Sphenoid bone:

垂体窝
Hypophyseal fossa

蝶窦
Sphenoidal sinus

犁骨:
Vomer:

鼻腭神经和
蝶腭动脉沟
Groove for
nasopalatine
nerve and
sphenopalatine
artery

腭骨:
Palatine bone:

鼻后棘
Posterior nasal spine

腭小孔
Lesser palatine foramen

水平板
Horizontal plate

腭大孔
Greater palatine foramen

额骨:
Frontal bone:

额窦
Frontal sinus

鼻棘
Nasal spine

鼻骨
Nasal bone

筛骨:
Ethmoid bone:

鸡冠
Crista galli

筛板
Cribriform plate

垂直板
Perpendicular plate

鼻中隔软骨
Septal cartilage

鼻翼大软骨内侧脚
Medial crus of
major alar cartilage

上颌骨:
Maxilla:

前鼻棘
Anterior nasal spine

切牙管
Incisive canal

腭突
Palatine process

牙槽突
Alveolar process

B. 黏膜特征
Mucosal features

咽扁桃体
Pharyngeal tonsil

鼻后孔
Choanae

咽鼓管圆枕
Torus tubarius

咽鼓管咽口
Opening of auditory
(pharyngotympanic)
tube

软腭:
Soft palate:

悬雍垂肌
Musculus uvulae

腭腺
Palatine glands

覆盖鼻中隔的黏膜
Mucosa covering
nasal septum

硬腭:
Hard palate:

上颌骨腭突
Palatine process of maxilla

腭骨水平板
Horizontal plate of palatine bone

A. 骨
Bones

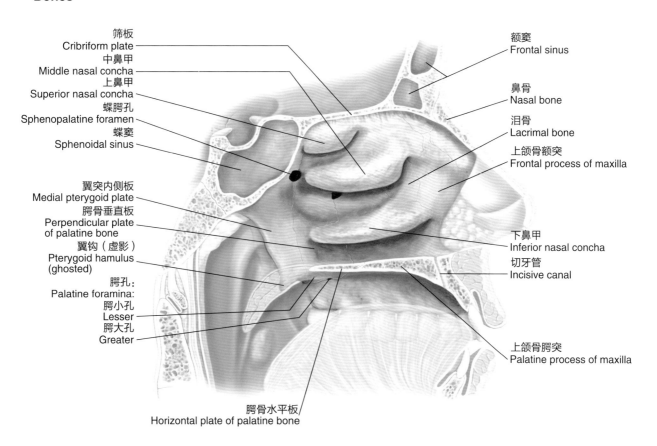

筛板
Cribriform plate

中鼻甲
Middle nasal concha

上鼻甲
Superior nasal concha

蝶腭孔
Sphenopalatine foramen

蝶窦
Sphenoidal sinus

翼突内侧板
Medial pterygoid plate

腭骨垂直板
Perpendicular plate
of palatine bone

翼钩（虚影）
Pterygoid hamulus
(ghosted)

腭孔：
Palatine foramina:
腭小孔
Lesser
腭大孔
Greater

额窦
Frontal sinus

鼻骨
Nasal bone

泪骨
Lacrimal bone

上颌骨额突
Frontal process of maxilla

下鼻甲
Inferior nasal concha

切牙管
Incisive canal

上颌骨腭突
Palatine process of maxilla

腭骨水平板
Horizontal plate of palatine bone

B. 中鼻道的骨
Bones of the middle meatus

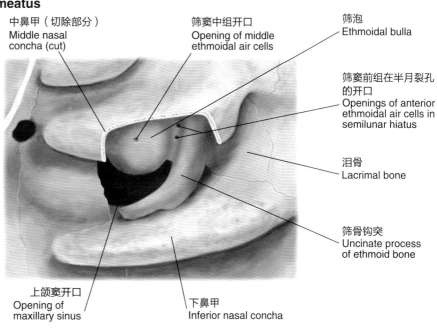

中鼻甲（切除部分）
Middle nasal
concha (cut)

筛窦中组开口
Opening of middle
ethmoidal air cells

筛泡
Ethmoidal bulla

筛窦前组在半月裂孔
的开口
Openings of anterior
ethmoidal air cells in
semilunar hiatus

泪骨
Lacrimal bone

筛骨钩突
Uncinate process
of ethmoid bone

上颌窦开口
Opening of
maxillary sinus

下鼻甲
Inferior nasal concha

图 7-52　鼻腔外侧壁 II　Lateral Wall of Nasal Cavity II

A. 鼻甲和鼻道
Nasal conchae and meatuses

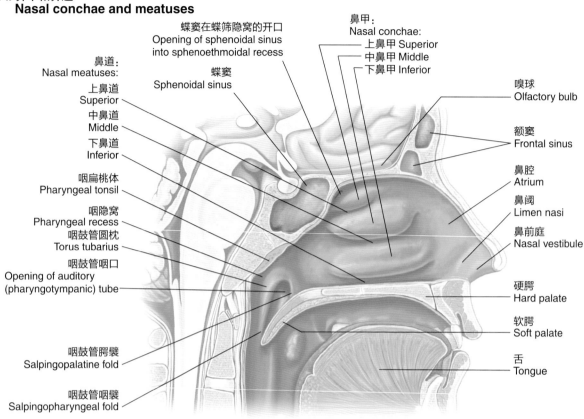

蝶窦在蝶筛隐窝的开口
Opening of sphenoidal sinus into sphenoethmoidal recess

蝶窦
Sphenoidal sinus

鼻甲：
Nasal conchae:
上鼻甲 Superior
中鼻甲 Middle
下鼻甲 Inferior

嗅球
Olfactory bulb

额窦
Frontal sinus

鼻腔
Atrium

鼻阈
Limen nasi

鼻前庭
Nasal vestibule

硬腭
Hard palate

软腭
Soft palate

舌
Tongue

鼻道：
Nasal meatuses:
上鼻道
Superior
中鼻道
Middle
下鼻道
Inferior

咽扁桃体
Pharyngeal tonsil

咽隐窝
Pharyngeal recess

咽鼓管圆枕
Torus tubarius

咽鼓管咽口
Opening of auditory (pharyngotympanic) tube

咽鼓管腭襞
Salpingopalatine fold

咽鼓管咽襞
Salpingopharyngeal fold

B. 鼻腔外侧壁的开口
Openings in the lateral wall of the nasal cavity

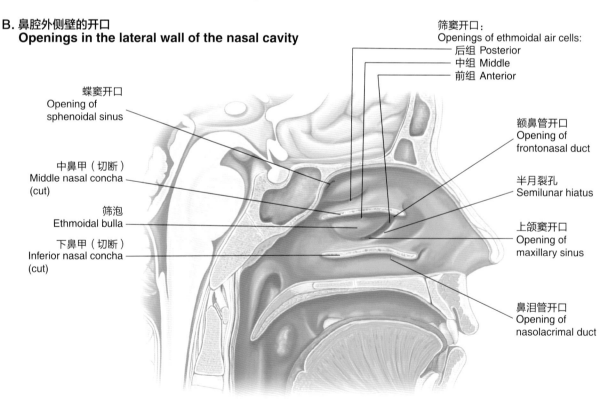

筛窦开口：
Openings of ethmoidal air cells:
后组 Posterior
中组 Middle
前组 Anterior

蝶窦开口
Opening of sphenoidal sinus

中鼻甲（切断）
Middle nasal concha (cut)

筛泡
Ethmoidal bulla

下鼻甲（切断）
Inferior nasal concha (cut)

额鼻管开口
Opening of frontonasal duct

半月裂孔
Semilunar hiatus

上颌窦开口
Opening of maxillary sinus

鼻泪管开口
Opening of nasolacrimal duct

A. 内侧面观
Medial view

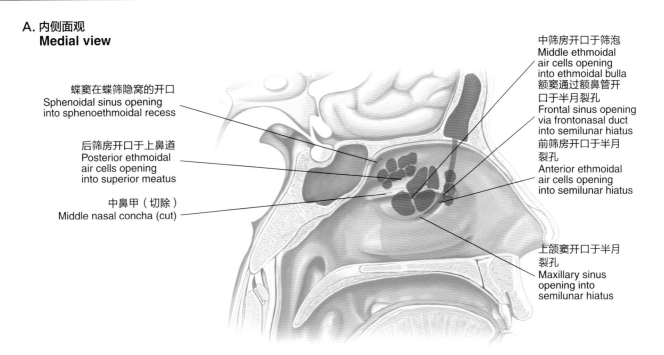

蝶窦在蝶筛隐窝的开口
Sphenoidal sinus opening
into sphenoethmoidal recess

后筛房开口于上鼻道
Posterior ethmoidal
air cells opening
into superior meatus

中鼻甲（切除）
Middle nasal concha (cut)

中筛房开口于筛泡
Middle ethmoidal
air cells opening
into ethmoidal bulla
额窦通过额鼻管开
口于半月裂孔
Frontal sinus opening
via frontonasal duct
into semilunar hiatus
前筛房开口于半月
裂孔
Anterior ethmoidal
air cells opening
into semilunar hiatus

上颌窦开口于半月
裂孔
Maxillary sinus
opening into
semilunar hiatus

B. 前面观
Anterior view

C. 外侧面观
Lateral view

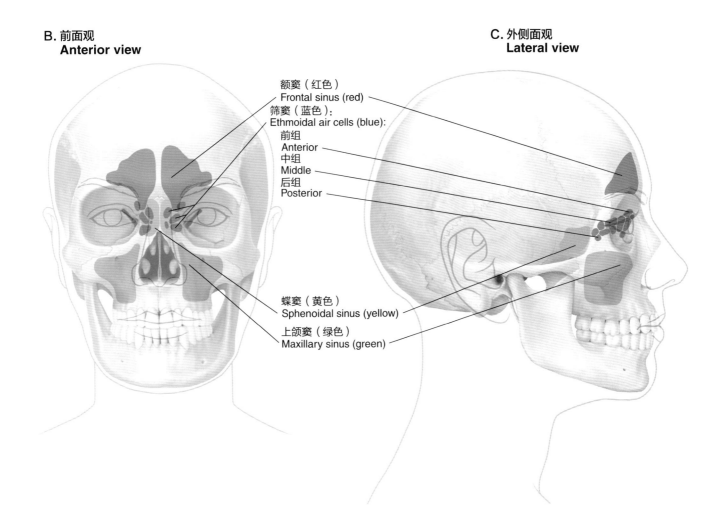

额窦（红色）
Frontal sinus (red)
筛窦（蓝色）:
Ethmoidal air cells (blue):
前组
Anterior
中组
Middle
后组
Posterior

蝶窦（黄色）
Sphenoidal sinus (yellow)
上颌窦（绿色）
Maxillary sinus (green)

A. 外侧壁的血液供应
Blood supply of lateral wall

筛后动脉鼻外侧支
Lateral nasal branches of posterior ethmoidal artery

筛前动脉:
Anterior ethmoidal artery:

鼻外侧支
Lateral nasal branch

鼻外支
External nasal branch

蝶腭动脉前中隔支（切断）
Anterior septal branch of anterior ethmoidal artery (cut)

筛后动脉中隔支（切断）
Septal branches of posterior ethmoidal artery (cut)

蝶腭动脉后中隔支（切断）
Posterior septal branch of sphenopalatine artery (cut)

面动脉鼻外侧支翼支
Alar branch of lateral nasal branch of facial artery

蝶腭动脉鼻后外侧支
Posterior lateral nasal branches of sphenopalatine artery

上颌动脉（切断）
Maxillary artery (cut)

蝶腭动脉
Sphenopalatine artery

腭降动脉（虚影）
Descending palatine artery (ghosted)

腭小动脉
Lesser palatine artery

腭大动脉
Greater palatine artery

B. 鼻中隔血液供应
Blood supply of nasal septum

面动脉上唇支的中隔支
Septal branch of superior labial branch of facial artery

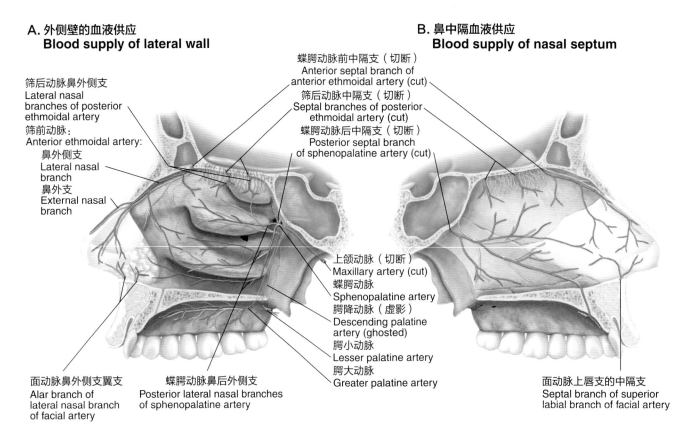

C. 外侧壁的神经
Nerves of lateral wall

筛前神经鼻内侧外支
Lateral internal nasal branch of anterior ethmoidal nerve

筛前神经鼻外支
External nasal branch of anterior ethmoidal nerve

眶下神经鼻内支
Internal nasal branches of infraorbital nerve

上颌神经后上鼻外侧支
Posterior superior lateral nasal branch of maxillary nerve

腭大神经后下鼻外侧支
Posterior inferior lateral nasal branch of greater palatine nerve

D. 鼻中隔的神经
Nerves of nasal septum

筛前神经鼻内侧内支（切断）
Medial internal branch of anterior ethmoidal nerve (cut)

嗅球和嗅束
Olfactory bulb and tract

嗅神经（CN I，切断）
Olfactory nerves (CN I, cut)

鼻腭神经（切断）
Nasopalatine nerve (cut)

上颌神经（虚影）
Maxillary nerve (ghosted)

翼管神经（虚影）
Nerve of the pterygoid canal (ghosted)

翼腭神经节（虚影）
Pterygopalatine ganglion (ghosted)

腭小神经
Lesser palatine nerve (cut)

腭大神经
Greater palatine nerve

鼻腭神经穿过切牙管
Nasopalatine nerve passing through incisive canal

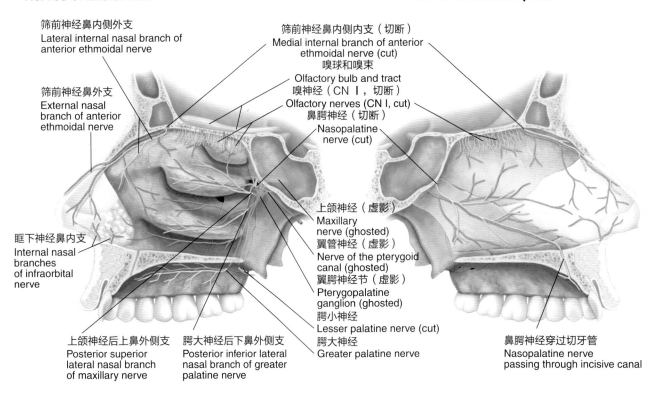

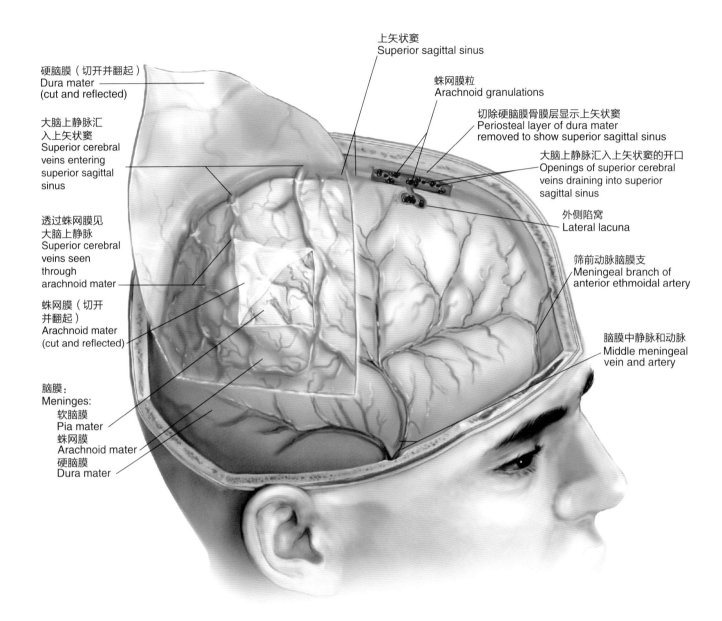

上矢状窦
Superior sagittal sinus

蛛网膜粒
Arachnoid granulations

切除硬脑膜骨膜层显示上矢状窦
Periosteal layer of dura mater
removed to show superior sagittal sinus

大脑上静脉汇入上矢状窦的开口
Openings of superior cerebral
veins draining into superior
sagittal sinus

外侧陷窝
Lateral lacuna

筛前动脉脑膜支
Meningeal branch of
anterior ethmoidal artery

脑膜中静脉和动脉
Middle meningeal
vein and artery

硬脑膜（切开并翻起）
Dura mater
(cut and reflected)

大脑上静脉汇
入上矢状窦
Superior cerebral
veins entering
superior sagittal
sinus

透过蛛网膜见
大脑上静脉
Superior cerebral
veins seen
through
arachnoid mater

蛛网膜（切开
并翻起）
Arachnoid mater
(cut and reflected)

脑膜：
Meninges:
软脑膜
Pia mater
蛛网膜
Arachnoid mater
硬脑膜
Dura mater

图 7-56　硬脑膜静脉窦，上面观　Dural Venous Sinuses, Superior View

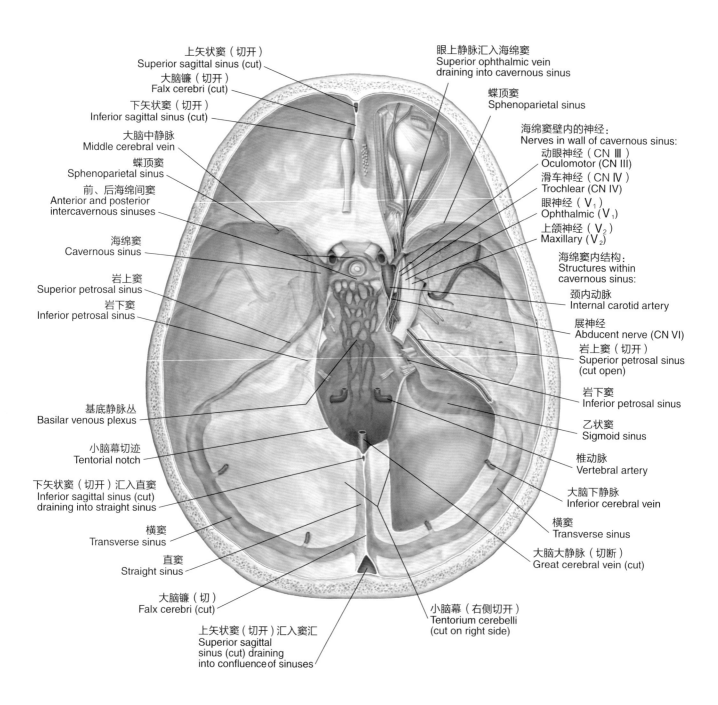

上矢状窦（切开）
Superior sagittal sinus (cut)

大脑镰（切开）
Falx cerebri (cut)

下矢状窦（切开）
Inferior sagittal sinus (cut)

大脑中静脉
Middle cerebral vein

蝶顶窦
Sphenoparietal sinus

前、后海绵间窦
Anterior and posterior
intercavernous sinuses

海绵窦
Cavernous sinus

岩上窦
Superior petrosal sinus

岩下窦
Inferior petrosal sinus

基底静脉丛
Basilar venous plexus

小脑幕切迹
Tentorial notch

下矢状窦（切开）汇入直窦
Inferior sagittal sinus (cut)
draining into straight sinus

横窦
Transverse sinus

直窦
Straight sinus

大脑镰（切）
Falx cerebri (cut)

上矢状窦（切开）汇入窦汇
Superior sagittal
sinus (cut) draining
into confluence of sinuses

眼上静脉汇入海绵窦
Superior ophthalmic vein
draining into cavernous sinus

蝶顶窦
Sphenoparietal sinus

海绵窦壁内的神经：
Nerves in wall of cavernous sinus:

动眼神经（CN Ⅲ）
Oculomotor (CN III)

滑车神经（CN Ⅳ）
Trochlear (CN IV)

眼神经（V_1）
Ophthalmic (V_1)

上颌神经（V_2）
Maxillary (V_2)

海绵窦内结构：
Structures within
cavernous sinus:

颈内动脉
Internal carotid artery

展神经
Abducent nerve (CN VI)

岩上窦（切开）
Superior petrosal sinus
(cut open)

岩下窦
Inferior petrosal sinus

乙状窦
Sigmoid sinus

椎动脉
Vertebral artery

大脑下静脉
Inferior cerebral vein

横窦
Transverse sinus

大脑大静脉（切断）
Great cerebral vein (cut)

小脑幕（右侧切开）
Tentorium cerebelli
(cut on right side)

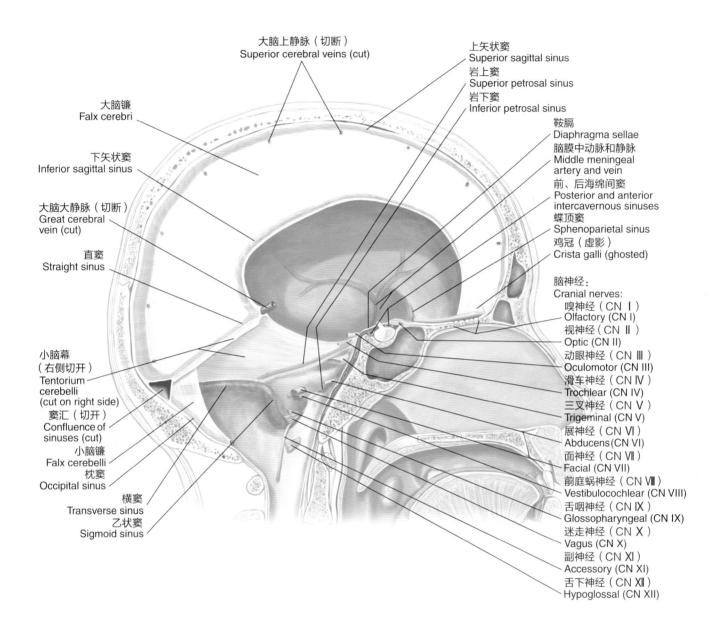

大脑上静脉（切断）
Superior cerebral veins (cut)

上矢状窦
Superior sagittal sinus
岩上窦
Superior petrosal sinus
岩下窦
Inferior petrosal sinus

鞍膈
Diaphragma sellae
脑膜中动脉和静脉
Middle meningeal
artery and vein
前、后海绵间窦
Posterior and anterior
intercavernous sinuses
蝶顶窦
Sphenoparietal sinus
鸡冠（虚影）
Crista galli (ghosted)

脑神经：
Cranial nerves:
嗅神经（CN Ⅰ）
Olfactory (CN I)
视神经（CN Ⅱ）
Optic (CN II)
动眼神经（CN Ⅲ）
Oculomotor (CN III)
滑车神经（CN Ⅳ）
Trochlear (CN IV)
三叉神经（CN Ⅴ）
Trigeminal (CN V)
展神经（CN Ⅵ）
Abducens(CN VI)
面神经（CN Ⅶ）
Facial (CN VII)
前庭蜗神经（CN Ⅷ）
Vestibulocochlear (CN VIII)
舌咽神经（CN Ⅸ）
Glossopharyngeal (CN IX)
迷走神经（CN Ⅹ）
Vagus (CN X)
副神经（CN Ⅺ）
Accessory (CN XI)
舌下神经（CN Ⅻ）
Hypoglossal (CN XII)

大脑镰
Falx cerebri

下矢状窦
Inferior sagittal sinus

大脑大静脉（切断）
Great cerebral
vein (cut)

直窦
Straight sinus

小脑幕
（右侧切开）
Tentorium
cerebelli
(cut on right side)

窦汇（切开）
Confluence of
sinuses (cut)

小脑镰
Falx cerebelli
枕窦
Occipital sinus

横窦
Transverse sinus
乙状窦
Sigmoid sinus

图 7-58　硬脑膜静脉窦，断面　Dural Venous Sinuses, Sectioned

A. 矢状断面
Sagittal section

大脑镰
Falx cerebri
上矢窦
Superior sagittal sinus
第三脑室脉络丛
Choroid plexus of 3rd ventricle
下矢窦
Inferior sagittal sinus

图 B 所在平面
Plane of section B

扣带回
Cingulate gyrus
胼胝体
Corpus callosum
透明隔
Septum pellucidum
穹隆
Fornix
前连合
Anterior commissure
第三脑室
3rd ventricle
前、后海绵间窦
Posterior and anterior intercavernous sinuses

大脑大静脉
Great cerebral vein

直窦
Straight sinus
小脑幕（切除）
Tentorium cerebelli (cut)
窦汇（切开）
Confluence of sinuses (cut)
小脑镰内的枕窦
Occipital sinus in falx cerebelli
小脑
Cerebellum
第四脑室
4th ventricle

垂体
Hypophysis
蝶窦
Sphenoidal sinus
基底动脉
Basilar artery
基底静脉丛
Basilar plexus

延髓和脊髓的中央管
Central canal of medulla oblongata and spinal cord
颈髓
Cervical spinal cord
延髓
Medulla oblongata
脑桥
Pons

B. 冠状断面
Coronal section

硬脑膜：
Dura mater:
骨膜层
Periosteal layer
脑膜层
Meningeal layer
蛛网膜
Arachnoid mater
蛛网膜下隙和蛛网膜小梁
Subarachnoid space and arachnoid trabeculae
软脑膜
Pia mater

静脉腔隙
Venous lacuna
板障静脉
Diploic vein

上矢状窦
Superior sagittal sinus
蛛网膜粒
Arachnoid granulation

头皮的层次：
Layers of the scalp:
皮肤
Skin
结缔组织
Connective tissue
帽状腱膜
Aponeurosis
疏松结缔组织
Loose connective tissue
骨外膜
Periosteum

大脑上静脉
Superior cerebral veins
大脑动脉
Cerebral artery

大脑半球
Cerebral hemisphere
胼胝体
Corpus callosum
透明隔
Septum pellucidum
大脑镰
Falx cerebri
侧脑室
Lateral ventricle
下矢窦
Inferior sagittal sinus

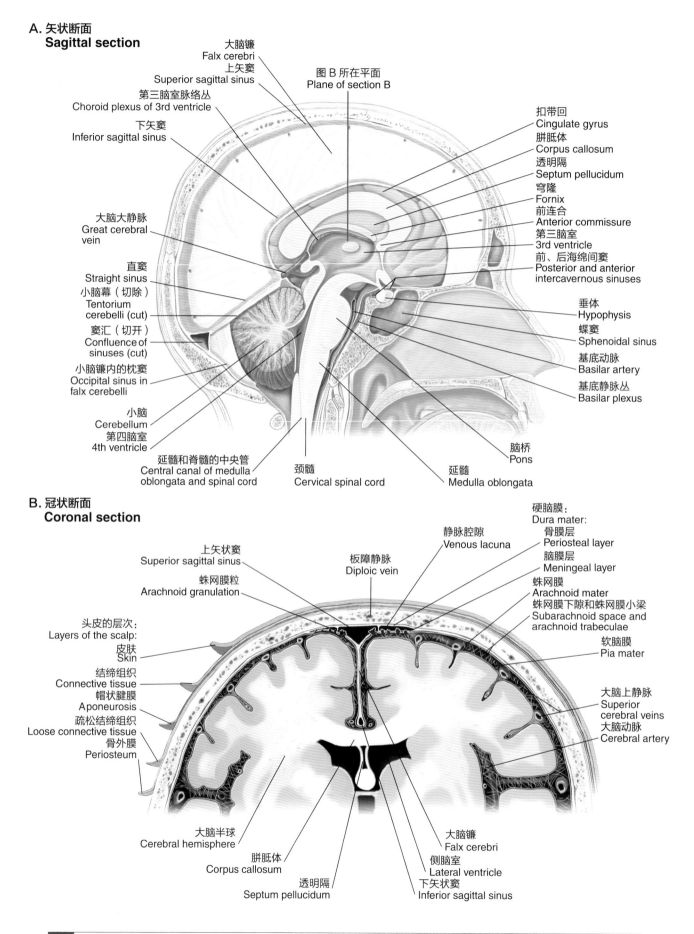

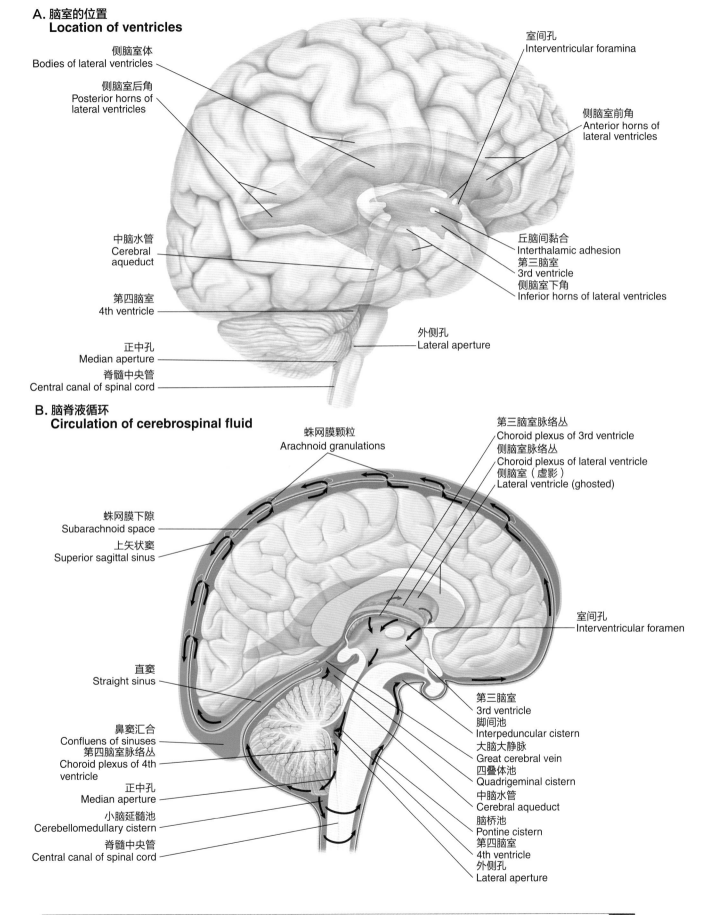

A. 脑室的位置
Location of ventricles

侧脑室体
Bodies of lateral ventricles

侧脑室后角
Posterior horns of
lateral ventricles

中脑水管
Cerebral
aqueduct

第四脑室
4th ventricle

正中孔
Median aperture

脊髓中央管
Central canal of spinal cord

室间孔
Interventricular foramina

侧脑室前角
Anterior horns of
lateral ventricles

丘脑间黏合
Interthalamic adhesion

第三脑室
3rd ventricle

侧脑室下角
Inferior horns of lateral ventricles

外侧孔
Lateral aperture

B. 脑脊液循环
Circulation of cerebrospinal fluid

蛛网膜颗粒
Arachnoid granulations

蛛网膜下隙
Subarachnoid space

上矢状窦
Superior sagittal sinus

直窦
Straight sinus

鼻窦汇合
Confluens of sinuses

第四脑室脉络丛
Choroid plexus of 4th
ventricle

正中孔
Median aperture

小脑延髓池
Cerebellomedullary cistern

脊髓中央管
Central canal of spinal cord

第三脑室脉络丛
Choroid plexus of 3rd ventricle

侧脑室脉络丛
Choroid plexus of lateral ventricle

侧脑室（虚影）
Lateral ventricle (ghosted)

室间孔
Interventricular foramen

第三脑室
3rd ventricle

脚间池
Interpeduncular cistern

大脑大静脉
Great cerebral vein

四叠体池
Quadrigeminal cistern

中脑水管
Cerebral aqueduct

脑桥池
Pontine cistern

第四脑室
4th ventricle

外侧孔
Lateral aperture

图 7-60　颅腔中的脑神经　Cranial Nerves in the Cranial Cavity

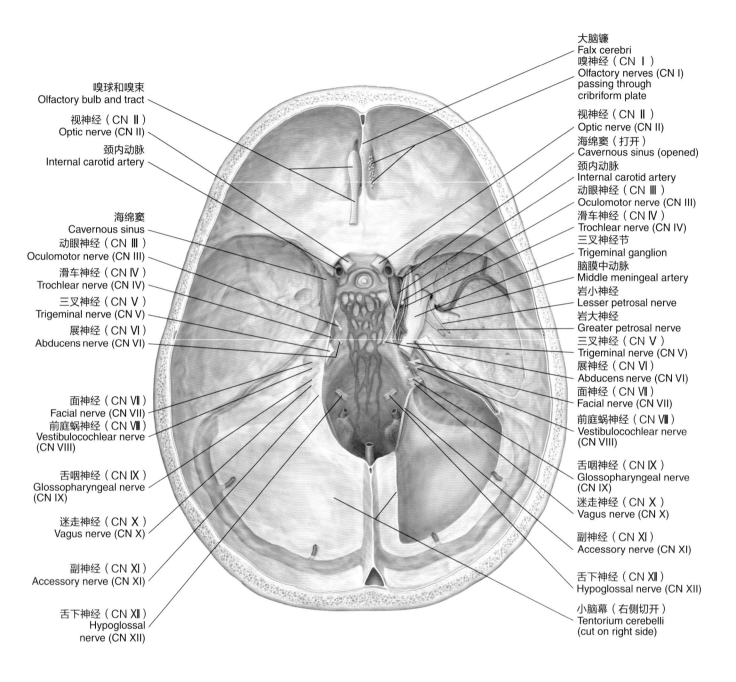

嗅球和嗅束
Olfactory bulb and tract

视神经（CN Ⅱ）
Optic nerve (CN II)

颈内动脉
Internal carotid artery

海绵窦
Cavernous sinus
动眼神经（CN Ⅲ）
Oculomotor nerve (CN III)
滑车神经（CN Ⅳ）
Trochlear nerve (CN IV)
三叉神经（CN Ⅴ）
Trigeminal nerve (CN V)
展神经（CN Ⅵ）
Abducens nerve (CN VI)

面神经（CN Ⅶ）
Facial nerve (CN VII)
前庭蜗神经（CN Ⅷ）
Vestibulocochlear nerve
(CN VIII)

舌咽神经（CN Ⅸ）
Glossopharyngeal nerve
(CN IX)

迷走神经（CN Ⅹ）
Vagus nerve (CN X)

副神经（CN Ⅺ）
Accessory nerve (CN XI)

舌下神经（CN Ⅻ）
Hypoglossal
nerve (CN XII)

大脑镰
Falx cerebri
嗅神经（CN Ⅰ）
Olfactory nerves (CN I)
passing through
cribriform plate

视神经（CN Ⅱ）
Optic nerve (CN II)
海绵窦（打开）
Cavernous sinus (opened)
颈内动脉
Internal carotid artery
动眼神经（CN Ⅲ）
Oculomotor nerve (CN III)
滑车神经（CN Ⅳ）
Trochlear nerve (CN IV)
三叉神经节
Trigeminal ganglion
脑膜中动脉
Middle meningeal artery
岩小神经
Lesser petrosal nerve
岩大神经
Greater petrosal nerve
三叉神经（CN Ⅴ）
Trigeminal nerve (CN V)
展神经（CN Ⅵ）
Abducens nerve (CN VI)
面神经（CN Ⅶ）
Facial nerve (CN VII)
前庭蜗神经（CN Ⅷ）
Vestibulocochlear nerve
(CN VIII)

舌咽神经（CN Ⅸ）
Glossopharyngeal nerve
(CN IX)
迷走神经（CN Ⅹ）
Vagus nerve (CN X)

副神经（CN Ⅺ）
Accessory nerve (CN XI)

舌下神经（CN Ⅻ）
Hypoglossal nerve (CN XII)

小脑幕（右侧切开）
Tentorium cerebelli
(cut on right side)

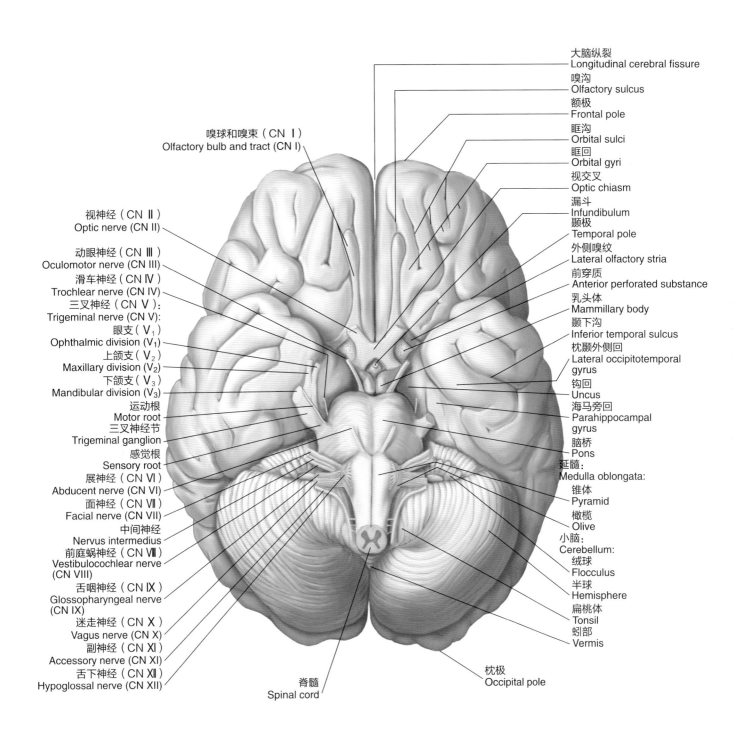

嗅球和嗅束（CN Ⅰ）
Olfactory bulb and tract (CN I)

视神经（CN Ⅱ）
Optic nerve (CN II)

动眼神经（CN Ⅲ）
Oculomotor nerve (CN III)

滑车神经（CN Ⅳ）
Trochlear nerve (CN IV)

三叉神经（CN Ⅴ）:
Trigeminal nerve (CN V):

眼支（ V_1 ）
Ophthalmic division (V_1)

上颌支（ V_2 ）
Maxillary division (V_2)

下颌支（ V_3 ）
Mandibular division (V_3)

运动根
Motor root

三叉神经节
Trigeminal ganglion

感觉根
Sensory root

展神经（CN Ⅵ）
Abducent nerve (CN VI)

面神经（CN Ⅶ）
Facial nerve (CN VII)

中间神经
Nervus intermedius

前庭蜗神经（CN Ⅷ）
Vestibulocochlear nerve
(CN VIII)

舌咽神经（CN Ⅸ）
Glossopharyngeal nerve
(CN IX)

迷走神经（CN Ⅹ）
Vagus nerve (CN X)

副神经（CN Ⅺ）
Accessory nerve (CN XI)

舌下神经（CN Ⅻ）
Hypoglossal nerve (CN XII)

脊髓
Spinal cord

大脑纵裂
Longitudinal cerebral fissure

嗅沟
Olfactory sulcus

额极
Frontal pole

眶沟
Orbital sulci

眶回
Orbital gyri

视交叉
Optic chiasm

漏斗
Infundibulum

颞极
Temporal pole

外侧嗅纹
Lateral olfactory stria

前穿质
Anterior perforated substance

乳头体
Mammillary body

颞下沟
Inferior temporal sulcus

枕颞外侧回
Lateral occipitotemporal
gyrus

钩回
Uncus

海马旁回
Parahippocampal
gyrus

脑桥
Pons

延髓：
Medulla oblongata:

锥体
Pyramid

橄榄
Olive

小脑：
Cerebellum:

绒球
Flocculus

半球
Hemisphere

扁桃体
Tonsil

蚓部
Vermis

枕极
Occipital pole

图 7-62　　大脑、脑干和小脑　Brain, Brainstem, and Cerebellum

A. 外侧面观
Lateral view

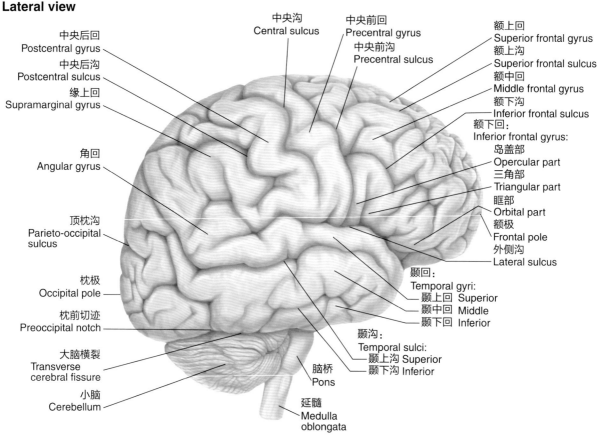

中央后回
Postcentral gyrus

中央后沟
Postcentral sulcus

缘上回
Supramarginal gyrus

角回
Angular gyrus

顶枕沟
Parieto-occipital
sulcus

枕极
Occipital pole

枕前切迹
Preoccipital notch

大脑横裂
Transverse
cerebral fissure

小脑
Cerebellum

中央沟
Central sulcus

中央前回
Precentral gyrus

中央前沟
Precentral sulcus

额上回
Superior frontal gyrus

额上沟
Superior frontal sulcus

额中回
Middle frontal gyrus

额下沟
Inferior frontal sulcus

额下回：
Inferior frontal gyrus:

岛盖部
Opercular part

三角部
Triangular part

眶部
Orbital part

额极
Frontal pole

外侧沟
Lateral sulcus

颞回：
Temporal gyri:
颞上回 Superior
颞中回 Middle
颞下回 Inferior

颞沟：
Temporal sulci:
颞上沟 Superior
颞下沟 Inferior

脑桥
Pons

延髓
Medulla
oblongata

B. 大脑半球的分叶
Lobes of the cerebral hemispheres

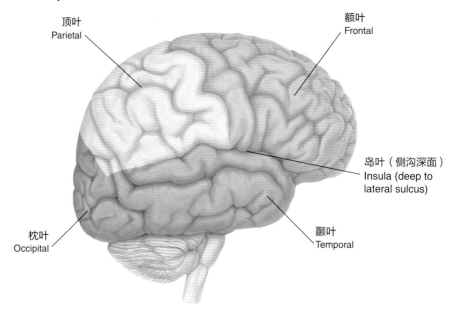

顶叶
Parietal

额叶
Frontal

岛叶（侧沟深面）
Insula (deep to
lateral sulcus)

枕叶
Occipital

颞叶
Temporal

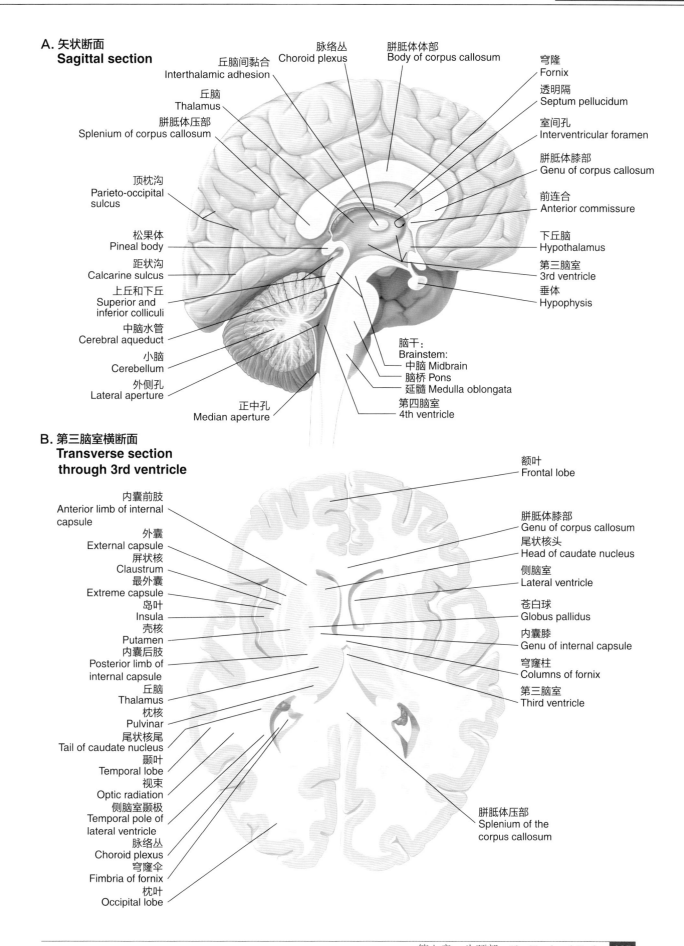

A. 矢状断面
Sagittal section

丘脑间黏合
Interthalamic adhesion

脉络丛
Choroid plexus

胼胝体体部
Body of corpus callosum

穹隆
Fornix

透明隔
Septum pellucidum

丘脑
Thalamus

胼胝体压部
Splenium of corpus callosum

室间孔
Interventricular foramen

胼胝体膝部
Genu of corpus callosum

顶枕沟
Parieto-occipital
sulcus

前连合
Anterior commissure

松果体
Pineal body

下丘脑
Hypothalamus

距状沟
Calcarine sulcus

第三脑室
3rd ventricle

上丘和下丘
Superior and
inferior colliculi

垂体
Hypophysis

中脑水管
Cerebral aqueduct

脑干：
Brainstem:
中脑 Midbrain
脑桥 Pons
延髓 Medulla oblongata

小脑
Cerebellum

外侧孔
Lateral aperture

正中孔
Median aperture

第四脑室
4th ventricle

B. 第三脑室横断面
Transverse section
through 3rd ventricle

额叶
Frontal lobe

内囊前肢
Anterior limb of internal
capsule

胼胝体膝部
Genu of corpus callosum

外囊
External capsule

尾状核头
Head of caudate nucleus

屏状核
Claustrum

侧脑室
Lateral ventricle

最外囊
Extreme capsule

苍白球
Globus pallidus

岛叶
Insula

内囊膝
Genu of internal capsule

壳核
Putamen

穹隆柱
Columns of fornix

内囊后肢
Posterior limb of
internal capsule

第三脑室
Third ventricle

丘脑
Thalamus

枕核
Pulvinar

尾状核尾
Tail of caudate nucleus

颞叶
Temporal lobe

视束
Optic radiation

侧脑室颞极
Temporal pole of
lateral ventricle

脉络丛
Choroid plexus

穹隆伞
Fimbria of fornix

枕叶
Occipital lobe

胼胝体压部
Splenium of the
corpus callosum

图 7-64　大脑底和脑干断面　**Base of Brain and Sectioned Brainstem**

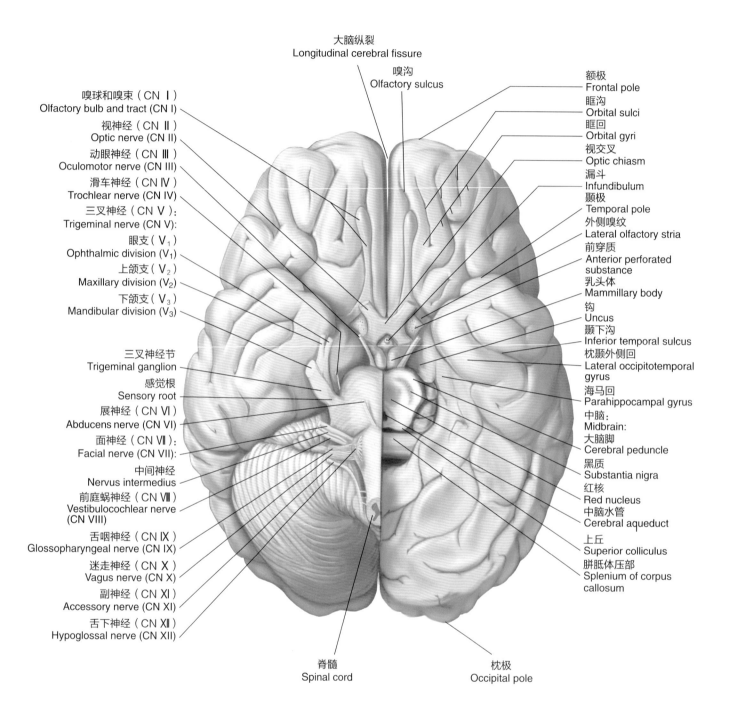

大脑纵裂
Longitudinal cerebral fissure

嗅沟
Olfactory sulcus

额极
Frontal pole

眶沟
Orbital sulci

眶回
Orbital gyri

视交叉
Optic chiasm

漏斗
Infundibulum

颞极
Temporal pole

外侧嗅纹
Lateral olfactory stria

前穿质
Anterior perforated substance

乳头体
Mammillary body

钩
Uncus

颞下沟
Inferior temporal sulcus

枕颞外侧回
Lateral occipitotemporal gyrus

海马回
Parahippocampal gyrus

中脑：
Midbrain:

大脑脚
Cerebral peduncle

黑质
Substantia nigra

红核
Red nucleus

中脑水管
Cerebral aqueduct

上丘
Superior colliculus

胼胝体压部
Splenium of corpus callosum

嗅球和嗅束（CN Ⅰ）
Olfactory bulb and tract (CN I)

视神经（CN Ⅱ）
Optic nerve (CN II)

动眼神经（CN Ⅲ）
Oculomotor nerve (CN III)

滑车神经（CN Ⅳ）
Trochlear nerve (CN IV)

三叉神经（CN Ⅴ）:
Trigeminal nerve (CN V):

眼支（V₁）
Ophthalmic division (V₁)

上颌支（V₂）
Maxillary division (V₂)

下颌支（V₃）
Mandibular division (V₃)

三叉神经节
Trigeminal ganglion

感觉根
Sensory root

展神经（CN Ⅵ）
Abducens nerve (CN VI)

面神经（CN Ⅶ）:
Facial nerve (CN VII):

中间神经
Nervus intermedius

前庭蜗神经（CN Ⅷ）
Vestibulocochlear nerve (CN VIII)

舌咽神经（CN Ⅸ）
Glossopharyngeal nerve (CN IX)

迷走神经（CN Ⅹ）
Vagus nerve (CN X)

副神经（CN Ⅺ）
Accessory nerve (CN XI)

舌下神经（CN Ⅻ）
Hypoglossal nerve (CN XII)

脊髓
Spinal cord

枕极
Occipital pole

A. 前面观
Anterior view

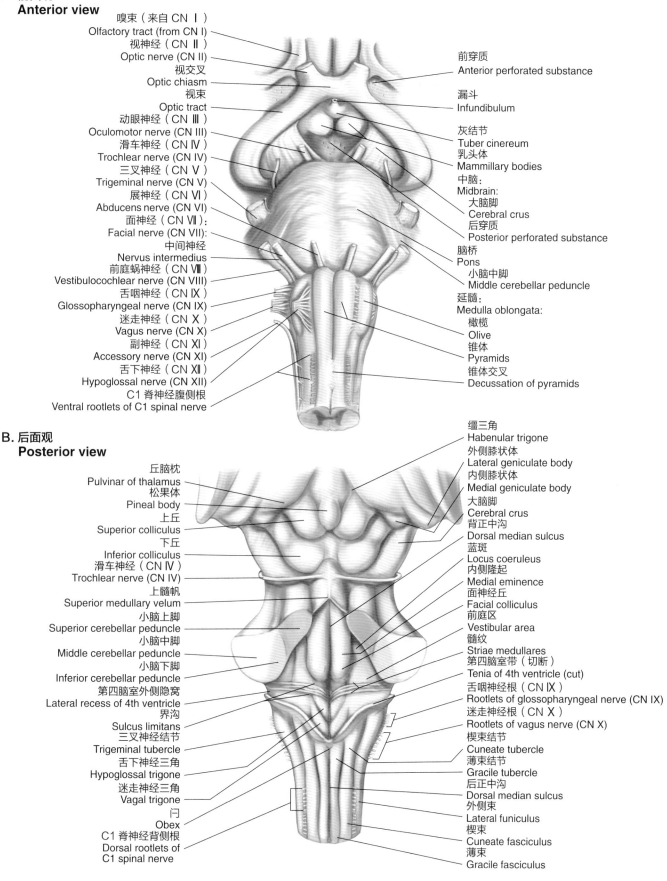

嗅束（来自 CN Ⅰ）
Olfactory tract (from CN I)
视神经（CN Ⅱ）
Optic nerve (CN II)
视交叉
Optic chiasm
视束
Optic tract
动眼神经（CN Ⅲ）
Oculomotor nerve (CN III)
滑车神经（CN Ⅳ）
Trochlear nerve (CN IV)
三叉神经（CN Ⅴ）
Trigeminal nerve (CN V)
展神经（CN Ⅵ）
Abducens nerve (CN VI)
面神经（CN Ⅶ）：
Facial nerve (CN VII):
中间神经
Nervus intermedius
前庭蜗神经（CN Ⅷ）
Vestibulocochlear nerve (CN VIII)
舌咽神经（CN Ⅸ）
Glossopharyngeal nerve (CN IX)
迷走神经（CN Ⅹ）
Vagus nerve (CN X)
副神经（CN Ⅺ）
Accessory nerve (CN XI)
舌下神经（CN Ⅻ）
Hypoglossal nerve (CN XII)
C1 脊神经腹侧根
Ventral rootlets of C1 spinal nerve

前穿质
Anterior perforated substance
漏斗
Infundibulum
灰结节
Tuber cinereum
乳头体
Mammillary bodies
中脑：
Midbrain:
大脑脚
Cerebral crus
后穿质
Posterior perforated substance
脑桥
Pons
小脑中脚
Middle cerebellar peduncle
延髓：
Medulla oblongata:
橄榄
Olive
锥体
Pyramids
锥体交叉
Decussation of pyramids

B. 后面观
Posterior view

丘脑枕
Pulvinar of thalamus
松果体
Pineal body
上丘
Superior colliculus
下丘
Inferior colliculus
滑车神经（CN Ⅳ）
Trochlear nerve (CN IV)
上髓帆
Superior medullary velum
小脑上脚
Superior cerebellar peduncle
小脑中脚
Middle cerebellar peduncle
小脑下脚
Inferior cerebellar peduncle
第四脑室外侧隐窝
Lateral recess of 4th ventricle
界沟
Sulcus limitans
三叉神经结节
Trigeminal tubercle
舌下神经三角
Hypoglossal trigone
迷走神经三角
Vagal trigone
闩
Obex
C1 脊神经背侧根
Dorsal rootlets of
C1 spinal nerve

缰三角
Habenular trigone
外侧膝状体
Lateral geniculate body
内侧膝状体
Medial geniculate body
大脑脚
Cerebral crus
背正中沟
Dorsal median sulcus
蓝斑
Locus coeruleus
内侧隆起
Medial eminence
面神经丘
Facial colliculus
前庭区
Vestibular area
髓纹
Striae medullares
第四脑室带（切断）
Tenia of 4th ventricle (cut)
舌咽神经根（CN Ⅸ）
Rootlets of glossopharyngeal nerve (CN IX)
迷走神经根（CN Ⅹ）
Rootlets of vagus nerve (CN X)
楔束结节
Cuneate tubercle
薄束结节
Gracile tubercle
后正中沟
Dorsal median sulcus
外侧束
Lateral funiculus
楔束
Cuneate fasciculus
薄束
Gracile fasciculus

图 7-66　**大脑的动脉　Arteries of the Brain**

A. 下面观
Inferior view

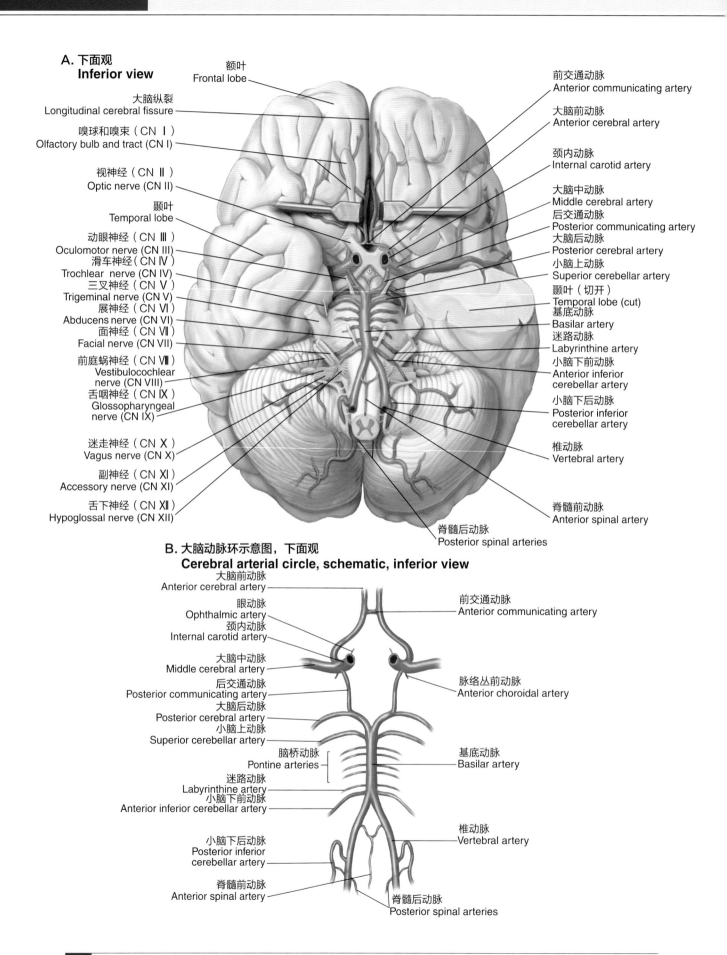

额叶
Frontal lobe

大脑纵裂
Longitudinal cerebral fissure

嗅球和嗅束（CN Ⅰ）
Olfactory bulb and tract (CN I)

视神经（CN Ⅱ）
Optic nerve (CN II)

颞叶
Temporal lobe

动眼神经（CN Ⅲ）
Oculomotor nerve (CN III)
滑车神经（CN Ⅳ）
Trochlear nerve (CN IV)
三叉神经（CN Ⅴ）
Trigeminal nerve (CN V)
展神经（CN Ⅵ）
Abducens nerve (CN VI)
面神经（CN Ⅶ）
Facial nerve (CN VII)
前庭蜗神经（CN Ⅷ）
Vestibulocochlear
nerve (CN VIII)
舌咽神经（CN Ⅸ）
Glossopharyngeal
nerve (CN IX)

迷走神经（CN Ⅹ）
Vagus nerve (CN X)

副神经（CN Ⅺ）
Accessory nerve (CN XI)

舌下神经（CN Ⅻ）
Hypoglossal nerve (CN XII)

前交通动脉
Anterior communicating artery

大脑前动脉
Anterior cerebral artery

颈内动脉
Internal carotid artery

大脑中动脉
Middle cerebral artery
后交通动脉
Posterior communicating artery
大脑后动脉
Posterior cerebral artery
小脑上动脉
Superior cerebellar artery
颞叶（切开）
Temporal lobe (cut)
基底动脉
Basilar artery
迷路动脉
Labyrinthine artery
小脑下前动脉
Anterior inferior
cerebellar artery

小脑下后动脉
Posterior inferior
cerebellar artery

椎动脉
Vertebral artery

脊髓前动脉
Anterior spinal artery

脊髓后动脉
Posterior spinal arteries

B. 大脑动脉环示意图，下面观
Cerebral arterial circle, schematic, inferior view

大脑前动脉
Anterior cerebral artery
眼动脉
Ophthalmic artery
颈内动脉
Internal carotid artery
大脑中动脉
Middle cerebral artery
后交通动脉
Posterior communicating artery
大脑后动脉
Posterior cerebral artery
小脑上动脉
Superior cerebellar artery
脑桥动脉
Pontine arteries
迷路动脉
Labyrinthine artery
小脑下前动脉
Anterior inferior cerebellar artery
小脑下后动脉
Posterior inferior
cerebellar artery
脊髓前动脉
Anterior spinal artery

前交通动脉
Anterior communicating artery

脉络丛前动脉
Anterior choroidal artery

基底动脉
Basilar artery

椎动脉
Vertebral artery

脊髓后动脉
Posterior spinal arteries

A. 侧面观
Lateral view

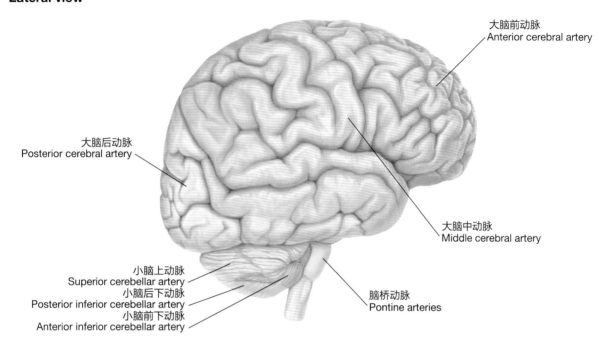

大脑前动脉
Anterior cerebral artery

大脑后动脉
Posterior cerebral artery

大脑中动脉
Middle cerebral artery

小脑上动脉
Superior cerebellar artery

小脑后下动脉
Posterior inferior cerebellar artery

小脑前下动脉
Anterior inferior cerebellar artery

脑桥动脉
Pontine arteries

B. 矢状面观
Sagittal view

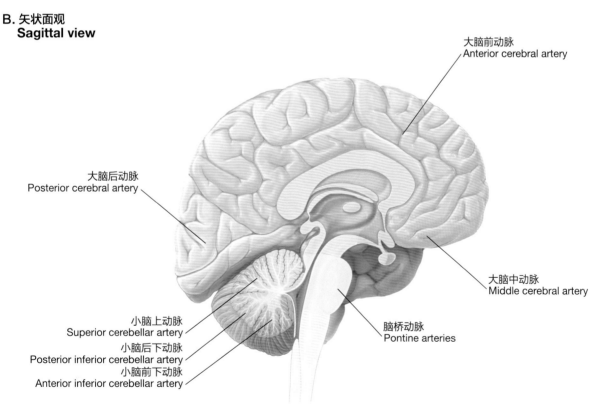

大脑前动脉
Anterior cerebral artery

大脑后动脉
Posterior cerebral artery

大脑中动脉
Middle cerebral artery

小脑上动脉
Superior cerebellar artery

小脑后下动脉
Posterior inferior cerebellar artery

小脑前下动脉
Anterior inferior cerebellar artery

脑桥动脉
Pontine arteries

图 7-68　　**眶，前面观 I　Orbit, Anterior View I**

A. 体表投影
Surface projection

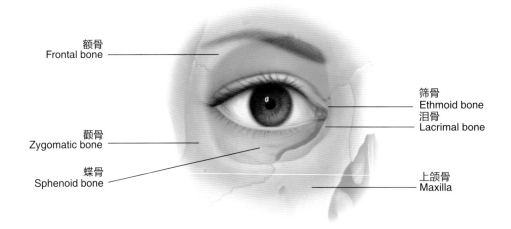

额骨
Frontal bone

筛骨
Ethmoid bone
泪骨
Lacrimal bone

颧骨
Zygomatic bone

蝶骨
Sphenoid bone

上颌骨
Maxilla

B. 肌和眶隔
Muscles and orbital septum

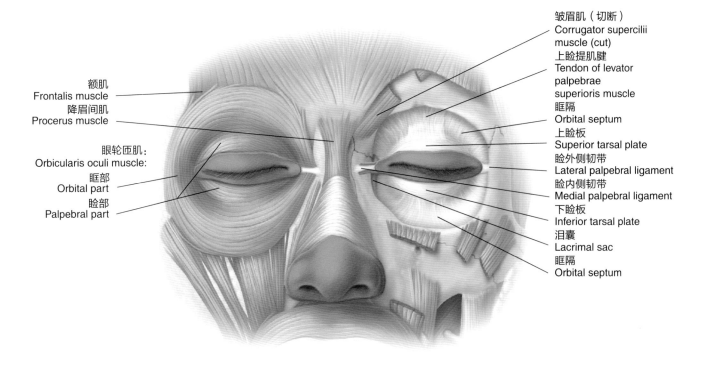

皱眉肌（切断）
Corrugator supercilii
muscle (cut)
上睑提肌腱
Tendon of levator
palpebrae
superioris muscle
眶隔
Orbital septum
上睑板
Superior tarsal plate
睑外侧韧带
Lateral palpebral ligament
睑内侧韧带
Medial palpebral ligament
下睑板
Inferior tarsal plate
泪囊
Lacrimal sac
眶隔
Orbital septum

额肌
Frontalis muscle
降眉间肌
Procerus muscle

眼轮匝肌：
Orbicularis oculi muscle:

眶部
Orbital part

睑部
Palpebral part

A. 眶的骨
Bones of the orbit

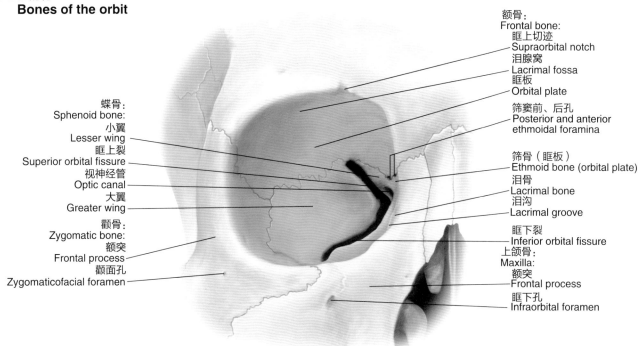

额骨：
Frontal bone:
眶上切迹
Supraorbital notch
泪腺窝
Lacrimal fossa
眶板
Orbital plate

筛窦前、后孔
Posterior and anterior ethmoidal foramina

筛骨（眶板）
Ethmoid bone (orbital plate)
泪骨
Lacrimal bone
泪沟
Lacrimal groove

眶下裂
Inferior orbital fissure
上颌骨：
Maxilla:
额突
Frontal process
眶下孔
Infraorbital foramen

蝶骨：
Sphenoid bone:
小翼
Lesser wing
眶上裂
Superior orbital fissure
视神经管
Optic canal
大翼
Greater wing

颧骨：
Zygomatic bone:
额突
Frontal process
颧面孔
Zygomaticofacial foramen

B. 骨性眶尖
Apex of bony orbit

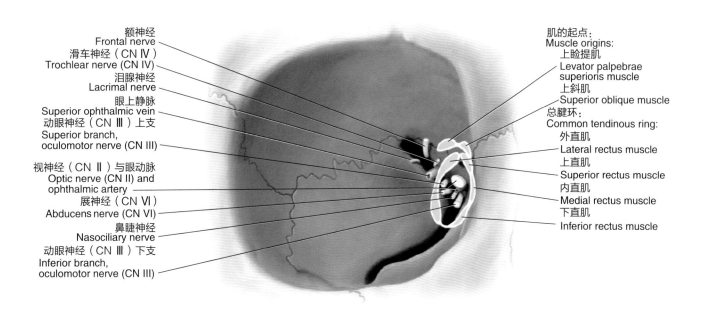

额神经
Frontal nerve
滑车神经（CN Ⅳ）
Trochlear nerve (CN Ⅳ)
泪腺神经
Lacrimal nerve
眼上静脉
Superior ophthalmic vein
动眼神经（CN Ⅲ）上支
Superior branch, oculomotor nerve (CN Ⅲ)

视神经（CN Ⅱ）与眼动脉
Optic nerve (CN Ⅱ) and ophthalmic artery
展神经（CN Ⅵ）
Abducens nerve (CN Ⅵ)
鼻睫神经
Nasociliary nerve
动眼神经（CN Ⅲ）下支
Inferior branch, oculomotor nerve (CN Ⅲ)

肌的起点：
Muscle origins:
上睑提肌
Levator palpebrae superioris muscle
上斜肌
Superior oblique muscle
总腱环：
Common tendinous ring:
外直肌
Lateral rectus muscle
上直肌
Superior rectus muscle
内直肌
Medial rectus muscle
下直肌
Inferior rectus muscle

图 7-70　眶，前面观Ⅲ　Orbit, Anterior View Ⅲ

A. 眼外肌
Extraocular muscles

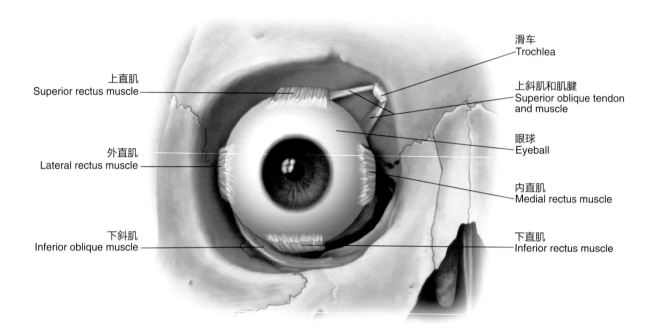

上直肌
Superior rectus muscle

外直肌
Lateral rectus muscle

下斜肌
Inferior oblique muscle

滑车
Trochlea

上斜肌和肌腱
Superior oblique tendon
and muscle

眼球
Eyeball

内直肌
Medial rectus muscle

下直肌
Inferior rectus muscle

B. 冠状断面
Coronal section

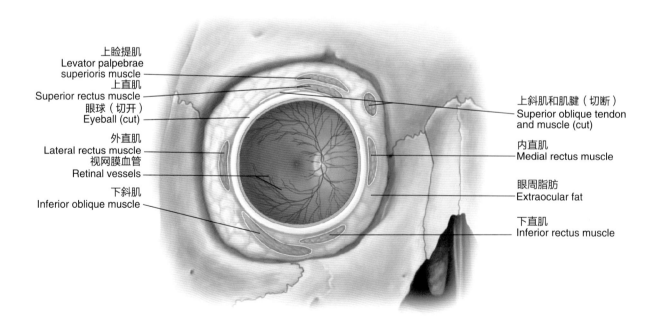

上睑提肌
Levator palpebrae
superioris muscle
上直肌
Superior rectus muscle
眼球（切开）
Eyeball (cut)

外直肌
Lateral rectus muscle
视网膜血管
Retinal vessels

下斜肌
Inferior oblique muscle

上斜肌和肌腱（切断）
Superior oblique tendon
and muscle (cut)

内直肌
Medial rectus muscle

眼周脂肪
Extraocular fat

下直肌
Inferior rectus muscle

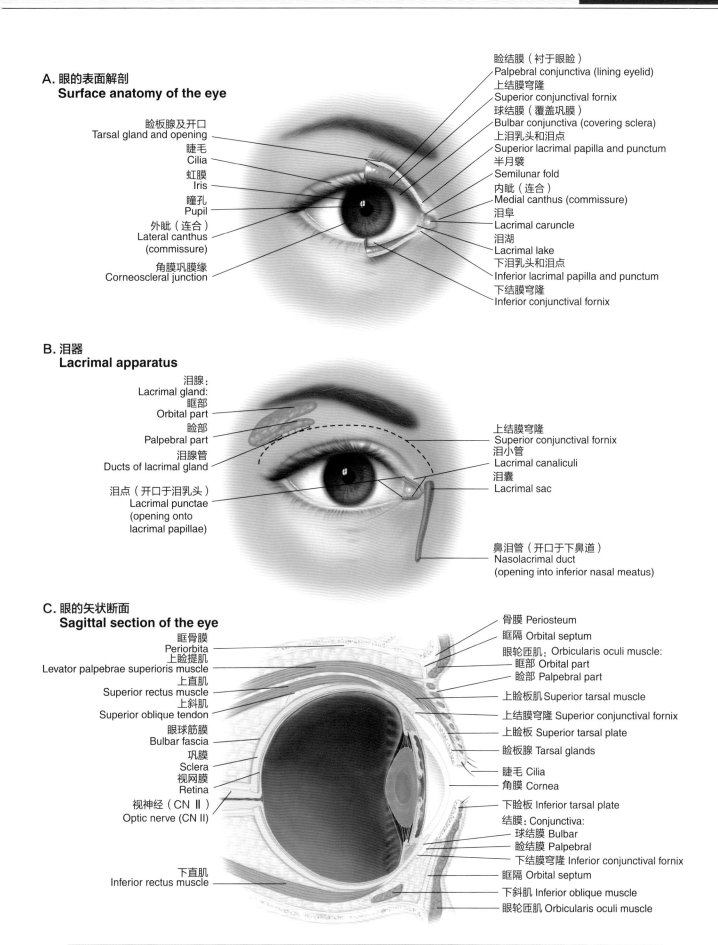

A. 眼的表面解剖
Surface anatomy of the eye

睑板腺及开口
Tarsal gland and opening

睫毛
Cilia

虹膜
Iris

瞳孔
Pupil

外眦（连合）
Lateral canthus
(commissure)

角膜巩膜缘
Corneoscleral junction

睑结膜（衬于眼睑）
Palpebral conjunctiva (lining eyelid)

上结膜穹隆
Superior conjunctival fornix

球结膜（覆盖巩膜）
Bulbar conjunctiva (covering sclera)

上泪乳头和泪点
Superior lacrimal papilla and punctum

半月襞
Semilunar fold

内眦（连合）
Medial canthus (commissure)

泪阜
Lacrimal caruncle

泪湖
Lacrimal lake

下泪乳头和泪点
Inferior lacrimal papilla and punctum

下结膜穹隆
Inferior conjunctival fornix

B. 泪器
Lacrimal apparatus

泪腺：
Lacrimal gland:

眶部
Orbital part

睑部
Palpebral part

泪腺管
Ducts of lacrimal gland

泪点（开口于泪乳头）
Lacrimal punctae
(opening onto
lacrimal papillae)

上结膜穹隆
Superior conjunctival fornix

泪小管
Lacrimal canaliculi

泪囊
Lacrimal sac

鼻泪管（开口于下鼻道）
Nasolacrimal duct
(opening into inferior nasal meatus)

C. 眼的矢状断面
Sagittal section of the eye

眶骨膜
Periorbita

上睑提肌
Levator palpebrae superioris muscle

上直肌
Superior rectus muscle

上斜肌
Superior oblique tendon

眼球筋膜
Bulbar fascia

巩膜
Sclera

视网膜
Retina

视神经（CN II）
Optic nerve (CN II)

下直肌
Inferior rectus muscle

骨膜 Periosteum

眶隔 Orbital septum

眼轮匝肌：Orbicularis oculi muscle:

眶部 Orbital part

睑部 Palpebral part

上睑板肌 Superior tarsal muscle

上结膜穹隆 Superior conjunctival fornix

上睑板 Superior tarsal plate

睑板腺 Tarsal glands

睫毛 Cilia

角膜 Cornea

下睑板 Inferior tarsal plate

结膜：Conjunctiva:

球结膜 Bulbar

睑结膜 Palpebral

下结膜穹隆 Inferior conjunctival fornix

眶隔 Orbital septum

下斜肌 Inferior oblique muscle

眼轮匝肌 Orbicularis oculi muscle

图 7-72　海绵窦　**Cavernous Sinus**

A. 上面观
Superior view

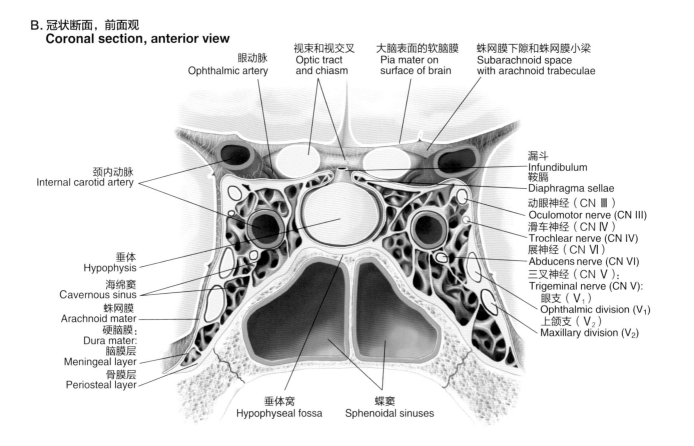

视神经（CN Ⅱ）
Optic nerve (CN II)

颈内动脉
Internal carotid artery

图 B 所在平面
Plane of section B

海绵窦
Cavernous sinus

动眼神经（CN Ⅲ）
Oculomotor nerve (CN III)

滑车神经（CN Ⅳ）
Trochlear nerve (CN IV)

三叉神经（CN Ⅴ）
Trigeminal nerve (CN V)

展神经（CN Ⅵ）
Abducens nerve (CN VI)

海绵窦壁切开显示：
Wall of cavernous
sinus opened to reveal:
动眼神经（CN Ⅲ）
Oculomotor nerve (CN III)
滑车神经（CN Ⅳ）
Trochlear nerve (CN IV)
三叉神经（CN Ⅴ）：
Trigeminal nerve (CN V):
眼支（V$_1$）
Ophthalmic division (V$_1$)
上颌支（V$_2$）
Maxillary division (V$_2$)
下颌支（V$_3$）
Mandibular division (V$_3$)

三叉神经节
Trigeminal ganglion

展神经（CN Ⅵ）
Abducens nerve (CN VI)

垂体 Hypophysis

B. 冠状断面，前面观
Coronal section, anterior view

眼动脉
Ophthalmic artery

视束和视交叉
Optic tract
and chiasm

大脑表面的软脑膜
Pia mater on
surface of brain

蛛网膜下隙和蛛网膜小梁
Subarachnoid space
with arachnoid trabeculae

颈内动脉
Internal carotid artery

垂体
Hypophysis

海绵窦
Cavernous sinus

蛛网膜
Arachnoid mater

硬脑膜：
Dura mater:
脑膜层
Meningeal layer
骨膜层
Periosteal layer

漏斗
Infundibulum
鞍膈
Diaphragma sellae

动眼神经（CN Ⅲ）
Oculomotor nerve (CN III)

滑车神经（CN Ⅳ）
Trochlear nerve (CN IV)

展神经（CN Ⅵ）
Abducens nerve (CN VI)

三叉神经（CN Ⅴ）：
Trigeminal nerve (CN V):
眼支（V$_1$）
Ophthalmic division (V$_1$)
上颌支（V$_2$）
Maxillary division (V$_2$)

垂体窝
Hypophyseal fossa

蝶窦
Sphenoidal sinuses

A. 第一层
Layer I

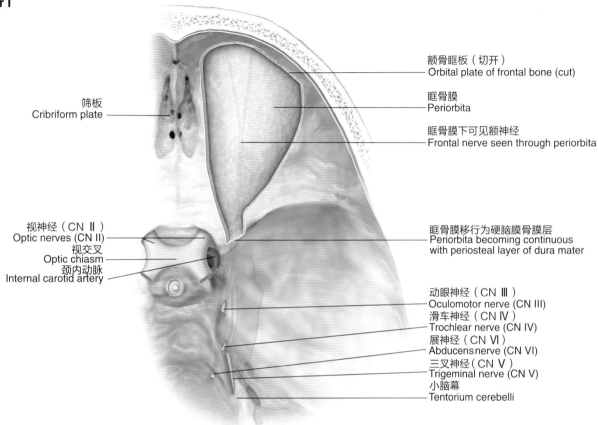

筛板
Cribriform plate

额骨眶板（切开）
Orbital plate of frontal bone (cut)

眶骨膜
Periorbita

眶骨膜下可见额神经
Frontal nerve seen through periorbita

视神经（CN Ⅱ）
Optic nerves (CN II)

视交叉
Optic chiasm

颈内动脉
Internal carotid artery

眶骨膜移行为硬脑膜骨膜层
Periorbita becoming continuous
with periosteal layer of dura mater

动眼神经（CN Ⅲ）
Oculomotor nerve (CN III)

滑车神经（CN Ⅳ）
Trochlear nerve (CN IV)

展神经（CN Ⅵ）
Abducens nerve (CN VI)

三叉神经（CN Ⅴ）
Trigeminal nerve (CN V)

小脑幕
Tentorium cerebelli

B. 第二层
Layer II

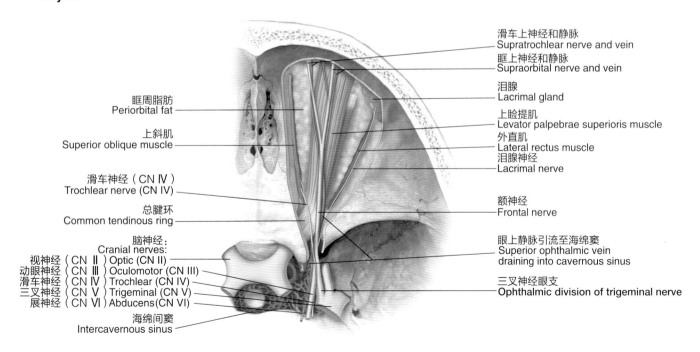

眶周脂肪
Periorbital fat

上斜肌
Superior oblique muscle

滑车神经（CN Ⅳ）
Trochlear nerve (CN IV)

总腱环
Common tendinous ring

脑神经：
Cranial nerves:
视神经（CN Ⅱ）Optic (CN II)
动眼神经（CN Ⅲ）Oculomotor (CN III)
滑车神经（CN Ⅳ）Trochlear (CN IV)
三叉神经（CN Ⅴ）Trigeminal (CN V)
展神经（CN Ⅵ）Abducens (CN VI)

海绵间窦
Intercavernous sinus

滑车上神经和静脉
Supratrochlear nerve and vein

眶上神经和静脉
Supraorbital nerve and vein

泪腺
Lacrimal gland

上睑提肌
Levator palpebrae superioris muscle

外直肌
Lateral rectus muscle

泪腺神经
Lacrimal nerve

额神经
Frontal nerve

眼上静脉引流至海绵窦
Superior ophthalmic vein
draining into cavernous sinus

三叉神经眼支
Ophthalmic division of trigeminal nerve

图 7-74　眶，上面观Ⅱ　Orbit, Superior View Ⅱ

A. 第三层
Layer III

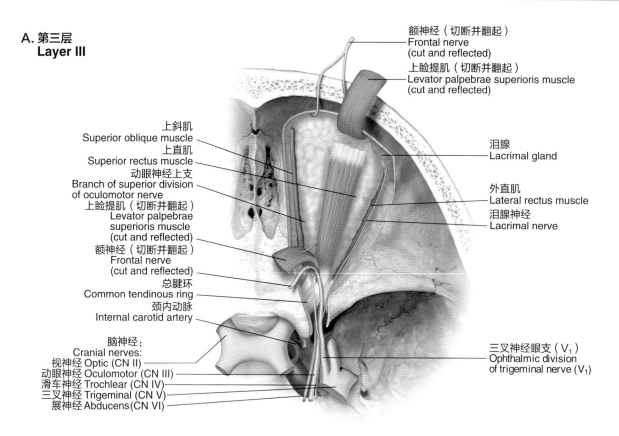

额神经（切断并翻起）
Frontal nerve
(cut and reflected)

上睑提肌（切断并翻起）
Levator palpebrae superioris muscle
(cut and reflected)

上斜肌
Superior oblique muscle
上直肌
Superior rectus muscle
动眼神经上支
Branch of superior division
of oculomotor nerve
上睑提肌（切断并翻起）
Levator palpebrae
superioris muscle
(cut and reflected)
额神经（切断并翻起）
Frontal nerve
(cut and reflected)
总腱环
Common tendinous ring
颈内动脉
Internal carotid artery

脑神经：
Cranial nerves:
视神经 Optic (CN II)
动眼神经 Oculomotor (CN III)
滑车神经 Trochlear (CN IV)
三叉神经 Trigeminal (CN V)
展神经 Abducens (CN VI)

泪腺
Lacrimal gland

外直肌
Lateral rectus muscle
泪腺神经
Lacrimal nerve

三叉神经眼支（V₁）
Ophthalmic division
of trigeminal nerve (V₁)

B. 第四层
Layer IV

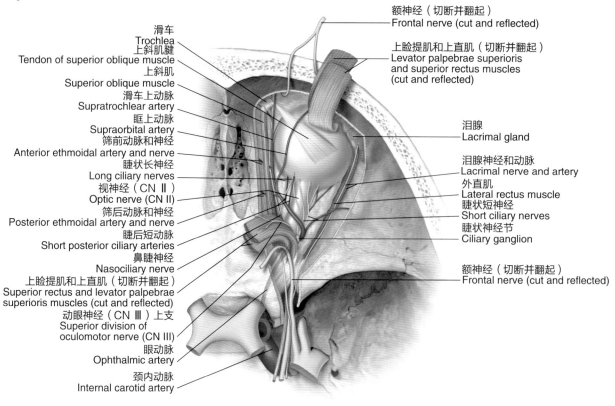

额神经（切断并翻起）
Frontal nerve (cut and reflected)

上睑提肌和上直肌（切断并翻起）
Levator palpebrae superioris
and superior rectus muscles
(cut and reflected)

滑车
Trochlea
上斜肌腱
Tendon of superior oblique muscle
上斜肌
Superior oblique muscle
滑车上动脉
Supratrochlear artery
眶上动脉
Supraorbital artery
筛前动脉和神经
Anterior ethmoidal artery and nerve
睫状长神经
Long ciliary nerves
视神经（CN Ⅱ）
Optic nerve (CN II)
筛后动脉和神经
Posterior ethmoidal artery and nerve
睫后短动脉
Short posterior ciliary arteries
鼻睫神经
Nasociliary nerve
上睑提肌和上直肌（切断并翻起）
Superior rectus and levator palpebrae
superioris muscles (cut and reflected)
动眼神经（CN Ⅲ）上支
Superior division of
oculomotor nerve (CN III)
眼动脉
Ophthalmic artery
颈内动脉
Internal carotid artery

泪腺
Lacrimal gland

泪腺神经和动脉
Lacrimal nerve and artery
外直肌
Lateral rectus muscle
睫状短神经
Short ciliary nerves
睫状神经节
Ciliary ganglion

额神经（切断并翻起）
Frontal nerve (cut and reflected)

A. 第五层
Layer V

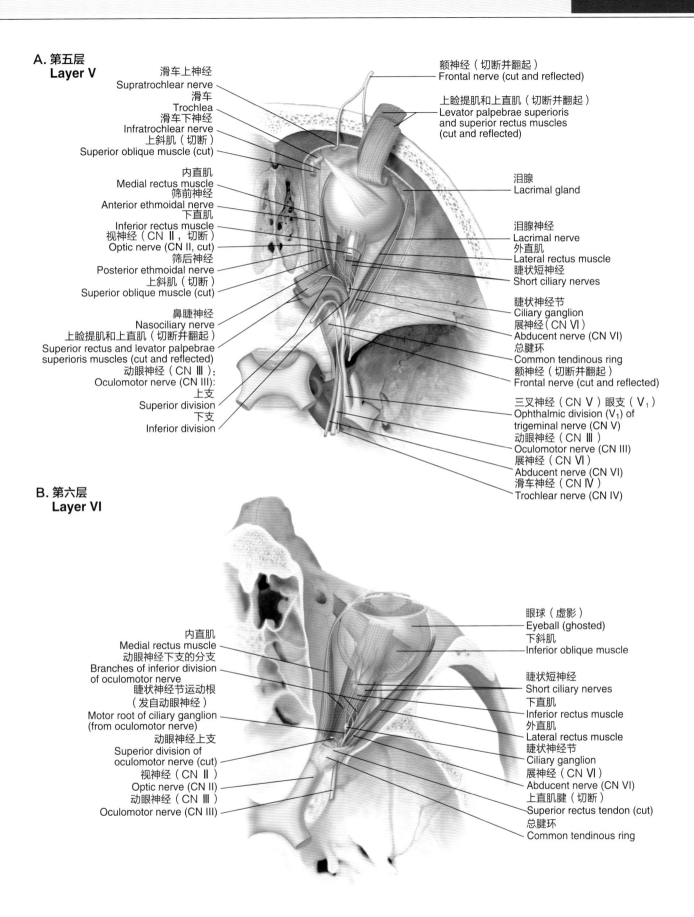

滑车上神经
Supratrochlear nerve
滑车
Trochlea
滑车下神经
Infratrochlear nerve
上斜肌（切断）
Superior oblique muscle (cut)

内直肌
Medial rectus muscle
筛前神经
Anterior ethmoidal nerve
下直肌
Inferior rectus muscle
视神经（CN Ⅱ，切断）
Optic nerve (CN II, cut)
筛后神经
Posterior ethmoidal nerve
上斜肌（切断）
Superior oblique muscle (cut)

鼻睫神经
Nasociliary nerve
上睑提肌和上直肌（切断并翻起）
Superior rectus and levator palpebrae
superioris muscles (cut and reflected)
动眼神经（CN Ⅲ）：
Oculomotor nerve (CN III):
上支
Superior division
下支
Inferior division

额神经（切断并翻起）
Frontal nerve (cut and reflected)
上睑提肌和上直肌（切断并翻起）
Levator palpebrae superioris
and superior rectus muscles
(cut and reflected)

泪腺
Lacrimal gland

泪腺神经
Lacrimal nerve
外直肌
Lateral rectus muscle
睫状短神经
Short ciliary nerves

睫状神经节
Ciliary ganglion
展神经（CN Ⅵ）
Abducent nerve (CN VI)
总腱环
Common tendinous ring
额神经（切断并翻起）
Frontal nerve (cut and reflected)
三叉神经（CN Ⅴ）眼支（V₁）
Ophthalmic division (V₁) of
trigeminal nerve (CN V)
动眼神经（CN Ⅲ）
Oculomotor nerve (CN III)
展神经（CN Ⅵ）
Abducent nerve (CN VI)
滑车神经（CN Ⅳ）
Trochlear nerve (CN IV)

B. 第六层
Layer VI

内直肌
Medial rectus muscle
动眼神经下支的分支
Branches of inferior division
of oculomotor nerve
睫状神经节运动根
（发自动眼神经）
Motor root of ciliary ganglion
(from oculomotor nerve)
动眼神经上支
Superior division of
oculomotor nerve (cut)
视神经（CN Ⅱ）
Optic nerve (CN II)
动眼神经（CN Ⅲ）
Oculomotor nerve (CN III)

眼球（虚影）
Eyeball (ghosted)
下斜肌
Inferior oblique muscle

睫状短神经
Short ciliary nerves
下直肌
Inferior rectus muscle
外直肌
Lateral rectus muscle
睫状神经节
Ciliary ganglion
展神经（CN Ⅵ）
Abducent nerve (CN VI)
上直肌腱（切断）
Superior rectus tendon (cut)
总腱环
Common tendinous ring

图 7-76　　眼球　Eyeball

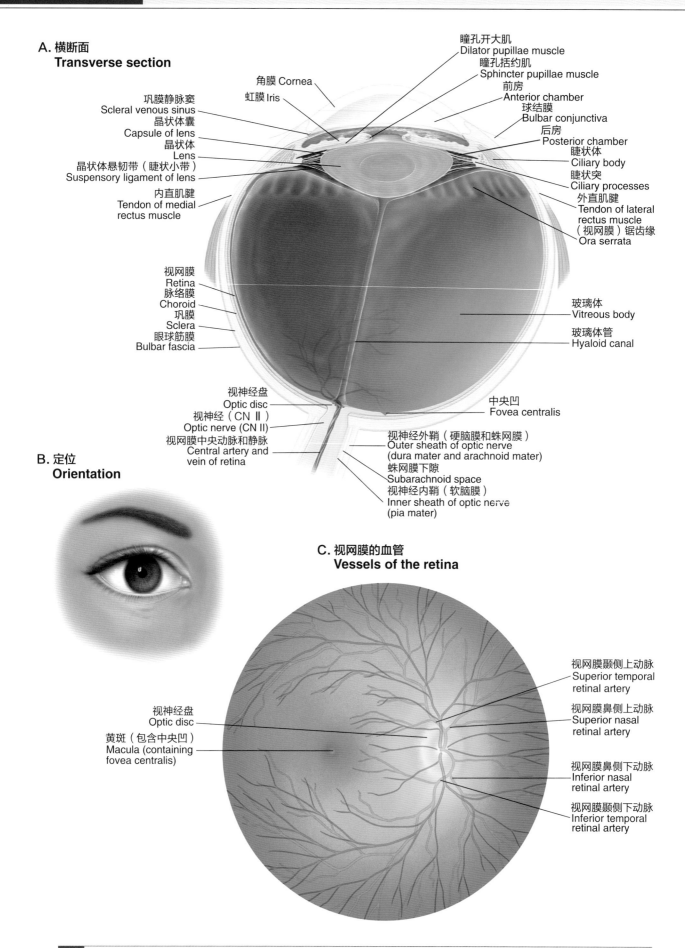

A. 横断面
Transverse section

瞳孔开大肌
Dilator pupillae muscle

瞳孔括约肌
Sphincter pupillae muscle

前房
Anterior chamber

球结膜
Bulbar conjunctiva

后房
Posterior chamber

睫状体
Ciliary body

睫状突
Ciliary processes

外直肌腱
Tendon of lateral rectus muscle

（视网膜）锯齿缘
Ora serrata

角膜 Cornea

虹膜 Iris

巩膜静脉窦
Scleral venous sinus

晶状体囊
Capsule of lens

晶状体
Lens

晶状体悬韧带（睫状小带）
Suspensory ligament of lens

内直肌腱
Tendon of medial rectus muscle

视网膜
Retina

脉络膜
Choroid

巩膜
Sclera

眼球筋膜
Bulbar fascia

玻璃体
Vitreous body

玻璃体管
Hyaloid canal

视神经盘
Optic disc

视神经（CN Ⅱ）
Optic nerve (CN II)

视网膜中央动脉和静脉
Central artery and vein of retina

中央凹
Fovea centralis

视神经外鞘（硬脑膜和蛛网膜）
Outer sheath of optic nerve (dura mater and arachnoid mater)

蛛网膜下隙
Subarachnoid space

视神经内鞘（软脑膜）
Inner sheath of optic nerve (pia mater)

B. 定位
Orientation

C. 视网膜的血管
Vessels of the retina

视神经盘
Optic disc

黄斑（包含中央凹）
Macula (containing fovea centralis)

视网膜颞侧上动脉
Superior temporal retinal artery

视网膜鼻侧上动脉
Superior nasal retinal artery

视网膜鼻侧下动脉
Inferior nasal retinal artery

视网膜颞侧下动脉
Inferior temporal retinal artery

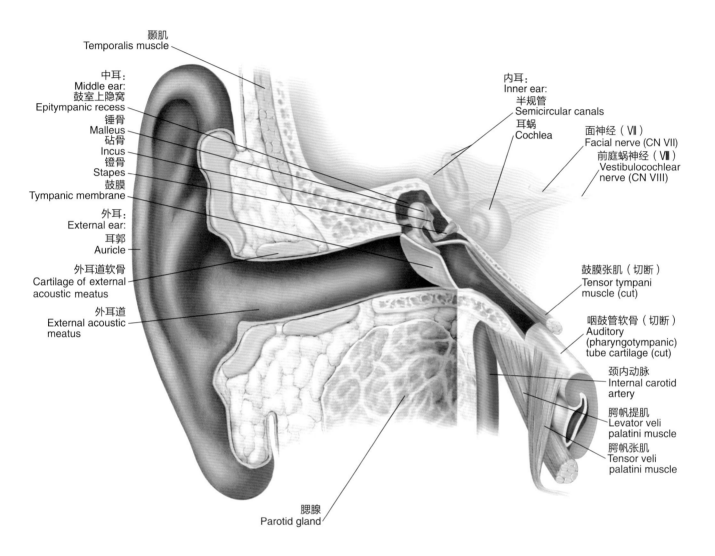

颞肌
Temporalis muscle

中耳：
Middle ear:
鼓室上隐窝
Epitympanic recess
锤骨
Malleus
砧骨
Incus
镫骨
Stapes
鼓膜
Tympanic membrane
外耳：
External ear:
耳郭
Auricle
外耳道软骨
Cartilage of external
acoustic meatus
外耳道
External acoustic
meatus

内耳：
Inner ear:
半规管
Semicircular canals
耳蜗
Cochlea

面神经（Ⅶ）
Facial nerve (CN VII)
前庭蜗神经（Ⅷ）
Vestibulocochlear
nerve (CN VIII)

鼓膜张肌（切断）
Tensor tympani
muscle (cut)

咽鼓管软骨（切断）
Auditory
(pharyngotympanic)
tube cartilage (cut)

颈内动脉
Internal carotid
artery

腭帆提肌
Levator veli
palatini muscle

腭帆张肌
Tensor veli
palatini muscle

腮腺
Parotid gland

图 7-78　　耳II　Ear II

A. 耳郭
Auricle

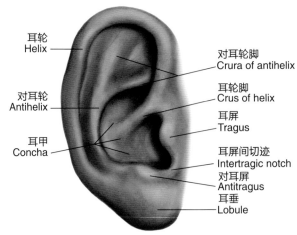

耳轮
Helix

对耳轮脚
Crura of antihelix

耳轮脚
Crus of helix

对耳轮
Antihelix

耳屏
Tragus

耳甲
Concha

耳屏间切迹
Intertragic notch

对耳屏
Antitragus

耳垂
Lobule

B. 鼓膜，外侧面观
Tympanic membrane, lateral view

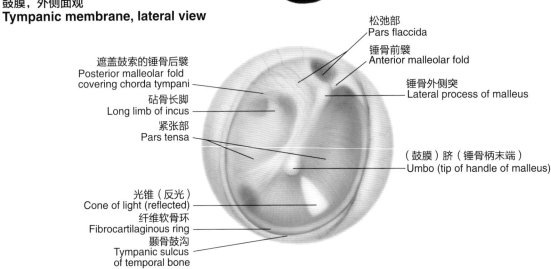

松弛部
Pars flaccida

锤骨前襞
Anterior malleolar fold

遮盖鼓索的锤骨后襞
Posterior malleolar fold
covering chorda tympani

锤骨外侧突
Lateral process of malleus

砧骨长脚
Long limb of incus

紧张部
Pars tensa

（鼓膜）脐（锤骨柄末端）
Umbo (tip of handle of malleus)

光锥（反光）
Cone of light (reflected)

纤维软骨环
Fibrocartilaginous ring

颞骨鼓沟
Tympanic sulcus
of temporal bone

C. 听小骨透过鼓膜观
Ossicles of ear seen through tympanic membrane

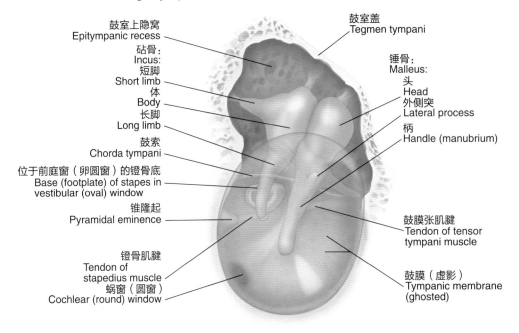

鼓室上隐窝
Epitympanic recess

鼓室盖
Tegmen tympani

砧骨：
Incus:
短脚
Short limb
体
Body
长脚
Long limb

锤骨：
Malleus:
头
Head
外侧突
Lateral process
柄
Handle (manubrium)

鼓索
Chorda tympani

位于前庭窗（卵圆窗）的镫骨底
Base (footplate) of stapes in
vestibular (oval) window

锥隆起
Pyramidal eminence

鼓膜张肌腱
Tendon of tensor
tympani muscle

镫骨肌腱
Tendon of
stapedius muscle
蜗窗（圆窗）
Cochlear (round) window

鼓膜（虚影）
Tympanic membrane
(ghosted)

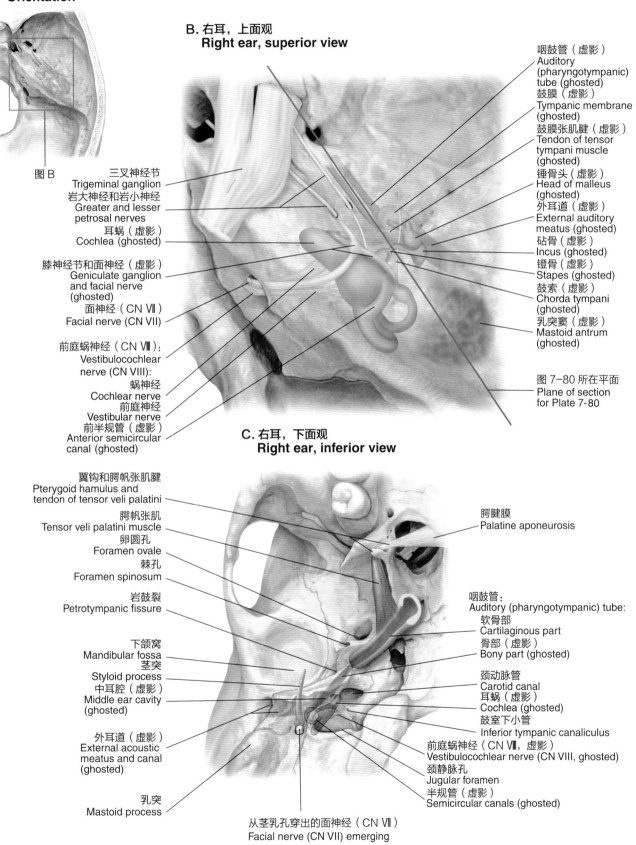

A. 定位
Orientation

图 B

B. 右耳，上面观
Right ear, superior view

咽鼓管（虚影）
Auditory (pharyngotympanic) tube (ghosted)

鼓膜（虚影）
Tympanic membrane (ghosted)

鼓膜张肌腱（虚影）
Tendon of tensor tympani muscle (ghosted)

锤骨头（虚影）
Head of malleus (ghosted)

外耳道（虚影）
External auditory meatus (ghosted)

砧骨（虚影）
Incus (ghosted)

镫骨（虚影）
Stapes (ghosted)

鼓索（虚影）
Chorda tympani (ghosted)

乳突窦（虚影）
Mastoid antrum (ghosted)

三叉神经节
Trigeminal ganglion

岩大神经和岩小神经
Greater and lesser petrosal nerves

耳蜗（虚影）
Cochlea (ghosted)

膝神经节和面神经（虚影）
Geniculate ganglion and facial nerve (ghosted)

面神经（CN Ⅶ）
Facial nerve (CN VII)

前庭蜗神经（CN Ⅷ）：
Vestibulocochlear nerve (CN VIII):

蜗神经
Cochlear nerve

前庭神经
Vestibular nerve

前半规管（虚影）
Anterior semicircular canal (ghosted)

图 7-80 所在平面
Plane of section for Plate 7-80

C. 右耳，下面观
Right ear, inferior view

翼钩和腭帆张肌腱
Pterygoid hamulus and tendon of tensor veli palatini

腭帆张肌
Tensor veli palatini muscle

卵圆孔
Foramen ovale

棘孔
Foramen spinosum

岩鼓裂
Petrotympanic fissure

下颌窝
Mandibular fossa

茎突
Styloid process

中耳腔（虚影）
Middle ear cavity (ghosted)

外耳道（虚影）
External acoustic meatus and canal (ghosted)

乳突
Mastoid process

从茎乳孔穿出的面神经（CN Ⅶ）
Facial nerve (CN VII) emerging

腭腱膜
Palatine aponeurosis

咽鼓管：
Auditory (pharyngotympanic) tube:

软骨部
Cartilaginous part

骨部（虚影）
Bony part (ghosted)

颈动脉管
Carotid canal

耳蜗（虚影）
Cochlea (ghosted)

鼓室下小管
Inferior tympanic canaliculus

前庭蜗神经（CN Ⅷ，虚影）
Vestibulocochlear nerve (CN VIII, ghosted)

颈静脉孔
Jugular foramen

半规管（虚影）
Semicircular canals (ghosted)

图 7-80　耳IV　Ear IV

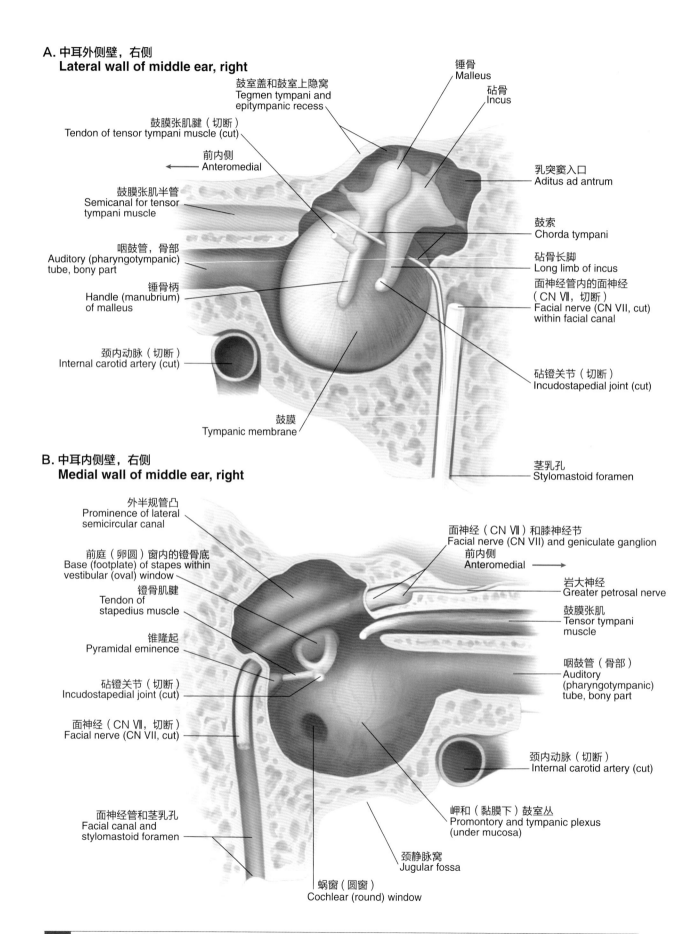

A. 中耳外侧壁，右侧
Lateral wall of middle ear, right

鼓室盖和鼓室上隐窝
Tegmen tympani and epitympanic recess

锤骨
Malleus

砧骨
Incus

鼓膜张肌腱（切断）
Tendon of tensor tympani muscle (cut)

前内侧
Anteromedial

乳突窦入口
Aditus ad antrum

鼓膜张肌半管
Semicanal for tensor tympani muscle

鼓索
Chorda tympani

咽鼓管，骨部
Auditory (pharyngotympanic) tube, bony part

砧骨长脚
Long limb of incus

锤骨柄
Handle (manubrium) of malleus

面神经管内的面神经
（CN VII，切断）
Facial nerve (CN VII, cut) within facial canal

颈内动脉（切断）
Internal carotid artery (cut)

砧镫关节（切断）
Incudostapedial joint (cut)

鼓膜
Tympanic membrane

茎乳孔
Stylomastoid foramen

B. 中耳内侧壁，右侧
Medial wall of middle ear, right

外半规管凸
Prominence of lateral semicircular canal

面神经（CN VII）和膝神经节
Facial nerve (CN VII) and geniculate ganglion

前内侧
Anteromedial

前庭（卵圆）窗内的镫骨底
Base (footplate) of stapes within vestibular (oval) window

岩大神经
Greater petrosal nerve

镫骨肌腱
Tendon of stapedius muscle

鼓膜张肌
Tensor tympani muscle

锥隆起
Pyramidal eminence

咽鼓管（骨部）
Auditory (pharyngotympanic) tube, bony part

砧镫关节（切断）
Incudostapedial joint (cut)

面神经（CN VII，切断）
Facial nerve (CN VII, cut)

颈内动脉（切断）
Internal carotid artery (cut)

面神经管和茎乳孔
Facial canal and stylomastoid foramen

岬和（黏膜下）鼓室丛
Promontory and tympanic plexus (under mucosa)

颈静脉窝
Jugular fossa

蜗窗（圆窗）
Cochlear (round) window

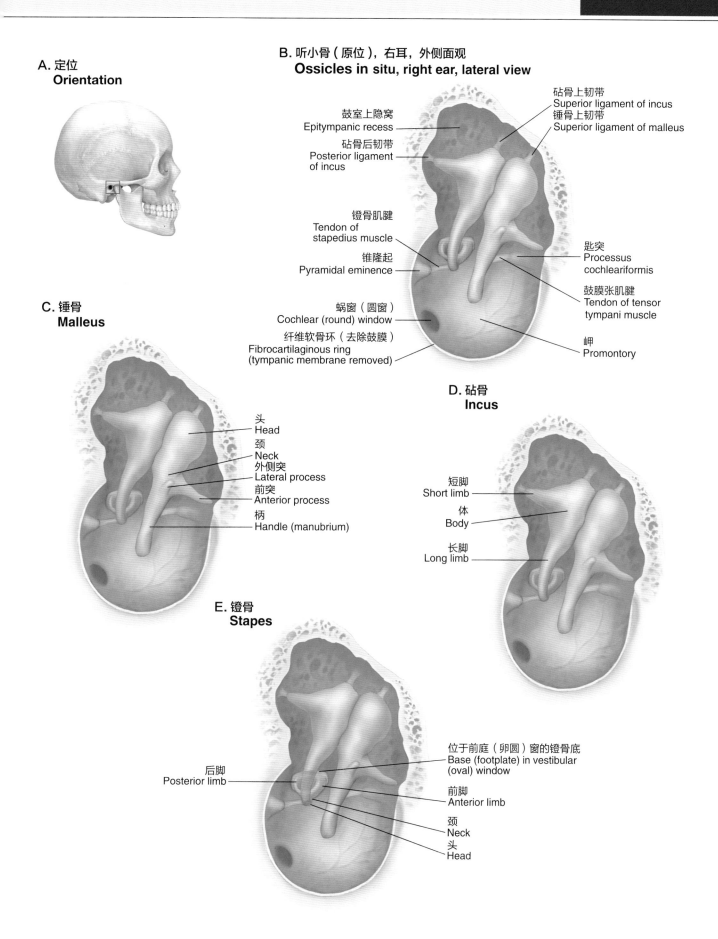

A. 定位
Orientation

B. 听小骨（原位），右耳，外侧面观
Ossicles in situ, right ear, lateral view

鼓室上隐窝
Epitympanic recess

砧骨后韧带
Posterior ligament
of incus

镫骨肌腱
Tendon of
stapedius muscle

锥隆起
Pyramidal eminence

蜗窗（圆窗）
Cochlear (round) window

纤维软骨环（去除鼓膜）
Fibrocartilaginous ring
(tympanic membrane removed)

砧骨上韧带
Superior ligament of incus
锤骨上韧带
Superior ligament of malleus

匙突
Processus
cochleariformis

鼓膜张肌腱
Tendon of tensor
tympani muscle

岬
Promontory

C. 锤骨
Malleus

头
Head
颈
Neck
外侧突
Lateral process
前突
Anterior process
柄
Handle (manubrium)

D. 砧骨
Incus

短脚
Short limb
体
Body
长脚
Long limb

E. 镫骨
Stapes

后脚
Posterior limb

位于前庭（卵圆）窗的镫骨底
Base (footplate) in vestibular
(oval) window

前脚
Anterior limb

颈
Neck
头
Head

图 7-82　耳Ⅵ　Ear Ⅵ

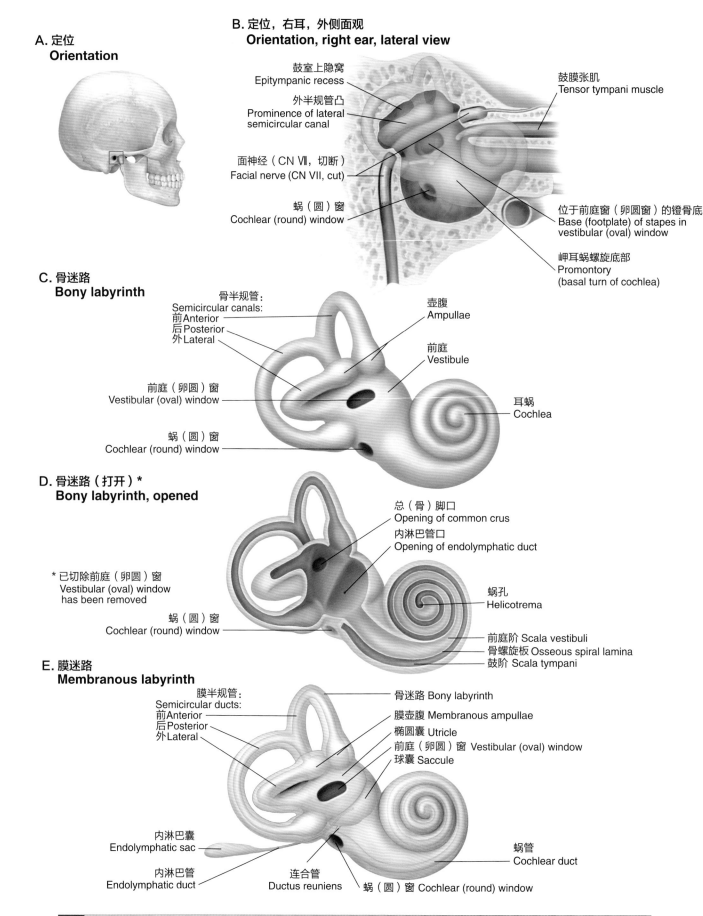

A. 定位
Orientation

B. 定位，右耳，外侧面观
Orientation, right ear, lateral view

鼓室上隐窝
Epitympanic recess

外半规管凸
Prominence of lateral
semicircular canal

面神经（CN Ⅶ，切断）
Facial nerve (CN Ⅶ, cut)

蜗（圆）窗
Cochlear (round) window

鼓膜张肌
Tensor tympani muscle

位于前庭窗（卵圆窗）的镫骨底
Base (footplate) of stapes in
vestibular (oval) window

岬耳蜗螺旋底部
Promontory
(basal turn of cochlea)

C. 骨迷路
Bony labyrinth

骨半规管：
Semicircular canals:
前 Anterior
后 Posterior
外 Lateral

前庭（卵圆）窗
Vestibular (oval) window

蜗（圆）窗
Cochlear (round) window

壶腹
Ampullae

前庭
Vestibule

耳蜗
Cochlea

D. 骨迷路（打开）*
Bony labyrinth, opened

* 已切除前庭（卵圆）窗
Vestibular (oval) window
has been removed

蜗（圆）窗
Cochlear (round) window

总（骨）脚口
Opening of common crus

内淋巴管口
Opening of endolymphatic duct

蜗孔
Helicotrema

前庭阶 Scala vestibuli
骨螺旋板 Osseous spiral lamina
鼓阶 Scala tympani

E. 膜迷路
Membranous labyrinth

膜半规管：
Semicircular ducts:
前 Anterior
后 Posterior
外 Lateral

内淋巴囊
Endolymphatic sac

内淋巴管
Endolymphatic duct

连合管
Ductus reuniens

骨迷路 Bony labyrinth
膜壶腹 Membranous ampullae
椭圆囊 Utricle
前庭（卵圆）窗 Vestibular (oval) window
球囊 Saccule

蜗管
Cochlear duct

蜗（圆）窗 Cochlear (round) window

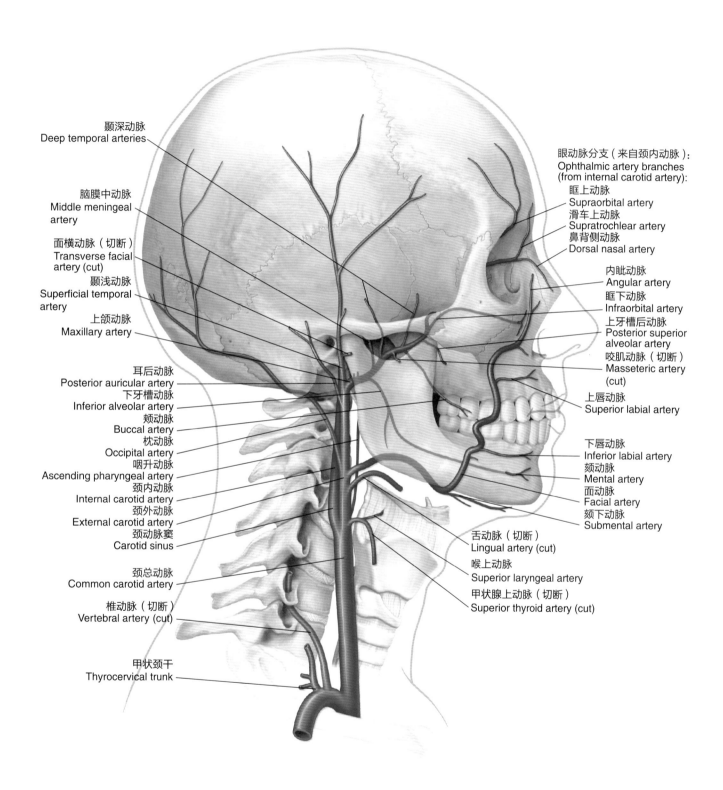

颞深动脉
Deep temporal arteries

脑膜中动脉
Middle meningeal artery

面横动脉（切断）
Transverse facial artery (cut)

颞浅动脉
Superficial temporal artery

上颌动脉
Maxillary artery

耳后动脉
Posterior auricular artery

下牙槽动脉
Inferior alveolar artery

颊动脉
Buccal artery

枕动脉
Occipital artery

咽升动脉
Ascending pharyngeal artery

颈内动脉
Internal carotid artery

颈外动脉
External carotid artery

颈动脉窦
Carotid sinus

颈总动脉
Common carotid artery

椎动脉（切断）
Vertebral artery (cut)

甲状颈干
Thyrocervical trunk

眼动脉分支（来自颈内动脉）：
Ophthalmic artery branches (from internal carotid artery):

眶上动脉
Supraorbital artery

滑车上动脉
Supratrochlear artery

鼻背侧动脉
Dorsal nasal artery

内眦动脉
Angular artery

眶下动脉
Infraorbital artery

上牙槽后动脉
Posterior superior alveolar artery

咬肌动脉（切断）
Masseteric artery (cut)

上唇动脉
Superior labial artery

下唇动脉
Inferior labial artery

颏动脉
Mental artery

面动脉
Facial artery

颏下动脉
Submental artery

舌动脉（切断）
Lingual artery (cut)

喉上动脉
Superior laryngeal artery

甲状腺上动脉（切断）
Superior thyroid artery (cut)

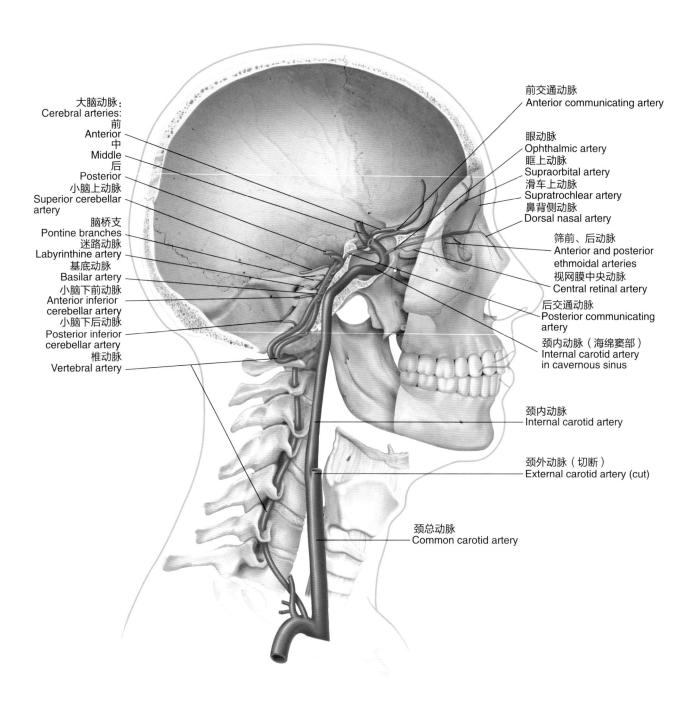

大脑动脉：
Cerebral arteries:
前
Anterior
中
Middle
后
Posterior
小脑上动脉
Superior cerebellar artery
脑桥支
Pontine branches
迷路动脉
Labyrinthine artery
基底动脉
Basilar artery
小脑下前动脉
Anterior inferior cerebellar artery
小脑下后动脉
Posterior inferior cerebellar artery
椎动脉
Vertebral artery

前交通动脉
Anterior communicating artery

眼动脉
Ophthalmic artery
眶上动脉
Supraorbital artery
滑车上动脉
Supratrochlear artery
鼻背侧动脉
Dorsal nasal artery

筛前、后动脉
Anterior and posterior ethmoidal arteries
视网膜中央动脉
Central retinal artery

后交通动脉
Posterior communicating artery
颈内动脉（海绵窦部）
Internal carotid artery in cavernous sinus

颈内动脉
Internal carotid artery

颈外动脉（切断）
External carotid artery (cut)

颈总动脉
Common carotid artery

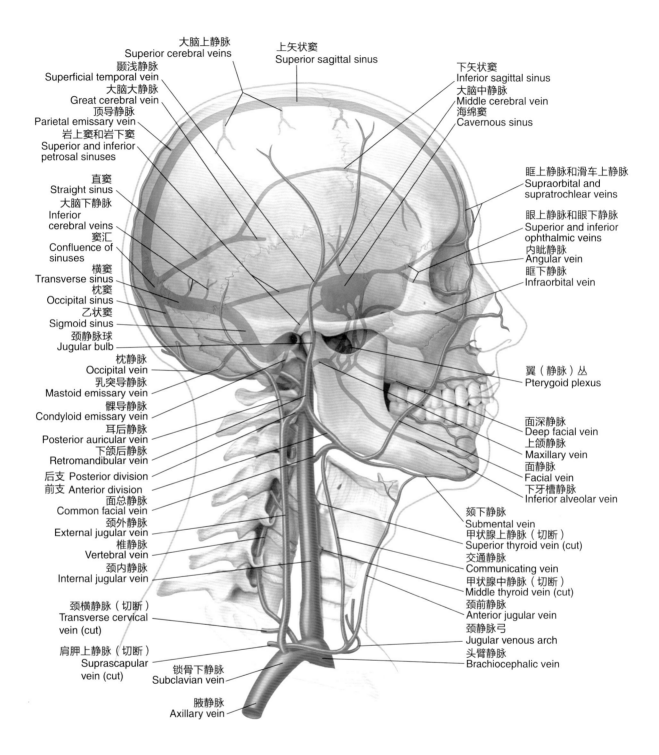

大脑上静脉
Superior cerebral veins

颞浅静脉
Superficial temporal vein

大脑大静脉
Great cerebral vein

顶导静脉
Parietal emissary vein

岩上窦和岩下窦
Superior and inferior
petrosal sinuses

直窦
Straight sinus

大脑下静脉
Inferior
cerebral veins

窦汇
Confluence of
sinuses

横窦
Transverse sinus

枕窦
Occipital sinus

乙状窦
Sigmoid sinus

颈静脉球
Jugular bulb

枕静脉
Occipital vein

乳突导静脉
Mastoid emissary vein

髁导静脉
Condyloid emissary vein

耳后静脉
Posterior auricular vein

下颌后静脉
Retromandibular vein

后支 Posterior division
前支 Anterior division

面总静脉
Common facial vein

颈外静脉
External jugular vein

椎静脉
Vertebral vein

颈内静脉
Internal jugular vein

颈横静脉（切断）
Transverse cervical
vein (cut)

肩胛上静脉（切断）
Suprascapular
vein (cut)

锁骨下静脉
Subclavian vein

腋静脉
Axillary vein

上矢状窦
Superior sagittal sinus

下矢状窦
Inferior sagittal sinus

大脑中静脉
Middle cerebral vein

海绵窦
Cavernous sinus

眶上静脉和滑车上静脉
Supraorbital and
supratrochlear veins

眼上静脉和眼下静脉
Superior and inferior
ophthalmic veins

内眦静脉
Angular vein

眶下静脉
Infraorbital vein

翼（静脉）丛
Pterygoid plexus

面深静脉
Deep facial vein

上颌静脉
Maxillary vein

面静脉
Facial vein

下牙槽静脉
Inferior alveolar vein

颏下静脉
Submental vein

甲状腺上静脉（切断）
Superior thyroid vein (cut)

交通静脉
Communicating vein

甲状腺中静脉（切断）
Middle thyroid vein (cut)

颈前静脉
Anterior jugular vein

颈静脉弓
Jugular venous arch

头臂静脉
Brachiocephalic vein

图 7-86 头颈部的淋巴 Lymphatics of the Head and Neck

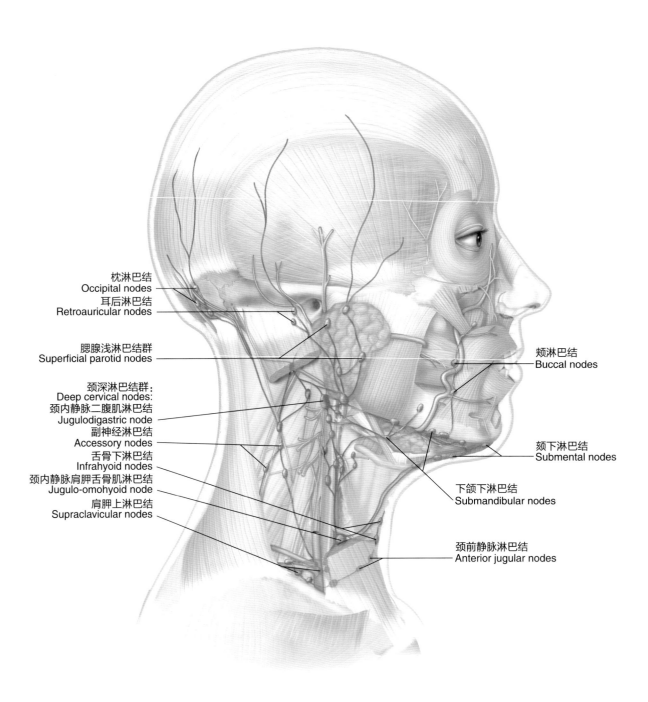

枕淋巴结
Occipital nodes

耳后淋巴结
Retroauricular nodes

腮腺浅淋巴结群
Superficial parotid nodes

颈深淋巴结群：
Deep cervical nodes:
颈内静脉二腹肌淋巴结
Jugulodigastric node
副神经淋巴结
Accessory nodes
舌骨下淋巴结
Infrahyoid nodes
颈内静脉肩胛舌骨肌淋巴结
Jugulo-omohyoid node
肩胛上淋巴结
Supraclavicular nodes

颊淋巴结
Buccal nodes

颏下淋巴结
Submental nodes

下颌下淋巴结
Submandibular nodes

颈前静脉淋巴结
Anterior jugular nodes

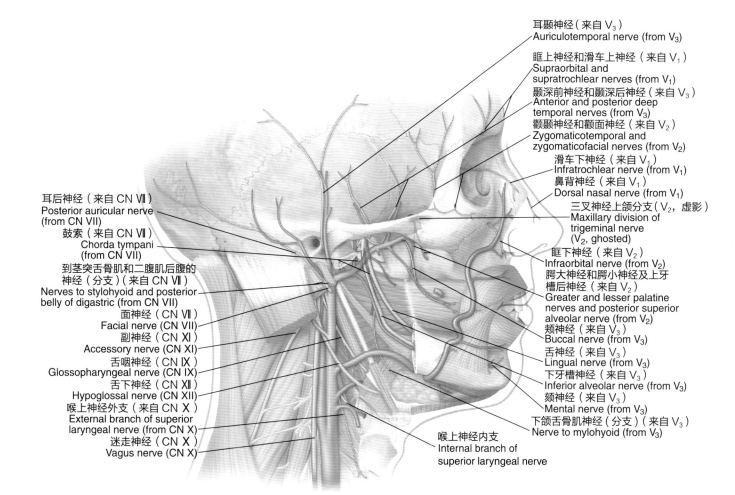

耳颞神经（来自 V₃）
Auriculotemporal nerve (from V₃)

眶上神经和滑车上神经（来自 V₁）
Supraorbital and supratrochlear nerves (from V₁)

颞深前神经和颞深后神经（来自 V₃）
Anterior and posterior deep temporal nerves (from V₃)

颧颞神经和颧面神经（来自 V₂）
Zygomaticotemporal and zygomaticofacial nerves (from V₂)

滑车下神经（来自 V₁）
Infratrochlear nerve (from V₁)

鼻背神经（来自 V₁）
Dorsal nasal nerve (from V₁)

三叉神经上颌分支（V₂，虚影）
Maxillary division of trigeminal nerve (V₂, ghosted)

眶下神经（来自 V₂）
Infraorbital nerve (from V₂)

腭大神经和腭小神经及上牙槽后神经（来自 V₂）
Greater and lesser palatine nerves and posterior superior alveolar nerve (from V₂)

颊神经（来自 V₃）
Buccal nerve (from V₃)

舌神经（来自 V₃）
Lingual nerve (from V₃)

下牙槽神经（来自 V₃）
Inferior alveolar nerve (from V₃)

颏神经（来自 V₃）
Mental nerve (from V₃)

下颌舌骨肌神经（分支）（来自 V₃）
Nerve to mylohyoid (from V₃)

耳后神经（来自 CN Ⅶ）
Posterior auricular nerve (from CN VII)

鼓索（来自 CN Ⅶ）
Chorda tympani (from CN VII)

到茎突舌骨肌和二腹肌后腹的神经（分支）（来自 CN Ⅶ）
Nerves to stylohyoid and posterior belly of digastric (from CN VII)

面神经（CN Ⅶ）
Facial nerve (CN VII)

副神经（CN Ⅺ）
Accessory nerve (CN XI)

舌咽神经（CN Ⅸ）
Glossopharyngeal nerve (CN IX)

舌下神经（CN Ⅻ）
Hypoglossal nerve (CN XII)

喉上神经外支（来自 CN Ⅹ）
External branch of superior laryngeal nerve (from CN X)

迷走神经（CN Ⅹ）
Vagus nerve (CN X)

喉上神经内支
Internal branch of superior laryngeal nerve

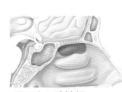

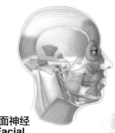

CN Ⅱ：视神经
CN II: Optic
纯感觉：视觉
Sensory only: vision

CN Ⅰ：嗅神经
CN I: Olfactory
纯感觉：嗅觉
Sensory only: smell

CN Ⅶ：面神经
CN VII: Facial
运动：面部表情肌、镫骨肌、二腹肌后腹、茎突舌骨肌；泪腺、下颌下腺和舌下腺的分泌
Motor: muscles of facial expression, stapedius, posterior belly of digastric, stylohyoid; secretomotor to lacrimal, submandibular, sublingual glands

CN Ⅲ：动眼神经
CN III: Oculomotor
纯运动：上睑提肌、上直肌，内直肌、下直肌、下斜肌、睫状肌、瞳孔括约肌
Motor only: levator palpebrae superioris, superior rectus, medial rectus, inferior rectus, inferior oblique, ciliary muscle, sphincter pupillae

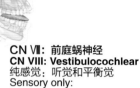

CN Ⅷ：前庭蜗神经
CN VIII: Vestibulocochlear
纯感觉：听觉和平衡觉
Sensory only: hearing and balance

感觉：舌前 2/3 的味觉，腭
Sensory: taste of anterior 2/3 of tongue, palate

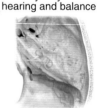

CN Ⅳ：滑车神经
CN IV: Trochlear
纯运动：上斜肌
Motor only: superior oblique

CN Ⅸ：舌咽神经
CN IX: Glossopharyngeal
运动：茎突咽肌，腮腺分泌
Motor: stylopharyngeus, secretomotor to parotid gland
感觉：咽、中耳、颈动脉窦，舌后 1/3 的味觉
Sensory: oropharynx, middle ear, carotid sinus, posterior 1/3 of tongue

CN Ⅴ：三叉神经
CN V: Trigeminal
运动：咀嚼肌、下颌舌骨肌、二腹肌前腹、鼓膜张肌、腭帆张肌
Motor: muscles of mastication mylohyoid, anterior belly of digastric, tensor tympani, tensor veli palatini
感觉：面部、鼻腔、口腔、牙
Sensory: face, nasal cavity, nasopharynx, oral cavity, teeth

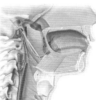

CN Ⅹ：迷走神经
CN X: Vagus
运动：软腭、咽、喉、支气管树、心、（结肠）脾曲以上的消化道，黏液腺分泌
Motor: soft palate, pharynx, larynx, bronchial tree, heart, GI tract to splenic flexure, secretomotor to mucous glands
感觉：咽、喉、颈动脉体、支气管树、胃肠道
Sensory: laryngopharynx, larynx, carotid body, bronchial tree, GI tract

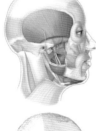

CN Ⅵ：展神经
CN VI: Abducens
纯运动：外直肌
Motor only: lateral rectus

CN Ⅻ：舌下神经
CN XII: Hypoglossal
纯运动：舌肌
Motor only: muscles of tongue

CN Ⅺ：副神经
CN XI: Accessory
纯运动：斜方肌，胸锁乳突肌
Motor only: trapezius, sternocleidomastoid

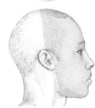

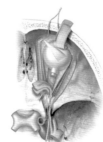

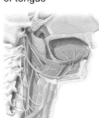

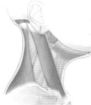

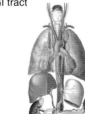

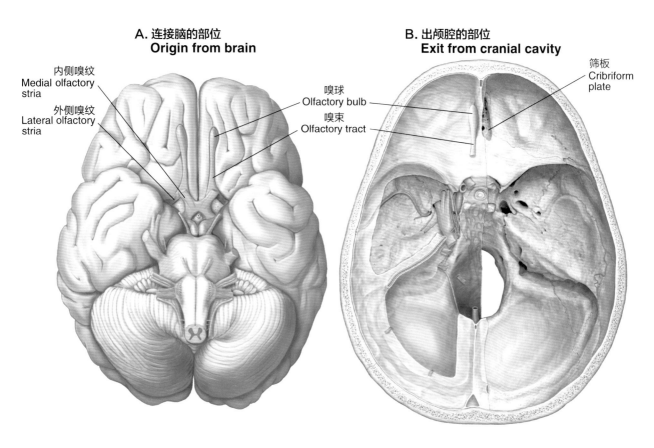

A. 连接脑的部位
Origin from brain

内侧嗅纹
Medial olfactory
stria

外侧嗅纹
Lateral olfactory
stria

B. 出颅腔的部位
Exit from cranial cavity

嗅球
Olfactory bulb

嗅束
Olfactory tract

筛板
Cribriform
plate

C. 感觉神经支配，矢状断面
Sensory innervation, sagittal section

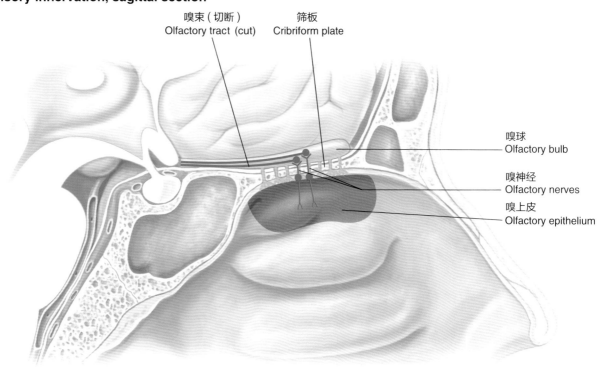

嗅束（切断）
Olfactory tract (cut)

筛板
Cribriform plate

嗅球
Olfactory bulb

嗅神经
Olfactory nerves

嗅上皮
Olfactory epithelium

图 7-90　视神经，CN Ⅱ　Optic Nerve, Cranial Nerve Ⅱ

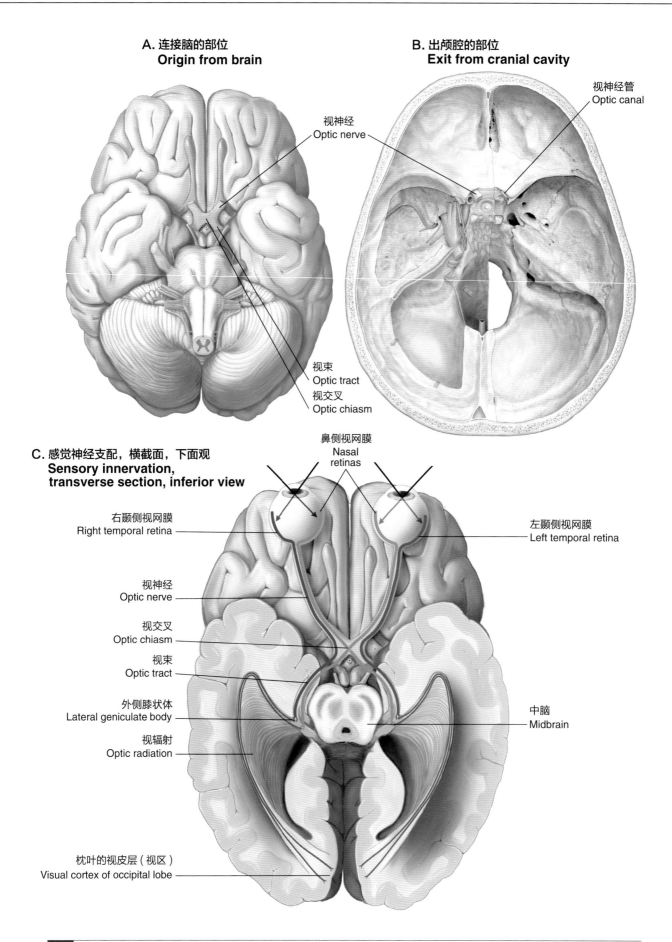

A. 连接脑的部位
Origin from brain

视神经
Optic nerve

视束
Optic tract

视交叉
Optic chiasm

B. 出颅腔的部位
Exit from cranial cavity

视神经管
Optic canal

C. 感觉神经支配，横截面，下面观
Sensory innervation,
transverse section, inferior view

鼻侧视网膜
Nasal
retinas

右颞侧视网膜
Right temporal retina

左颞侧视网膜
Left temporal retina

视神经
Optic nerve

视交叉
Optic chiasm

视束
Optic tract

外侧膝状体
Lateral geniculate body

中脑
Midbrain

视辐射
Optic radiation

枕叶的视皮层（视区）
Visual cortex of occipital lobe

A. 连接脑的部位
Origin from brain

B. 出颅腔的部位
Exit from cranial cavity

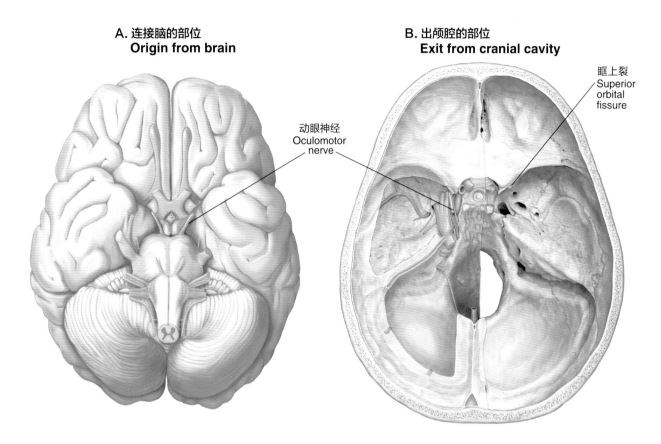

动眼神经
Oculomotor
nerve

眶上裂
Superior
orbital
fissure

C. 支配的骨骼肌
Skeletal muscle innervation

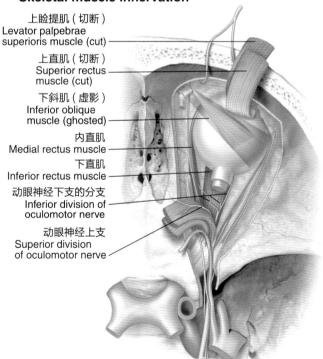

上睑提肌（切断）
Levator palpebrae
superioris muscle (cut)

上直肌（切断）
Superior rectus
muscle (cut)

下斜肌（虚影）
Inferior oblique
muscle (ghosted)

内直肌
Medial rectus muscle

下直肌
Inferior rectus muscle

动眼神经下支的分支
Inferior division of
oculomotor nerve

动眼神经上支
Superior division
of oculomotor nerve

D. 副交感神经支配
Parasympathetic innervation

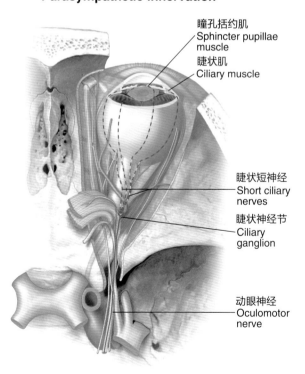

瞳孔括约肌
Sphincter pupillae
muscle

睫状肌
Ciliary muscle

睫状短神经
Short ciliary
nerves

睫状神经节
Ciliary
ganglion

动眼神经
Oculomotor
nerve

图 7-92　　滑车神经，CN Ⅳ　Trochlear Nerve, Cranial Nerve IV

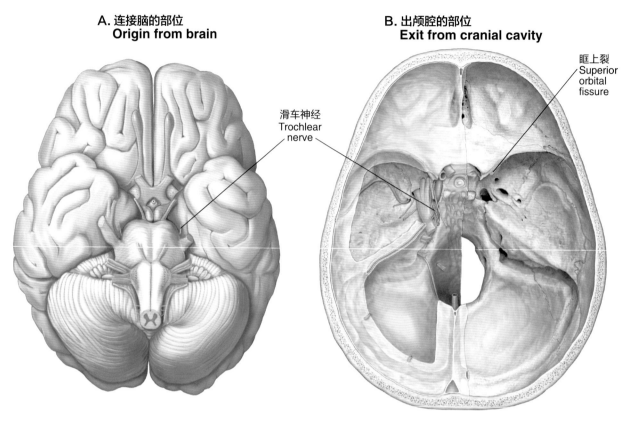

A. 连接脑的部位
Origin from brain

B. 出颅腔的部位
Exit from cranial cavity

眶上裂
Superior
orbital
fissure

滑车神经
Trochlear
nerve

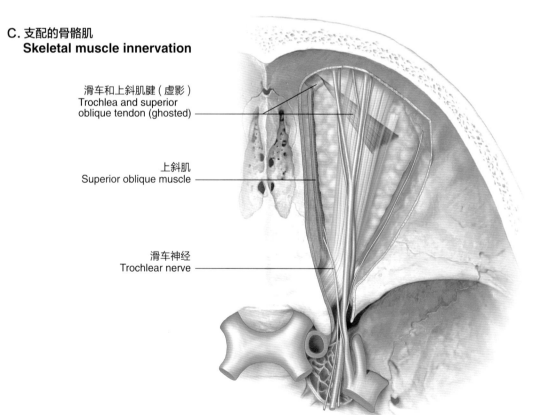

C. 支配的骨骼肌
Skeletal muscle innervation

滑车和上斜肌腱（虚影）
Trochlea and superior
oblique tendon (ghosted)

上斜肌
Superior oblique muscle

滑车神经
Trochlear nerve

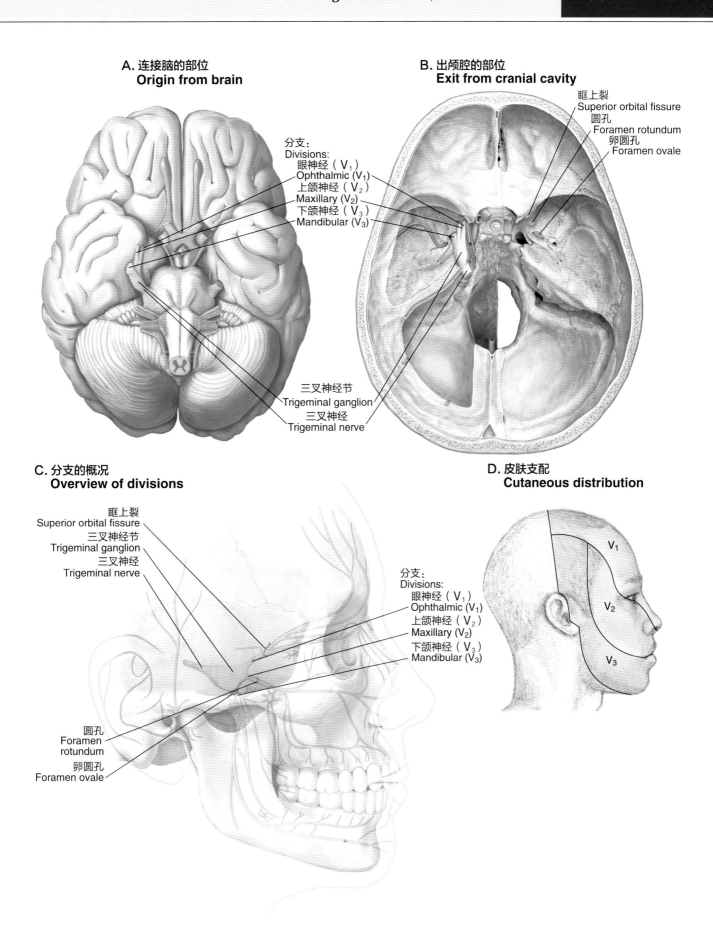

A. 连接脑的部位
Origin from brain

分支：
Divisions:
　眼神经（V₁）
　Ophthalmic (V₁)
　上颌神经（V₂）
　Maxillary (V₂)
　下颌神经（V₃）
　Mandibular (V₃)

三叉神经节
Trigeminal ganglion
三叉神经
Trigeminal nerve

B. 出颅腔的部位
Exit from cranial cavity

眶上裂
Superior orbital fissure
圆孔
Foramen rotundum
卵圆孔
Foramen ovale

C. 分支的概况
Overview of divisions

眶上裂
Superior orbital fissure
三叉神经节
Trigeminal ganglion
三叉神经
Trigeminal nerve

分支：
Divisions:
　眼神经（V₁）
　Ophthalmic (V₁)
　上颌神经（V₂）
　Maxillary (V₂)
　下颌神经（V₃）
　Mandibular (V₃)

圆孔
Foramen rotundum
卵圆孔
Foramen ovale

D. 皮肤支配
Cutaneous distribution

V₁
V₂
V₃

图 7-94 三叉神经的眼神经（V₁） Ophthalmic Division of Trigeminal Nerve (V₁)

A. 感觉支配
Sensory innervation

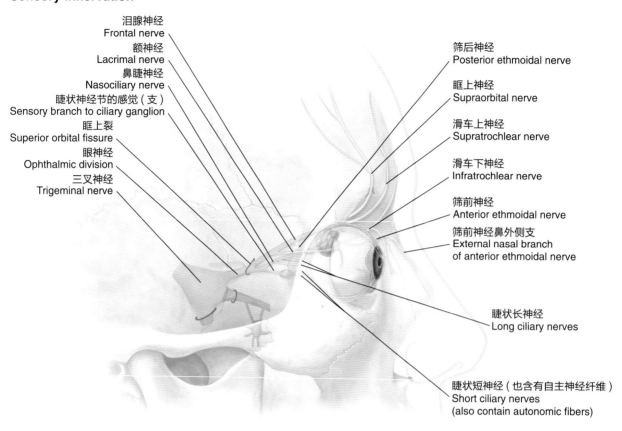

泪腺神经
Frontal nerve

额神经
Lacrimal nerve

鼻睫神经
Nasociliary nerve

睫状神经节的感觉（支）
Sensory branch to ciliary ganglion

眶上裂
Superior orbital fissure

眼神经
Ophthalmic division

三叉神经
Trigeminal nerve

筛后神经
Posterior ethmoidal nerve

眶上神经
Supraorbital nerve

滑车上神经
Supratrochlear nerve

滑车下神经
Infratrochlear nerve

筛前神经
Anterior ethmoidal nerve

筛前神经鼻外侧支
External nasal branch
of anterior ethmoidal nerve

睫状长神经
Long ciliary nerves

睫状短神经（也含有自主神经纤维）
Short ciliary nerves
(also contain autonomic fibers)

B. 皮肤支配
Cutaneous distribution

C. 含副交感神经的分支
Branches that carry parasympathetic innervation

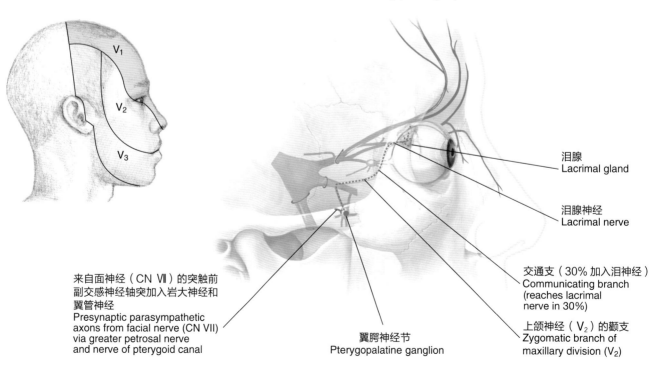

V₁

V₂

V₃

来自面神经（CN Ⅶ）的突触前
副交感神经轴突加入岩大神经和
翼管神经
Presynaptic parasympathetic
axons from facial nerve (CN VII)
via greater petrosal nerve
and nerve of pterygoid canal

翼腭神经节
Pterygopalatine ganglion

泪腺
Lacrimal gland

泪腺神经
Lacrimal nerve

交通支（30% 加入泪神经）
Communicating branch
(reaches lacrimal
nerve in 30%)

上颌神经（V₂）的颧支
Zygomatic branch of
maxillary division (V₂)

A. 感觉支配
Sensory innervation

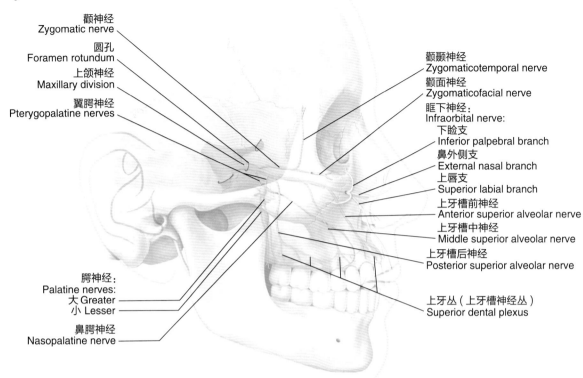

颧神经
Zygomatic nerve

圆孔
Foramen rotundum

上颌神经
Maxillary division

翼腭神经
Pterygopalatine nerves

颧颞神经
Zygomaticotemporal nerve

颧面神经
Zygomaticofacial nerve

眶下神经：
Infraorbital nerve:

下睑支
Inferior palpebral branch

鼻外侧支
External nasal branch

上唇支
Superior labial branch

上牙槽前神经
Anterior superior alveolar nerve

上牙槽中神经
Middle superior alveolar nerve

上牙槽后神经
Posterior superior alveolar nerve

上牙丛（上牙槽神经丛）
Superior dental plexus

腭神经：
Palatine nerves:
大 Greater
小 Lesser

鼻腭神经
Nasopalatine nerve

B. 皮肤支配
Cutaneous distribution

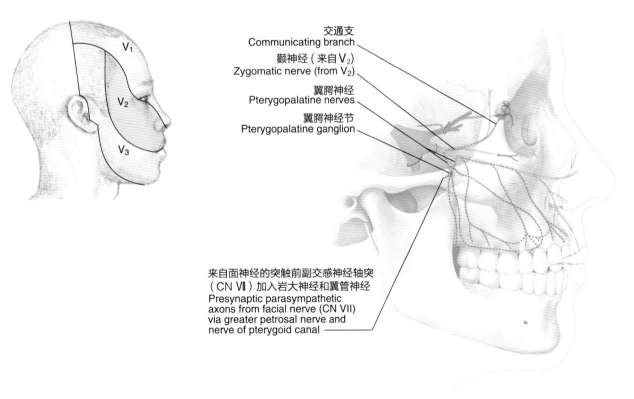

V_1

V_2

V_3

C. 含副交感神经的分支
Branches that carry parasympathetic innervation

交通支
Communicating branch

颧神经（来自 V_2）
Zygomatic nerve (from V_2)

翼腭神经
Pterygopalatine nerves

翼腭神经节
Pterygopalatine ganglion

来自面神经的突触前副交感神经轴突
（CN Ⅶ）加入岩大神经和翼管神经
Presynaptic parasympathetic
axons from facial nerve (CN VII)
via greater petrosal nerve and
nerve of pterygoid canal

A. 感觉支配
Sensory innervation

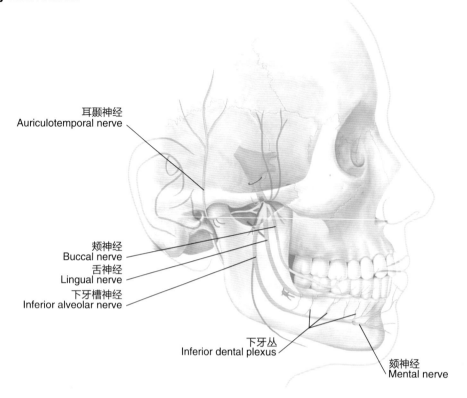

耳颞神经
Auriculotemporal nerve

颊神经
Buccal nerve

舌神经
Lingual nerve

下牙槽神经
Inferior alveolar nerve

下牙丛
Inferior dental plexus

颏神经
Mental nerve

B. 皮肤支配
Cutaneous distribution

V₁

V₂

V₃

C. 含副交感神经的分支
Branches that carry parasympathetic innervation

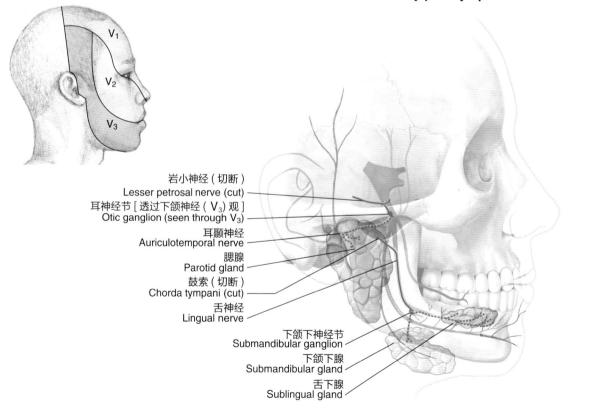

岩小神经（切断）
Lesser petrosal nerve (cut)

耳神经节［透过下颌神经（V₃）观］
Otic ganglion (seen through V₃)

耳颞神经
Auriculotemporal nerve

腮腺
Parotid gland

鼓索（切断）
Chorda tympani (cut)

舌神经
Lingual nerve

下颌下神经节
Submandibular ganglion

下颌下腺
Submandibular gland

舌下腺
Sublingual gland

A. 支配的骨骼肌 I
Skeletal muscle innervation I

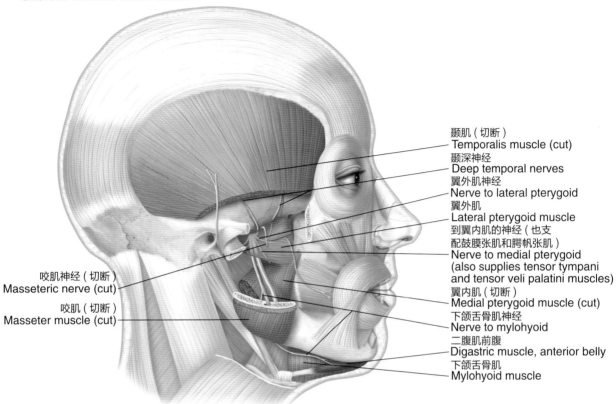

颞肌（切断）
Temporalis muscle (cut)

颞深神经
Deep temporal nerves

翼外肌神经
Nerve to lateral pterygoid

翼外肌
Lateral pterygoid muscle

到翼内肌的神经（也支
配鼓膜张肌和腭帆张肌）
Nerve to medial pterygoid
(also supplies tensor tympani
and tensor veli palatini muscles)

翼内肌（切断）
Medial pterygoid muscle (cut)

下颌舌骨肌神经
Nerve to mylohyoid

二腹肌前腹
Digastric muscle, anterior belly

下颌舌骨肌
Mylohyoid muscle

咬肌神经（切断）
Masseteric nerve (cut)

咬肌（切断）
Masseter muscle (cut)

B. 支配的骨骼肌 II
Skeletal muscle innervation II

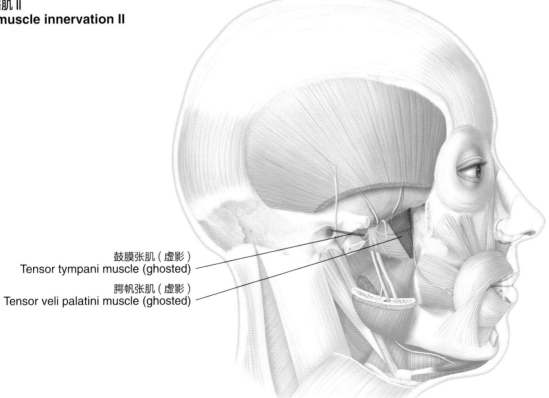

鼓膜张肌（虚影）
Tensor tympani muscle (ghosted)

腭帆张肌（虚影）
Tensor veli palatini muscle (ghosted)

图 7-98　　展神经，CN Ⅵ　Abducens Nerve, Cranial Nerve Ⅵ

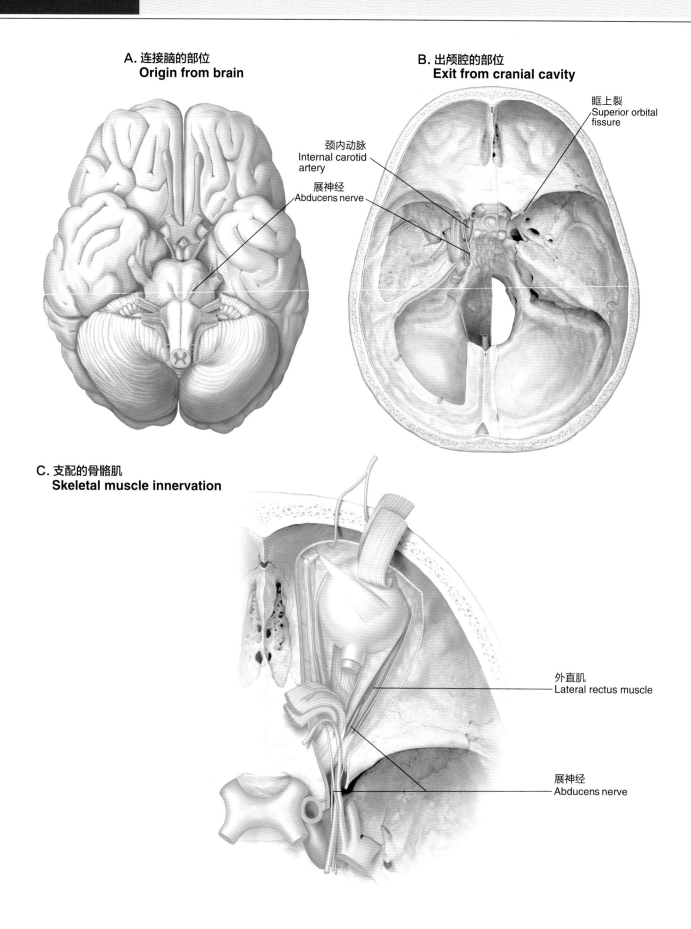

A. 连接脑的部位
Origin from brain

B. 出颅腔的部位
Exit from cranial cavity

眶上裂
Superior orbital fissure

颈内动脉
Internal carotid artery

展神经
Abducens nerve

C. 支配的骨骼肌
Skeletal muscle innervation

外直肌
Lateral rectus muscle

展神经
Abducens nerve

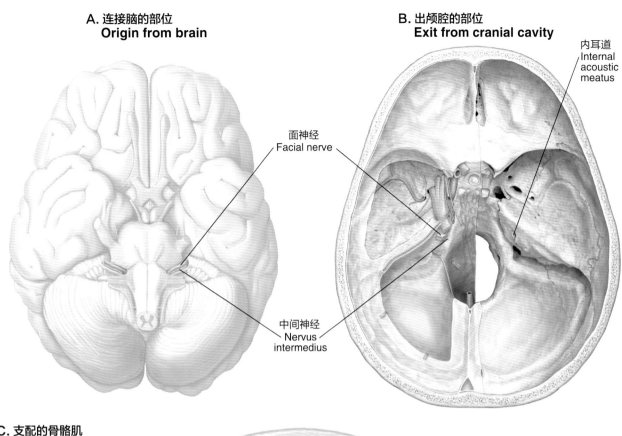

A. 连接脑的部位
Origin from brain

面神经
Facial nerve

中间神经
Nervus
intermedius

B. 出颅腔的部位
Exit from cranial cavity

内耳道
Internal
acoustic
meatus

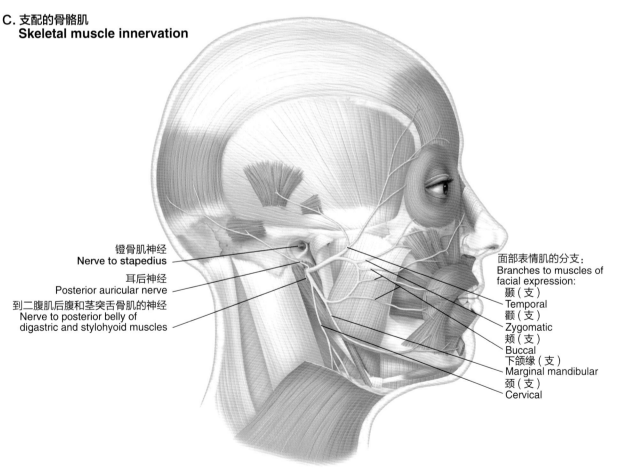

C. 支配的骨骼肌
Skeletal muscle innervation

镫骨肌神经
Nerve to stapedius

耳后神经
Posterior auricular nerve

到二腹肌后腹和茎突舌骨肌的神经
Nerve to posterior belly of
digastric and stylohyoid muscles

面部表情肌的分支：
Branches to muscles of
facial expression:
颞（支）
Temporal
颧（支）
Zygomatic
颊（支）
Buccal
下颌缘（支）
Marginal mandibular
颈（支）
Cervical

图 7-100　面神经，CN Ⅶ，Ⅱ　Facial Nerve, Cranial Nerve VII, II

A. 感觉支配
Sensory innervation

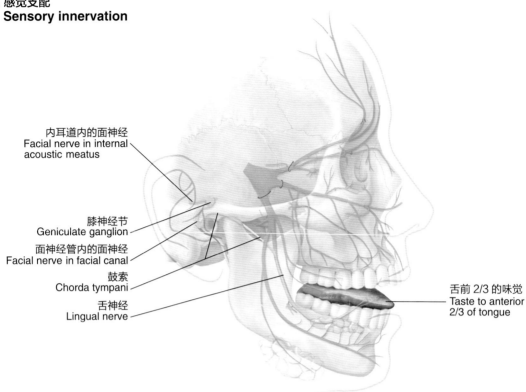

内耳道内的面神经
Facial nerve in internal
acoustic meatus

膝神经节
Geniculate ganglion

面神经管内的面神经
Facial nerve in facial canal

鼓索
Chorda tympani

舌神经
Lingual nerve

舌前 2/3 的味觉
Taste to anterior
2/3 of tongue

B. 副交感神经分布
Parasympathetic innervation

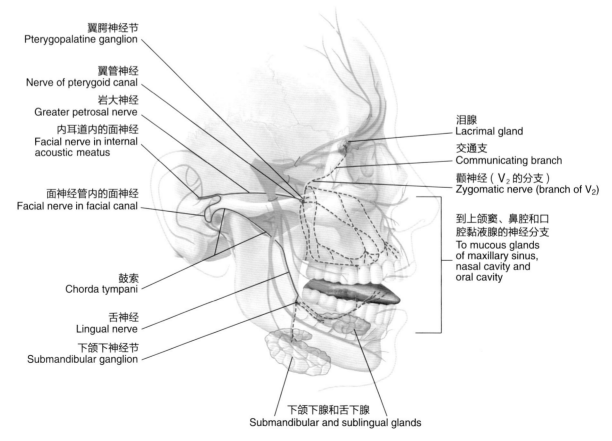

翼腭神经节
Pterygopalatine ganglion

翼管神经
Nerve of pterygoid canal

岩大神经
Greater petrosal nerve

内耳道内的面神经
Facial nerve in internal
acoustic meatus

面神经管内的面神经
Facial nerve in facial canal

鼓索
Chorda tympani

舌神经
Lingual nerve

下颌下神经节
Submandibular ganglion

泪腺
Lacrimal gland

交通支
Communicating branch

颧神经（ V₂ 的分支 ）
Zygomatic nerve (branch of V₂)

到上颌窦、鼻腔和口
腔黏液腺的神经分支
To mucous glands
of maxillary sinus,
nasal cavity and
oral cavity

下颌下腺和舌下腺
Submandibular and sublingual glands

A. 连接脑的部位
Origin from brain

B. 出颅腔的部位
Exit from cranial cavity

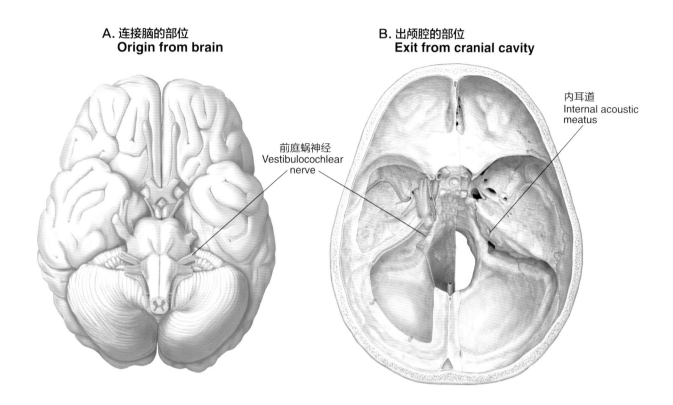

内耳道
Internal acoustic
meatus

前庭蜗神经
Vestibulocochlear
nerve

C. 感觉神经分布
Sensory innervation

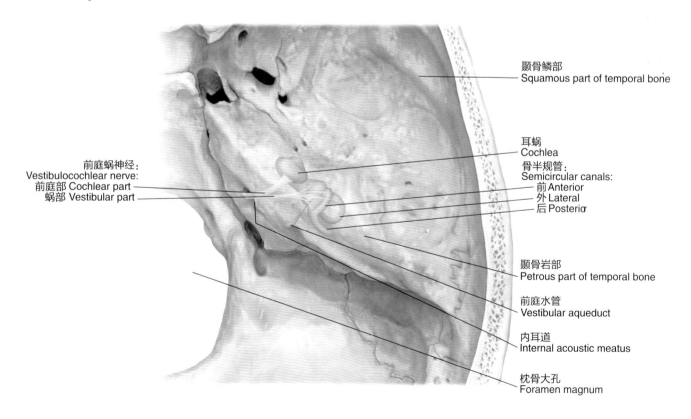

颞骨鳞部
Squamous part of temporal bone

耳蜗
Cochlea

骨半规管：
Semicircular canals:
前 Anterior
外 Lateral
后 Posterior

前庭蜗神经：
Vestibulocochlear nerve:
前庭部 Cochlear part
蜗部 Vestibular part

颞骨岩部
Petrous part of temporal bone

前庭水管
Vestibular aqueduct

内耳道
Internal acoustic meatus

枕骨大孔
Foramen magnum

图 7-102　舌咽神经，CN IX　Glossopharyngeal Nerve, Cranial Nerve IX

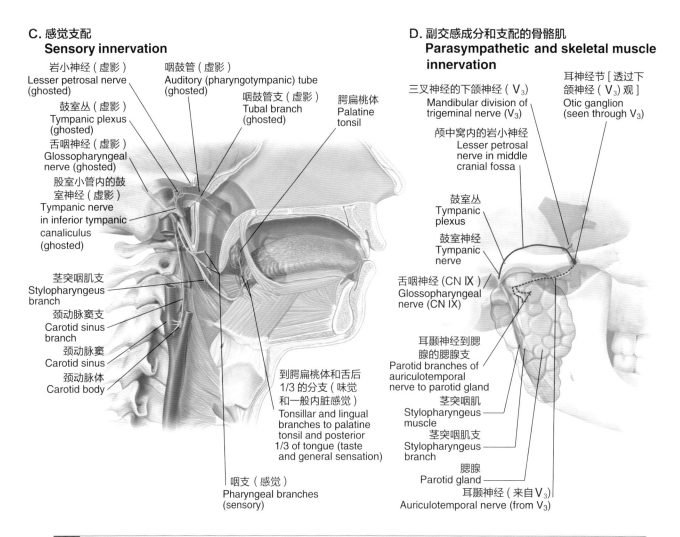

A. 连接脑的部位
Origin from brain

舌咽神经
Glossopharyngeal nerve

B. 出颅腔的部位
Exit from cranial cavity

颈静脉孔
Jugular foramen

C. 感觉支配
Sensory innervation

岩小神经（虚影）
Lesser petrosal nerve (ghosted)

咽鼓管（虚影）
Auditory (pharyngotympanic) tube (ghosted)

咽鼓管支（虚影）
Tubal branch (ghosted)

腭扁桃体
Palatine tonsil

鼓室丛（虚影）
Tympanic plexus (ghosted)

舌咽神经（虚影）
Glossopharyngeal nerve (ghosted)

股室小管内的鼓室神经（虚影）
Tympanic nerve in inferior tympanic canaliculus (ghosted)

茎突咽肌支
Stylopharyngeus branch

颈动脉窦支
Carotid sinus branch

颈动脉窦
Carotid sinus

颈动脉体
Carotid body

到腭扁桃体和舌后1/3 的分支（味觉和一般内脏感觉）
Tonsillar and lingual branches to palatine tonsil and posterior 1/3 of tongue (taste and general sensation)

咽支（感觉）
Pharyngeal branches (sensory)

D. 副交感成分和支配的骨骼肌
Parasympathetic and skeletal muscle innervation

三叉神经的下颌神经（V₃）
Mandibular division of trigeminal nerve (V₃)

耳神经节 [透过下颌神经（V₃）观]
Otic ganglion (seen through V₃)

颅中窝内的岩小神经
Lesser petrosal nerve in middle cranial fossa

鼓室丛
Tympanic plexus

鼓室神经
Tympanic nerve

舌咽神经（CN IX）
Glossopharyngeal nerve (CN IX)

耳颞神经到腮腺的腮腺支
Parotid branches of auriculotemporal nerve to parotid gland

茎突咽肌
Stylopharyngeus muscle

茎突咽肌支
Stylopharyngeus branch

腮腺
Parotid gland

耳颞神经（来自V₃）
Auriculotemporal nerve (from V₃)

A. 连接脑的部位
Origin from brain

B. 出颅腔的部位
Exit from cranial cavity

迷走神经
Vagus nerve

颈静脉孔
Jugular
foramen

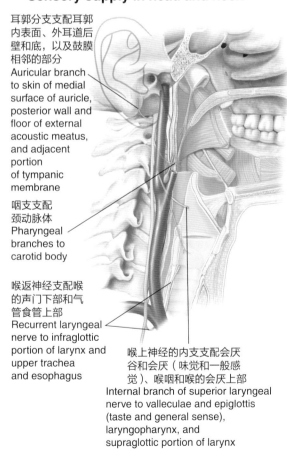

C. 头颈部感觉支配
Sensory supply in head and neck

耳郭分支支配耳郭内表面、外耳道后壁和底，以及鼓膜相邻的部分
Auricular branch to skin of medial surface of auricle, posterior wall and floor of external acoustic meatus, and adjacent portion of tympanic membrane

咽支支配颈动脉体
Pharyngeal branches to carotid body

喉返神经支配喉的声门下部和气管食管上部
Recurrent laryngeal nerve to infraglottic portion of larynx and upper trachea and esophagus

喉上神经的内支支配会厌谷和会厌（味觉和一般感觉）、喉咽和喉的会厌上部
Internal branch of superior laryngeal nerve to valleculae and epiglottis (taste and general sense), laryngopharynx, and supraglottic portion of larynx

D. 支配的骨骼肌
Skeletal musde innervation

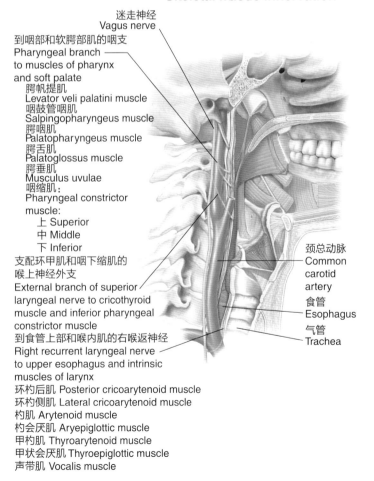

迷走神经
Vagus nerve

到咽部和软腭部肌的咽支
Pharyngeal branch to muscles of pharynx and soft palate
腭帆提肌
Levator veli palatini muscle
咽鼓管咽肌
Salpingopharyngeus muscle
腭咽肌
Palatopharyngeus muscle
腭舌肌
Palatoglossus muscle
腭垂肌
Musculus uvulae
咽缩肌：
Pharyngeal constrictor muscle:
上 Superior
中 Middle
下 Inferior
支配环甲肌和咽下缩肌的喉上神经外支
External branch of superior laryngeal nerve to cricothyroid muscle and inferior pharyngeal constrictor muscle
到食管上部和喉内肌的右喉返神经
Right recurrent laryngeal nerve to upper esophagus and intrinsic muscles of larynx
环杓后肌 Posterior cricoarytenoid muscle
环杓侧肌 Lateral cricoarytenoid muscle
杓肌 Arytenoid muscle
杓会厌肌 Aryepiglottic muscle
甲杓肌 Thyroarytenoid muscle
甲状会厌肌 Thyroepiglottic muscle
声带肌 Vocalis muscle

颈总动脉
Common carotid artery
食管
Esophagus
气管
Trachea

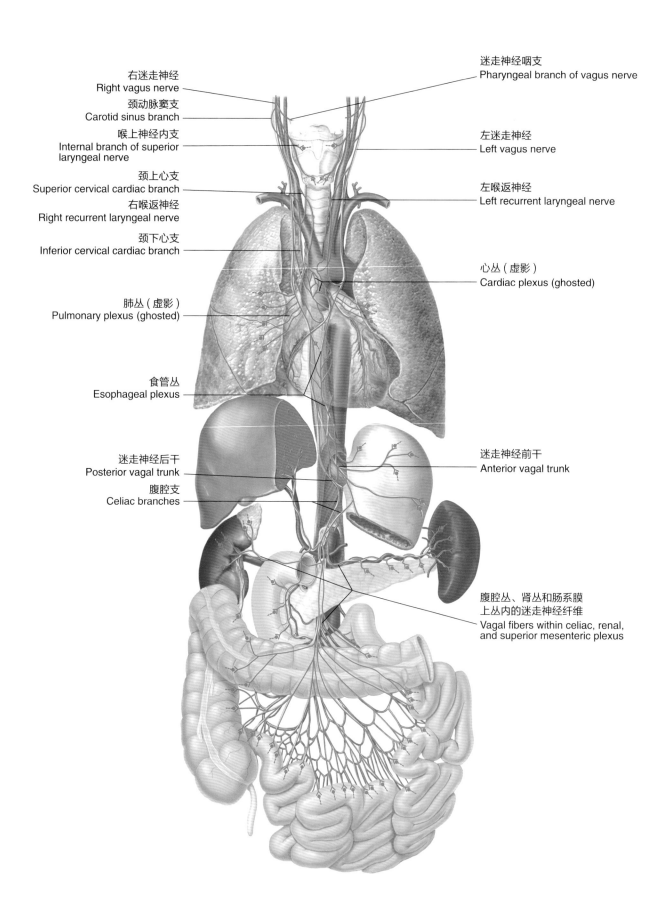

右迷走神经
Right vagus nerve

颈动脉窦支
Carotid sinus branch

喉上神经内支
Internal branch of superior
laryngeal nerve

颈上心支
Superior cervical cardiac branch

右喉返神经
Right recurrent laryngeal nerve

颈下心支
Inferior cervical cardiac branch

肺丛（虚影）
Pulmonary plexus (ghosted)

食管丛
Esophageal plexus

迷走神经后干
Posterior vagal trunk

腹腔支
Celiac branches

迷走神经咽支
Pharyngeal branch of vagus nerve

左迷走神经
Left vagus nerve

左喉返神经
Left recurrent laryngeal nerve

心丛（虚影）
Cardiac plexus (ghosted)

迷走神经前干
Anterior vagal trunk

腹腔丛、肾丛和肠系膜
上丛内的迷走神经纤维
Vagal fibers within celiac, renal,
and superior mesenteric plexus

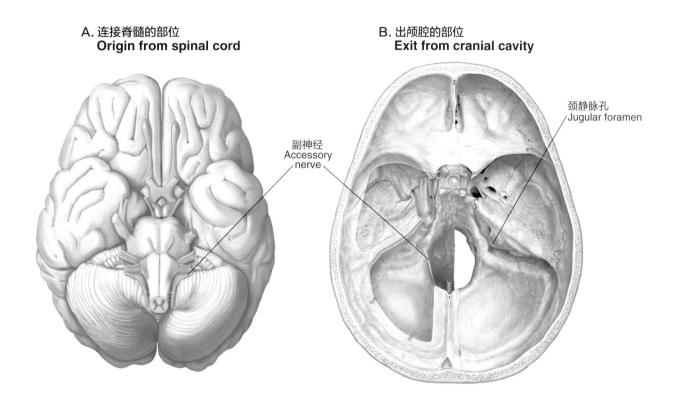

A. 连接脊髓的部位
Origin from spinal cord

副神经
Accessory
nerve

B. 出颅腔的部位
Exit from cranial cavity

颈静脉孔
Jugular foramen

C. 支配的骨骼肌
Skeletal muscle innervation

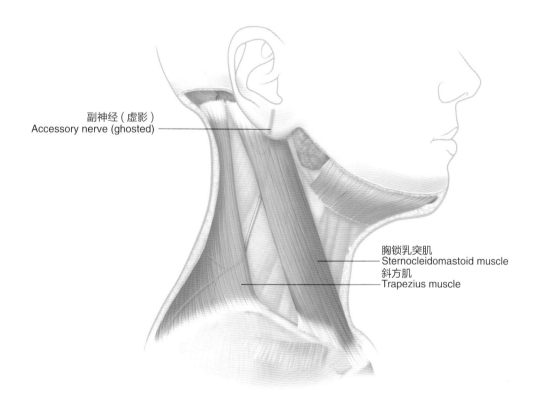

副神经（虚影）
Accessory nerve (ghosted)

胸锁乳突肌
Sternocleidomastoid muscle
斜方肌
Trapezius muscle

图 7-106   舌下神经，CN XII   Hypoglossal Nerve, Cranial Nerve XII

A. 连接脑的部位
Origin from brain

B. 出颅腔的部位
Exit from cranial cavity

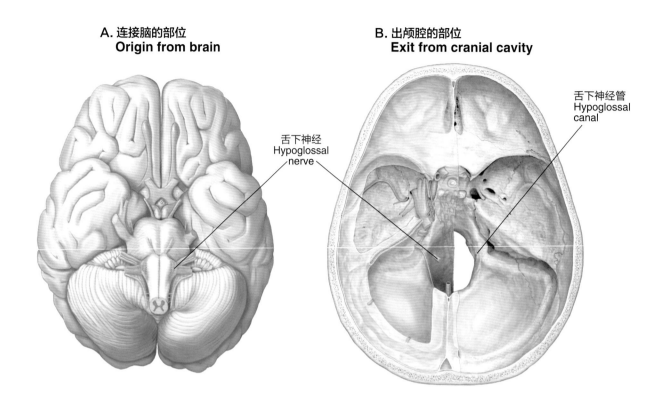

舌下神经
Hypoglossal
nerve

舌下神经管
Hypoglossal
canal

C. 支配的骨骼肌
Skeletal muscle innervation

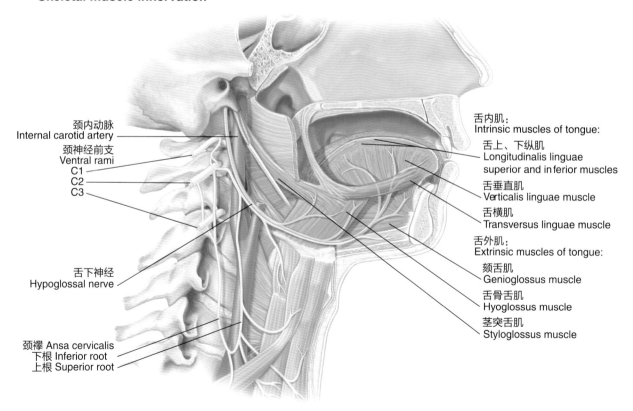

颈内动脉
Internal carotid artery

颈神经前支
Ventral rami
C1
C2
C3

舌下神经
Hypoglossal nerve

颈襻 Ansa cervicalis
下根 Inferior root
上根 Superior root

舌内肌：
Intrinsic muscles of tongue:

舌上、下纵肌
Longitudinalis linguae
superior and inferior muscles

舌垂直肌
Verticalis linguae muscle

舌横肌
Transversus linguae muscle

舌外肌：
Extrinsic muscles of tongue:

颏舌肌
Genioglossus muscle

舌骨舌肌
Hyoglossus muscle

茎突舌肌
Styloglossus muscle

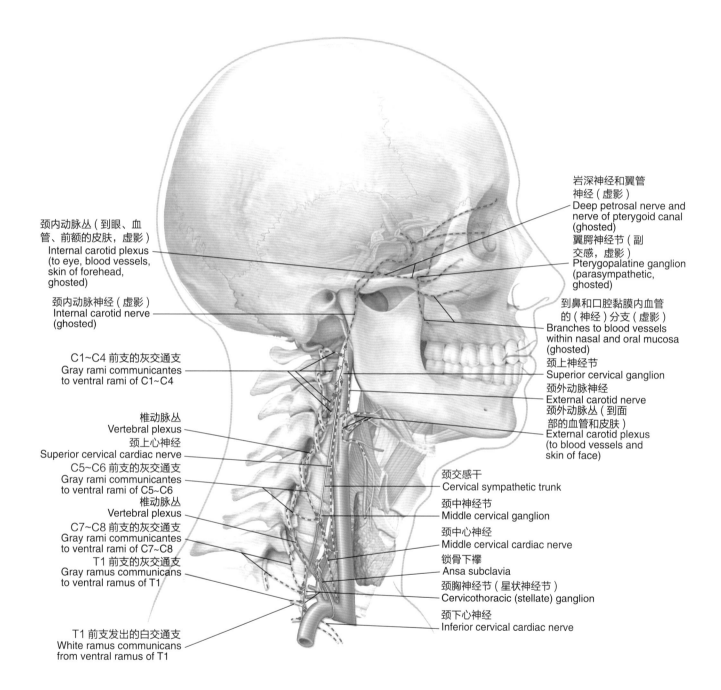

颈内动脉丛（到眼、血管、前额的皮肤，虚影）
Internal carotid plexus (to eye, blood vessels, skin of forehead, ghosted)

颈内动脉神经（虚影）
Internal carotid nerve (ghosted)

C1~C4 前支的灰交通支
Gray rami communicantes to ventral rami of C1~C4

椎动脉丛
Vertebral plexus

颈上心神经
Superior cervical cardiac nerve

C5~C6 前支的灰交通支
Gray rami communicantes to ventral rami of C5~C6

椎动脉丛
Vertebral plexus

C7~C8 前支的灰交通支
Gray rami communicantes to ventral rami of C7~C8

T1 前支的灰交通支
Gray ramus communicans to ventral ramus of T1

T1 前支发出的白交通支
White ramus communicans from ventral ramus of T1

岩深神经和翼管神经（虚影）
Deep petrosal nerve and nerve of pterygoid canal (ghosted)

翼腭神经节（副交感，虚影）
Pterygopalatine ganglion (parasympathetic, ghosted)

到鼻和口腔黏膜内血管的（神经）分支（虚影）
Branches to blood vessels within nasal and oral mucosa (ghosted)

颈上神经节
Superior cervical ganglion

颈外动脉神经
External carotid nerve

颈外动脉丛（到面部的血管和皮肤）
External carotid plexus (to blood vessels and skin of face)

颈交感干
Cervical sympathetic trunk

颈中神经节
Middle cervical ganglion

颈中心神经
Middle cervical cardiac nerve

锁骨下襻
Ansa subclavia

颈胸神经节（星状神经节）
Cervicothoracic (stellate) ganglion

颈下心神经
Inferior cervical cardiac nerve

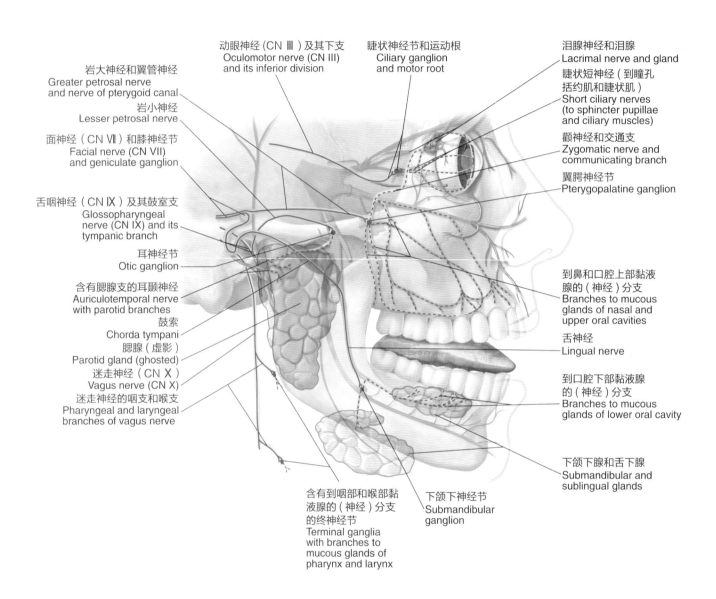

岩大神经和翼管神经
Greater petrosal nerve
and nerve of pterygoid canal

岩小神经
Lesser petrosal nerve

面神经（CN Ⅶ）和膝神经节
Facial nerve (CN VII)
and geniculate ganglion

舌咽神经（CN Ⅸ）及其鼓室支
Glossopharyngeal
nerve (CN IX) and its
tympanic branch

耳神经节
Otic ganglion

含有腮腺支的耳颞神经
Auriculotemporal nerve
with parotid branches

鼓索
Chorda tympani

腮腺（虚影）
Parotid gland (ghosted)

迷走神经（CN Ⅹ）
Vagus nerve (CN X)

迷走神经的咽支和喉支
Pharyngeal and laryngeal
branches of vagus nerve

动眼神经（CN Ⅲ）及其下支
Oculomotor nerve (CN III)
and its inferior division

睫状神经节和运动根
Ciliary ganglion
and motor root

泪腺神经和泪腺
Lacrimal nerve and gland

睫状短神经（到瞳孔
括约肌和睫状肌）
Short ciliary nerves
(to sphincter pupillae
and ciliary muscles)

颧神经和交通支
Zygomatic nerve and
communicating branch

翼腭神经节
Pterygopalatine ganglion

到鼻和口腔上部黏液
腺的（神经）分支
Branches to mucous
glands of nasal and
upper oral cavities

舌神经
Lingual nerve

到口腔下部黏液腺
的（神经）分支
Branches to mucous
glands of lower oral cavity

下颌下腺和舌下腺
Submandibular and
sublingual glands

下颌下神经节
Submandibular
ganglion

含有到咽部和喉部黏
液腺的（神经）分支
的终神经节
Terminal ganglia
with branches to
mucous glands of
pharynx and larynx

头颈肌群						
名称	起点	止点	主要作用	神经支配	动脉	注释
颅顶肌 （图 7-33）	额肌：帽状腱膜；枕肌：上项线	额肌：眉毛处的皮肤；枕肌：帽状腱膜	上提眉和皱眉	额肌：面神经（CN Ⅶ）的颞支；枕肌：面神经（CN Ⅶ）耳后支	额肌：眶上动脉和滑车上动脉；枕肌：枕动脉	额肌和枕肌是颅顶肌的 2 个肌腹；也称为枕额肌
额肌 （图 7-33）	帽状腱膜	眉毛区的皮肤	上提眉和皱眉	面神经（CN Ⅶ）的颞支	眶上动脉和滑车上动脉	额肌是颅顶肌的前腹
枕肌 （图 7-32 和图 7-33）	上项线	帽状腱膜	向后拉头皮；上提眉	面神经（CN Ⅶ）的耳后支	枕动脉	枕肌是颅顶肌的后腹
颈阔肌 （图 7-32）	覆盖胸大肌和三角肌的筋膜	下颌骨下缘和面下部皮肤	拉口角向下；辅助下拉下颌骨	面神经（CN Ⅶ）的颈支	面动脉、颈横动脉、肩胛上动脉	
二腹肌 （图 7-37）	前腹：下颌骨的二腹肌窝；后腹：颞骨的乳突切迹	借中间腱上的纤维环止于舌骨体	上提舌骨；下拉下颌骨	前腹：三叉神经（CN Ⅴ）下颌支发出的下颌舌骨肌神经；后腹：面神经（CN Ⅶ）	枕动脉、舌动脉	构成下颌三角的两个边
茎突舌骨肌 （图 7-24 和图 7-38）	茎突后缘	在二腹肌的中间腱处分叉止于舌骨体	上提和后拉舌骨	面神经（CN Ⅶ）	枕动脉、舌动脉	面神经穿茎乳孔后即发支支配茎突舌骨肌和二腹肌后腹
下颌舌骨肌 （图 7-24 和图 7-37）	下颌骨的下颌舌骨肌线	中缝和舌骨体	上提舌骨和舌，下拉下颌骨	下颌舌骨肌神经由三叉神经（CN Ⅴ）下颌支的下牙槽支发出	舌动脉、枕动脉	下颌舌骨肌神经也支配二腹肌前腹
肩胛舌骨肌 （图 7-13 和图 7-15）	下腹：肩胛骨上缘的肩胛切迹内侧；上腹：中间腱	下腹：中间腱；上腹：茎突舌骨肌外侧的舌骨下缘	下拉 / 稳定舌骨	颈襻	甲状腺上动脉、颈横动脉、肩胛上动脉	肩胛舌骨肌的中间腱借筋膜吊腱连于锁骨
胸骨舌骨肌 （图 7-15 和图 7-16）	胸骨柄后面和锁骨的胸骨端	舌骨下缘，肩胛舌骨肌止点内侧	下拉 / 稳定舌骨	颈襻	甲状腺上动脉	胸骨舌骨肌位于胸骨甲状肌和甲状舌骨肌浅面
胸骨甲状肌 （图 7-15 和图 7-16）	胸骨柄后面胸骨舌骨肌起点下方	甲状软骨的斜线	下拉 / 稳定喉的甲状软骨	颈襻	甲状腺上动脉	胸骨甲状肌位于胸骨舌骨肌深面
甲状舌骨肌 （图 7-15 和图 7-16）	甲状软骨的斜线	甲状软骨的下缘	上提喉；下拉 / 稳定舌骨	C1 和 C2 脊神经纤维与舌下神经（CN Ⅻ）在颈襻上根前方发出的分支	甲状腺上动脉	甲状舌骨肌位于胸骨舌骨肌深面
胸锁乳突肌 （图 7-15 和图 7-16）	胸骨头：胸骨柄前面；锁骨头：锁骨内侧 1/3	乳突和上项线的外侧半	拉同侧乳突向下；下颌转向对侧	脊副神经（CN Ⅺ），感觉支来自 C2 和 C3（本体感觉）	枕动脉	深面有颈动脉鞘结构位
前斜角肌 （图 7-18A 及 B，图 7-20 和图 7-21）	C3~C6 横突前结节	第 1 肋的前斜角肌结节	上提第 1 肋；屈曲和侧弯颈部	臂丛，C5~C7	颈升动脉、颈横动脉和颈深动脉	呼吸肌；前斜角肌止于锁骨下静脉后方，锁骨下动脉和臂丛根的前方

续表

头颈肌群						
名称	起点	止点	主要作用	神经支配	动脉	注释
中斜角肌（图 7-18A 及 B，图 7-20 和图 7-21）	C2~C7 横突后结节	第 1 肋上面，锁骨下动脉后方	上提第 1 肋；屈曲和侧弯颈部	臂丛，C3~C8	颈横动脉和颈深动脉	呼吸肌（吸气）；有肩胛背神经和胸长神经穿过
后锯肌（图 7-18A 及 B，图 7-20 和图 7-21）	C5~C7 横突后结节	第 2 肋外侧面	上提第 2 肋；屈曲和侧弯颈部	臂丛，C7~C8	颈横动脉和颈深动脉	呼吸肌（吸气）
咽上缩肌（图 7-22）	翼突内侧板、翼突钩、翼突下颌缝、上颌骨的下颌舌骨肌线	咽结节和咽中缝	收缩咽腔	迷走神经（CN X）借咽丛支配	咽升动脉	
咽中缩肌（图 7-22）	舌骨大角和小角，茎突舌骨韧带下部	咽中缝	收缩咽腔	迷走神经（CN X）借咽丛支配	咽升动脉	
咽下缩肌（图 7-22）	甲状软骨的斜线、环状软骨外面	咽中缝	收缩咽腔	迷走神经（CN X）借咽丛支配，有喉上神经和喉返神经参与	甲状腺上动脉	位于 3 块咽缩肌中的最外层
茎突咽肌（图 7-22）	茎突内侧面	甲状软骨上缘和咽壁	上提喉	舌咽神经（CN IX）	咽升动脉	茎突咽肌受舌咽神经（CN IX）支配，是唯一一块不受迷走神经（CN X）支配的咽肌
降口角肌（图 7-32 和图 7-33A）	上颌骨的斜线	口角	拉口角向下	面神经（CN VII）的下颌缘支和颊支	下唇动脉	"皱眉"肌
提上唇肌（图 7-32 和图 7-33A）	眶下缘	上唇皮肤	提上唇	面神经（CN VII）的颊支	上唇动脉	
颧大肌（图 7-32 和图 7-33A）	颧骨外上面	口角部皮肤	向外侧上提和拉口角	面神经（CN VII）的颧支和颊支	面动脉和颊动脉	微笑肌
口轮匝肌（图 7-32 和图 7-33A）	唇及唇周的皮肤和筋膜	唇部皮肤和筋膜	缩小口唇	面神经（CN VII）的颊支	唇上动脉和唇下动脉	
颊肌（图 7-32）	翼突下颌缝、下颌骨、磨牙外侧的上颌骨	口角和上下唇外侧部	拉口角向外；使颊贴近牙齿	面神经（CN VII）的颊支	颊动脉	虽然颊肌是重要的咀嚼肌，但是受面神经支配，不受 V_3 发出的颊神经（感觉神经）支配

头颈肌群						
名称	起点	止点	主要作用	神经支配	动脉	注释
环杓后肌（图7-31）	环状软骨板的后面	杓状软骨的肌突	拉肌突向后，外展声襞	来自迷走神经（CN X）的喉返神经发出的喉下神经	喉上动脉和喉下动脉	环杓后肌是唯一的声襞外展肌
杓横机（图7-31）	环状软骨板的后面	对侧杓状软骨后面	拉杓状软骨靠拢，内收声襞	来自迷走神经（CN X）的喉返神经发出的喉下神经	喉上动脉和喉下动脉	杓肌被认为是1块肌，分为斜部和横部
杓斜肌（图7-31）	杓状软骨的肌突	对侧杓状软骨后面，靠近尖部	拉杓状软骨靠拢，内收声襞	来自迷走神经（CN X）的喉返神经发出的喉下神经	喉上动脉和喉下动脉	杓肌被认为是1块肌，分为斜部和横部
甲杓肌（图7-30）	甲状软骨内面前方	杓状软骨后缘	拉杓状软骨向前，放松和内收声襞	来自迷走神经（CN X）的喉返神经发出的喉下神经	喉上动脉和喉下动脉	甲杓肌被认为是甲状会厌肌；最内侧的肌纤维止于声韧带上，这部分肌称为声带肌
环杓侧肌（图7-30）	环状软骨弓	杓状软骨的肌突	拉杓状软骨的肌突向前，转动杓状软骨使声襞内收	来自迷走神经（CN X）的喉返神经发出的喉下神经	喉上动脉和喉下动脉	环杓后肌的拮抗肌；供应喉部的动脉在喉内吻合营养黏膜和肌
环甲肌（图7-29）	环状软骨弓	甲状软骨下缘	拉甲状软骨向前，使声带伸长	喉上神经外支，是迷走神经（CN X）的分支	喉上动脉和喉下动脉	这是喉固有肌中唯一不受喉返神经支配的肌；所有其他肌都受喉返神经的喉下支支配
咬肌（图7-34）	颧骨弓和颧骨	下颌支外侧面和下颌角	上提下颌骨	三叉神经（CN V）下颌支发出的咬肌神经	咬肌动脉	有力的咀嚼肌
颞肌（图7-34和图7-38）	颞窝和颞筋膜	冠突和下颌支的前面	上提下颌骨；后拉下颌骨（后部纤维）	三叉神经（CN V）下颌支发出的颞深神经前后支	颞深动脉前、后支	有力的咀嚼肌
翼外肌（图7-38）	上头：蝶骨大翼；下头：翼突外侧板的外面	上头：颞下颌关节的关节盘和关节囊；下头：下颌颈	伸长下颌骨；张口	三叉神经（CN V）下颌支发出的翼外肌支	上颌动脉	咀嚼肌中唯一的张口肌；翼外肌的上头止于颞下颌关节的关节盘，有时也称为蝶骨关节盘肌
翼内肌（图7-38）	翼突外侧板内面、腭骨锥突、上颌结节	下颌支内侧面和下颌角	上提和伸长下颌骨	三叉神经（CN V）下颌支发出的翼内肌支	上颌动脉	翼内肌在与下颌支的位置和功能上与咬肌镜像
颏舌骨肌（图7-42和图7-45）	下颌骨的颏棘	舌骨体	上提舌骨；降下颌骨	C1脊神经腹侧主支加入舌下神经	面动脉和舌动脉	甲状舌骨肌和颏舌骨肌接受与舌下神经远端伴行的颈襻上支支配

续表

头颈肌群

名称	起点	止点	主要作用	神经支配	动脉	注释
颏舌肌 （图 7-42 和图 7-45）	颏联合内面的颏棘	扇形展开止于舌尖到舌底	伸舌（下部纤维）；降舌（中部纤维）	舌下神经（CN XII）	舌动脉	舌的固有肌；舌下神经支配除腭舌肌［与大部分腭肌和咽肌一样，受迷走神经（CN X）支配］以外的全部舌肌
舌骨舌肌 （图 7-45）	舌骨大角上缘和舌骨体	与舌固有肌编织在一起	降舌两侧，后拉舌	舌下神经（CN XII）	舌动脉	舌固有肌之一
茎突舌肌 （图 7-23 和图 7-45）	茎突	舌的两侧	后拉和上提舌	舌下神经（CN XII）	咽升动脉和舌动脉	舌固有肌之一
眼轮匝肌 （图 7-33，图 7-64 和图 7-65）	眶部：眶内侧缘和眼睑内侧韧带；眼睑部：眼睑内侧韧带	眶部：外侧颊部皮肤；眼睑部：眼睑缝外侧	闭眼	面神经（CN XII）颞支和颧支	眶上动脉、滑车上动脉、眶下动脉	眨眼反射时激活的随意肌
上睑提肌 （图 7-65 和图 7-68）	视神经管上方的眶尖	上睑的皮肤和筋膜以及上睑板	提上睑	动眼神经（CN III）和交感神经（支配上睑板部分）	眼动脉	止于上睑板的肌纤维称上睑板肌，属平滑肌；支配的交感神经损伤会引起轻度上睑下垂
上直肌 （图 7-66，图 7-69 和图 7-70A）	眶尖的总腱环	眼球巩膜的上面	上提和外展眼球；将虹膜上极转向内侧	动眼神经（CN III）上支	眼动脉	
下直肌 （图 7-66 和图 7-70）	眶尖的总腱环	眼球巩膜的下面	下压和内收眼球；将虹膜上极转向外侧	动眼神经（CN III）下支	眼动脉	
内直肌 （图 7-66 和图 7-70）	眶尖的总腱环	眼球巩膜的内侧面	内收眼球	动眼神经（CN III）下支	眼动脉	
外直肌 （图 7-66，图 7-68B，图 7-69 和图 7-70）	眶尖的总腱环	眼球巩膜的外侧面	外展眼球	展神经（CN VI）	眼动脉	
上斜肌 （图 7-66，图 7-68B，图 7-69 和图 7-70A）	视神经管上方的眶尖	眼球后方巩膜的上面	下压和外展眼球；将虹膜上极转向内侧	滑车神经（CN IV）	眼动脉	经过纤维软骨滑车
下斜肌 （图 7-66 和图 7-70B）	眶底的泪沟外侧	眼球巩膜下面，下直肌下方	上提和外展眼球；将虹膜上极转向外侧	动眼神经（CN III）下支	眼动脉	
瞳孔括约肌 （图 7-71）	环绕虹膜	环绕虹膜	收缩瞳孔	动眼神经（CN III）的副交感纤维，在睫状神经节换元	睫状前、后动脉	

头颈肌群						
名称	起点	止点	主要作用	神经支配	动脉	注释
睫状肌 （图 7-71）	径向纤维：巩膜 突； 环状纤维：环绕 虹膜根部	径向纤维：睫状 突，环状纤维： 环绕虹膜根部	放松调节晶状体 的悬韧带（近 视力）	动眼神经（CN Ⅲ） 的副交感纤维，在 睫状神经节换元	睫状前、后动 脉	
瞳孔开大肌 （图 7-65 和 图 7-71）	虹膜外缘	虹膜内缘	扩大瞳孔	睫状短神经内的交感 纤维，在颈上交感 神经节换元	睫状前、后动 脉	
镫骨肌 （图 7-73 和 图 7-75）	锥隆起的壁	镫骨颈	抑制镫骨的震动	面神经（CN Ⅶ）	迷路动脉	包绕除肌腱外的 整个镫骨
鼓膜张肌 （图 7-73 和 图 7-75）	咽鼓管软骨部和 邻近的蝶骨大 翼	锤骨柄	抑制鼓膜的震动	三叉神经（CN Ⅴ） 下颌支发出的翼内 肌支	上颌动脉的鼓 室支	V₃ 支配 2 块张 肌（鼓膜张肌 和腭帆张肌）
腭帆提肌 （图 7-23 和 图 7-27）	颞骨岩尖部和咽 鼓管软骨部内 面	软腭的肌与筋 膜；腭腱膜	上提软腭	迷走神经（CN Ⅹ） 经咽丛	咽升动脉和腭 降动脉	第 4 咽弓的衍生 物
腭帆张肌 （图 7-23 和 图 7-27）	咽鼓管软骨部的 外侧壁	腭腱膜	开放咽鼓管；紧 张软腭	三叉神经（CN Ⅴ） 的下颌支	咽升动脉和腭 降动脉	记住：V₃ 支配 2 块张肌（鼓膜 张肌和腭帆张 肌）；迷走神 经（CN Ⅹ） 支配其他腭肌

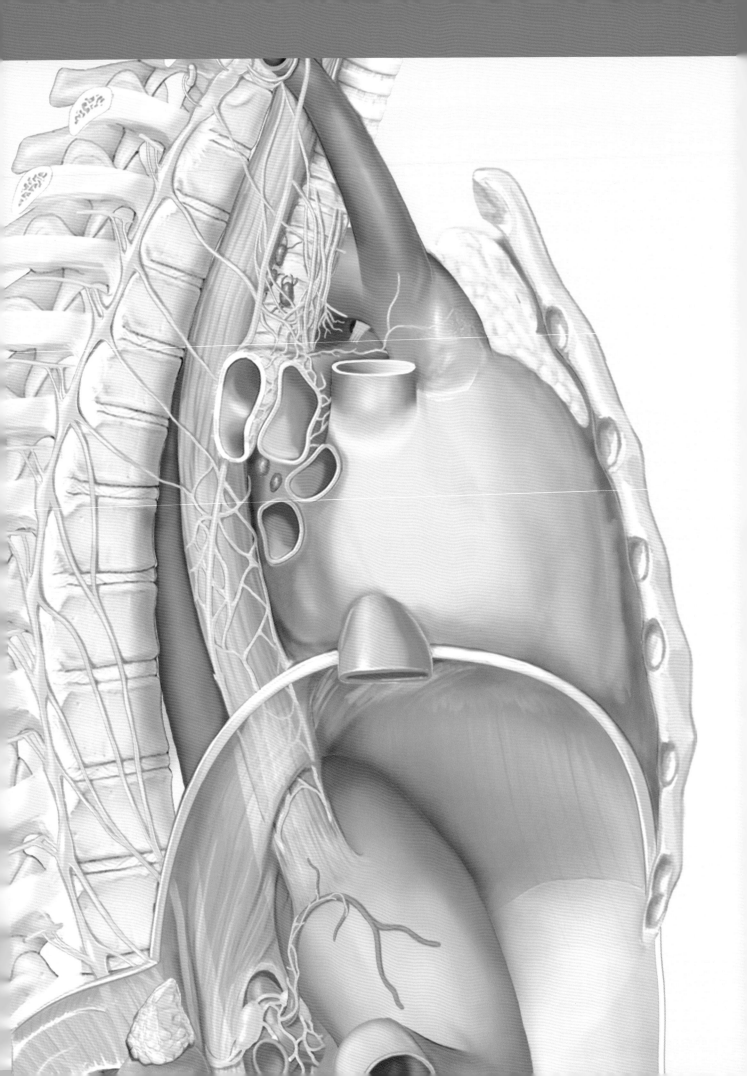

第八章 自主神经系统
CHAPTER 8 | The Autonomic Nervous System

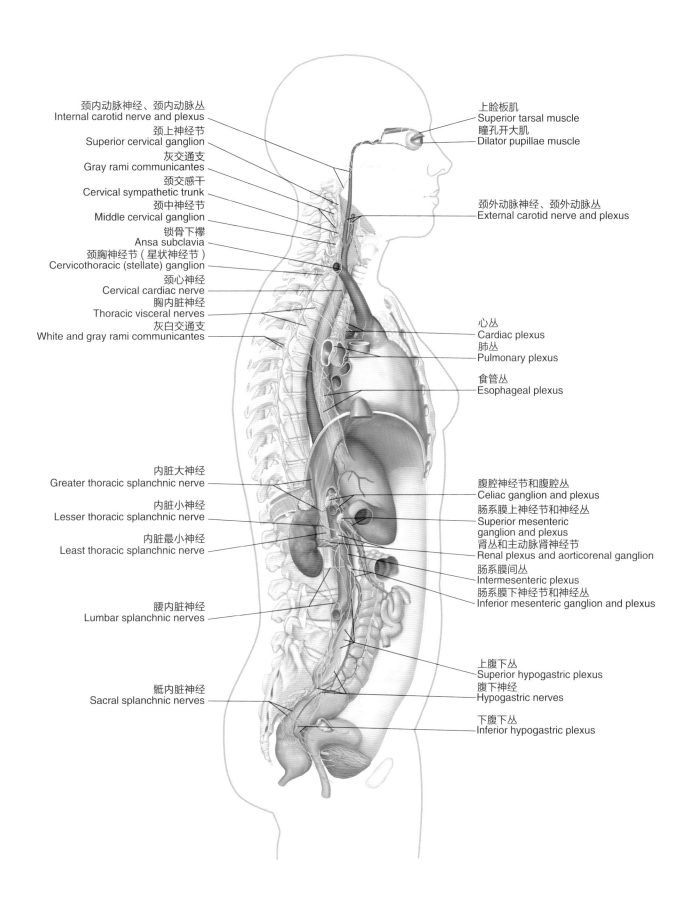

颈内动脉神经、颈内动脉丛
Internal carotid nerve and plexus

颈上神经节
Superior cervical ganglion

灰交通支
Gray rami communicantes

颈交感干
Cervical sympathetic trunk

颈中神经节
Middle cervical ganglion

锁骨下襻
Ansa subclavia

颈胸神经节（星状神经节）
Cervicothoracic (stellate) ganglion

颈心神经
Cervical cardiac nerve

胸内脏神经
Thoracic visceral nerves

灰白交通支
White and gray rami communicantes

内脏大神经
Greater thoracic splanchnic nerve

内脏小神经
Lesser thoracic splanchnic nerve

内脏最小神经
Least thoracic splanchnic nerve

腰内脏神经
Lumbar splanchnic nerves

骶内脏神经
Sacral splanchnic nerves

上睑板肌
Superior tarsal muscle

瞳孔开大肌
Dilator pupillae muscle

颈外动脉神经、颈外动脉丛
External carotid nerve and plexus

心丛
Cardiac plexus

肺丛
Pulmonary plexus

食管丛
Esophageal plexus

腹腔神经节和腹腔丛
Celiac ganglion and plexus

肠系膜上神经节和神经丛
Superior mesenteric ganglion and plexus

肾丛和主动脉肾神经节
Renal plexus and aorticorenal ganglion

肠系膜间丛
Intermesenteric plexus

肠系膜下神经节和神经丛
Inferior mesenteric ganglion and plexus

上腹下丛
Superior hypogastric plexus

腹下神经
Hypogastric nerves

下腹下丛
Inferior hypogastric plexus

图 8-02 交感神经系统组成 I Components of the Sympathetic Nervous System I

A. 节前神经元胞体的位置
Location of presynaptic cell bodies

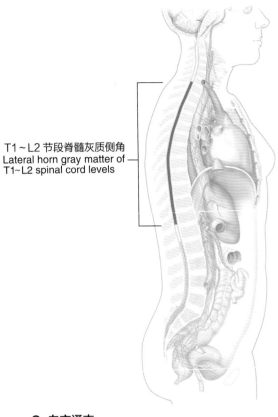

T1~L2 节段脊髓灰质侧角
Lateral horn gray matter of
T1~L2 spinal cord levels

B. 交感干
Sympathetic trunk

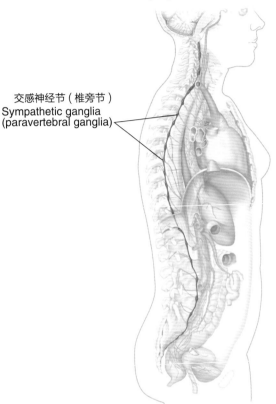

交感神经节（椎旁节）
Sympathetic ganglia
(paravertebral ganglia)

C. 白交通支
White rami communicantes

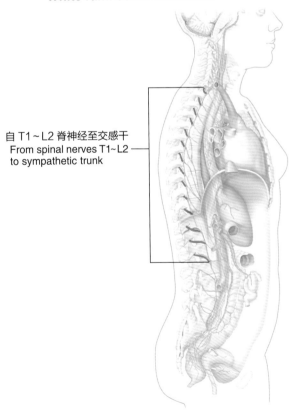

自 T1~L2 脊神经至交感干
From spinal nerves T1~L2
to sympathetic trunk

D. 灰交通支
Gray rami communicantes

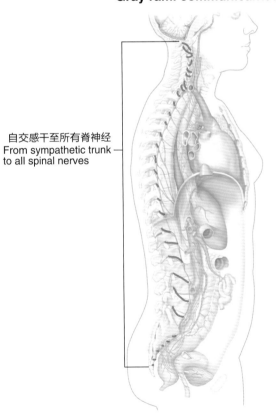

自交感干至所有脊神经
From sympathetic trunk
to all spinal nerves

A. 含有交感神经纤维的神经
Nerves that carry sympathetic fibers

颈内动脉神经
Internal carotid nerve

颈外动脉神经
External carotid nerve

颈心神经
Cervical cardiac nerves

胸内脏神经
Thoracic visceral nerves

胸内脏神经
Thoracic splanchnic nerves

内脏大神经 Greater
内脏小神经 Lesser
内脏最小神经 Least

腰内脏神经
Lumbar splanchnic nerves

骶内脏神经
Sacral splanchnic nerves

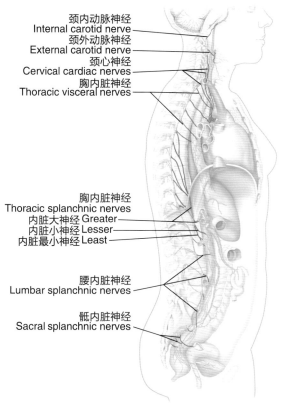

B. 主动脉前神经节（椎前节）
Preaortic ganglia

腹腔神经节
Celiac ganglion

肠系膜上神经节
Superior mesenteric
ganglion

主动脉肾神经节
Aorticorenal ganglion

肠系膜下神经节
Inferior mesenteric
ganglion

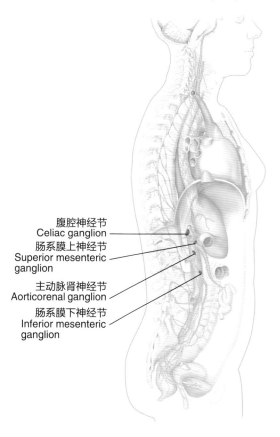

C. 含有交感神经节后纤维的神经丛
Plexuses that carry postsynaptic sympathetic fibers

颈内动脉丛
Internal carotid plexus

颈外动脉丛
External carotid plexus

肺丛
Pulmonary plexus

心丛
Cardiac plexus

腹腔丛
Celiac plexus

肠系膜上丛
Superior mesenteric plexus

肠系膜间丛
Intermesenteric plexus

肠系膜下丛
Inferior mesenteric plexus

肾丛
Renal plexus

上腹下丛
Superior hypogastric plexus

腹下神经
Hypogastric nerves

下腹下丛（盆丛）
Inferior hypogastric (pelvic) plexus:

直肠丛
Rectal plexus

子宫阴道丛
Uterovaginal plexus

膀胱丛
Vesical plexus

前列腺丛
Prostatic plexus

D. 男性骨盆
Male pelvis

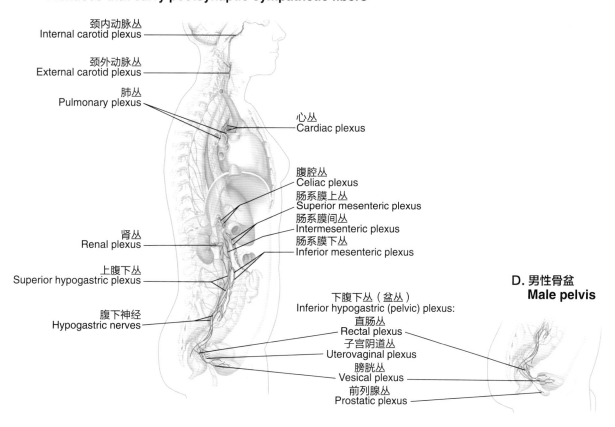

图 8-04　　交感干的位置　Position of Sympathetic Trunks

A. 外侧面观
Lateral view

B. 前面观
Anterior view

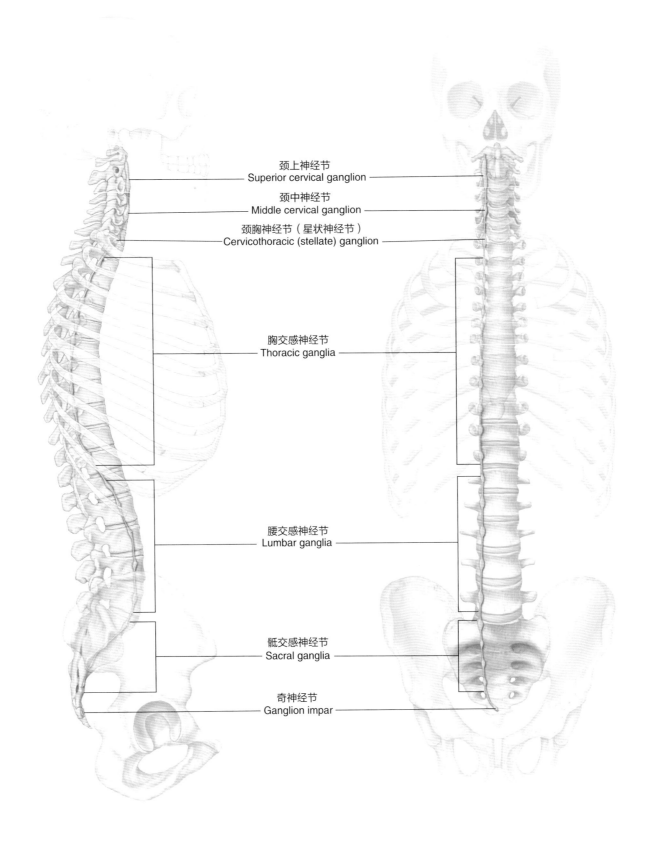

颈上神经节
Superior cervical ganglion

颈中神经节
Middle cervical ganglion

颈胸神经节（星状神经节）
Cervicothoracic (stellate) ganglion

胸交感神经节
Thoracic ganglia

腰交感神经节
Lumbar ganglia

骶交感神经节
Sacral ganglia

奇神经节
Ganglion impar

A. C1~C8 节段
C1~C8 levels

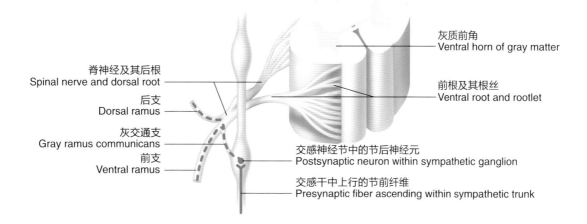

灰质前角
Ventral horn of gray matter

脊神经及其后根
Spinal nerve and dorsal root

前根及其根丝
Ventral root and rootlet

后支
Dorsal ramus

灰交通支
Gray ramus communicans

前支
Ventral ramus

交感神经节中的节后神经元
Postsynaptic neuron within sympathetic ganglion

交感干中上行的节前纤维
Presynaptic fiber ascending within sympathetic trunk

B. T1~L2 节段
B. T1~L2 levels

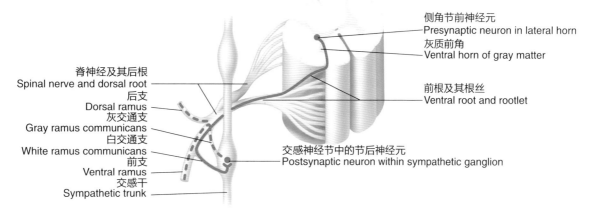

侧角节前神经元
Presynaptic neuron in lateral horn

灰质前角
Ventral horn of gray matter

脊神经及其后根
Spinal nerve and dorsal root

后支
Dorsal ramus

灰交通支
Gray ramus communicans

白交通支
White ramus communicans

前支
Ventral ramus

交感干
Sympathetic trunk

前根及其根丝
Ventral root and rootlet

交感神经节中的节后神经元
Postsynaptic neuron within sympathetic ganglion

C. L3~Co 节段
C. L3~Co levels

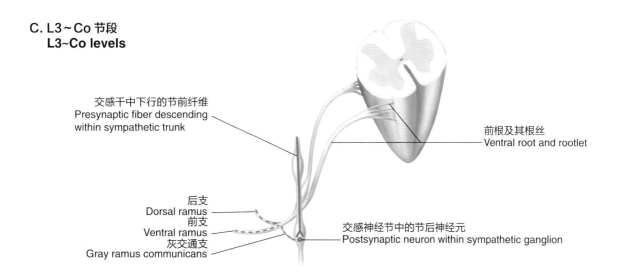

交感干中下行的节前纤维
Presynaptic fiber descending within sympathetic trunk

前根及其根丝
Ventral root and rootlet

后支
Dorsal ramus

前支
Ventral ramus

灰交通支
Gray ramus communicans

交感神经节中的节后神经元
Postsynaptic neuron within sympathetic ganglion

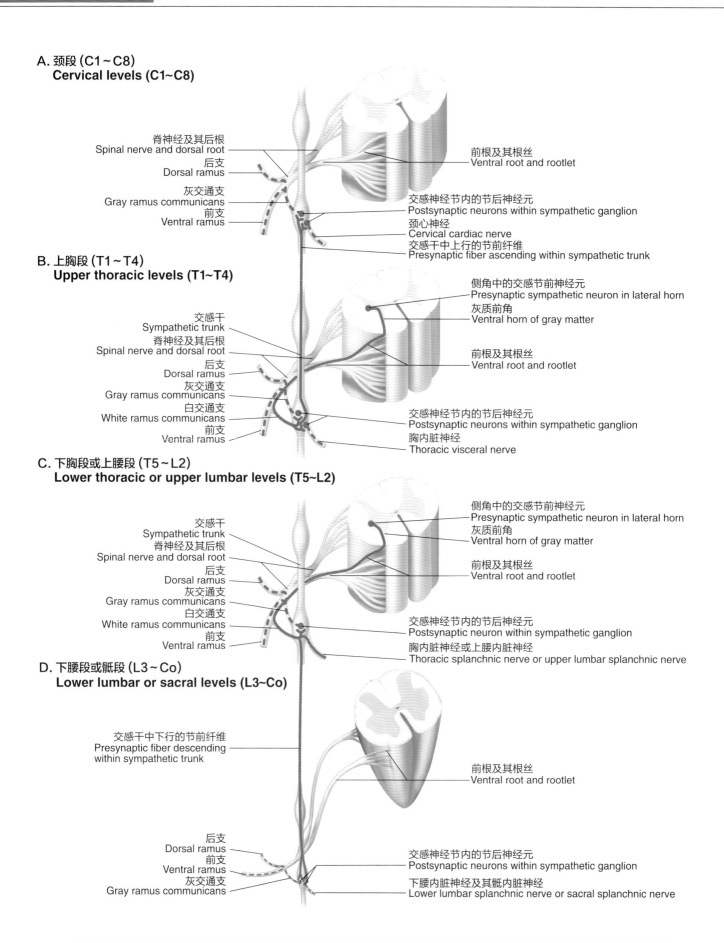

A. 颈段 (C1~C8)
Cervical levels (C1~C8)

脊神经及其后根
Spinal nerve and dorsal root

后支
Dorsal ramus

灰交通支
Gray ramus communicans

前支
Ventral ramus

前根及其根丝
Ventral root and rootlet

交感神经节内的节后神经元
Postsynaptic neurons within sympathetic ganglion

颈心神经
Cervical cardiac nerve

交感干中上行的节前纤维
Presynaptic fiber ascending within sympathetic trunk

B. 上胸段 (T1~T4)
Upper thoracic levels (T1~T4)

交感干
Sympathetic trunk

脊神经及其后根
Spinal nerve and dorsal root

后支
Dorsal ramus

灰交通支
Gray ramus communicans

白交通支
White ramus communicans

前支
Ventral ramus

侧角中的交感节前神经元
Presynaptic sympathetic neuron in lateral horn

灰质前角
Ventral horn of gray matter

前根及其根丝
Ventral root and rootlet

交感神经节内的节后神经元
Postsynaptic neurons within sympathetic ganglion

胸内脏神经
Thoracic visceral nerve

C. 下胸段或上腰段 (T5~L2)
Lower thoracic or upper lumbar levels (T5~L2)

交感干
Sympathetic trunk

脊神经及其后根
Spinal nerve and dorsal root

后支
Dorsal ramus

灰交通支
Gray ramus communicans

白交通支
White ramus communicans

前支
Ventral ramus

侧角中的交感节前神经元
Presynaptic sympathetic neuron in lateral horn

灰质前角
Ventral horn of gray matter

前根及其根丝
Ventral root and rootlet

交感神经节内的节后神经元
Postsynaptic neuron within sympathetic ganglion

胸内脏神经或上腰内脏神经
Thoracic splanchnic nerve or upper lumbar splanchnic nerve

D. 下腰段或骶段 (L3~Co)
Lower lumbar or sacral levels (L3~Co)

交感干中下行的节前纤维
Presynaptic fiber descending within sympathetic trunk

前根及其根丝
Ventral root and rootlet

后支
Dorsal ramus

前支
Ventral ramus

灰交通支
Gray ramus communicans

交感神经节内的节后神经元
Postsynaptic neurons within sympathetic ganglion

下腰内脏神经及其骶内脏神经
Lower lumbar splanchnic nerve or sacral splanchnic nerve

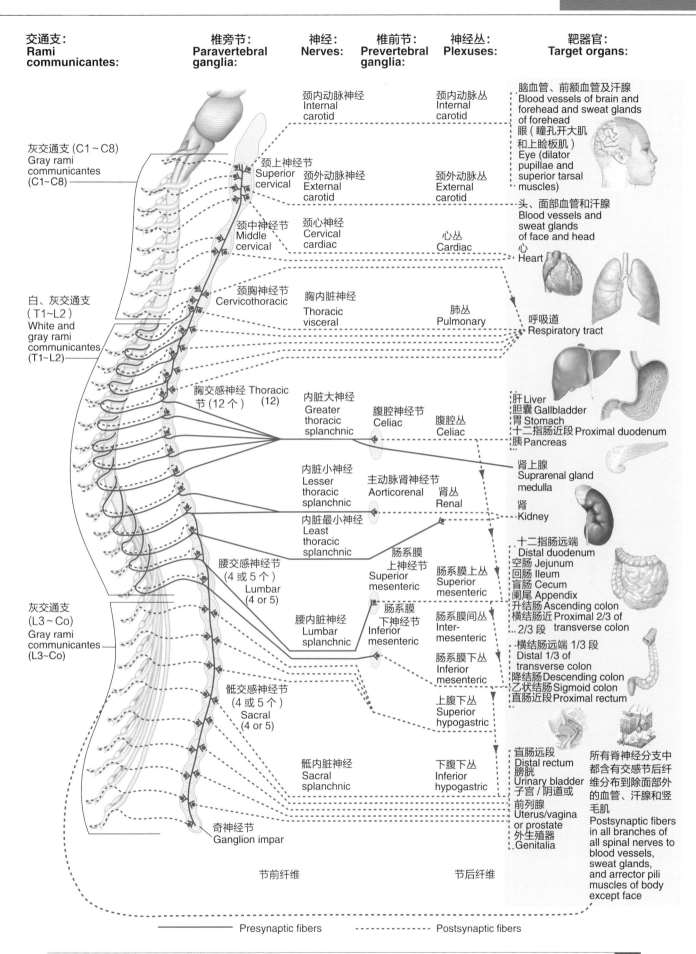

交通支：
Rami
communicantes:

椎旁节：
Paravertebral
ganglia:

神经：
Nerves:

椎前节：
Prevertebral
ganglia:

神经丛：
Plexuses:

靶器官：
Target organs:

灰交通支（C1～C8）
Gray rami
communicantes
(C1~C8)

白、灰交通支
（T1~L2）
White and
gray rami
communicantes
(T1~L2)

灰交通支
（L3～Co）
Gray rami
communicantes
(L3~Co)

颈内动脉神经
Internal
carotid

颈上神经节
Superior
cervical

颈外动脉神经
External
carotid

颈中神经节
Middle
cervical

颈心神经
Cervical
cardiac

颈胸神经节
Cervicothoracic

胸内脏神经
Thoracic
visceral

胸交感神经
节（12 个）Thoracic
(12)

内脏大神经
Greater
thoracic
splanchnic

腹腔神经节
Celiac

内脏小神经
Lesser
thoracic
splanchnic

主动脉肾神经节
Aorticorenal

内脏最小神经
Least
thoracic
splanchnic

腰交感神经节
（4 或 5 个）
Lumbar
(4 or 5)

腰内脏神经
Lumbar
splanchnic

肠系膜
上神经节
Superior
mesenteric

肠系膜
下神经节
Inferior
mesenteric

骶交感神经节
（4 或 5 个）
Sacral
(4 or 5)

骶内脏神经
Sacral
splanchnic

奇神经节
Ganglion impar

颈内动脉丛
Internal
carotid

颈外动脉丛
External
carotid

心丛
Cardiac

肺丛
Pulmonary

腹腔丛
Celiac

肾丛
Renal

肠系膜上丛
Superior
mesenteric

肠系膜间丛
Inter-
mesenteric

肠系膜下丛
Inferior
mesenteric

上腹下丛
Superior
hypogastric

下腹下丛
Inferior
hypogastric

脑血管、前额血管及汗腺
Blood vessels of brain and
forehead and sweat glands
of forehead
眼（瞳孔开大肌
和上睑板肌）
Eye (dilator
pupillae and
superior tarsal
muscles)

头、面部血管和汗腺
Blood vessels and
sweat glands
of face and head
心
Heart

呼吸道
Respiratory tract

肝 Liver
胆囊 Gallbladder
胃 Stomach
十二指肠近段 Proximal duodenum
胰 Pancreas

肾上腺
Suprarenal gland
medulla

肾
Kidney

十二指肠远端
Distal duodenum
空肠 Jejunum
回肠 Ileum
盲肠 Cecum
阑尾 Appendix
升结肠 Ascending colon
横结肠近 Proximal 2/3 of
2/3 段　transverse colon

横结肠远端 1/3 段
Distal 1/3 of
transverse colon
降结肠 Descending colon
乙状结肠 Sigmoid colon
直肠近段 Proximal rectum

直肠远段
Distal rectum
膀胱
Urinary bladder
子宫 / 阴道或
Uterus/vagina
or prostate
外生殖器
Genitalia

所有脊神经分支中
都含有交感节后纤
维分布到除面部外
的血管、汗腺和竖
毛肌
Postsynaptic fibers
in all branches of
all spinal nerves to
blood vessels,
sweat glands,
and arrector pili
muscles of body
except face

节前纤维

节后纤维

———— Presynaptic fibers　　- - - - - - Postsynaptic fibers

图 8-08　牵涉痛的定位　**Locations of Referred Pain**

A. 前面观
Anterior view

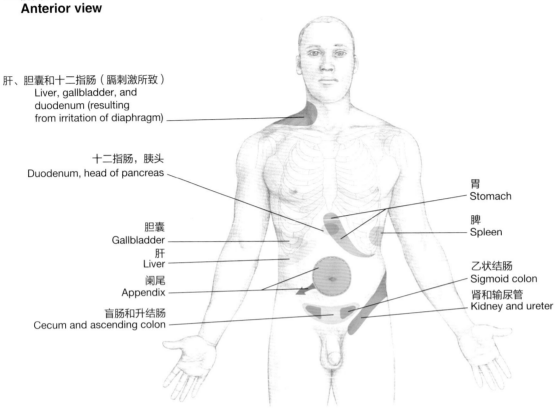

肝、胆囊和十二指肠（膈刺激所致）
Liver, gallbladder, and
duodenum (resulting
from irritation of diaphragm)

十二指肠，胰头
Duodenum, head of pancreas

胆囊
Gallbladder

肝
Liver

阑尾
Appendix

盲肠和升结肠
Cecum and ascending colon

胃
Stomach

脾
Spleen

乙状结肠
Sigmoid colon

肾和输尿管
Kidney and ureter

B. 后面观
Posterior view

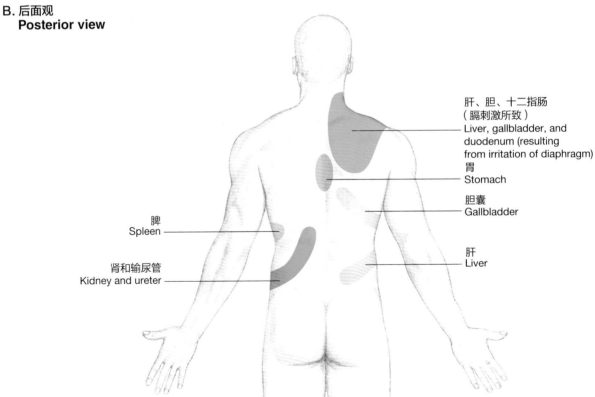

肝、胆、十二指肠
（膈刺激所致）
Liver, gallbladder, and
duodenum (resulting
from irritation of diaphragm)

胃
Stomach

胆囊
Gallbladder

肝
Liver

脾
Spleen

肾和输尿管
Kidney and ureter

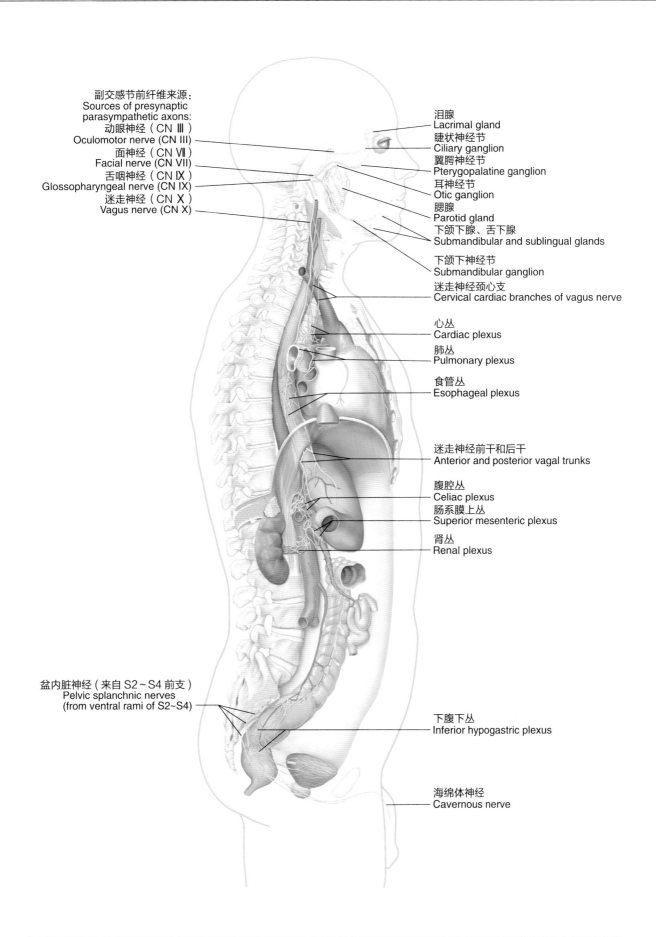

副交感节前纤维来源：
Sources of presynaptic parasympathetic axons:
动眼神经（CN Ⅲ）
Oculomotor nerve (CN III)
面神经（CN Ⅶ）
Facial nerve (CN VII)
舌咽神经（CN Ⅸ）
Glossopharyngeal nerve (CN IX)
迷走神经（CN Ⅹ）
Vagus nerve (CN X)

泪腺
Lacrimal gland
睫状神经节
Ciliary ganglion
翼腭神经节
Pterygopalatine ganglion
耳神经节
Otic ganglion
腮腺
Parotid gland
下颌下腺、舌下腺
Submandibular and sublingual glands
下颌下神经节
Submandibular ganglion
迷走神经颈心支
Cervical cardiac branches of vagus nerve
心丛
Cardiac plexus
肺丛
Pulmonary plexus
食管丛
Esophageal plexus
迷走神经前干和后干
Anterior and posterior vagal trunks
腹腔丛
Celiac plexus
肠系膜上丛
Superior mesenteric plexus
肾丛
Renal plexus

盆内脏神经（来自 S2～S4 前支）
Pelvic splanchnic nerves
(from ventral rami of S2~S4)

下腹下丛
Inferior hypogastric plexus

海绵体神经
Cavernous nerve

A. 副交感节前神经元的位置
Location of presynaptic parasympathetic cell bodies

脑干
Brainstem

S2~S4 脊髓节段灰质侧角
Lateral horn gray matter of spinal cord segments S2~S4

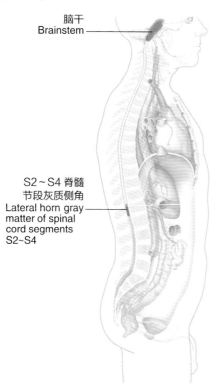

B. 含副交感节前纤维的神经
Nerves that carry presynaptic parasympathetic fibers

动眼神经 (CN III)
Oculomotor nerve (CN III)
面神经 (CN VII)
Facial nerve (CN VII)
舌咽神经 (CN IX)
Glossopharyngeal nerve (CN IX)
迷走神经 (CN X)
Vagus nerve (CN X)

迷走神经干
Vagal trunks
前干 Anterior
后干 Posterior

盆内脏神经
Pelvic splanchnic nerves

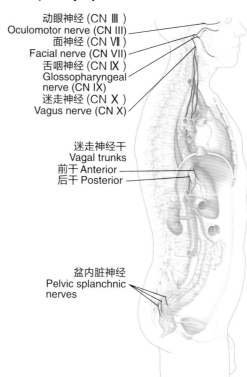

C. 含副交感节前纤维的神经丛
Plexuses that carry presynaptic parasympathetic fibers

心丛
Cardiac plexus
肺丛
Pulmonary plexus
食管丛
Esophageal plexus

腹腔丛
Celiac plexus
肾丛
Renal plexus
肠系膜上神经丛
Superior mesenteric plexus

下腹下丛（盆丛）
Inferior hypogastric (pelvic) plexus
直肠丛 Rectal plexus
膀胱丛 Vesical plexus
前列腺/子宫阴道丛 Prostatic/uterovaginal plexus

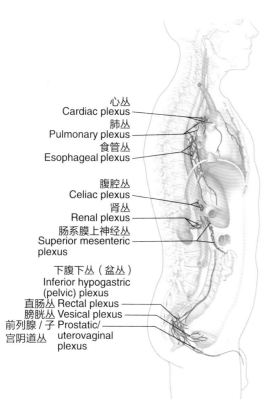

D. 副交感节后神经元的位置
Location of postsynaptic parasympathetic cell bodies

头部副交感神经节
Cranial parasympathetic ganglia
睫状神经节 Ciliary
耳神经节 Otic
翼腭神经节 Pterygopalatine
下颌下神经节 Submandibular

器官内节
In the organ innervated
呼吸道 Respiratory tract
心 Heart
消化道 GI tract
肾盂 Renal pelvis
输尿管 Ureter
膀胱 Bladder
前列腺、子宫和阴道 Prostate/uterus and vagina
勃起组织 Erectile tissues

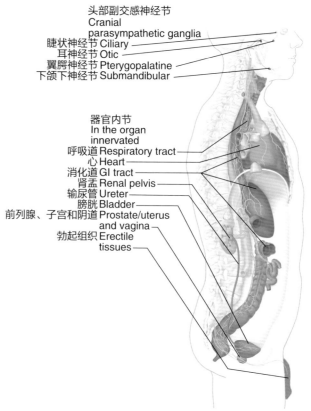

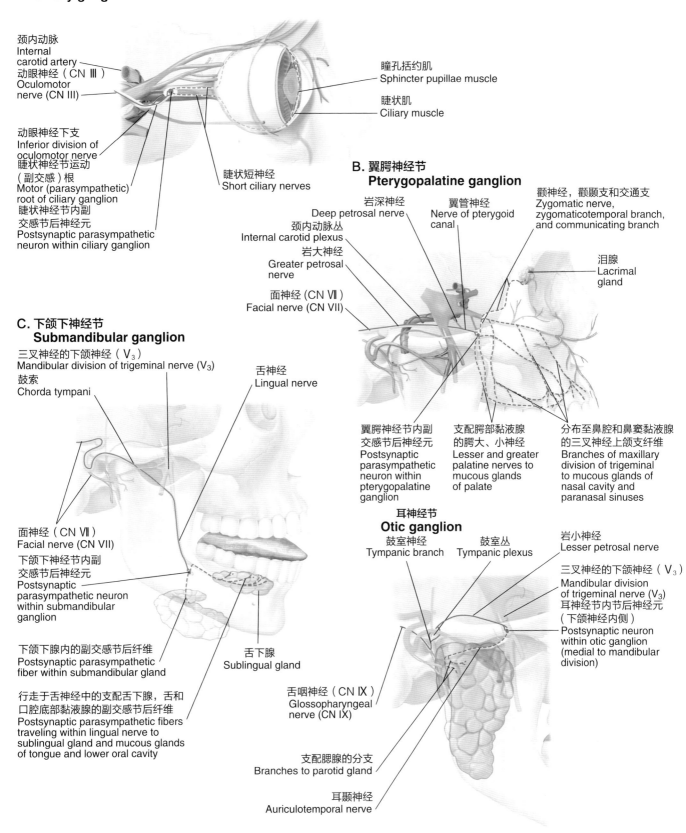

A. 睫状神经节 Ciliary ganglion

颈内动脉
Internal carotid artery

动眼神经（CN Ⅲ）
Oculomotor nerve (CN III)

动眼神经下支
Inferior division of oculomotor nerve

睫状神经节运动（副交感）根
Motor (parasympathetic) root of ciliary ganglion

睫状神经节内副交感节后神经元
Postsynaptic parasympathetic neuron within ciliary ganglion

瞳孔括约肌
Sphincter pupillae muscle

睫状肌
Ciliary muscle

睫状短神经
Short ciliary nerves

B. 翼腭神经节 Pterygopalatine ganglion

岩深神经
Deep petrosal nerve

颈内动脉丛
Internal carotid plexus

岩大神经
Greater petrosal nerve

面神经（CN Ⅶ）
Facial nerve (CN VII)

翼管神经
Nerve of pterygoid canal

颧神经，颧颞支和交通支
Zygomatic nerve, zygomaticotemporal branch, and communicating branch

泪腺
Lacrimal gland

翼腭神经节内副交感节后神经元
Postsynaptic parasympathetic neuron within pterygopalatine ganglion

支配腭部黏液腺的腭大、小神经
Lesser and greater palatine nerves to mucous glands of palate

分布至鼻腔和鼻窦黏液腺的三叉神经上颌支纤维
Branches of maxillary division of trigeminal to mucous glands of nasal cavity and paranasal sinuses

C. 下颌下神经节 Submandibular ganglion

三叉神经的下颌神经（V₃）
Mandibular division of trigeminal nerve (V₃)

鼓索
Chorda tympani

舌神经
Lingual nerve

面神经（CN Ⅶ）
Facial nerve (CN VII)

下颌下神经节内副交感节后神经元
Postsynaptic parasympathetic neuron within submandibular ganglion

下颌下腺内的副交感节后纤维
Postsynaptic parasympathetic fiber within submandibular gland

行走于舌神经中的支配舌下腺，舌和口腔底部黏液腺的副交感节后纤维
Postsynaptic parasympathetic fibers traveling within lingual nerve to sublingual gland and mucous glands of tongue and lower oral cavity

舌下腺
Sublingual gland

耳神经节 Otic ganglion

鼓室神经
Tympanic branch

鼓室丛
Tympanic plexus

岩小神经
Lesser petrosal nerve

三叉神经的下颌神经（V₃）
Mandibular division of trigeminal nerve (V₃)

耳神经节内节后神经元（下颌神经内侧）
Postsynaptic neuron within otic ganglion (medial to mandibular division)

舌咽神经（CN Ⅸ）
Glossopharyngeal nerve (CN IX)

支配腮腺的分支
Branches to parotid gland

耳颞神经
Auriculotemporal nerve

图 8-12　头部以下的副交感神经通路　Parasympathetic Pathways Below the Head

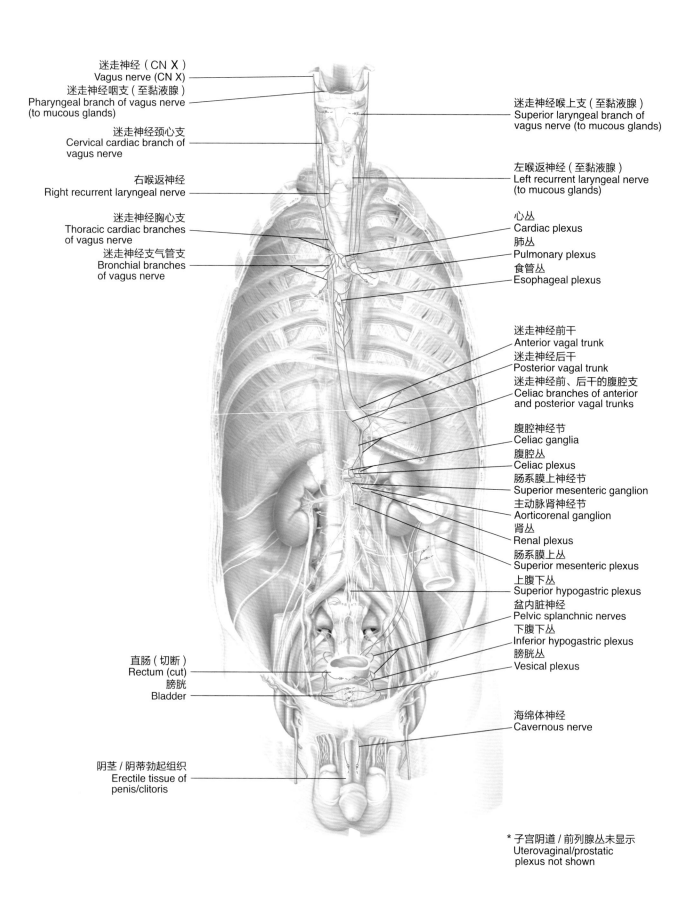

迷走神经（CN X）
Vagus nerve (CN X)

迷走神经咽支（至黏液腺）
Pharyngeal branch of vagus nerve
(to mucous glands)

迷走神经颈心支
Cervical cardiac branch of
vagus nerve

右喉返神经
Right recurrent laryngeal nerve

迷走神经胸心支
Thoracic cardiac branches
of vagus nerve

迷走神经支气管支
Bronchial branches
of vagus nerve

迷走神经喉上支（至黏液腺）
Superior laryngeal branch of
vagus nerve (to mucous glands)

左喉返神经（至黏液腺）
Left recurrent laryngeal nerve
(to mucous glands)

心丛
Cardiac plexus

肺丛
Pulmonary plexus

食管丛
Esophageal plexus

迷走神经前干
Anterior vagal trunk

迷走神经后干
Posterior vagal trunk

迷走神经前、后干的腹腔支
Celiac branches of anterior
and posterior vagal trunks

腹腔神经节
Celiac ganglia

腹腔丛
Celiac plexus

肠系膜上神经节
Superior mesenteric ganglion

主动脉肾神经节
Aorticorenal ganglion

肾丛
Renal plexus

肠系膜上丛
Superior mesenteric plexus

上腹下丛
Superior hypogastric plexus

盆内脏神经
Pelvic splanchnic nerves

下腹下丛
Inferior hypogastric plexus

膀胱丛
Vesical plexus

直肠（切断）
Rectum (cut)

膀胱
Bladder

海绵体神经
Cavernous nerve

阴茎 / 阴蒂勃起组织
Erectile tissue of
penis/clitoris

* 子宫阴道 / 前列腺丛未显示
Uterovaginal/prostatic
plexus not shown

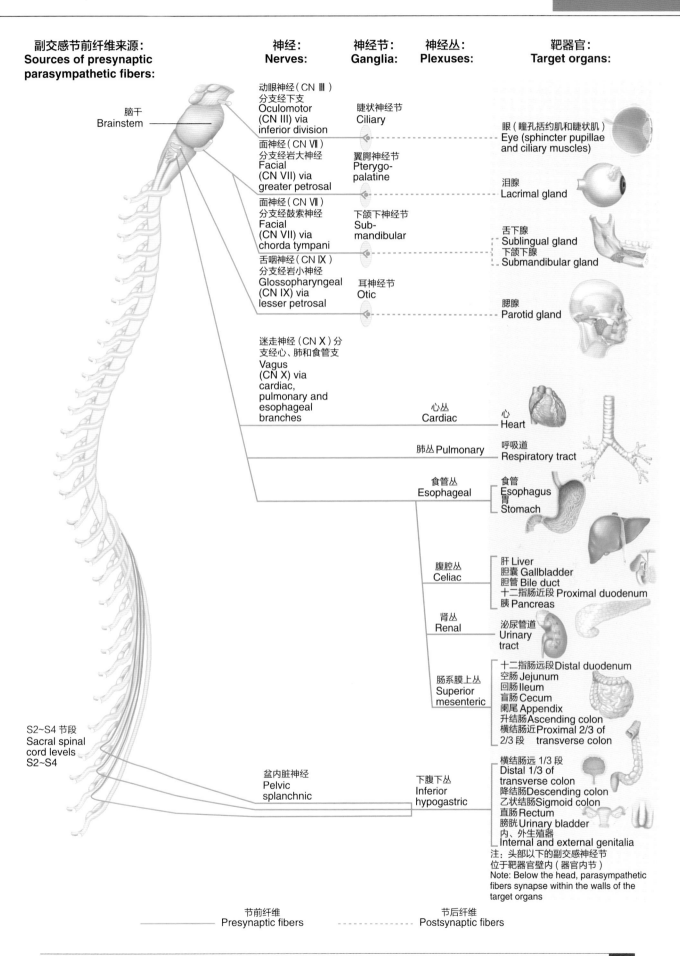

副交感节前纤维来源：
Sources of presynaptic parasympathetic fibers:

神经：
Nerves:

神经节：
Ganglia:

神经丛：
Plexuses:

靶器官：
Target organs:

脑干
Brainstem

动眼神经（CN Ⅲ）分支经下支
Oculomotor (CN III) via inferior division

睫状神经节
Ciliary

眼（瞳孔括约肌和睫状肌）
Eye (sphincter pupillae and ciliary muscles)

面神经（CN Ⅶ）分支经岩大神经
Facial (CN VII) via greater petrosal

翼腭神经节
Pterygo-palatine

泪腺
Lacrimal gland

面神经（CN Ⅶ）分支经鼓索神经
Facial (CN VII) via chorda tympani

下颌下神经节
Sub-mandibular

舌下腺
Sublingual gland
下颌下腺
Submandibular gland

舌咽神经（CN Ⅸ）分支经岩小神经
Glossopharyngeal (CN IX) via lesser petrosal

耳神经节
Otic

腮腺
Parotid gland

迷走神经（CN Ⅹ）分支经心、肺和食管支
Vagus (CN X) via cardiac, pulmonary and esophageal branches

心丛
Cardiac

心
Heart

肺丛 Pulmonary

呼吸道
Respiratory tract

食管丛
Esophageal

食管
Esophagus
胃
Stomach

腹腔丛
Celiac

肝 Liver
胆囊 Gallbladder
胆管 Bile duct
十二指肠近段 Proximal duodenum
胰 Pancreas

肾丛
Renal

泌尿管道
Urinary tract

肠系膜上丛
Superior mesenteric

十二指肠远段 Distal duodenum
空肠 Jejunum
回肠 Ileum
盲肠 Cecum
阑尾 Appendix
升结肠 Ascending colon
横结肠近 Proximal 2/3 of
2/3 段　transverse colon

S2~S4 节段
Sacral spinal cord levels S2~S4

盆内脏神经
Pelvic splanchnic

下腹下丛
Inferior hypogastric

横结肠远 1/3 段
Distal 1/3 of transverse colon
降结肠 Descending colon
乙状结肠 Sigmoid colon
直肠 Rectum
膀胱 Urinary bladder
内、外生殖器
Internal and external genitalia

注：头部以下的副交感神经节位于靶器官壁内（器官内节）
Note: Below the head, parasympathetic fibers synapse within the walls of the target organs

节前纤维
——————— Presynaptic fibers

节后纤维
- - - - - - - Postsynaptic fibers

图 8-14　四肢和体壁的自主神经　Autonomics of the Limbs and Body Wall

A. 传递交感纤维到四肢和体壁的神经
Nerves carrying sympathetic fibers to the limbs and body wall

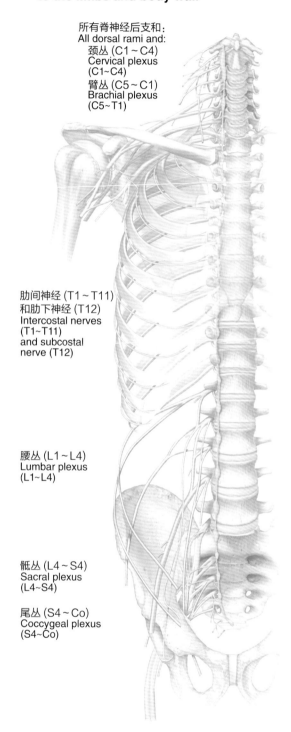

所有脊神经后支和:
All dorsal rami and:
颈丛 (C1～C4)
Cervical plexus
(C1～C4)
臂丛 (C5～C1)
Brachial plexus
(C5～T1)

肋间神经 (T1～T11)
和肋下神经 (T12)
Intercostal nerves
(T1～T11)
and subcostal
nerve (T12)

腰丛 (L1～L4)
Lumbar plexus
(L1～L4)

骶丛 (L4～S4)
Sacral plexus
(L4～S4)

尾丛 (S4～Co)
Coccygeal plexus
(S4～Co)

B. C1～C8 节段交感神经分布
Sympathetic pathways at C1~C8 levels

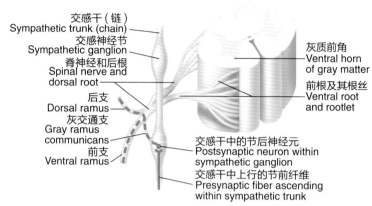

交感干（链）
Sympathetic trunk (chain)
交感神经节
Sympathetic ganglion
脊神经和后根
Spinal nerve and
dorsal root
后支
Dorsal ramus
灰交通支
Gray ramus
communicans
前支
Ventral ramus

灰质前角
Ventral horn
of gray matter
前根及其根丝
Ventral root
and rootlet

交感干中的节后神经元
Postsynaptic neuron within
sympathetic ganglion
交感干中上行的节前纤维
Presynaptic fiber ascending
within sympathetic trunk

C. T1～L2 节段交感神经分布
Sympathetic pathways at T1~L2 levels

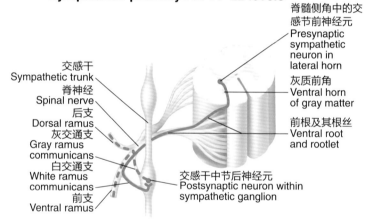

交感干
Sympathetic trunk
脊神经
Spinal nerve
后支
Dorsal ramus
灰交通支
Gray ramus
communicans
白交通支
White ramus
communicans
前支
Ventral ramus

脊髓侧角中的交
感节前神经元
Presynaptic
sympathetic
neuron in
lateral horn
灰质前角
Ventral horn
of gray matter
前根及其根丝
Ventral root
and rootlet

交感干中节后神经元
Postsynaptic neuron within
sympathetic ganglion

D. L3～Co 节段交感神经分布
Sympathetic pathways at L3~Co levels

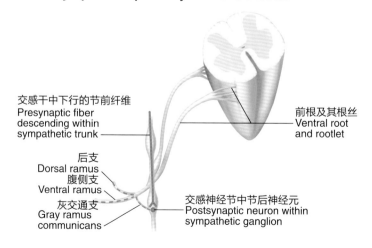

交感干中下行的节前纤维
Presynaptic fiber
descending within
sympathetic trunk

后支
Dorsal ramus
腹侧支
Ventral ramus
灰交通支
Gray ramus
communicans

前根及其根丝
Ventral root
and rootlet

交感神经节中节后神经元
Postsynaptic neuron within
sympathetic ganglion

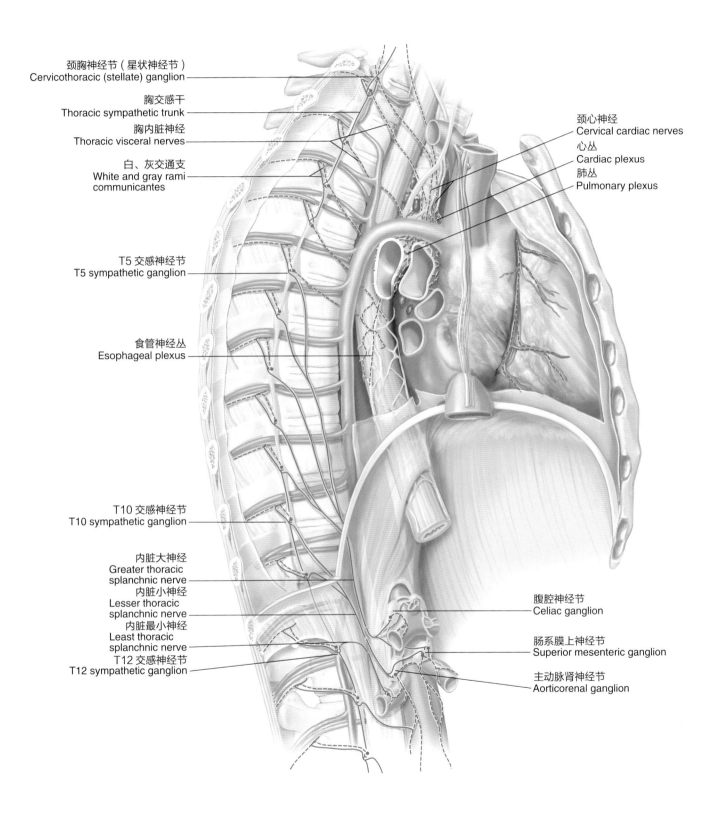

颈胸神经节（星状神经节）
Cervicothoracic (stellate) ganglion

胸交感干
Thoracic sympathetic trunk

胸内脏神经
Thoracic visceral nerves

白、灰交通支
White and gray rami
communicantes

T5 交感神经节
T5 sympathetic ganglion

食管神经丛
Esophageal plexus

T10 交感神经节
T10 sympathetic ganglion

内脏大神经
Greater thoracic
splanchnic nerve

内脏小神经
Lesser thoracic
splanchnic nerve

内脏最小神经
Least thoracic
splanchnic nerve

T12 交感神经节
T12 sympathetic ganglion

颈心神经
Cervical cardiac nerves

心丛
Cardiac plexus

肺丛
Pulmonary plexus

腹腔神经节
Celiac ganglion

肠系膜上神经节
Superior mesenteric ganglion

主动脉肾神经节
Aorticorenal ganglion

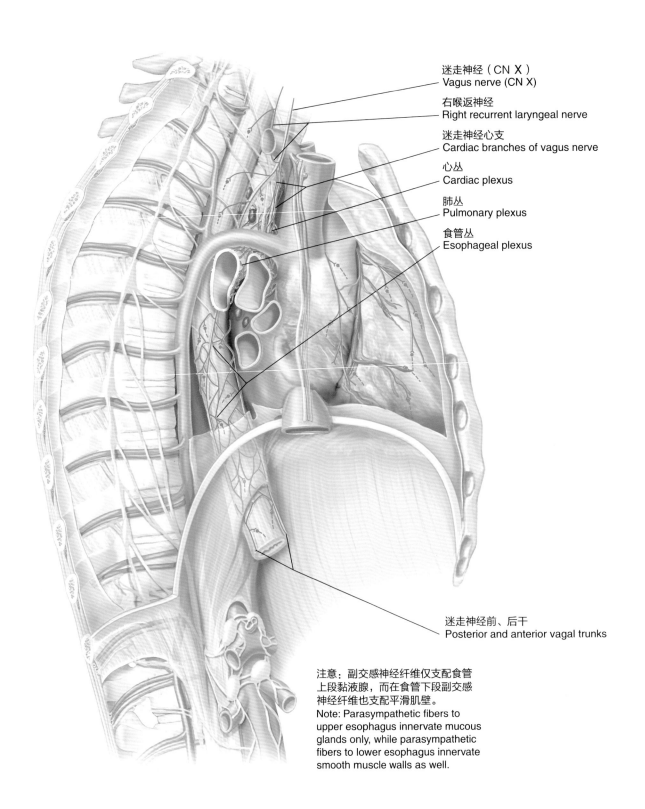

迷走神经（CN X）
Vagus nerve (CN X)

右喉返神经
Right recurrent laryngeal nerve

迷走神经心支
Cardiac branches of vagus nerve

心丛
Cardiac plexus

肺丛
Pulmonary plexus

食管丛
Esophageal plexus

迷走神经前、后干
Posterior and anterior vagal trunks

注意：副交感神经纤维仅支配食管
上段黏液腺，而在食管下段副交感
神经纤维也支配平滑肌壁。
Note: Parasympathetic fibers to
upper esophagus innervate mucous
glands only, while parasympathetic
fibers to lower esophagus innervate
smooth muscle walls as well.

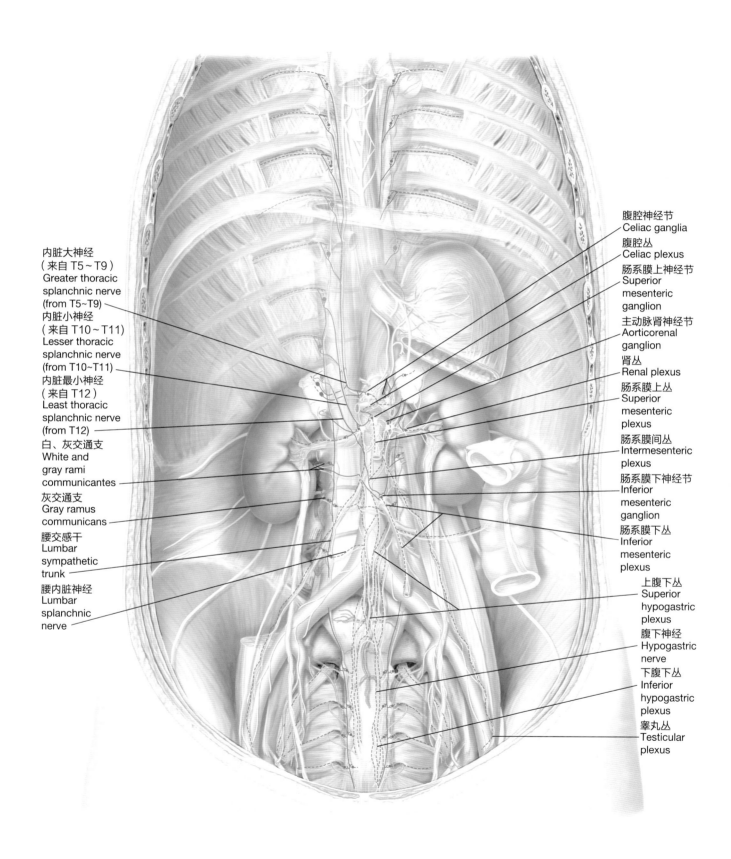

内脏大神经
（来自 T5～T9）
Greater thoracic
splanchnic nerve
(from T5~T9)

内脏小神经
（来自 T10～T11）
Lesser thoracic
splanchnic nerve
(from T10~T11)

内脏最小神经
（来自 T12）
Least thoracic
splanchnic nerve
(from T12)

白、灰交通支
White and
gray rami
communicantes

灰交通支
Gray ramus
communicans

腰交感干
Lumbar
sympathetic
trunk

腰内脏神经
Lumbar
splanchnic
nerve

腹腔神经节
Celiac ganglia

腹腔丛
Celiac plexus

肠系膜上神经节
Superior
mesenteric
ganglion

主动脉肾神经节
Aorticorenal
ganglion

肾丛
Renal plexus

肠系膜上丛
Superior
mesenteric
plexus

肠系膜间丛
Intermesenteric
plexus

肠系膜下神经节
Inferior
mesenteric
ganglion

肠系膜下丛
Inferior
mesenteric
plexus

上腹下丛
Superior
hypogastric
plexus

腹下神经
Hypogastric
nerve

下腹下丛
Inferior
hypogastric
plexus

睾丸丛
Testicular
plexus

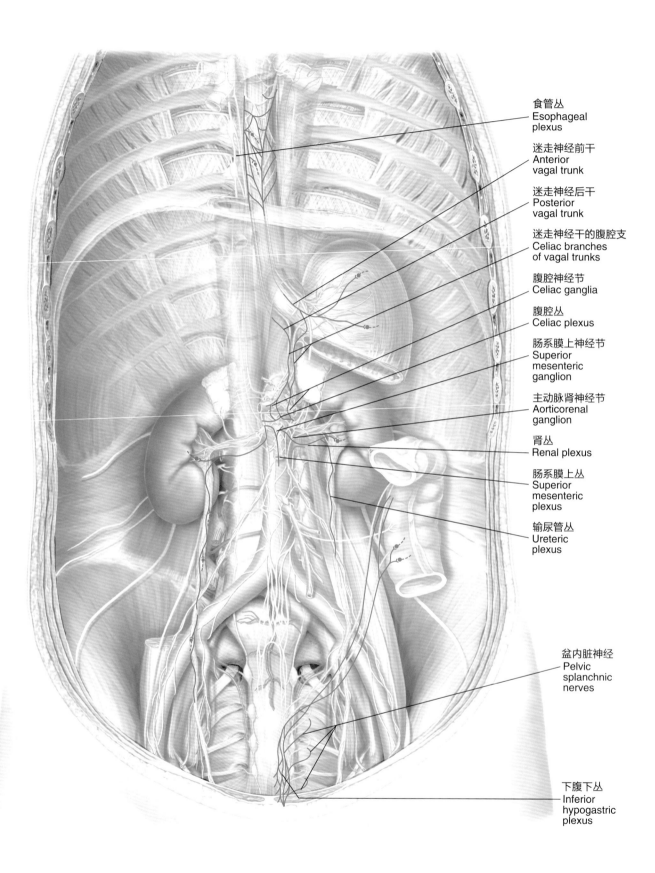

食管丛
Esophageal
plexus

迷走神经前干
Anterior
vagal trunk

迷走神经后干
Posterior
vagal trunk

迷走神经干的腹腔支
Celiac branches
of vagal trunks

腹腔神经节
Celiac ganglia

腹腔丛
Celiac plexus

肠系膜上神经节
Superior
mesenteric
ganglion

主动脉肾神经节
Aorticorenal
ganglion

肾丛
Renal plexus

肠系膜上丛
Superior
mesenteric
plexus

输尿管丛
Ureteric
plexus

盆内脏神经
Pelvic
splanchnic
nerves

下腹下丛
Inferior
hypogastric
plexus

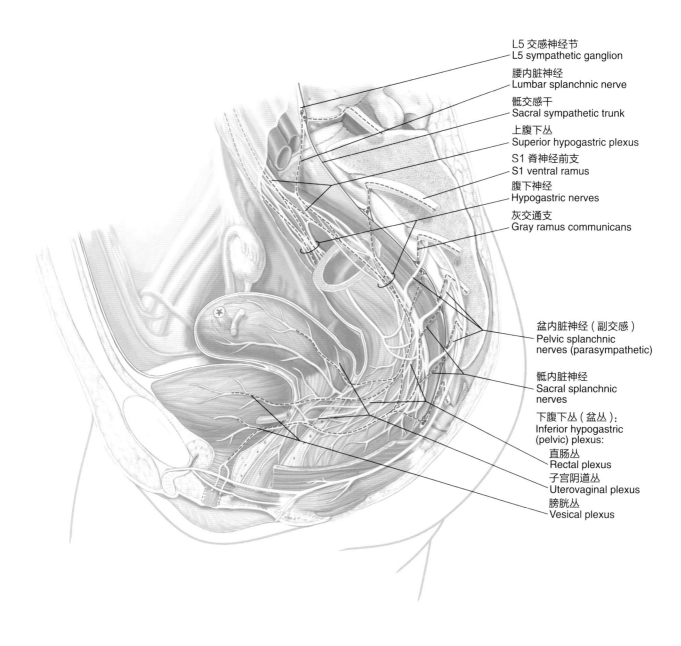

L5 交感神经节
L5 sympathetic ganglion

腰内脏神经
Lumbar splanchnic nerve

骶交感干
Sacral sympathetic trunk

上腹下丛
Superior hypogastric plexus

S1 脊神经前支
S1 ventral ramus

腹下神经
Hypogastric nerves

灰交通支
Gray ramus communicans

盆内脏神经（副交感）
Pelvic splanchnic nerves (parasympathetic)

骶内脏神经
Sacral splanchnic nerves

下腹下丛（盆丛）：
Inferior hypogastric (pelvic) plexus:

直肠丛
Rectal plexus

子宫阴道丛
Uterovaginal plexus

膀胱丛
Vesical plexus

图 8-20

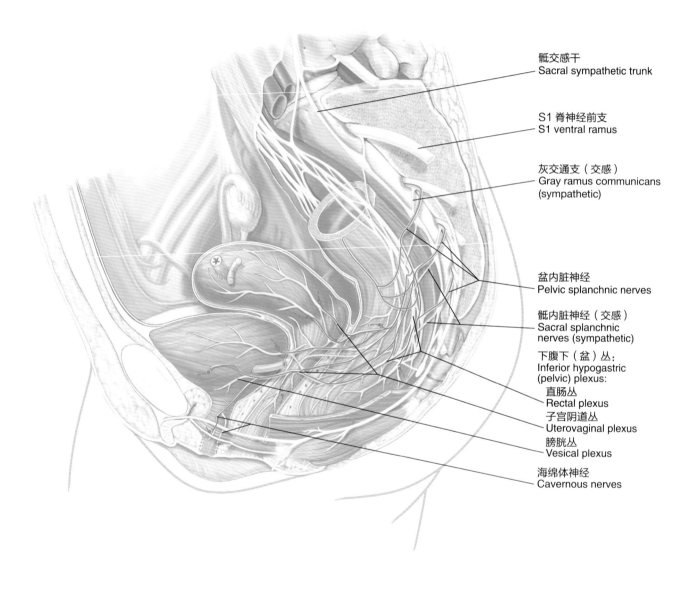

骶交感干
Sacral sympathetic trunk

S1 脊神经前支
S1 ventral ramus

灰交通支（交感）
Gray ramus communicans
(sympathetic)

盆内脏神经
Pelvic splanchnic nerves

骶内脏神经（交感）
Sacral splanchnic
nerves (sympathetic)

下腹下（盆）丛：
Inferior hypogastric
(pelvic) plexus:

直肠丛
Rectal plexus

子宫阴道丛
Uterovaginal plexus

膀胱丛
Vesical plexus

海绵体神经
Cavernous nerves

女性盆腔自主神经，副交感神经通路
Autonomics of the Pelvis, Parasympathetic Pathways, Female

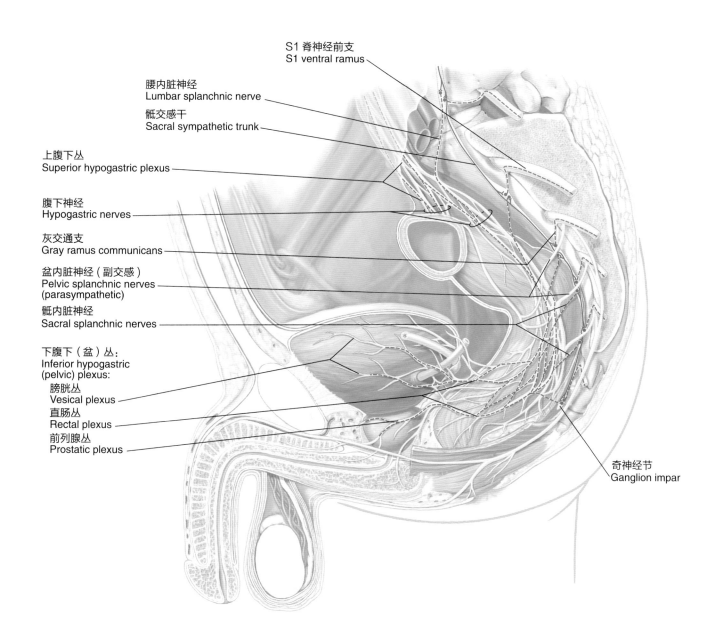

S1 脊神经前支
S1 ventral ramus

腰内脏神经
Lumbar splanchnic nerve

骶交感干
Sacral sympathetic trunk

上腹下丛
Superior hypogastric plexus

腹下神经
Hypogastric nerves

灰交通支
Gray ramus communicans

盆内脏神经（副交感）
Pelvic splanchnic nerves
(parasympathetic)

骶内脏神经
Sacral splanchnic nerves

下腹下（盆）丛：
Inferior hypogastric
(pelvic) plexus:

　膀胱丛
　Vesical plexus

　直肠丛
　Rectal plexus

　前列腺丛
　Prostatic plexus

奇神经节
Ganglion impar

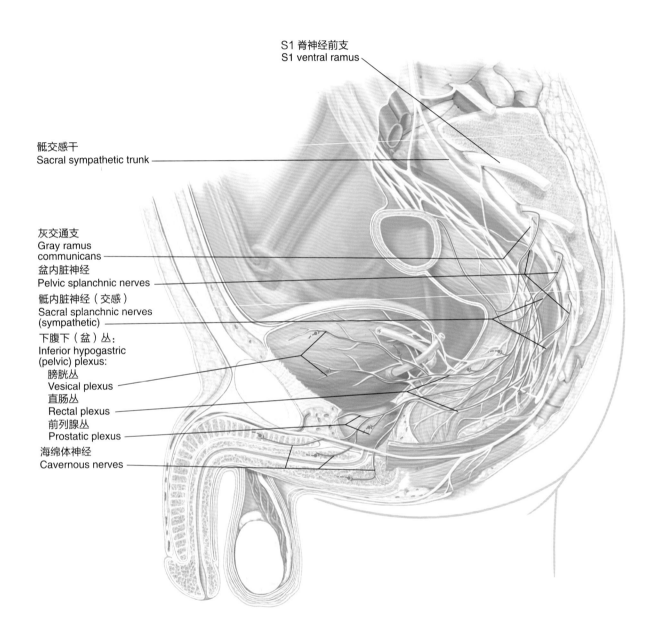

S1 脊神经前支
S1 ventral ramus

骶交感干
Sacral sympathetic trunk

灰交通支
Gray ramus
communicans

盆内脏神经
Pelvic splanchnic nerves

骶内脏神经（交感）
Sacral splanchnic nerves
(sympathetic)

下腹下（盆）丛：
Inferior hypogastric
(pelvic) plexus:

　膀胱丛
　Vesical plexus

　直肠丛
　Rectal plexus

　前列腺丛
　Prostatic plexus

海绵体神经
Cavernous nerves

男性盆腔自主神经，副交感神经通路
Autonomics of the Pelvis, Parasympathetic Pathways, Male

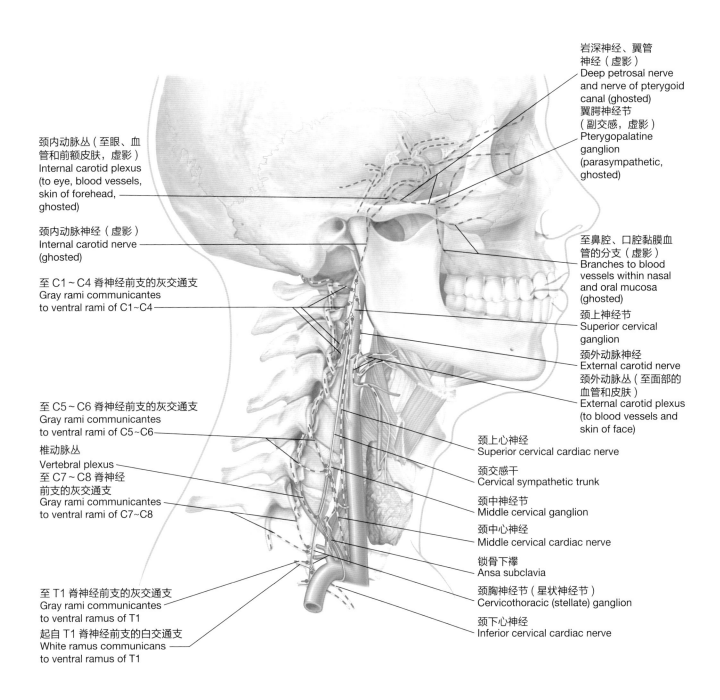

岩深神经、翼管神经（虚影）
Deep petrosal nerve and nerve of pterygoid canal (ghosted)

翼腭神经节（副交感，虚影）
Pterygopalatine ganglion (parasympathetic, ghosted)

颈内动脉丛（至眼、血管和前额皮肤，虚影）
Internal carotid plexus (to eye, blood vessels, skin of forehead, ghosted)

颈内动脉神经（虚影）
Internal carotid nerve (ghosted)

至 C1～C4 脊神经前支的灰交通支
Gray rami communicantes to ventral rami of C1~C4

至鼻腔、口腔黏膜血管的分支（虚影）
Branches to blood vessels within nasal and oral mucosa (ghosted)

颈上神经节
Superior cervical ganglion

颈外动脉神经
External carotid nerve

颈外动脉丛（至面部的血管和皮肤）
External carotid plexus (to blood vessels and skin of face)

颈上心神经
Superior cervical cardiac nerve

颈交感干
Cervical sympathetic trunk

至 C5～C6 脊神经前支的灰交通支
Gray rami communicantes to ventral rami of C5~C6

椎动脉丛
Vertebral plexus

至 C7～C8 脊神经前支的灰交通支
Gray rami communicantes to ventral rami of C7~C8

颈中神经节
Middle cervical ganglion

颈中心神经
Middle cervical cardiac nerve

锁骨下襻
Ansa subclavia

至 T1 脊神经前支的灰交通支
Gray rami communicantes to ventral ramus of T1

起自 T1 脊神经前支的白交通支
White ramus communicans to ventral ramus of T1

颈胸神经节（星状神经节）
Cervicothoracic (stellate) ganglion

颈下心神经
Inferior cervical cardiac nerve

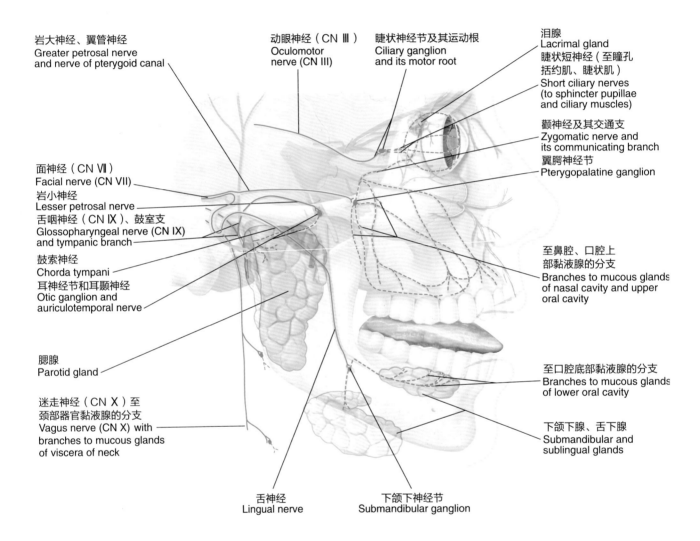

岩大神经、翼管神经
Greater petrosal nerve
and nerve of pterygoid canal

动眼神经（CN Ⅲ）
Oculomotor
nerve (CN III)

睫状神经节及其运动根
Ciliary ganglion
and its motor root

泪腺
Lacrimal gland

睫状短神经（至瞳孔
括约肌、睫状肌）
Short ciliary nerves
(to sphincter pupillae
and ciliary muscles)

颧神经及其交通支
Zygomatic nerve and
its communicating branch

翼腭神经节
Pterygopalatine ganglion

面神经（CN Ⅶ）
Facial nerve (CN VII)

岩小神经
Lesser petrosal nerve

舌咽神经（CN Ⅸ）、鼓室支
Glossopharyngeal nerve (CN IX)
and tympanic branch

鼓索神经
Chorda tympani

耳神经节和耳颞神经
Otic ganglion and
auriculotemporal nerve

至鼻腔、口腔上
部黏液腺的分支
Branches to mucous glands
of nasal cavity and upper
oral cavity

腮腺
Parotid gland

至口腔底部黏液腺的分支
Branches to mucous glands
of lower oral cavity

迷走神经（CN Ⅹ）至
颈部器官黏液腺的分支
Vagus nerve (CN X) with
branches to mucous glands
of viscera of neck

下颌下腺、舌下腺
Submandibular and
sublingual glands

舌神经
Lingual nerve

下颌下神经节
Submandibular ganglion